TOPICS IN
CLINICAL UROLOGY

DIAGNOSIS AND MANAGEMENT OF MALE SEXUAL DYSFUNCTION

TOPICS IN CLINICAL UROLOGY

Series Editors
Martin I. Resnick, M.D.
Jack S. Elder, M.D.

New Techniques in Reconstructive Urology
Jack W. McAninch, M.D.

Complications of Interventional Techniques
Culley C. Carson III, M.D.

Pediatric Urology for the General Urologist
Jack S. Elder, M.D.

New Diagnostic Tests
Martin I. Resnick, M.D.
J. Patrick Spirnak, M.D.

New Developments in the Management of Urolithiasis
James E. Lingeman, M.D.
Glenn M. Preminger, M.D.

Medical and Surgical Management of Prostate Cancer
Richard G. Middleton, M.D.

Techniques for Ablation of Benign and Malignant Prostate Tissue
Joseph A. Smith, Jr., M.D.
Douglas F. Milam, M.D.

Evaluation and Treatment of Urinary Incontinence
Jerry G. Blaivas, M.D.

Diagnosis and Management of Male Sexual Dysfunction
John J. Mulcahy, M.D., Ph.D.

TOPICS IN CLINICAL UROLOGY

DIAGNOSIS AND MANAGEMENT OF MALE SEXUAL DYSFUNCTION

John J. Mulcahy, M.D., Ph.D.
Professor of Urology
Department of Urology
Indiana University Medical Center
Indianapolis, Indiana

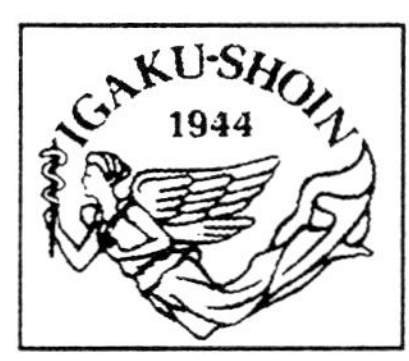

IGAKU-SHOIN   NEW YORK · TOKYO

Published and distributed by

IGAKU-SHOIN Medical Publishers, Inc.
One Madison Avenue, New York, New York   10010

IGAKU-SHOIN Ltd.,
5-24-3 Hongo, Bunkyo-ku, Tokyo 113-91.

Library of Congress Cataloging-in-Publication Data

Diagnosis and management of male sexual dysfunction / [edited by] John J.
  Mulcahy.
      p.   cm.—(Topics in clinical urology)
      Includes bibliographical references and index.
      1. Impotence.   2. Premature ejaculation.   3. Generative organs, Male—
Diseases.   I. Mulcahy, John J. (John Joseph), 1941-   . II. Series.
      [DNLM: 1. Sexual Disorders—diagnosis.   2. Sex Disorders—therapy.
   3. Impotence.   4. Penile Erection.
   WJ 709 D5358 1997]
   RC889.D526   1997
   616.6′9—dc20
   DNLM/DLC
   for Library of Congress   96-22329
                                                                         CIP

ISBN: 0-89640-322-X   (New York)
ISBN: 4-260-14322-0   (Tokyo)

Printed and bound in the U.S.A.
10 9 8 7 6 5 4 3 2 1

PREFACE

Advances in the understanding of erectile physiology and the medical management of erectile dysfunction have mushroomed in the past decade. As less aggressive treatments become available and are widely promulgated by the media, more patients are willing and anxious to come forward and pursue therapy for this problem. In addition, as life expectancy increases, more of the population will experience waning erectile abilities. Physicians and other health care professionals involved in the treatment of erectile dysfunction must be prepared to deal with this problem.

The scope of this monograph is a comprehensive overview of the field of male sexual dysfunction. The incidence, pathophysiology, diagnosis, and treatment of erectile abnormalities and premature ejaculation are covered by the movers and shakers in each category. The technique of performing various tests, the limitations, results, and indications are put in proper perspective.

The material is up-to-date, and each of the contributors has a unique expertise in the area designated. The urologist and health care provider with a special interest in male sexual disorders will find the information presented to be new in many respects and to be a reinforcement of concepts, techniques, and treatment plans already well established in other instances. The thrust of the monograph is a practical nuts-and-bolts presentation for the physician in the trenches dealing with male sexuality on a day-to-day basis. It is designed to be of use in frequently encountered clinical situations, to aid the practitioner in selecting and performing the appropriate diagnostic tests that will delineate the sexual aberration so it can be treated in the most subjectively satisfying way for the patient.

John J. Mulcahy, M.D., Ph.D.

DEDICATION

To my family
RaeAnne, Lori, Maureen, Mike, and Mark

CONTRIBUTORS

Stanley E. Althof, Ph.D.
Associate Professor of Urology
Case Western Reserve University
School of Medicine
University Hospitals of Cleveland
Cleveland, OH
and
Center for Sexual and Marital Health
Beachwood, OH

Alexandru E. Benet, M.D.
Clinical Fellow in Sexual Dysfunction
Albert Einstein College of Medicine
New York, NY

Gregory A. Broderick, M.D.
Associate Professor of Urology
University of Pennsylvania School of
   Medicine
Philadelphia, PA

Culley C. Carson, III, M.D.
Professor of Urology and
Chief of the Division of Urology
University of North Carolina School of
   Medicine
Chapel Hill, NC

James J. Chang, M.D.
Resident, Department of Urology
University of California at San
   Francisco
San Francisco, CA

James A. Daitch, M.D.
Resident, Department of Urology
Cleveland Clinic Foundation
Cleveland, OH

Irwin Goldstein, M.D.
Professor of Urology
Boston University School of Medicine
Boston, MA

Wayne J.G. Hellstrom, M.D.
Associate Professor of Urology
Tulane University School of Medicine
New Orleans, LA

Jonathan Jaspan, M.D.
Professor of Medicine
Tulane University School of Medicine
New Orleans, LA

Milton M. Lakin, M.D.
Head, Section of Medical Urology
Cleveland Clinic Foundation
Cleveland, OH

Stephen B. Levine, M.D.
Professor of Psychiatry
Case Western Reserve University
School of Medicine
University Hospitals of Cleveland
Cleveland, OH
and
Center for Sexual and Marital Health
Beachwood, OH

Ronald W. Lewis, M.D.
Professor and Chief, Division of
  Urology
Medical College of Georgia
Augusta, GA

Tom F. Lue, M.D.
Professor of Urology
University of California at San
  Francisco
San Francisco, CA

Arnold Melman, M.D.
Professor and Chairman
Department of Urology
Albert Einstein College of Medicine
New York, NY

Ignacio Moncada Iribarren, M.D.
Department of Urology
Hospital General Universitario
  Gregorio Marañón
Madrid, Spain

Drogo K. Montague, M.D.
Head, Section of Prosthetic Surgery
Cleveland Clinic Foundation
Cleveland, OH
Professor of Urology
Ohio State University
Columbus, OH

John J. Mulcahy, M.D., Ph.D.
Professor of Urology
Indiana University School of Medicine
Indianapolis, IN

John Mulhall, M.D.
Instructor, Department of Urology
Loyola University School of Medicine
Maywood, IL

Harin Padma-Nathan, M.D.
Assistant Professor, Department of
  Urology
University of Southern California
Director, The Male Clinic
Los Angeles, CA

Jamil Rehman, M.D.
Research Fellow in Urology
Albert Einstein College of Medicine
New York, NY

Iñigo Saenz de Tejada, M.D.
Departamento de Investigacion
Hospital Ramon y Cajal
Madrid, Spain

Allen D. Seftel, M.D.
Assistant Professor, Department of
  Urology
Case Western Reserve University
School of Medicine
University Hospitals of Cleveland
Cleveland VA Medical Center
Cleveland, OH

Todd L. VandenBerg, M.D.
Resident in Urology
Tulane University School of Medicine
New Orleans, LA

Steven K. Wilson, M.D.
Clinical Associate Professor of Urology
University of Arkansas
Little Rock, AK

CONTENTS

1

Epidemiology of Erectile Dysfunction

John P. Mulhall

Irwin Goldstein

Erectile dysfunction, which has replaced the term *impotence* since the National Institutes of Health (NIH) consensus conference in 1988, is defined as the consistent inability to obtain or maintain a penile erection sufficient for satisfactory sexual relations.[1] Of note, in contradistinction to prior definitions, the concepts of vaginal penetration and percentage of failed attempts have been removed from the definition.[2] Erectile impairment is a condition with profound psychologic consequences and may interfere with a man's overall well-being, self-esteem, and interpersonal relationships.[3] Its incidence has been conservatively estimated at between 10 and 20 million men.[4,5] Furthermore, it has been shown that erectile problems account for 400,000 outpatient physician visits, 30,000 hospital admissions, and an annual financial outlay by our health industry of 146 million dollars.[6] These figures, from a 1985 survey, have most probably increased given the increasing media exposure of this problem, the resultant reduced patient reticence to present himself, the FDA approval of prostaglandin E_1 (PGE_1), and the widespread acceptance of a variety of therapeutic modalities, including intracavernosal injection therapy and vacuum erection devices.

Unfortunately, until recently, hard epidemiologic data has been lacking. Prior to the Massachusetts Male Aging Study (MMAS) (*vide infra*), epidemiologic studies had suffered from a number of inherent problems, including failure to standardize methods of study population selection, variation in the definition of impotence, and failure to stratify patient populations by age and, physiologic correlates.[7] Furthermore, little study has been conducted on the referral patterns of patients, reasons for patient presentation, sources of patient information, and patient knowledge bases.

EPIDEMIOLOGIC STUDIES

Kinsey's report in 1948 was the first study to address the occurence of sexual dysfunction in the general population.[8] Results from this study, based on the detailed interview of 12,000 males, stratified for age, education, and occupation, indicated an increasing rate of impotence with age. Its prevalence was cited as less than 1% in men under 19 yr of age, 3% of men under 45 yr, 7% less than 55 yr, and 25% by the age of 75 yr. In 1979, Gebhard reanalyzed the Kinsey data and in a cohort of over 5,000 men, 42% admitted to erectile difficulties.[9]

Other studies performed on subjects derived from general populations have suffered from two major problems, the use of nonrepresentative samples due to the method of sampling and the unknown value of the instrument used in the study.[10] Ard, in 1977, reported on the sexual behavior of 161 couples married for greater than 20 yr and noted a 3% incidence of erectile problems.[11] In 1978, Frank studied 100 volunteer couples, reportedly normal, who were married and sexually active, with a mean age of 37 yr.[12] Forty percent of men reported difficulty with either erection of ejaculation. A year later, Nettelbladt found that 40% of randomly selected, sexually active males (mean age 31 yr) noted some degree of erectile problems.[13] Other studies have reported a variable incidence of erectile impairment, from 3% to 40%.[10,14,15] The Baltimore Longitudinal Study of Aging cited erectile impairment as being present in 8% of men 55 yr or less, 25% of 65-yr-olds, 55% of 75-yr-olds and 75% of 80-yr-old.[16] The Charleston Heart Study Cohort reported on sexual activity rather than erectile dysfunction.[17] It reported a 30% incidence of inactivity between the ages of 66–69 yr. In subjects over 80 yr of age this figure rose to 60%.

Subjects obtained from medical health statistics have also been analyzed for the occurrence of erectile difficulties. In an analysis of family practice patients, Schein noted a prevalence of erectile difficulties of 27% in 212 patients with a mean age of 35 yr.[18] Mulligan cited a 6-fold increase in erectile problems in middle-aged men with self-reported poor health, and a 40-fold increase in similar patients over 70 yr of age.[19] In a cohort of 50-yr-old men undergoing a nutritional and general health screening, Morley found a 27% incidence of impotence.[20] This finding is in keeping with other data from Masters and Johnson[2] and Slag,[21] inferring that men with medical conditions have a higher incidence of erectile dysfunction.

In an analysis of 100 consecutive new patients to an impotence clinic, Mulhall reviewed patient referral patterns, knowledge base, and expectations.[22] Seventy-five percent of patients were referred by another physician, most commonly a primary care physician. Self-referral and partner referral each accounted for only 10% of patients. The mean duration of erectile dysfunction among this cohort was 3 yr. Patients under 50 yr of age presented a mean of 16 months earlier than those older than 50 yr. The most common reason for delaying presentation was embarrassment, accounting for 65% of patients' primary reason for procrastination. Other major reasons for delay in presentation included fear (15%) and lack of partner (10%). On assessment of patient knowledge, 45% of patients had no knowledge of any form of therapy for impotence, while the best known form of therapy was the penile prosthesis (25%). Sixteen percent of patients used the media as their primary source of information while the majority relied on a physician for information (60%) prior to presenting to the impotence clinician. With regard to patient expectations, 67% had a primary goal of obtaining useful erections again and 70% agreed on first encounter to consider intracavernosal therapy while 92% said they would agree to psychologic counselling if they were advised to do so by the physician. These data underline a number of points with regard to the impotent patient: the majority are referred for evaluation by primary care physicians, younger patients tend to present earlier, embarrassment continues to be a major problem for these men and delays their presentation, a significant number of men use the media for educational purposes, and in general, patient knowledge base remains poor.

MASSACHUSETTS MALE AGING STUDY (MMAS)

This was a cross-sectional, community-based, random-sample, multidisciplinary epidemiologic survey of aging and health in men aged 40–70 yr.[7] The study was conducted between 1987 and 1989, in and around Boston. The responses of 1,290 subjects were evaluated following the administration of a detailed, comprehensive questionnaire-based instrument. This work represents the largest work since the Kinsey report in 1948.[8] The MMAS differed from prior studies in both size and content. It included four groups of intervening variables (confounders) that could be related to sexual function: health status and medical care use, sociodemographic data, psychosocial and lifestyle characteristics.

All data were collected at the subject's home by trained interviewers. The multidisciplinary approach included gerontologists, behavioral scientists, endocrinologists, and sexual dysfunction clinicians. The study design allowed precise estimation of key parameters while controlling for potentially important confounders and permitted identification of statistically predictive risk factors. The sample group was as close to the general population as could be achieved. The population studied were a free-living, noninstitutionalized group, only a fraction of whom was sick and interacting with the health system.

The MMAS instrument contained 23 questions, nine of which related to erectile capability. A subjective assessment of erectile potency was made as opposed to a more concretely defined erectile dysfunction state. A calibration study was conducted to discriminate different potency profiles.[23] Potency was divided into four grades: not impotent, minimally impotent, moderately impotent, and completely impotent.

The overall rate of any degree of impotence in the MMAS was 52%, including 17% minimally impotent, 25% moderately impotent, and 10% completely impotent. The overall probability of impotence, of any degree, at 40 yr was 39% and at 70 yr 67%. Extrapolating these data, there would be 30 million men in the United States with some form of erectile impairment. The conditions that were associated with impotence in this study included diabetes, hypertension, heart disease, untreated ulcer disease, arthritis, cardiac medications (including vasodilators and antihypertensive agents) cigarette smoking, hypoglycemic agents, and depression.

VASCULAR RISK FACTORS

The association between vascular disease and erectile dysfunction has been recognized and well documented. Indeed, alterations in the vascular hemodynamics (whether arterial insufficiency or corporo-veno-occlusive dysfunction) are believed to be the most common cause of organic erectile dysfunction.[24] Such vascular disease as myocardial infarction, coronary artery bypass surgery, cerebral vascular accidents, peripheral vascular disease, and hypertension have all been shown to have a higher incidence of impotence compared to the general population without documented vasculopathies. Myocardial infarction (MI) and cororonary artery bypass surgery have been associated with erectile difficulties in 64%[25] and 57%[26] respectively. Furthermore, in a group of 130 impotent men, the incidence of MI was 8 times higher in men with abnormal penile-brachial indices (PBI) than in those with normal PBI (12% versus 1.5%).[27] In men with peripheral vascular disease (PVD), the incidence of erectile dysfunction has been estimated at 80%.[28] This figure is 10% in untreated hypertensive males.[29]

Diabetes with its related vasculopathy is associated with a higher incidence of impotence at all ages compared to the general population. The prevalence of impotence in all-comer diabetics has been variably estimated at between 35% and 75%.[3] Erectile difficulties may be the harbinger of diabetes, this phenomenon occurring in 12% of newly diagnosed diabetics.[30] The incidence of impotence in diabetics is age-dependent and is higher in men with juvenile-onset diabetes compared to adult-onset diabetics.[31,32] Of those diabetic men who will develop impotence, 50% will do so within 5–10 yr of the diagnosis of their diabetes.[33,34] When combined with hypertensive disease, impotence in diabetics is even more prevalent.[35]

As the number of vascular risk factors (such as cigarette smoking, hypertension, cardiac disease, hyperlipidemia, and diabetes) increases, so too does the likelihood of erectile dysfunction.[36] This finding was confirmed in Virag's analysis of 400 impotent men, demonstrating that 80% of these men had physiologic abnormalities and that vascular risk factors were more common in this group compared to the general population.[28]

HORMONES AND ERECTILE DYSFUNCTION

While androgens are essential to the growth and differentiation of the male genital tract the development of secondary sexual characteristics, and the presence of libido, their role in the erectile process remains unclear.[31,37–41] At this time, the nature of an appropriate hormonal investigation—whether a complete hormone panel is required for every patient or whether a single testosterone determination constitutes effective screening—remains debated.[21,42] Indeed, disagreement exists on whether free or total testosterone levels are more important in the evaluation of the impotent male.[43] Nevertheless, endocrinopathies probably account for between 3% and 6% of all organic erectile dysfunction and those endocrinopathies that may lead to impotence include hypogonadism, hypothyroidism, hyperprolactinemia, diabetes mellitus, adrenal disorders, chronic liver disease, chronic renal failure and AIDS.[44]

DRUG-INDUCED ERECTILE DYSFUNCTION

Drug associated erectile dysfunction is common and the list of medications that can induce erectile dysfunction is significant (Table 1.1).[45] Medication-induced impo-

TABLE 1.1. Medications Associated with Erectile Dysfunction

Antihypertensives	Diuretics
	Beta-blockers
	Ganglion-blockers
	Calcium-channel blockers
	Spironolactone
Cardiac	Digoxin
	Antilipidemics
Psychotropics	Tricyclic antidepressants
	Phenothiazines
	Butyrophenones
	Monoamine oxidase inhibitors
	Selective sertonin-reuptake inhibitors
	Lithium
Hormones	Estrogen
	Progesterone
	Antiandrogens
	Luteinizing hormone-releasing hormone (LHRH) agonists
	5α-Reductase inhibitors
Anticonvulsants	
H_2 Antagonists	
Miscellaneous	Metoclopramide
	Baclofen
	Alcohol
	Opiates
	Amphetamines

tence has been estimated to occur in up to 25% of patients in a medical outpatient clinic.[21] Antihypertensive agents are associated with erectile difficulties, depending upon the specific agents in 4% to 40% of patients.[45–49] They induce impotence either by actions at the central level (clonidine), by direct actions at the corporal level (calcium channel blockers), or by purely dropping systemic blood pressure upon which the patient has relied to maintain an intracorporal pressure sufficient for the development of penile rigidity.

Several medications cause impotence based on their antiandrogen actions, for example estrogens, luteinizing hormone-releasing hormone (LHRH) agonists, H_2 antagonists, and spironolactone.[50–52] Digoxin induces erectile difficulties via blockade of the NA-K-ATPase pump resulting in a net increase in intracellular Ca and subsequent increased tone in the corporal smooth muscle.[52a] The psychotropic medications alter central nervous system (CNS) mechanisms [53–56] Chronic use of recreational drugs has been associated with erectile dysfunction.[57–60] Other agents affect erection through, unknown mechanisms. Ultimately, it is essential to define a mechanism for each medication suspected of causing impotence. Furthermore, the diagnosis of drug-induced erectile dysfunction must be predicated upon reproducibility of the problem with administration of medication and cessation of the problem upon its discontinuation.[45]

TRAUMA

Pelvic trauma, in particular injuries to the perineum and pelvic fractures, is associated with erectile dysfunction. In an analysis of patients presenting to a university-based practice, Goldstein reported that 35 of the patients seen had erectile dysfunction resulting from trauma. Furthermore, the pathophysiologic mechanisms for the development of such impotence has been previously postulated.[60a] In recent years it has been recognized that a disproportionate number of young men with erectile difficulties have a history of bicycling accidents. Disruption of the prostato-membranous urethra, as seen in severe pelvic fractures, has been reported to be associated with up to a 50% incidence of impotence.[61]

Urologic surgery of a variety of types has been implicated in erectile dysfunction. The operations that have been reported to cause erectile dysfunction include radical prostatectomy, retropubic and perineal, whether nerve-sparing or not,[62–66] transurethral resection of the prostate (TURP),[67,68] internal urethrotomy,[67,68] perineal urethroplasty,[69] and pelvic exenterative procedures.[70]

PSYCHOLOGIC CORRELATES

Until 15 yr ago impotence was believed to be the result of psychologic issues in the majority of men. Various workers have demonstrated the association between depression and erectile dysfunction.[71–73] The presence of erectile dysfunction correlated with marital discord in 25% of couples.[74] In the MMAS, psychologic factors associated with erectile problems included depression, anger, and low levels of dominance.[7]

CHRONIC ILLNESS

Apart from the factors already outlined (vascular risk factors, endocrinopathies, and psychologic problems) that may lead to impotence, the following conditions may induce erectile problems.

Renal Failures

Up to 40% of men suffering from chronic renal failure have some form of erectile dysfunction.[75] The mechanism by which impotence results in this disorder is probably multifactorial, involving endocrinologic (hypogonadism, hyperprolactinemia), neuropathic (diabetes-induced nephropathy), and vascular factors. Hatzichristou investigated the vascular etiologies in a cohort of men with chronic renal failure who had undergone hemodynamic evaluation and found an inordinately high incidence of corporo-veno-occulusive dysfunction.[75a] The role of renal transplantation in the development of erectile dysfunction in these patients is variable. In some, transplant improves the renal function to the point where the patient's erectile function also improves[76,77] and in others, particularly those men who had received two transplants, the erectile function may deteriorate further.[78]

Neurologic Disorders

Neurogenic erectile dysfunction may be caused by disorders such as. stroke,[16] brain and spinal tumors, cerebral infection, Alzheimer's disease, temporal lobe epilepsy, and multiple sclerosis (MS).[79] Agarwal cited an 85% incidence of impotence in a group of men following stroke,[80] while Goldstein noted 71% of men with MS were affected by erectile difficulties.[81] More recently, it has been recognized that autoimmune deficiency syndrome (AIDS) has been associated with an autonomic neuropathy that may cause neurogenic erectile dysfunction.[82]

Pulmonary Diseases

Fletcher noted a 30% incidence of impotence in men with chronic obstructive pulmonary disease (COPD), all of whom had normal peripheral and penile pulses by Doppler assessment, suggesting that COPD was the primary etiologic factor.[83]

Systemic Disorders

Apart from diseases already mentioned (diabetes, vascular diseases, renal failure), some other disorders are associated with impotence. Scleroderma may result in erectile dysfunction as a result of the small vessel vasculopathy that it causes.[84] Chronic liver disease has been associated with erectile impairment in up to 50% of patients with this disorder. This incidence is somewhat dependent on the etiology of the liver dysfunction, alcoholic liver disease having a higher incidence than nonalcoholic.[85]

REFERENCES

1. NIH Consensus Conference: Impotence. NIH Consensus Development Panel on Impotence. *JAMA* 270:83–87, 1993.

2. Masters W, Johnson V: *Human Sexual Inadequacy*. Boston, Little Browr. Co., 1970.

3. Krane RJ, Goldstein I, Saenz de Tejada I: Impotence. *N Engl Med J* 321:1648–1659, 1989.

4. Furlow WL: Prevalence of impotence in the United States. *Med Aspects Hum Sex* 19:13, 1985.

5. Shabigh R, Fishman IJ, Scott, FB: Evaluation of erectile impotence. *Urology* 32:83, 1988.

6. National Center for Health Statistics DHSS 87-1751: National Hospital Discharge Survey. Bethesda, MD, 1989.

7. Feldman HA, Goldstein I, Hatzichristou DG, Krane RJ, McKinlay JB: Impotence and

its medical and psychological correlates: results of Massachusetts male aging study. *J Urol* 151:54–61, 1994.

8. Kinsey AC, Pomeroy WB, Martin CE: *Sexual Behavior in the Human Male* Philadelphia, W. B. Saunders, 1948.

9. Gebhard PH, Johnson AB: *The Kinsey Data: Marginal Tabulations of the 1938–1963 Interviews Conducted by the Institute for Sex Research.* Philadelphia, W. B. Saunders, 1972.

10. Spector IP, Carey MP: Incidence and prevalence of the sexual dysfunctions. *Arch Sex Behav* 19:389, 1990.

11. Ard BN: Sex in lasting marriages: a longitudinal study. *J Sex Res* 13:274, 1977.

12. Frank E, Anderson C, Rubinstein D: Frequency of sexual dysfunction in normal couples. *N Engl J Med* 299:111, 1978.

13. Nettelbladt P, Uddenberg N: Sexual dysfunction and sexual satisfaction in 58 Swedish men. *J Psychosom Res* 23:141, 1979.

14. Diokno AC, Brown MB, Herzog AR: Sexual function in the elderly. *Arch Intern Med* 150:197, 1990.

15. Reading AE, Wiest WM: An analysis of self-reported sexual behaviour in a sample of normal males. *Arch Sex Behav* 13:69, 1984.

16. Morley JE: Impotence. *Am J Med* 80:897, 1985.

17. Keil JE, Sutherlan SE, Knapp RG, et al: Self-reported sexual functioning in elderly blacks and whites. The Charleston Heart Study experience. *J Aging Health* 4:112, 1992.

18. Schein M, Zyzanski SJ, Levine S, et al: The frequency of sexual problems among family practice patients. *Fam Pract Res J* 7:122, 1988.

19. Mulligan T, Retchin SM, Chincilli VM: The role of aging and chronic disease in sexual dysfunction. *J Am Geriatr Soc* 36:520, 1988.

20. Morley JE: Impotence in older men. *Hosp Pract* 4:139, 1988.

21. Slag MF, Morley JE, Elson JK, et al: Impotence in medical clinic outpatients. *JAMA* 249:1736, 1983.

22. Mulhall JP, Graydon RJ: Characteristics of men presenting for impotence evaluation (*Submitted*).

23. Feldman HA, Goldstein I, Hatzichristou DG, Krane RJ, McKinlay JB: Impotence and its psychosocial correlates: Results of the Massachusetts Male aging study. *J Urol* 151:54, 1994.

24. Junemann KP, Persson-Junemann C, Alken P: Pathophysiology of erectile dysfunction. *Semin Urol* 8:80, 1990.

25. Wabrek AJ, Burchell RC: Male sexual dysfunction associated with coronary heart disease. *Arch Sex Behav* 9:69, 1980.

26. Gundle GJ, Bozman BR, Tate S, et al: Psychosocial outcome after aortocoronary artery surgery. *Am J Psych* 137:1591, 1980.

27. Morley JE, Korenman SG, Mooradian AD, Kaiser FE: Sexual dysfunction in the elderly male. *J Am Geriatr Soc* 35:1014, 1987.

28. Virag R, Bouilly P, Frydman D: Is impotence an arterial disorder? A study of arterial risk factors in 400 impotent men. *Lancet* 1:181, 1985.

29. Oaks WW, Moyer JH: Sex and hypertension. *Med Aspects Hum Sex* 6:128, 1972.

30. Whitehead ED, Klyde BJ: Diabetes-related impotence in the elderly. *Clin Geriatr Med* 6:771, 1990.

31. Lehman TP, Jacobs JA: Etiology of diabetic impotence. *J Urol* 129:291, 1983.

32. McCulloch DK, Campbell IW, Wu FC, Prescott RJ, Clarke BF: The prevalence of diabetic impotence. *Diabetologia* 18:279, 1980.

33. Rubin A, Babbott D: Impotence and diabetes mellitus. *JAMA* 168 498, 1958.

34. Kaiser FEK, Korenman SG: Impotence in diabetic men. *Am J Med* 85:147, 1988.

35. Zemel P: Sexual dysfunction in the diabetic patient with hypertension. *Am J Cardiol* 61:27H, 1988.

36. Shabsigh R, Fishman I, Schum C, Dunn JK: Cigarette smoking and other vascular risk factors in vasculogenic impotence. *Urology* 38:227, 1991.

37. Nickel JC, Morales A, Conra M, et al: Endocrine dysfunction in impotence: incidence, significance, and cost-effective screening. *J Urol* 132:40, 1984.

38. Spark RR, White RA, Connolly PB: Impotence is not always psychogenic: newer insights into the hypothalamic-pituitary-gonadal dysfunction. *JAMA* 243:750, 1980.

39. Maatman TJ, Montague DK: Routine endocrine screening in impotence. *Urology* 27:499, 1986.

40. Korenman SG, Morley JE, Mooradian AD, et al: Secondary hypogonadism in older men: its relation to impotence. *J Clin Endocrinol Metab* 71:963. 1990.

41. Bancroft J, Wu FCW: Changes in erectile responsiveness during androgen replacement therapy. *Arch Sex Behav* 12:59, 1983.

42. Foster RS, Mulcahy N, Callaghan JT, et al: Role of serum prolactin determination in evaluation of the impotent patient. *Urology* 36:499, 1990.

43. Morales A, Johnston B, Heaton J: Oral androgens in the treatment of hypogonadal impotent men. *J Urol* 128:1115–1117, 1994.

44. Zonszein J: Diagnosis and management of endocrine disorders of erectile dysfunction. *Urol Clin North Am* 22:789–802, 1995.

45. Wein AJ, Van Arsdalen K: Drug-induced male sexual dysfunction. *Urol Clin North Am* 15:23, 1988.

46. Goldstein I, Krane RJ: Drug-induced sexual dysfunction. *World J Urol* 1:239, 1983.

47. Seagraves RT, Madsen R, Carter CS, et al: Erectile dysfunction associated with pharmacologic agents. In Seagraves RT, Schoenberg HW (eds): *Diagnosis and Treatment of Erectile Disturbances*. New York, Plenum, 1985, p 22.

48. Neri A, Aygen M, Zuckerman Z, et al: Subjective assessment of sexual dysfunction of patients on long-term administration of digoxin. *Arch Sex Behav* 9:343, 1980.

49. Horowitz JD, Gobel AJ: Drugs and impaired sexual function. *Drugs* 18:206, 1979.

50. Pont A, Williams PL, Azhar S, et al: Ketoconazole blocks testosterone synthesis. *Arch Intern Med* 142:2137, 1982.

51. Greenblatt DJ, Koch-Weser J: Gynecomastia and impotence: complication of spironolactone. *JAMA* 223:83, 1983.

52. Jones CD, Langman MJ, Lawson DH, et al: Post-marketing surveillance of the safety of cimetidine: 12 month morbidity report. *Q J Med* 54:253, 1985.

52a. Gupta S, Daley J, Pabby A, et al: A new mechanism for Digoxin—associated impotence in vitro and in vivo study. *J Urol* 155:621A.

53. Yassa R: Sexual disorders in the course of clomipramine therapy. *Can J Psych* 27:148, 1982.

54. Mitchell JE, Popkin MK: Antidepressant drug therapy and sexual dysfunction in men: a review. *J Clin Psychopharmacol* 3:76, 1983.

55. Mathew RJ, Weinman ML, Thapar R, et al: Somatic symptoms in depression and anti-depressants. *J Clin Psych* 44:10, 1983.

56. Blay S, Ferraz MP, Calil HM: Lithium-induced male sexual impairment. *J Clin Psych* 43:497, 1982.

57. Whalley LJ: Sexual adjustment of male alcoholics. *Acta Psychiatr Scand* 56:281, 1978.

58. Mirin SM, Meyer RE, Mendelsohn JH, et al: Opiate use and sexual function. *Am J Psychiatry* 137:909, 1980.

59. Melman A, Gordon G, Warner T: Evaluation of sexual dysfunction in men with severe chronic alcoholism. *J Urol* 133:187A, 1985.

60. Cicero TJ, Bell RD, West WG, et al: Function of the male sex organs in heroin and methadone users. *N Engl J Med* 292:882, 1975.

60a. Mumarriz R, Quingwei RY, Goldstein I: Blunt trauma: The pathophysiology of hemo-dynamic injury leading to erectile dysfunction *J Urol* 153:1831, 1995.

61. Dhabuwala CB, Hamid S, Katsikas DM, et al: Impotence following delayed repair of prostatomembranous urethral disruption. *J Urol* 144:677, 1990.

62. Mulhall JP, Graydon RJ: Hemodynamics of erectile dysfunction following nerve-sparing radical retropubic prostatectomy. *Int J Imp Res* (*in press*).

63. Quinlan DM, Epstein JI, Carter BS, et al: Sexual function following radical prostatec-tomy: influence of preservation of neurovascular bundles. *J Urol* 145:998, 1991.

64. Walsh PC, Lepor H, Eggleston JC: Radical prostatectomy with preservation of sexual function: anatomical and pathological considerations. *Prostate* 4:473, 1983.

65. Finkle AL, Taylor SP: Sexual potency after radical prostatectomy. *J Urol* 125:350, 1981.

66. Fowler JE, Clayton M, Sharifi R, et al: Early experience with Walsh technique of radical retropubic prostatectomy. *Urology* 29:242, 1987.

67. Lindner A, Golomb J, Korczak D, et al: Effects of prostatectomy on sexual function. *Urology* 37:26, 1991.

68. Gilling PJ, Wright WL, Gray JM: Factors associated with sexual dysfunction following transurethral resection of the prostate. *N Z Med J* 101:484, 1988.

69. Benet AE, Abarbanel J, Lask DM, et al: Surgical management of long urethral strictures. *J Urol* 143:917, 1990.

70. Lue TF: Impotence after radical pelvic surgery: physiology and management. *Urol Int* 46:259, 1991.

71. LoPiccolo J: Management of psychogenic erectile dysfunction. In Tanagho EA, Lue TF, McClure RD (eds): *Contemporary Management of Impotence and Infertility*. Baltimore, Williams & Wilkins, 1988, p 133.

72. Hengevelt MW: Erectile disorders: a psychosexual review. In Jonas U, Thon WF, Stief CG (eds): *Erectile Dysfunction*. Berlin, Springer-Verlag, 1991, p 207.

73. Thase ME, Reynolds CF, Jennings JR, et al: Nocturnal penile tumescence is diminished in depressed men. *Biol Psychiatry* 24:33, 1988.

74. Rust J, Golombok S, Collier J: Marital problems and sexual dysfunction: how are they related? *Br J Psychiatry* 152:629, 1988.

75. Abrams HS, Hester LR, Sheridan WF, et al: Sexual functioning in men with chronic renal failure. *J Nerv Ment Dis* 160:220, 1975.

75a Kaufman JM, Hatzichristou DG, Mulhall JP: Impotence and chronic renal failure. A study of the hemodynamic pathophysiology *J Urol* 151:612, 1994.

76. Glass CA, Fielding DM, Evans C, et al: Factors related to sexual functioning in males undergoing hemodialysis and with kidney transplants. *Arch Sex Behav* 16:189, 1987.

77. Salvatierra O, Fortman JL, Belzer FO: Sexual function of males before and after renal transplantation. *Urology* 5:64, 1975.

78. Gittes RF, Waters WB: Sexual impotence: the overlooked complication of a second renal transplant. *J Urol* 121:719, 1979.

79. Lilius HG, Valtonen EJ, Wikstrom J: Sexual problems in patients suffering from multiple sclerosis. *J Chronic Dis* 29:643, 1976.

80. Agarwal A, Jain DC: Male sexual dysfunction after stroke. *J Assoc Phys India* 37:505, 1989.

81. Goldstein I, Siroky MB, Sax DS, et al: Neurourologic abnormalities in multiple sclerosis. *J Urol* 128:541, 1982.

82. Welby SB, Rogerson SJ, Beeching NJ: Autonomic neuropathy is common in human immunodeficiency virus infection. *J Infect* 23:123, 1991.

83. Fletcher EC, Martin RJ: Sexual dysfunction and erectile impotence in chronic obstructive pulmonary disease. *Chest* 81:413, 1982.

84. Nowlin NS, Brick JE, Weaver DJ, et al: Impotence in scleroderma. *Ann Intern Med* 104:794, 1986.

85. Cornely CM, Schade RR, Van Thiel DH, et al: Chronic advanced liver disease and impotence: cause and effect? *Hepatology* 4:1227, 1984.

2

Anatomy and Physiology of Erection

Ignacio Moncada Iribarren
Iñigo Saenz de Tejada

ANATOMY OF THE PENIS

The penis comprises the urethra and three erectile bodies: two corpora and the corpus spongiosum wrapped by a fascial sheath called Buck's fascia (Fig. 2.1). It is a thick elastic layer firmly attached to the underlying tunica albuginea. Surrounding this fascia there is Colles' fascia or superficial penile fascia, which is continuous with Scarpa's fascia of the lower abdominal wall and the dartos fascia of the scrotum. Above this fascia there is the skin.[1]

The skin over the penis is remarkably movable and expandable to accommodate erection. Such flexibility and lack of adherence makes it highly susceptible to edema. Along with its thinness, the absence of fat beneath if accounts for its darker color. Distally, the skin of the penis is attached to the glans to form the prepuce or foreskin.

Proximally, the body of the penis is suspended from the linea alba and attached to the pubic bone by two ligamentous attachments that are continuous with Buck's fascia: the suspensory ligament, which extends from the pubic symphysis to Buck's fascia, just superior to the hilum of the penis; and the fundiform ligament, which lies distal to the suspensory ligament, arising from the lower part of the linea alba and passes on either side of the penis, coming together, inferiorly, as part of the scrotal septum. Proximal to the suspensory ligament, the right and left corpora cavernosa diverge forming the crura that reach the ischial tuberosities on either side. The crura are covered by the ischiocavernous muscle which may play a role in the final rigid phase of the erection (Fig. 2.2).

The corpus spongiosum surrounds the urethra which traverses the length of the penis within this structure, lying in the ventral groove formed by both corpora cavernosa in the pendulous portion of the penis. At its proximal section, it expands to form the bulb, which is attached to the inferior layer of the urogenital diaphragm. At this part of the penis, where both corpora split to form the crura, the bulbar urethra continues superiorly, passes through the urogenital diaphragm, reaches the prostatic gland, passing through it and reaches the bladder. Distally, the corpus

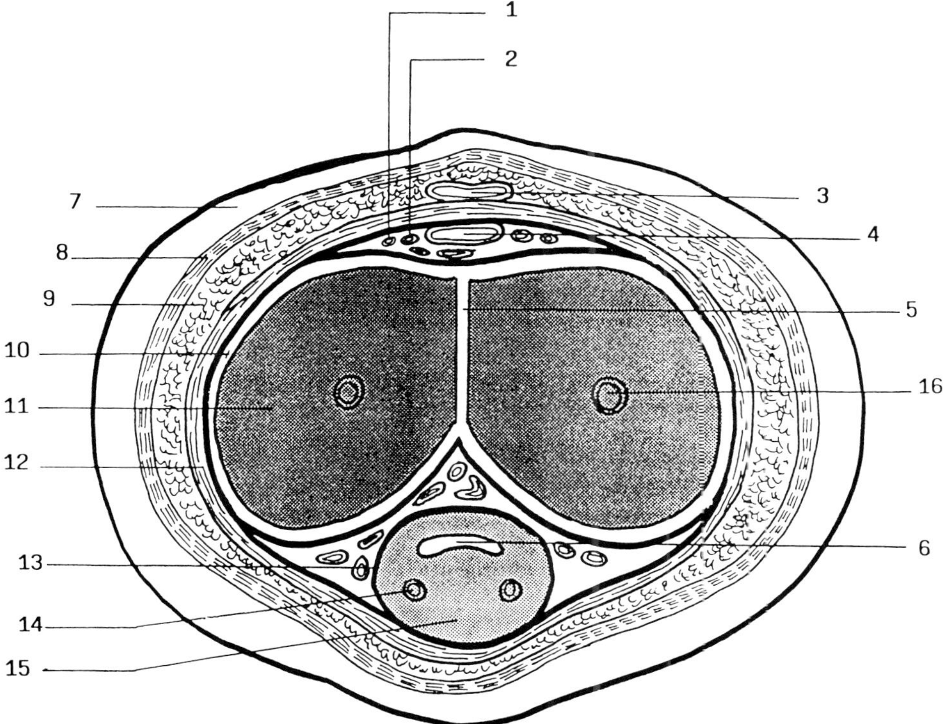

Fig. 2.1. Cross-section of the body of the penis. 1. Dorsal artery. 2. Dorsal nerve. 3. Superficial dorsal vein. 4. Deep dorsal vein. 5. Intercavernous midline septum. 6. Urethra. 7. Skin. 8. Dartos. 9. Subcutaneous cellular tissue. 10. Tunica albuginea. 11. Corpus cavernosum erectile tissue. 12. Buck's fascia. 13. Corpus spongiosum albuginea. 14. Urethral artery. 15. Corpus spongiosum.

spongiosum expands forming the glans penis. The spongiosum is composed of sinusoidal spaces of larger size than those of the cavernosal bodies and with less smooth muscle. There is practically no tunica albuginea and only a minimal amount of fibrous tissue between the sinusoids and the epidermis.

The corpora cavernosa are paired cylinders, dorsally located, which constitute the bulk of the penis. Both corpora cavernosa communicate for three-quarters of their length. Although in the simian the corpora cavernosa unite to form a single structure, in the human they remain as two separate tubular structures that connect freely through a common perforated midline septum composed of multiple strands of elastic tissue similar to that making up the tunica albuginea.[2] From a physiologic point of view, the corpora cavernosa may be considered a single blood space.

Each corpus cavernosum is encased with a thick fibrous sheath, the tunica albuginea, forming a white coat. Two layers may be identified: an outer longitudinal and an inner circular coat. Ventrally, the tunica albuginea forms a groove for the corpus spongiosum. Ventromedially, the tunica is thinner as the outer coat becomes attenuated, leaving only the inner coat. This difference in the thickness of the tunica explains the higher possibility of perforation at that site during the insertion of a penile prosthesis which may cause injury to the urethra.[3]

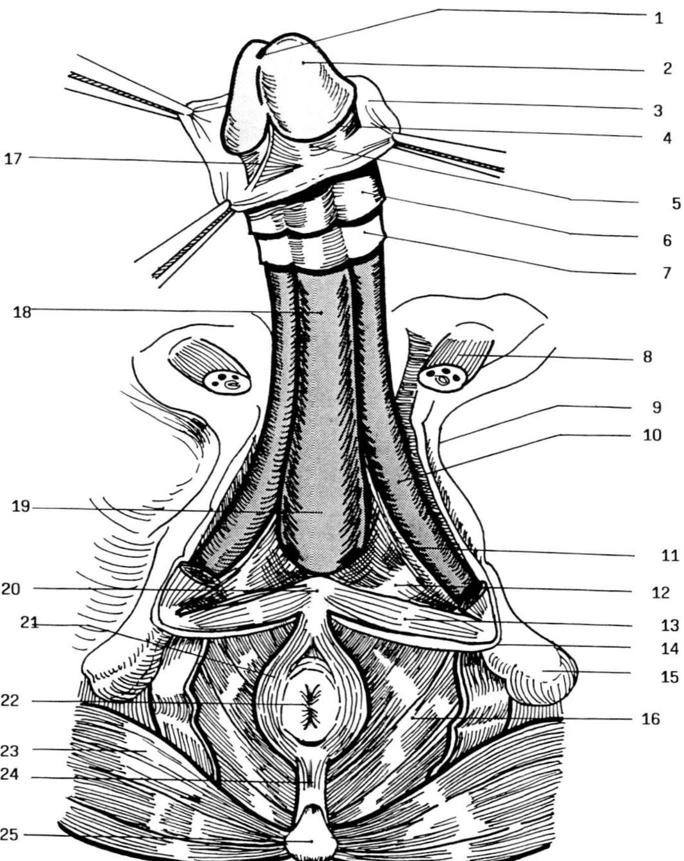

Fig. 2.2. Anatomy of the perineum, the crura, and the corpus spongiosum. 1. Urethral meatus. 2. Glans penis. 3. Foreskin. 4. Corona glandis. 5. Balanopreputial sulcus. 6. Dartos fascia or Colles' fascia. 7. Deep fascia or Buck's fascia. 8. Spermatic cord. 9. Ischiopubic ramus. 10. Left crura. 11. Ischiocavernous muscle. 12. Fascia of the urogenital diaphragm. 13. Transversus perinei muscle. 14. Insertion of the left crura. 15. Ischial tuberosity. 16. Levator ani. 17. Frenulum. 18. Corpus spongiosum. 19. Bulb of penis. 20. Central tendon of the perineum. 21. External anal sphincter. 22. Anus. 23. Gluteus maximus. 24. Anococcygeal ligament. 25. Coccyx.

The erectile tissue is composed of multiple lacunar spaces, interconnected and lined by vascular endothelium. The trabeculae are the walls of these spaces and are formed by smooth muscle (approximately 45%) and a fibroelastic framework of, mainly, collagen.[4]

VASCULAR ANATOMY

Arterial Vascularization

Blood supply to the deep structures of the penis is derived, mainly, from the internal pudendal artery, a branch of the hypogastric or internal iliac artery. The hypogastric artery divides on each side to form the inferior gluteal artery and the internal pudendal artery. In the pelvis, the internal pudendal artery passes beneath the sacroespinous ligament and over the sacrotuberous ligament and gives off the perineal artery in the Alcock's canal, where it runs under the superficial transverse perineal muscle and the symphysis. After giving off the perineal artery, it becomes the common penile artery. This artery pierces the urogenital diaphragm along the medial margin of the inferior ramus of the ischium behind the superficial transverse perineal muscle near the bulb of the urethra and gives off four terminal branches before reaching the corpora cavernosa: bulbar, urethral, dorsal, and cavernosal arteries (Fig. 2.3).[5]

The cavernosal artery or deep artery of the penis pierces the tunica entering each corpus cavernosum at the hilum of the penis, where the two corpora come together, running near the center of each corpus along the two-thirds of the length of the penile shaft. It gives off numerous terminal branches called helicine arteries. These muscular arteries are corkscrew-shaped and open directly into the lacunar spaces (Fig. 2.4). There is a strong smooth muscle surrounding these resistance arteries that acts as a sphincter: in flaccidity this muscle is contracted allowing only small amounts of blood into the lacunar spaces. After the proper stimulus this muscle relaxes, and the arteries dilate and straighten, increasing blood flow and pressure to the lacunar spaces. Occasionally the cavernosal arteries divide into two or three branches inside the corpus cavernosum and in 30% of cases there are communications between both cavernosal arteries and in some instances connections with dorsal arteries are also present.[6] Cavernosal arteries offer the main blood supply to the corpora cavernosa.

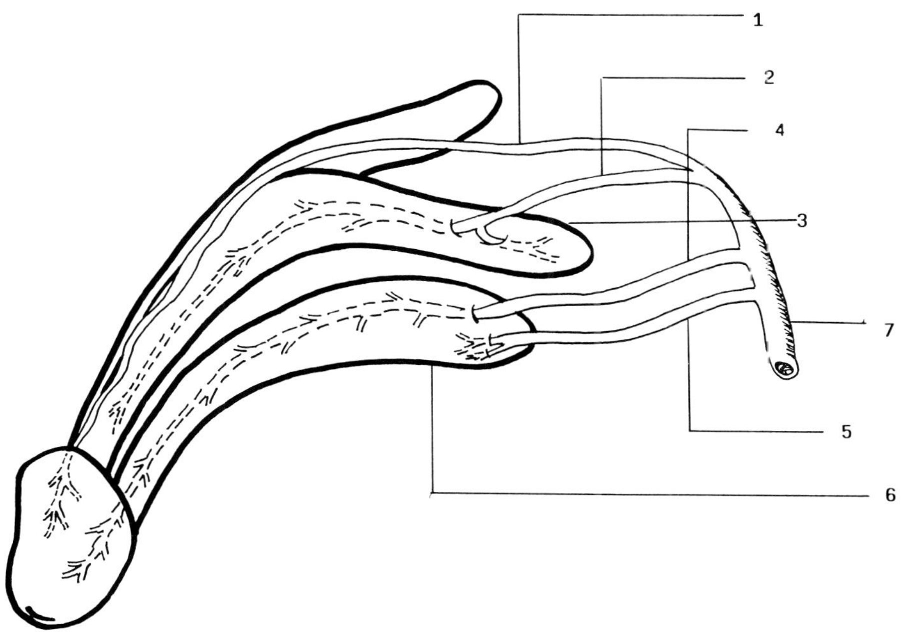

Fig. 2.3. Arterial supply to the penis. 1. Dorsal artery. 2. Cavernous artery. 3. Corpus cavernosum. 4. Urethral artery. 5. Bulbar artery. 6. Corpus spongiosum. 7. Pudendal artery.

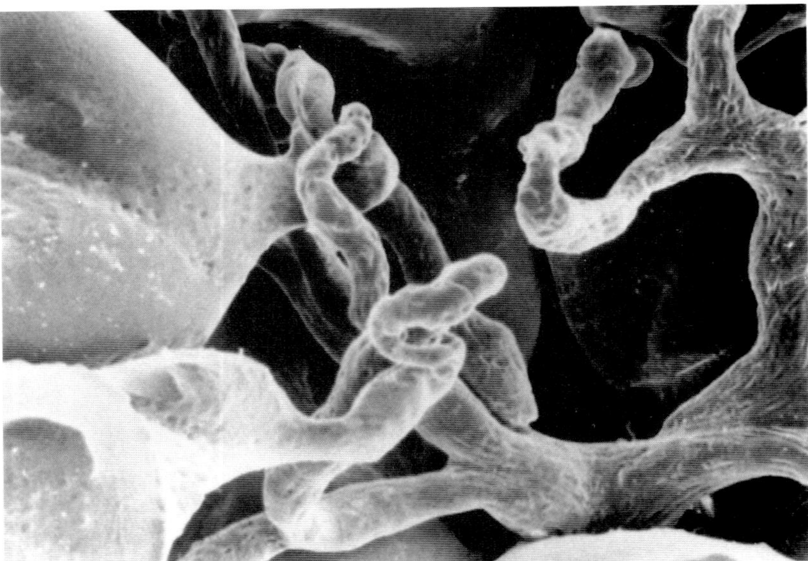

Fig. 2.4. Scanning electron-microscopic study of a cast of penile microcirculation. It shows an helicine artery opening directly into a lacunar space. Helicine arteries regulate the amount of blood entering into the lacunar spaces acting as a sphincter. After the proper stimulus, the muscle surrounding the artery relaxes, increasing the blood flow and pressure to the lacunar spaces. (Courtesy of Dr. Yoshiaki Banya).

The dorsal artery is a terminal branch of the internal pudendal artery. It travels along the dorsal surface of each corpus beneath the Buck's fascia between the deep dorsal vein (medially) and the dorsal nerves (laterally), reaching the glans penis. Along its course it gives off as many as ten circumflex branches that accompany the circumflex veins around the lateral surface of the corpora. These arteries contribute to the blood supply to the urethra and its terminal branches provide blood to the glans and account for glans congestion during the erection.[7]

The bulbar artery is a short blood vessel that enters the urethral bulb to irrigate the urethra in its most proximal portion and the Cowper's glands. The urethral artery runs along the corpus spongiosum providing the blood supply of the penile urethra and corpus spongiosum. Sometimes, bulbar and urethral arteries have a common origin from a bulbourethral artery.[5,7]

The penile skin and the prepuce are irrigated by branches of the external pudendal artery. The inferior external pudendal artery, a branch of the first portion of the femoral artery, divides in each side into two branches, one running dorsolaterally and the other ventrolaterally to the penis, within the dartos fascia. These four main branches give multiple collateral that anastomose to one another forming a penile subdermal arterial plexus.[5]

Venous Drainage

Three systems drain venous blood from the penis: superficial, intermediate, and deep (Fig. 2.5).

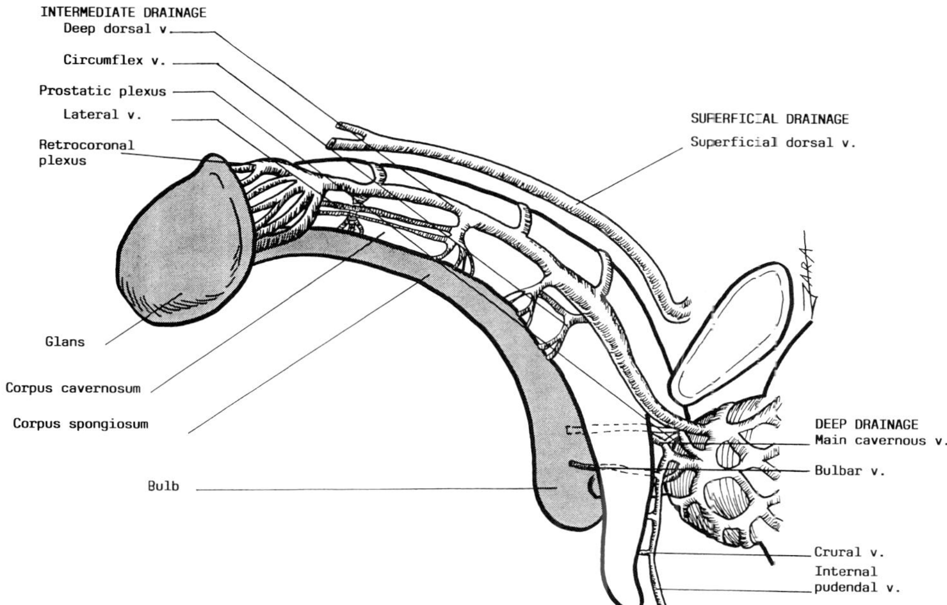

Fig. 2.5. Penile venous drainage.

The superficial system drains blood from multiple superficial veins of skin and subcutaneous tissue above Buck's fascia. These veins drain into the superficial dorsal vein that usually drains into the left external pudendal branch of the internal saphenous vein or, more rarely, into the right saphenous vein. Sometimes the superficial dorsal vein exists as two separate trunks, each draining into its corresponding saphenous veins.

The intermediate venous system lies beneath Buck's fascia and is comprised by the deep dorsal vein and the circumflex veins (Fig. 2.6). This system drains blood from the glans, corpus spongiosum, and two distal thirds of the corpora cavernosa. Veins emerging from the glans penis form a retrocoronal plexus which drains into the deep dorsal vein. This vein runs as a single trunk in a groove between both corpora. It enters the pelvis through the suspensory ligament to drain into the periprostatic or Santorini's plexus.

The deep drainage system is comprised of the cavernosal veins and the crural veins. Emissary veins in the proximal third of the penis join to form one or two cavernosal veins that originate in the hilum of the penis, on the dorsomedial surface of each corpus cavernosum, and pass between the bulb and the crus of the penis, to drain into the pudendal vein. In addition to the cavernous veins, there are 3 to 4 small crural veins which join to form a large channel that drains into the internal pudendal vein.

Drainage of the corpora cavernosa is by the way of venules located at the periphery of the erectile tissue forming a network under the tunica albuginea (Fig. 2.7). These venules coalesce to form the emissary veins which pierce the tunica and drain either directly into the deep dorsal vein or by the way of the circumflex veins. Compression and elongation of the subtunical venules by the expansion of the trabecular

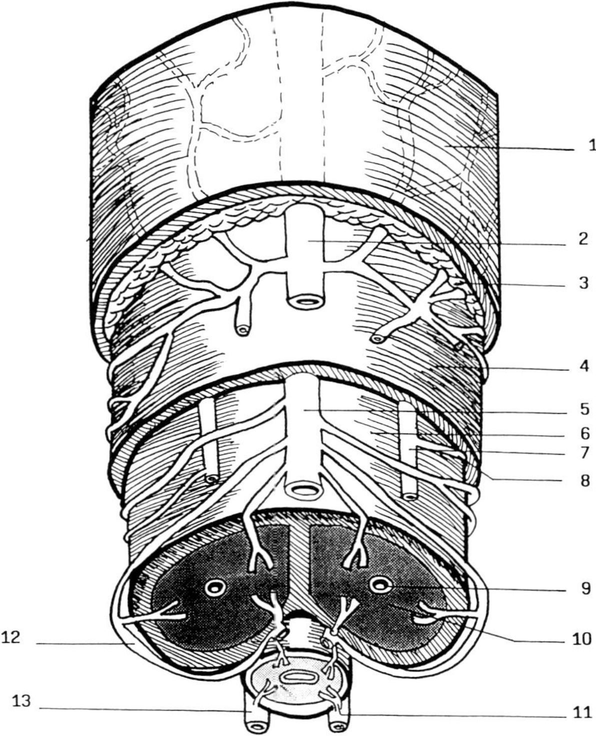

Fig. 2.6. Vascularization of the penis. Superficial and intermediate venous systems are separated by Buck's fascia. Dorsal artery is also beneath the Buck's fascia. 1. Dartos. 2. Superficial dorsal vein. 3. Subcutaneous cellular tissue. 4. Buck's fascia or deep fascia. 5. Deep dorsal vein. 6. Tunica albuginea. 7. Dorsal artery. 8. Collateral branch of the dorsal artery. 9. Cavernous artery or deep artery. 10. Corpus cavernosum erectile tissue. 11. Urethral veins. 12. Circumflex veins. 13. Bulbourethral veins.

structures against the tunica secondarily to the change in penile volume during the erection, causes a dramatic increase in the resistance to blood outflow from the corpora. This is known as the corporo-veno-occlusive mechanism which is triggered by the relaxation of trabecular smooth muscle.[8] This mechanism allows the maintenance of high intracavernosal pressure with low maintenance flow and is so efficient that outflow resistance increases one hundred fold compared to flaccidity (Fig. 2.8). Once erection has been established, only 1 to 5 ml of blood are needed to maintain intracavernosal pressures within a physiologic range (60 and 100 mm Hg).[9]

Lymphatic System

The lymphatic drainage of the penis is to the superficial and deep inguinal lymph nodes of the femoral triangle which, in turn, drain into the external and common iliac lymph nodes. However, the lymphatic drainage of the posterior urethra is to the internal iliac lymph nodes. Drainage from the anterior urethra is also to the inguinal lymph nodes.[7]

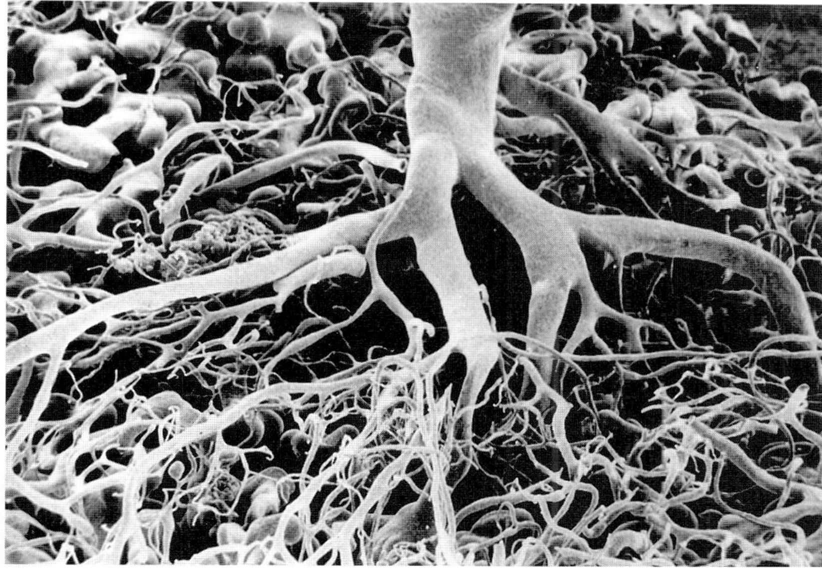

Fig. 2.7. Scanning electron-microscopic study of a cast of the venous system of the corpus. A dense plexus of venules that drain the lacunar spaces can be seen beneath the tunica albuginea. These veins coalesce to form the emissary veins. (Courtesy of Dr. Yoshiaki Banya).

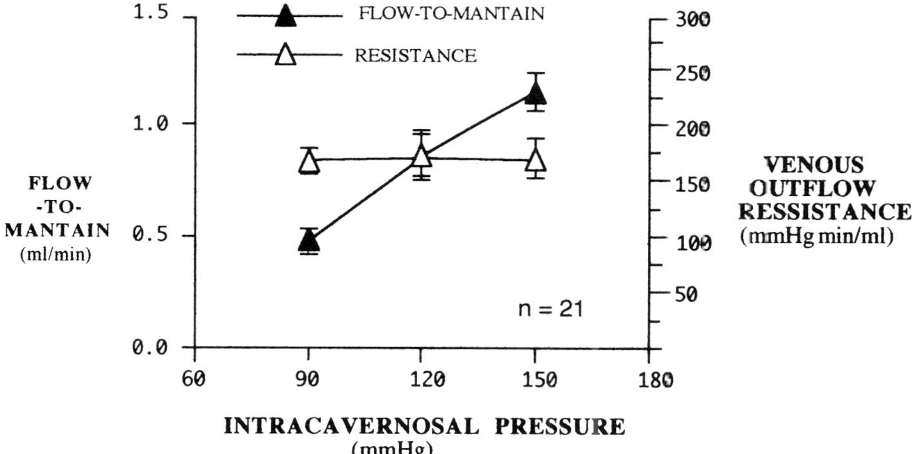

Fig. 2.8. Flow-to-maintain and venous outflow resistance compared to intracavernosal pressure. Flow-to-maintain values increase linearly with increasing intracavernous pressures, whereas venous outflow resistance values are constant indicating complete trabecular smooth muscle relaxation. From Hatzichristou et al.[21]

NEUROANATOMY

Three groups of peripheral nerves have a role in erectile function: thoracolumbar sympathetic, lumbosacral parasympathetic, and lumbosacral somatic.[10,11]

Peripheral Nerves

The thoracolumbar sympathetic center is located in the intermediolateral gray matter of the tenth thoracic to the second lumbar spinal cord segments. Preganglionic fibers abandon the spinal cord through the spinal nerves to the paravertebral sympathetic chain where they make synaptic connections at different levels, mainly at the superior hypogastric plexus, which lies on the great vessels at the level of third lumbar to the first sacral vertebrae. Occasionally preganglionic fibers reach this plexus via lumbar splanchnic nerves. The superior hypogastric plexus divides into two hypogastric nerves that join in the pelvis plexus. These nerves have postganglionic fibers coming from the hypogastric plexus and preganglionic fibers that will make synapsis in the pelvic plexus. Postganglionic fibers from the hypogastric and pelvic plexus and from the paravertebral ganglionar chain join to form the cavernous nerve which enters the penis near the posterolateral side of the prostate (Fig. 2.9).

The sacral parasympathetic center, the so-called "sacral erection center," is located in the intermediolateral gray matter of the spinal cord from the second to the fourth sacral segments.[11,12] The sacral preganglionic nerves constitute the pelvic

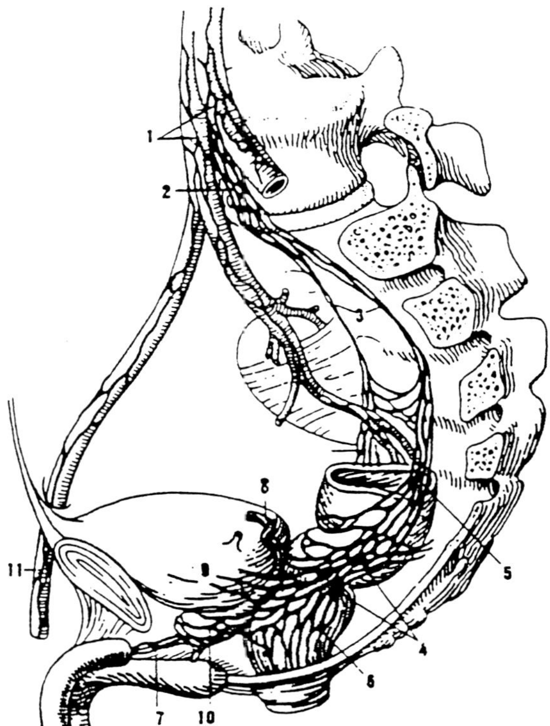

Fig. 2.9. Efferent innervation to the penis. 1. Inferior mesenteric plexus. 2. Superior hypogastric plexus. 3. Hypogastric nerves. 4. Pelvic plexus. 5. Pelvic nerve. 6. Rectal plexus. 7. Cavernous nerve. 8. Left ureter. 9. Bladder. 10. Neural bundle at the lateral aspect of the prostate. 11. Spermatic nerve.

nerve or nervi erigentes that reach the pelvic plexus. This plexus serves as a relay within which preganglionic fibers make synapsis with the postganglionic fibers that innervate the penis through the cavernous nerve.

The cavernous nerve, containing sympathetic and parasympathetic postganglionic fibers, leaves the pelvis between the transverse perineal muscles and the membranous urethra passing beneath the arch of the pubic bone to supply each corpus cavernosum. Two branches may be found. One is the lesser cavernous nerve that supplies the erectile tissue of the corpus spongiosum as well as the penile urethra. The outer branch, the greater cavernous nerve, stays beneath the prostatic venous plexus and enters the corpora cavernosa around the cavernous vessels in the hilum of the penis. The cavernous nerve runs with branches of the prostatovesicular artery and veins as the so-called neurovascular bundle. It passes anterior to Denonvilliers' fascia between the posterolateral surface of the prostate and the rectum to lie above the endopelvic fascia and under Santorini's venous plexus. As it passes posterolaterally to the prostate, the bundle gives off fine branches to supply the prostatic capsule (Fig. 2.9). At the prostatic apex the nerve passes very near to the urethral lumen at the 3 and 9 o'clock positions and enter the penile crura more anteriorly, at 1 and 11 o'clock. It is the main nerve responsible for providing signal transmission to the erectile tissue eliciting relaxation of smooth muscle and, thus, erection. The knowledge of this neuroanatomy of erection has stimulated strategies for the preservation of potency in operations like radical prostatectomy normally associated with a high rate of postoperative impotence.[12,13]

Somatic innervation depends on the pudendal nerve which is comprised of motor efferent fibers innervating the ischiocavernosal and bulbocavernosal muscles, as well as sensory fibers from the penis and perineal skin. Pudendal motor neurons are located in the Onuf's nucleus in the second, third, and fourth segments of the sacral cord. The pudendal nerve enters the perineum with the internal pudendal vessels through the lesser sciatic notch at the posterior border of the ischiorectal fossa and

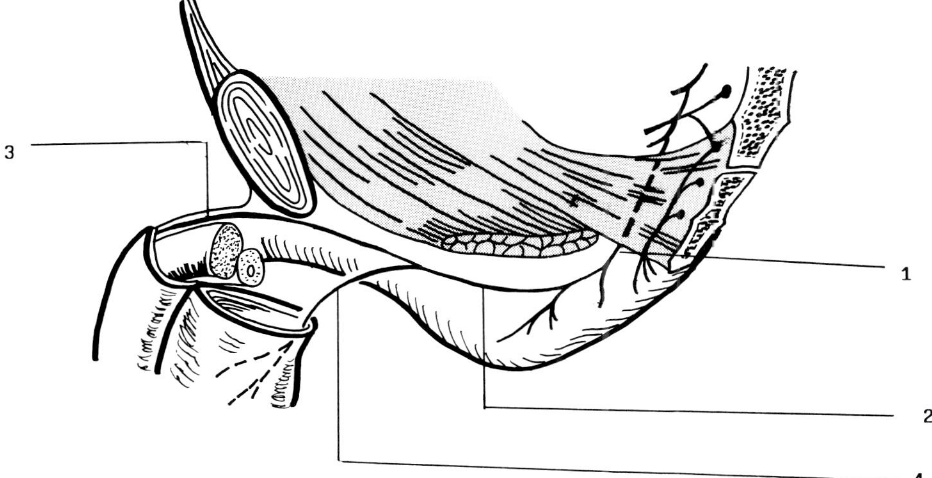

Fig. 2.10. Pudendal innervation. 1. Pelvic nerve. 2. Pudendal nerve. 3. Dorsal nerve of the penis. 4. Urethral fibers.

runs in the fibrofascial sheath of Alcock's canal toward the posterior aspect of the perineal membrane. There it gives off the perineal nerve with branches to the posterior part of the scrotum and the rectal nerve to the inferior rectal area (Fig. 2.10).

The dorsal nerve of the penis arises as the last branch of the pudendal nerve. Distally the nerve runs along the dorsal penile shaft lateral to the dorsal artery. Multiple fascicles fan out from the dorsal nerve, supplying proprioceptive and sensory nerve terminals on the surface of the tunica albuginea and sensory terminals in the skin and glans penis. Deep dorsal vein, dorsal arteries, and dorsal nerves constitute the neurovascular bundle of the penis, a structure that must be handled very carefully when penile surgery is to be done, as its damage may cause anesthesia to the glans and penile shaft as well as necrosis of the glans if there is not enough arterial supply by urethral arteries.[14]

The functional significance of the somatomotor system is not clear in humans. Patients with spinal cord injuries and paralysis of the pelvic floor can have erections, suggesting that perineal musculature is not needed for the erection.[15] On the other hand, it has been shown that glans stimulation is followed by contractions of ischiocavernous muscles provoking suprasystolic intracavernosal pressures. Tactile stimulation of the penis during sexual intercourse triggers this bulbocavernous reflex permitting the penis to reach a high level of rigidity for penetration.

Central Mechanisms

Penile erections are elicited by local sensory stimulation of the frenulum, glans penis, and penile skin (reflexogenic erections) and by central psychogenic stimuli received by or generated within the brain (psychogenic erections). Reflexogenic and psychogenic erectile mechanisms probably act synergistically in the control of penile erection.[8] Reflexogenic erections are mediated by a spinal reflex pathway in which the afferent limb consists of sensory receptors in the penile skin and the glans, and the dorsal nerve that joins the pudendal nerve to reach the sacral spinal cord. The efferent limb arises in the sacral parasympathetic center and contributes fibers to the pelvic nerve, which enter the erectile tissue as the cavernosal nerve.

The pathways for psychogenic erections are less well understood. They initiate in supraspinal centers by auditive, olfactory, imaginative, or visual stimuli. It is clear that psychogenic stimuli to the brain may also inhibit erections. Therefore the brain must exert an important modulator influence over spinal reflex pathways that control penile erection.

Diverse areas of the brain have the potential for modulating penile erection. This is predictable on the basis of the elevated number of stimuli that are known to elicit erectile responses. The anatomic regions are not completely known but it appears that the thalamic nuclei, the rhinencephalon, and the limbic structures are involved in the modulation of psychogenic penile erections. Messages from diverse regions are integrated in the medial preoptic–anterior hypothalamic area.[15] The cortico-subcortical region of the limbic system is implicated in the integration of inhibitory and facilitator signals connecting to the medial preoptic–anterior hypothalamic area. Efferent pathways from the medial preoptic–anterior area enter the medial forebrain bundle and then pass caudally into the midbrain tegmental region near the lateral part of the substantia nigra. Caudal to the midbrain the efferent pathway travels in the ventrolateral part of the pons and medulla reaching the spinal centers via the lateral funiculus of the spinal cord.

In contrast to the well-established role of the hypothalamus–spinal autonomic pathways in the mediation of sexual responses, the function of higher centers is less clear. It has been postulated that three systems are involved in penile erection: the gyrus rectus, the cyngulate gyrus, and the hippocampus and hippocampal projections to the septum.[10,11]

The spinal cord is a major site for the regulation of erectile and antierectile outflows, and the coordination of autonomic with somatic pathways. In patients with spinal cord injuries above sacral segments, the stimulus of penile receptors triggers an erection via the sacral spinal reflex. These patients have poor quality erections with premature detumescence because of the absence of supraspinal control.[16] On the other hand, lesions of the sacral segments of the spinal cord, the sacral roots, the pelvic or the pudendal nerves abolish reflexogenic erections.

PHYSIOLOGY OF ERECTION

Hemodynamics of Erection

The penis, during erection, acts as a capacitor, accumulating blood under pressure.[9] Cavernous and helicine arteries are contracted in the flaccid state creating a large pressure gradient between the cavernosal artery and the lacunar spaces, which is necessary to maintain the flaccid state of the penis. The peak flow velocity is not detectable below 15 cm/sec.[17] In physiologic conditions either the cavernosal or helicine resistance arteries are contracted, thus, a state of low flow and low pressure exists in the penis. Color Doppler studies of cavernosal arteries in humans show an inner diameter of 0.5 mm in the cavernous arteries at the base of the penis. Dilatation of cavernosal and helicine arteries (the resistance vessels of the corpora) is the first event leading to penile erection. In a healthy potent man, a twofold dilatation of the cavernous artery to a 1-mm diameter and a peak flow velocity of over 30 cm/sec can be detected.[18] High flow enters the corpora cavernosa during both diastolic and systolic phases. The dilated blood vessels allow transmission of systemic pressure to the corpora. Progressively, the penis begins to show a change in volume and fullness and the intracavernosal pressure begins to rise.

Relaxation of the trabecular smooth muscle increases the compliance of the tissue enabling the dilatation of the lacunar spaces with expansion of the erectile tissue against the tunica albuginea. Plastic casts of the penile vessels have demonstrated elongation and compression of subtunical venules because of the change in volume of the penis and the expansion of the erectile tissue against the tunica albuginea. Hemodynamically, the elongation and compression of the venules results in a large increase in the resistance to the passage of flow through these vessels, which is the functional basis of the corporo-veno-occlusive mechanism.[10] Therefore this mechanism is regulated by the tone of the trabecular smooth muscle. When the smooth muscle is contracted, there is low resistance to outflow allowing for the easy evacuation of the corporal bodies, contributing to the maintenance of penile flaccidity. Conversely, following smooth muscle relaxation, there is a large increase in outflow resistance: approximately 100-fold compared to the flaccid state.

The penis rapidly expands and elongates to its maximal capacity. When the compliance limit for the fibroelastic elements of the penis has been reached, the intracavernosal pressure increases rapidly. When it rises above the diastolic pressure, inflow occurs only in the systolic phase.[19] The intracavernosal pressure equilibrates at a pressure approximating the cavernosal artery systolic occlusion pressure less the loss of pressure from corporal drainage. The arterial pressure rather than arterial flow appears to govern penile rigidity under physiologic conditions.[10]

Penile rigidity expresses the basic mechanical parameter of the quality of the erectile response.[20] Although intracavernosal pressure has been recognized as the main component for penile rigidity, the widely varying magnitude of intracavernosal pressures associated with penile rigidity has made it apparent that there are additional contributory factors. The importance of the architecture and the geometry of the penis to its function has been demonstrated in several studies. Recently, an engineering investigation of penile hemodynamic and structural-dynamic relationships has analytically described the link between penile buckling forces and their underlying constituents.[21] The major factors associated with penile rigidity were: high values of intracavernosal pressure (pressure was related to rigidity in an exponential fashion); high values of penile aspect ratio or relatively large diameter and short length penile geometry; and high expandability of erectile tissue, implying the ability to achieve maximal volume at low pressure values during pressure loading.

Ultrastructure and General Properties of Smooth Muscle

Smooth muscle of the penis is, thus, a key determinant of the hemodynamic events that govern penile erection. We will review the ultrastructure and general properties of smooth muscle and then the mechanisms for the regulation of its contractility.

Approximately 45% of cavernosal volume is smooth muscle.[22] Alterations in the relative quantities and structure of the cytoskeleton and contractile proteins may be responsible for changes in the passive and active characteristics of penile smooth muscle. Passive mechanical properties of cavernosal tissue depend on the relative proportion between muscular and nonmuscular components, particularly collagen, and on the orientation of smooth muscle.[2,23] Active mechanical properties of smooth muscle depend on adequate levels of agonists (neurotransmitters, hormones, and endothelium-derived factors), adequate expression of receptors, integrity of transduction mechanisms, calcium homeostasis, interactions with contractile proteins, as well as intercellular communication between smooth muscle cells (gap junctions).[23]

Ultrastructural examination of a smooth muscle cell reveals thin, thick, and intermediate filamentous structures.[23] Thin filaments are mainly composed of actin. Thick filaments are formed of myosin. Intermediate filaments contain either desmin or vimentin. Each type of filament has a specific function.

Following phosphorylation of myosin by adenosine 5′-triphosphate (ATP), attachments form between the globular heads of a light chain of myosin and actin. These attachments are known as cross-bridges and provide a contractile tone to the smooth muscle.[24] For the maintenance of this tone there is a near zero expenditure of energy, in other words, ATP for myosin phosphorylation. This prolonged maintenance of tone has been attributed to the formation of a latch state during which cross-bridges between actin and myosin are dephosphorylated while attached, yet have a more reduced detachment rate than phosphorylated cross-bridges. This state of tone demands a high concentration of cytoplasmatic free calcium.

Adequate Ca^{2+} homeostasis is required for the regulation of smooth muscle tone. Three different mechanisms are involved: influx of extracellular Ca^{2+} through voltage-regulated channels; activation of membrane-bound receptors that allow extracellular Ca^{2+} to enter the cell through receptor-operated channels; and activation of specific signaling pathways relying on intracellular release of Ca^{2+} from sarcoplasmic reticulum.

Relaxation of smooth muscle is viewed as a "resetting" of contractile machinery, by the resumption of a precontractile state accomplished by lowering cytosolic Ca^{2+} or by a decrease in sensitivity of the contractile machinery to Ca^{2+} (Fig. 2.11). There are various mechanisms whereby cytosolic Ca^{2+} can be reduced and relaxation achieved, but in general, all pathways depend upon the accumulation of the cyclic nucleotides adenosine $3':5'$-cyclic phosphate (cAMP) and cyclic guanosine monophosphate (cGMP), or activation of K-channels with hyperpolarization of cellular membrane. Recently, activation of Na^+/K^+ adenosine triphosphatase (ATPase) by nitric oxide has been shown to be involved in relaxation of trabecular

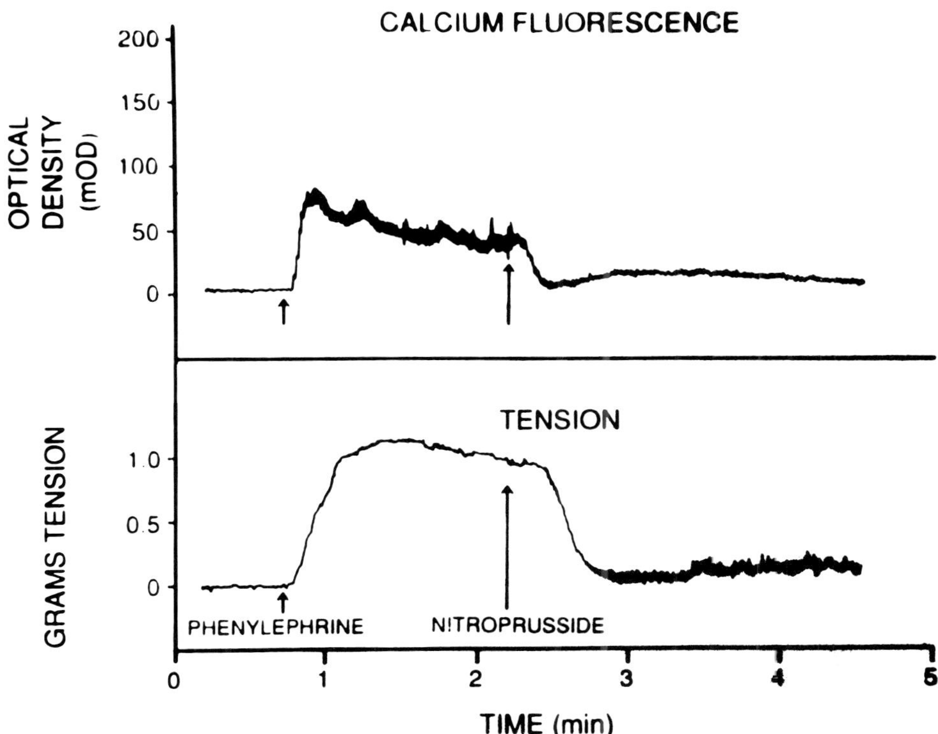

Fig. 2.11. Contraction of smooth muscle by phenylephrine causes an increase in calcium fluorescence that disappears after relaxation with nitroprusside. (Courtesy of Dr. Robert Levin).

smooth muscle.[25] Since Na^+/K^+-ATPase is electrogenic, its stimulation would cause hyperpolarization. Hyperpolarization will prevent the opening of voltage-dependent calcium channels.[26] Many relaxants or neurotransmitters activate guanylate cyclase which catalyzes the conversion of guanosine triphosphate (GTP) to cGMP that subsequently triggers relaxation by lowering cytosolic Ca^{2+} (Fig. 2.12). This pathway is activated by nitric oxide and nitrovasodilators (nitroprusside or nitroglycerine). Other muscle relaxants act by way of a cAMP-dependent mechanism, like prostaglandin E or vasoactive intestinal polypeptide (VIP). These substances react with membrane receptors coupled to a GS type G-protein that stimulates adenylate-cyclase, that catalyses the accumulation of cAMP. Other smooth muscle relaxants, like papaverine, exert its effect through phosphodiesterase inhibition inducing the accumulation of either cAMP and/or cGMP depending on its selectivity.[27]

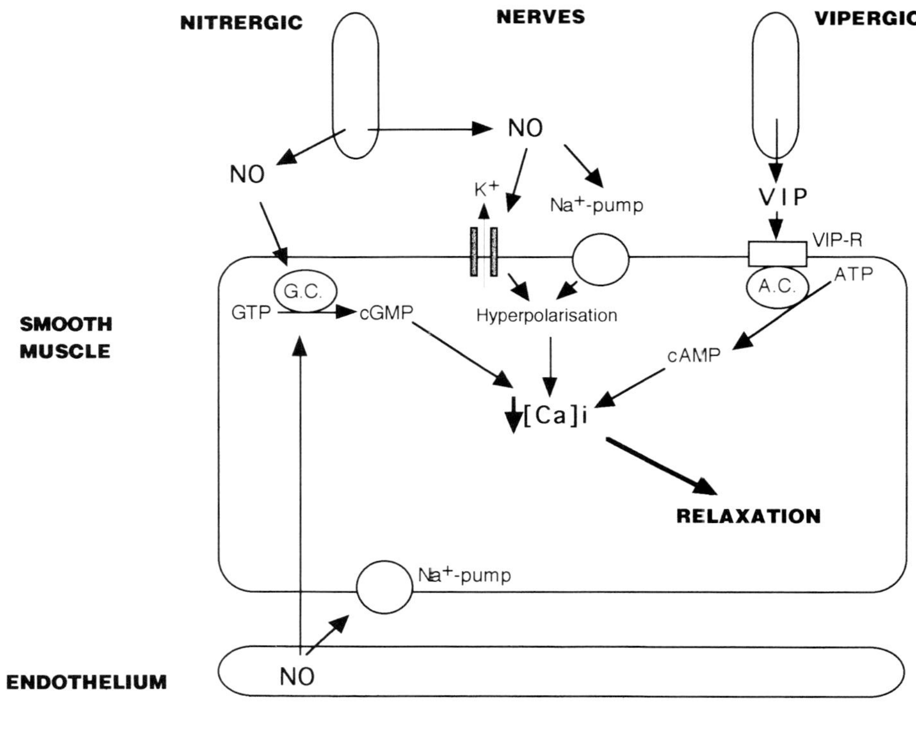

Fig. 2.12. Relaxation mechanisms in penile smooth muscle. Nitrergic nerves act via the accumulation of cGMP, decreasing the concentration of intracellular calcium eliciting relaxation of the smooth muscle cell. NO may act also via the Na pump or potassium channels hyperpolarizing the plasmatic membrane. Vipergic nerves act via the accumulation of cAMP, decreasing the concentration of intracellular calcium. Endothelium-derived NO act in the same way as nitrergic nerves.

Coordination of Smooth Muscle Response

It seems clear that in a tissue, as is the penis, where a scant autonomous innervation exists, the coordination of tissue responses will depend to a large extent on intercellular communications through gap junctions.[28] Gap junctions are a diverse group of intercellular channels formed of six homologous membrane-spanning proteins from each cell, known as conexins, that join to provide aqueous intercellular channels and, thus, partial cytoplasmic continuity between adjacent cells. The major protein component of gap junctions of penile smooth cells is conexin43.[29] The junctions allow the intercellular passage of current carrying ions and second messenger molecules such as inositol triphosphate and calcium ions and are an important pathway for coordination of cellular activation and syncytial smooth muscle responses of penile smooth cells.[30]

Mechanism for the Regulation of Penile Smooth Muscle Contractility

There are two principal types of control of the tone of penile smooth muscle: (a) neurogenic control in which adrenergic, cholinergic nerves and nonadrenergic, noncholinergic (NANC) neuroeffector systems play a role, and (b) endothelial control by substances released by the endothelium lining penile arteries and lacunar spaces.[31] (Fig. 2.13).

Neurogenic Control

Adrenergic mechanisms: The presence of adrenergic nerves has been demonstrated in cavernosal and helicine arteries, as well as in cavernosal smooth muscle of humans.[26] Sympathetic stimulation causes detumescence of the erect penis. This effect is locally mediated by adrenergic nerves. Adrenergic agonists induce contraction of corpus cavernosum strips in vitro, and intracavernosal injection of these agents in vivo causes detumescence of the erect penis. The presence of both α_1- and α_2-adrenergic receptor subtypes in corpus cavernosum tissue has been reported,[32] but the contraction of the trabecular smooth muscle to the noradrenaline seems to be mediated predominantly by the activation of α_1 receptors.[33,34] Recent pharmacologic and functional studies have suggested the presence of more than one α_1 receptor subtype in human corpus cavernosum. In situ hybridization analysis and ribonuclease (RNase) protection assays of messenger RNA (mRNA) isolated from whole tissue demonstrated the presence of mRNA transcripts for three α_1-AR receptor subtypes (α_{1d}, α_{1b}, and α_{1a}).[34] α_2-receptors can also be stimulated by nerve-released norepinephrine (penile arteries) but also by circulating catecholamines (penile arteries and trabecular smooth muscle). This is the rationale for the use of ohimbine, an α_2 blocker, in the treatment of psychogenic impotence associated with an excess of circulating catecholamines.

Cholinergic nerves: Erection is initiated by a sacral parasympathetic nerve input, the preganglionic neurotransmitter of which is acetylcholine. Because of this fact, it was initially assumed that postganglionic cholinergic dilator nerves opposed the constrictor effects of adrenergic nerves. However, recent studies have shown that the dilator neurogenic response is mediated by a NANC neurotransmitter, the chemical

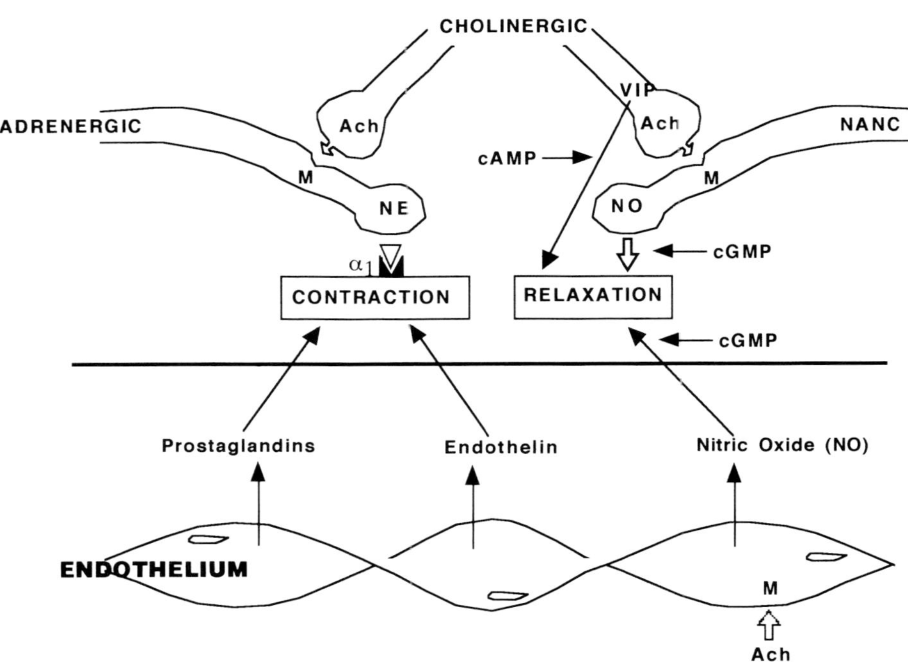

Fig. 2.13. Schematic representation of the mechanisms that control trabecular penile smooth muscle contractility. Neurogenic mechanisms involve three neuroeffector systems: adrenergic (constrictor); cholinergic (dilator); and vasoactive substances such as endothelium-derived nitric oxide, endothelin, and prostaglandins may also contribute to the control of trabecular smooth muscle tone. Ach = acetylcholine; VIP = vasoactive intestinal polypeptide; M = muscarinic receptor; NANC = nonadrenergic noncholinergic; NO = nitric oxide. From Saenz de Tejada.[31]

nature of which has now been defined as nitric oxide or a nitric oxide producing substance. While cholinergic nerves do not mediate corpus cavernosum relaxation via postjunctional receptors in the trabecular smooth muscle, they do act as modulators for other neuroeffectors systems. Acetylcholine, released from cholinergic terminals, has been suggested to stimulate prejunctional muscarinic receptors of adjacent adrenergic nerve endings, and thereby contribute to relaxation by inhibiting the release of norepinephrine.[33,35] In addition, cholinergic nerves enhance NANC relaxation by a yet unidentified mechanism. The vasodilator effects of acetylcholine are due to the stimulation of muscarinic receptors in the endothelium, which in turn releases nitric oxide that relaxes the underlying smooth muscle. In the absence of endothelium, acetylcholine causes either no effect or elicits contraction of trabecular smooth muscle.

Nonadrenergic, noncholinergic neuroeffector system: As mentioned above, the principal neurotransmitter mediating trabecular smooth muscle relaxation is characterized as a NANC neurotransmitter. This is supported by the fact that the intracavernosal injection of the muscarinic receptor blocker atropine does not block penile erection.[36-37] In vitro, transmural electrical stimulation of isolated corpus cavernosum causes a frequency-dependent neurogenic relaxation that is blocked by the neurotoxin tetrodotoxin, but that is resistant to adrenergic and cholinergic blockers.[35]

The 28 amino acid peptide VIP has been proposed by several investigators as the NANC inhibitory neurotransmitter in the trabecular smooth muscle, supported by the observation that VIP-immunoreactive fibers densely innervate penile arteries and the trabecular smooth muscle and VIP elicits relaxation of trabecular smooth muscle in vitro.[18,32] Some VIP-immunoreactive fibers also contain cholinesterase, suggesting a VIP and acetylcholine cotransmission.[38] However, the inability of VIP to elicit an erection when injected intracavernosally indicates that probably VIP is not the main NANC mediator of penile smooth muscle relaxation. Furthermore, several investigations have demonstrated that NANC-mediated relaxation of corpus cavernosum causes the release of nitric oxide and the accumulation of cGMP, questioning the role of VIP as principal neurotransmitter in the erection.[39]

Nitric oxide synthase has been localized by immunohistochemistry in the peripheral autonomic nerves innervating vascular and nonvascular smooth muscle.[40] Transmural electrical stimulation of human corpus cavernosum tissue, in which the endothelium has been mechanically or chemically disrupted, and in the presence of muscarinic and adrenergic blockade, elicits NANC neurogenic relaxation.[43] This response is significantly attenuated or blocked by substances that interfere with the synthesis or the effects of nitric oxide. In vivo, the administration of nitric oxide synthase inhibitors (NG-methyl-L-arginine, NG-nitro-L-arginine) inhibits pelvic nerve stimulated erection in the rat, rabbit, and dog.[44–46] These experiments strongly support the possibility that nitric oxide or a nitric oxide–like substance mediates NANC-mediated relaxation in trabecular smooth muscle. After blockade of adrenergic nerves and inhibition of cholinergic responses, a NANC relaxation of penile arteries to electrical field stimulation, similar to that observed in trabecular smooth muscle, is found. This relaxation involves mainly nitric oxide or a nitric oxide–like substance from nitrergic nerves. It has been also observed that relaxation that follows electrical stimulation of NANC nerve endings, in these arteries, is blocked by inhibitors of nitric oxide synthase.[41] Furthermore, relaxation of penile arteries by nitric oxide is inhibited by charybdotoxin, pointing to the role of calcium-activated potassium channels in this process.[42] Nitric oxide would stimulate the accumulation of cyclic GMP followed by increases in open probability of Ca^{2+}-activated K^+-channels and hyperpolarization leading to relaxation of penile arteries.[42]

Endothelial Control

Endothelium-derived relaxing factor: Vascular endothelium, when it is activated by chemical stimuli (acetylcholine, bradykinin) or physical stimuli (sheer stress), releases a relaxing factor that diffuses to the underlying smooth muscle, causing its relaxation. This paracrine mechanism for the control of the vascular tone was described by Furchgott in 1980 in the aorta of the rabbit.[47] A similar mechanism, in which the lacunar endothelium releases a substance that relaxes the trabecular muscle, has been demonstrated in human and experimental animal cavernous tissue. The mechanical or chemical disruption of the lacunar space endothelium completely eliminates the dilator effects of acetylcholine or bradykinin, two endothelium-dependent vasodilators.[43,48] The relaxing factor derived from the endothelium that lines the lacunar spaces has the chemical properties of nitric oxide.[49] It is also known that vasodilator drugs that are nitric oxide donors like nitroglycerine and nitroprusside elicit relaxation smooth muscle and erection when injected into the penis.

Endothelium-derived nitric oxide diffuses the smooth muscle where it stimulates soluble guanylate cyclase, with accumulation of cGMP and subsequent relaxation of trabecular smooth muscle.[39,50] Endothelium-dependent relaxation is blocked by nitric oxide synthase inhibitors (NG-monomethyl-L-arginine, NG-nitro-L-arginine), by guanylate cyclase blockers (methylene blue), and by nitric oxide scavengers (oxyhemoglobin). In penile arteries, the endothelium-dependent relaxation to acetylcholine and bradykinin is only partly inhibited in the presence of an inhibitor of nitric oxide synthase. The endothelium-dependent relaxing mechanisms of penile resistance arteries thus seem to be different from those observed in the trabecular smooth muscle.

Endothelin: Endothelin-1, discovered by Yanagisawa and collaborators in 1988, is a member of the endothelin family of peptides which includes two other members: endothelin-2 and endothelin-3. Endothelin-1 is a potent vasoconstrictor that, in addition, has been shown to have growth factor activity, stimulating mitogenesis in fibroblasts, smooth muscle, and endothelial cells.[51–53]

Endothelin-1 is synthesized by corpus cavernosum endothelium and elicits strong sustained contractions of corpus cavernosum smooth muscle.[54–55] This has led to the speculation that endothelin may contribute to the maintenance of penile flaccidity by providing a sustained tone to the smooth muscle.

Prostaglandins: Prostaglandins including PGF_2-α, PGE_2, and PGI_2, as well as thromboxane A_2, are synthesized in the corpus cavernosum tissue and cultured endothelial cells derived from this tissue.[56–57] PGE is the only endogenous prostaglandin that induces relaxation of the trabecular smooth muscle. The precise role of prostaglandins in penile erection is unknown. PGE may play an important role in the regulation of the extracellular matrix of the corpus cavernosum; in particular of collagen synthesis and turnover. During erection there is a state of blood stasis in the corpora. The anti–platelet-aggregating effects of PGI_2, released upon smooth muscle relaxation by the endothelium, may be important in preventing coagulation of blood.

Regulation of the Synthesis of Nitric Oxide

In human subjects, measurement of intracavernosal oxygen tension (Po_2) in blood drawn from corpus cavernosum in the flaccid state is comparable to that of venous blood (25–43 mm Hg). At this low oxygen tension, nitric oxide synthesis is inhibited, preventing the relaxation of trabecular smooth muscle. The synthesis of nitric oxide is mediated by nitric oxide synthase which, in addition to L-arginine, requires molecular oxygen as a substrate. Erection causes oxygen tension to rise rapidly to arterial levels (Po_2 ~ 100 mm Hg) (Fig. 2.14). Recent investigations have shown that corpus cavernosum strips, exposed to arterial-like Po_2, relaxed to the endothelium-dependent dilator acetylcholine and to electrical stimulation of the autonomic dilator nerves.[58] These nitric oxide–mediated responses were progressively inhibited as a function of decreasing Po_2 to levels measured in the flaccid penis.

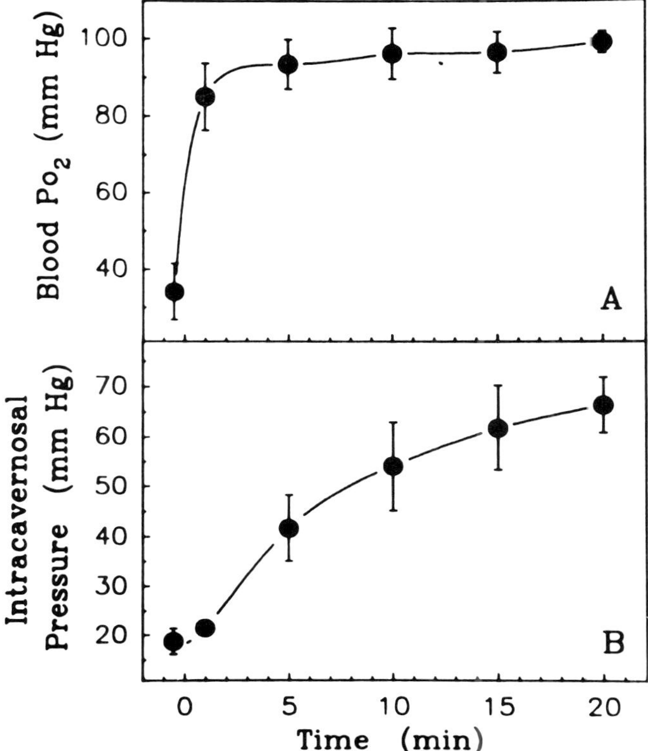

Fig. 2.14. In vivo measurements of intracavernosal blood Po$_2$ **A**: and pressure **B**: in humans. Patients (n = 10) were injected with papaverine and phentolamine at time 0 and intracavernosal pressure was monitored. Blood samples were drawn at the indicated time, and Po$_2$ values were immediately measured. Basal values were obtained just before drug injection. Values are expressed as mean ± SD. From Kim et al.[58]

REFERENCES

1. Tobin CE, Benjamin JA: Anatomical study and clinical consideration of the fasciae limiting urinary extravasation from the penile urethra. *Surg Gyn Obstet* 79:195–204, 1944.

2. Goldstein AMB, Meehan JP, Morrow JW, et al: The fibrous skeleton of the corpora cavernosa and its probable function in penile erection. *Br J Urol* 57:574–578, 1985.

3. Paick J, Lue T: Anatomy of the penis. In Hashmat A, Das S (eds): *The Penis.* Philadelphia, Lea & Febiger, 1993, p 12.

4. Goldstein AMB, Padma-Nathan H: The microarchitecture of the intracavernosal smooth muscle and the cavernosal fibrous skeleton. *J Urol* 144:1144–1146, 1990.

5. Breza J, Aboseif SR, Orvis BR, et al: Detailed anatomy of penile neurovascular structures: surgical significance. *J Urol* 141:437–443, 1989.

6. Wegner HEH, Andresen R, Knispel HH, et al: Evaluation of penile arteries with color-coded duplex sonography: prevalence and possible therapeutic implications of connections between dorsal and cavernous arteries in impotent men. *J Urol* 153:1469–1471, 1995.

7. Devine CJ, Angermeier KW: Anatomy of the penis and male perineum. *AUA Update Series* Vol XII, lesson 2, 1994.

8. Krane RJ, Goldstein I, Saenz de Tejada I: Impotence. *N Engl J Med* 321:1648–1659, 1989.

9. Saenz de Tejada I, Moroukian P, Tessier J, et al: Trabecular smooth muscle modulates the capacitor function of the penis. Studies on a rabbit model. *Am J Physiol* 261:H1078–H1085, 1991.

10. De Groat WC, Steers W: Neuroanatomy and neurophysiology of penile erection. In Tanagho EA, Lue TF, McClure D (eds): *Contemporary Management of Impotence and Infertility*. Baltimore, Williams & Wilkins, 1988.

11. Steers WD: Neural control of penile erection. *Semin Urol* 8:866–879, 1990.

12. Lue TF, Takamura T, Schmidt RA, et al: Neuroanatomy of penile erection: its relevance to iatrogenic impotence. *J Urol* 131:273–280, 1984.

13. Walsh PC, Donker PJ: Impotence following radical prostatectomy: insight into etiology and prevention. *J Urol* 128:492–497, 1982.

14. Amarenco G, Casanova JM: Lesion of the nerve of the penis in Peyronie's disease. *Prog Urol* 1:906–910, 1991.

15. Mallick HN, Manchanda SK, Mohan Kumar V: Sensory modulation of the medial pre-optic area neuronal activity by dorsal penile stimulation in rats. *J Urol* 151:759–762, 1994.

16. Andersson KE, Wagner G: Physiology of penile erection. *Physiol Rev* 75:191–236, 1995.

17. Moncada I, Concejo J, Escribano G, et al: Eco-Doppler duplex asociado a inyección intracavernosa de prostaglandina E 1 en el diagnóstico de la impotencia. *Arch Esp Urol* 45:45–51, 1992.

18. Lue TF, Tanagho EA: Physiology of erection and pharmacological management of impotence. *J Urol* 137:829–836, 1987.

19. Fournier GR, Juenemann KP, Lue TF, Tanagho EA: Mechanisms of venous occlusion during canine penile erection: an anatomic demonstration. *J Urol* 137:163–167, 1987.

20. Lavoisier P, Proulx J, Courtois F, de Carufel F, Durandl L-G: Relationship between perineal muscle contractions, penile tumescence, and penile rigidity during nocturnal erections. *J Urol* 139:176–179, 1988.

21. Hatzichristou DG, Saenz de Tejada I, Kupferman S, et al: In vivo assessment of tra-becular smooth muscle tone, its application in pharmacocavernosometry, and analysis of intracavernosal pressure determinants. *J Urol* 153:1126–1135, 1995.

22. Wespes E, Goes PM, Schiffmann S, et al: Computerized analysis of smooth muscle fibers in potent and impotent patients. *J Urol* 146:1015–1017, 1991.

23. Steers WD: Smooth muscle physiology. *AUA Update Series* Lesson 30, 1994.

24. Hai CM, Murphy RA: Crossbridge phosphorylation and regulation of the latch state in smooth muscle. *Am J Physiol* 255:C86–C94, 1988.

25. Andersson KE, Holmquist F: Mechanisms for contraction and relaxation of human penile smooth muscle. *Int J Impot Res* 2:209–229, 1990.

26. Andersson KE: Pharmacology of lower urinary tract smooth muscles and penile erectile tissues. *Pharmacol Rev* 45:253–309, 1993.

27. Kamm K, Stull J: Regulation of smooth muscle contractile elements by second messen-gers. *Ann Rev Physiol* 51:299–313, 1989.

28. Christ GJ, Moreno AP, Parker ME, et al: Intercellular communication through gap junc-tions: a potential role in pharmacomechanical coupling and syncytial tissue contraction

in vascular smooth muscle isolated from the human corpus cavernosum. *Life Sci* 49:PL195–200, 1991.

29. Campos de Carvallo AC, Roy C, Moreno AP, et al: Gap junctions of conexin43 are found between smooth muscle cells of human corpus cavernosum. *J Urol* 149:1568–1575, 1993.

30. Christ GJ, Brink PR, Melman A, et al: The role of gap junctions and ion channels in the modulation of electrical and chemical signals in human corpus cavernosum. *Int J Impot Res* 5:77–96, 1993.

31. Saenz de Tejada Y: Mechanisms for the regulation of penile smooth muscle contractility. In Lue T (ed): *World Book of Impotence*. London, Smith-Gordon, 1992.

32. Levin RM, Wein AJ: Adrenergic alpha receptors outnumber beta receptors in human penile corpus cavernosum. *Invest Urol* 18:225–226, 1980.

33. Saenz de Tejada I, Kim N, Lagan I, et al: Regulation of adrenergic activity in penile corpus cavernosum. *J Urol* 142:1117–1121, 1989.

34. Traish AM, Toselli P, Gupta S, et al: Identification of alpha 1-adrenergic receptor subtypes in human corpus cavernosum tissue and in cultured trabecular smooth muscle cells. *Receptor* (*in press*).

35. Saenz de Tejada I, Blanco R, Goldstein I, et al: Cholinergic neurotransmission in human corpus cavernosum. I. Responses of isolated tissue. *Am J Physiol* 261(*Heart Circ Physiol* 30):H468–H472, 1988.

36. Brindley GS: Pilot experiments on the actions of drugs injected into the human corpus cavernosum penis. *Br J Pharmacol* 87:495, 1986.

37. Wagner G, Brindley GS: Effect of atropine and alpha blockers on human penile erection. In Zorgniotti AW, Rossi G (eds): *Vasculogenic Impotence*. Springfield, Charles C Thomas, 1980, p 77.

38. Ottesen B, Wagner G, Virag R, et al: Penile erection: a possible role for vasoactive intestinal polypeptide as a neurotransmitter. *BMJ* 1:9, 1980.

39. Ignarro LJ, Bush PA, Buga GM, Wood KS, Fukuto JM, Rajfer J: Nitric oxide and cyclic GMP formation upon electrical stimulation cause relaxation of corpus cavernosum smooth muscle. *Biochem Biophys Res Commun* 170:843–850, 1990.

40. Bredt DS, Hwang PM, Snyder SH: Localization of nitric oxide synthase indicating a neural role for nitric oxide. *Nature* 347:768, 1990.

41. Blanco R, Saenz de Tejada I, Goldstein I, et al: Cholinergic neurotransmission in human corpus cavernosum. II. Acetycholine synthesis. *Am J Physiol* 254(*Heart Circ Physiol* 23):H468, 1988.

42. Simonsen U, Prieto D, Saenz de Tejada, et al: Involvement of nitric oxide in the non-adrenergic non-cholinergic neurotransmission of horse deep penile arteries: role of charybdotoxin-sensitive K^+-channels. *Br J Pharmacol* 116:2582–2590, 1995.

43. Kim N, Azadzoi KM, Goldstein I, Saenz de Tejada I: A nitric oxide–like factor mediates nonadrenergic noncholinergic neurogenic relaxation of penile corpus cavernosum smooth muscle. *J Clin Invest* 88:112–118, 1991.

44. Holmquist F, Stief CG, Jonas U, et al: Effects of nitric oxide synthase inhibitor Ng-nitro-L-arginine on the erectile response to cavernosus nerve stimulation in the rabbit. *Acta Physiol Scand* 143:299–304, 1991.

45. Trigo-Rocha F, Aronson WJ, Hohenfellner M, et al: Nitric oxide and cyclic guanosine monophosphate: mediators of pelvic nerve–stimulated erection in dogs. *Am J Physiol* 264:H419–H422, 1993.

46. Burnett AL, Lowenstein CJ, Bredt DS, et al: Nitric oxide: a physiologic mediator of penile erection. *Science* 257:401–403, 1992.

47. Furchgott RF, Zawadski JV: The obligatory role of endothelial cell in the relaxation of arterial smooth muscle by acetylcholine. *Nature* 288:373, 1980.

48. Kimoto Y, Kessler R, Constantinou CE: Endothelium dependent relaxation of human corpus cavernosum by bradykinin. *J Urol* 144:1015, 1990.

49. Azadzoi KM, Kim N, Brown ML, et al: Endothelium derived nitric oxide and cyclo-oxygenase products modulate corpus cavernosum smooth muscle tone. *J Urol* 147:220–225, 1992.

50. Vane JR, Anggard EE, Botting RM: Regulatory functions of the vascular endothelium. *N Engl J Med* 323:27, 1990.

51. Inoue K, Yanagisawa M, Kimura S, et al: The human endothelin family: three structurally and pharmacologically distinct isopeptides predicted by three separate genes. *Proc Natl Acad Sci USA* 86:2863, 1989.

52. Hirata Y, Takagi Y, Fukuda Y, et al: Endothelin is a potent mitogen for rat vascular smooth muscle cells. *Atherosclerosis* 78:225, 1989.

53. Muldoon LL, Rodland KD, Forsythe ML, et al: Stimulation of phosphatidylinositol hydrolysis, diacylglycerol release, and gene expression in response to endothelin, a potent new agonist for fibroblasts and smooth muscle cells. *J Biol Chem* 264:8529, 1989.

54. Saenz de Tejada I, Carson MP, de las Morenas A, Goldstein I, Traish AM: Endothelin: localization, synthesis, activity and receptor types in human penile corpus cavernosum. *Am J Physiol* 261:H1078–H1085, 1991.

55. Holmquist F, Andersson K-E, Hedlund H: Actions of endothelin on isolated corpus cavernosum from rabbit and man. *Acta Physiol Scand* 139:113, 1990.

56. Jeremy JY, Morgan RJ, Mikjalidis DP: Prostacyclin synthesis by the corpora cavernosa of the human penis: evidence for muscarinic control and pathological implications. *Prostaglandins Leukot Med* 23:211, 1986.

57. Saenz de Tejada I, Carson MP, Taylor L, et al: Prostaglandin production by human corpus cavernosum endothelial cells (HCC EC) in culture. *J Urol* 139:252A (abstract 358), 1988.

58. Kim N, Vardi Y, Padma-Nathan H, et al: Oxygen tension regulates the nitric oxide pathway. Physiological role in penile erection. *J Clin Invest* 91:3006–3012, 1993.

3

Hormonal Evaluation and Treatment of the Patient with Sexual Dysfunction

Todd L. VandenBerg
Jonathan Jaspan
Wayne J. G. Hellstrom

In 1948, Kinsey reported that 1.9% of 40-yr-old men had some degree of impotence. By the age of 70 yr, this incidence had increased to 27.4% in Kinsey's study. More recent studies from Michigan and Massachusetts have reported erectile difficulties in about 35% of married men older than 60, and complete impotence in approximately 15% of men 70 and above.[1] It is believed that 20 to 30 million American men have differing degrees of erectile dysfunction, with hormonal abnormalities estimated to be found in 1.7% to 35% of these persons.[2,3]

Sexual dysfunction comprises a wide variety of disorders. These include loss of libido, erectile difficulties, inability to achieve orgasm, and ejaculation disorders. Libido is influenced by psychological factors and is regulated partly by sex hormones. Erection involves both reflex and psychic mechanisms. Psychogenic erection involves the higher brain centers and is influenced by testosterone.

Androgens play critical roles during embryogenesis, development, and maintenance of male sex organs and secondary sex characteristics. Testosterone maintains libido, virilization, potency, secondary sex characteristics, and preserves muscle and bone mass in adult men.[4]

Many men with sexual dysfunction will initially be screened by their primary care physician. The complexity of the erectile and ejaculatory process, however, often behooves evaluation and treatment by a specialist. Not long ago, most physicians, including specialists, treated hormonal-related erectile dysfunction empirically with testosterone replacement, without appropriate laboratory evaluation. The current, preferred method involves a logical approach based upon laboratory findings. But even among specialists, there is no uniform agreement on exactly what constitutes proper workup and therapy. This chapter reviews male sexual endocrinology and associated abnormalities, and provides the practitioner with an up-to-date, practical, and effective approach for diagnosing and managing men with hormon related sexual disorders.

ENDOCRINOLOGY OF SEXUAL FUNCTION

Hypothalamic–Pituitary–Gonadal Axis

The hypothalamus receives messages from both the central nervous system and testes, which regulate the synthesis and secretion of gonadotropin-releasing hormone (GnRH).[5,6] Pulsatile secretion of GnRH is essential for proper synthesis and release of leutinizing hormone (LH) and follicle-stimulating hormone (FSH) by the anterior pituitary.[7] Animal studies have demonstrated that testosterone has an important role in the negative feedback of LH and FSH. Both LH and FSH can be maintained at normal levels with testosterone replacement after castration.[8] However, this role of testosterone in man may not be that clear. Frequently, FSH is not normalized in oligospermic men by androgen replacement.

LH and FSH then go on to bind to receptors on Leydig and Sertoli cells, respectively, and activate cellular metabolism. Testosterone, produced by the testes, inhibits LH secretion via a negative feedback loop. Testosterone is metabolized in the peripheral tissues to dihydrotestosterone (DHT) or estradiol. Androgens and estrogens can independently affect LH secretion. Some studies have suggested that estrogens may act primarily at the level of the pituitary, while androgens exert their effect at the hypothalamic level.[9]

Feedback control of FSH secretion is more controversial. FSH levels increase after castration. Secretion of inhibin, from the Sertoli cells, in association with spermatogenesis, is hypothesized to be the effector for this FSH feedback system[10] (Fig. 3.1).

Androgen Physiology

Leydig cells secrete testosterone in a diurnal pattern in response to LH surges. Testosterone peaks in the early morning and reaches its nadir in the early evenings.[10]

An intratesticular control system exists for regulating testosterone production. Exogenous LH administration has been shown to downregulate LH receptors in the testes.[11] Large doses of GnRH or its analogues also downregulate LH receptors or inhibit LH secretion directly.[12] (This clinical application is used to medically castrate men with advanced prostate cancer.) Estrogens inhibit testosterone production by inhibiting enzymes involved in testosterone synthesis.[13] Exogenous testosterone can override the effect of LH and suppress endogenous testosterone production. This constitutes the so-called intratesticular ultrashort feedback loop.[14]

Steroid-binding proteins modulate androgen function. In normal men, 40% to 50% of testosterone is bound to sex-hormone-binding globulin (SHBG). The remainder is either unbound or free (about 2%) or bound to albumin or other proteins.[6] It was once believed that the physiologically active (bioavailable) testosterone was the free form. However, studies have demonstrated that enhanced rates of dissociation of androgen from binding proteins occur in the microcirculation. SHBG binds with greater affinity to androgens versus estrogens and has been shown to modify hormonal concentrations. Additionally, SHBG levels are increased by estrogens and decreased by androgens.[7] Because of the continuous equilibrium

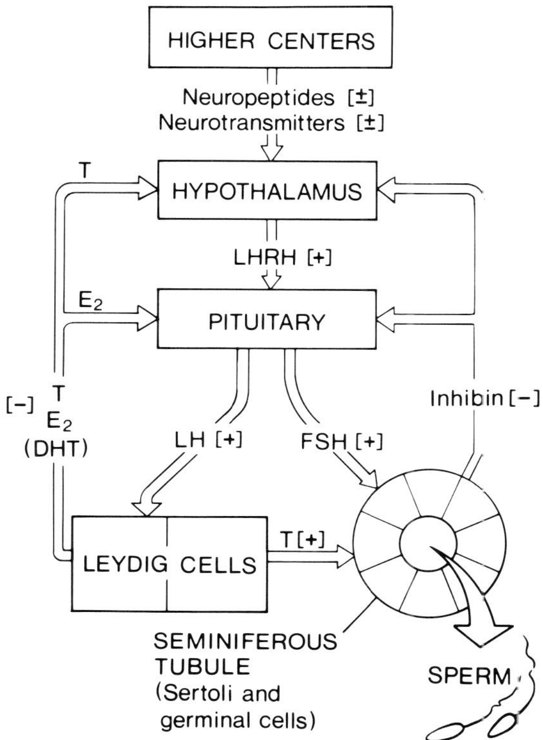

Fig. 3.1. Hypothalamic-pituitary-gonadal axis. LH = luteinizing hormone; FSH = follicle-stimulating hormone; T = testosterone; DHT = dihydrotestosterone; E_2 = estradiol; LHRH = LH-releasing hormone; + = positive influence; − = negative influence. From McClure,[33] with permission.

between new secretion, binding, and dissociation of testosterone, these findings suggest a more important role for protein-bound testosterone.

Androgens act on target organs via binding to specific cytoplasmic receptor proteins.[6] As testosterone leaves the circulation and enters the target cells, it may be converted to DHT by the 5α-reductase enzyme. Testosterone or DHT can then bind to the cellular receptor protein in tissues, such as brain, prostate, and penis. Although the precise interaction between testosterone and these target tissues is not entirely clear and is currently the topic of intense investigation, there is good evidence that testosterone is essentially a prohormone and most of its biologic action occurs after peripheral conversion.

Placebo-controlled clinical studies of hypogonadal men have demonstrated that androgen replacement increases sexual activity and interest. Implantation of testosterone in certain regions of the brain of castrate rats restores normal sexual behavior. Other studies using castrate animal models confirm that the primary site of testosterone action is the cerebrum.[15-17]

It has been demonstrated that hypogonadal men exhibit less erectile activity during nocturnal penile tumescence (NPT) testing and fewer daytime erections. Testosterone replacement corrected these abnormalities. However, erectile response to erotic stimulation and fantasy was not impaired in these hypogonadal men. These observations support the concept that the primary function of androgens on male sexual function is to enhance libido and not directly mediate penile erection.

Prolactin

The relationship between prolactin and gonadotropins is complex.[15,16] Serum LH is inappropriately low in men with hyperprolactinemia and testosterone deficiency, suggesting that the hypothalamic–pituitary axis fails to respond appropriately to reduced testosterone levels. Elevated prolactin also inhibits GnRH. However, patients with prolactin-secreting tumors will respond to an exogenous infusion of GnRH with an increase in LH levels.[1,18] There is, in addition, a direct inhibitory effect of prolactin on testicular secretion of testosterone. Thus, prolactin may cause primary, secondary, or tertiary hypogonadism.

In addition to preventing androgen secretion via the hypothalamic–pituitary axis, elevated serum prolactin levels influence the central nervous system. Accordingly, most hyperprolactinemic men are impotent and have markedly decreased serum testosterone levels. However, sexual function and libido return to normal in those receiving androgen replacement therapy, but only after prolactin levels are normalized. These findings suggest that the primary effect of hyperprolactinemia is diminished libido and that the associated impotence is secondary or psychogenic.

HORMONAL-RELATED SEXUAL DYSFUNCTION

Congenital Disorders

Patients who do not produce androgens during sexual development will usually not have normal libido, erectile or sexual function. This form of hypogonadism is rare, and often such men will seek medical attention for abnormal growth or sexual development.

Clinical manifestations of congenital androgen deficiency appear at various times. Severe primary sexual abnormalities will become apparent early in life. Conversely, the clinical findings of those with Klinefelter's syndrome, the most common cause of hypergonadotropic hypogonadism, are usually witnessed at puberty. Men with this syndrome exhibit delayed puberty, eunuchoidal features, gynecomastia, and atrophic testes. Less common genetic disorders associated with hypergonadotropic hypogonadism include ataxia telangiectasia, Werner syndrome, and Weinstein syndrome. Kallman's syndrome and "fertile" eunuch syndrome are examples of conditions associated with hypogonadotropic hypogonadism. Those with Prader-Labhart-Willi and Laurence-Moon-Biedl syndromes may present as primary or secondary hypogonadism (Table 3.1).

Hemochromatosis

Hemochromatosis is an autosomal recessive disorder involving progressive accumulation of iron in a variety of tissues, including the testes and pituitary gland. Over time, permanent tissue damage occurs. Therefore, these patients usually present with

TABLE 3.1. Hormonal-related Sexual Dysfunction

Congenital disorders
    Hemochromatosis
    Androgens and aging
    Acquired hypogonadism
Systemic disorders
    Acute illness
    Acquired immunodeficiency syndrome
    Liver disease
    Renal failure
    Sickle cell disease
    Nutritional disorders
Medications
Specific endocrinopathies
    Hyperprolactinemia
    Pituitary and hypothalamic diseases
    Thyroid disease
    Adrenal disease
    Autoimmune disease
    Estrogen excess
    Diabetes mellitus

this disorder later in life, around 40 to 60 yr of age. The iron accumulation within the pituitary causes a selective gonadotropin deficiency, but other pituitary functions are preserved. Deposition of iron within the testes is directly gonadotoxic.

Middle-aged men who present with decreased libido, erectile dysfunction, bronzed skin, hepatosplenomegaly, arthralgias, and diabetes need to be investigated for hemochromatosis. Iron testing will reveal an elevated serum iron and abnormally high transferrin saturation. Magnetic resonance imaging (MRI) can be helpful in demonstrating excessive amounts of ferric ion in these individuals.

Androgens and Aging

Anecdotal and clinical observations, along with extensive analysis of cross-sectional data, demonstrate a decrease in sexual activity and erectile function with age. Between the ages of 40 to 70, the prevalence of complete erectile impotence triples from 5% to 15% (Fig. 3.2). In men with heart disease, diabetes, hypertension, and who smoke, the prevalence is even greater. Ejaculation frequency peaks in the mid teens, then gradually declines.[1] Protracted refractory periods are common in the elderly. In elderly men, sexual performance decreases at a faster rate than sexual desire. A significant correlation between serum testosterone (free or total) and diminished sexual function has not been found, suggesting a multifactorial cause.

As men age, increased production of SHBG by the liver decreases the amount of free testosterone. LH secretion remains inappropriately low due to impaired hypothalamic–pituitary function, compounding the problem of low free testosterone. Supplementation therapy with testosterone in these aging, hypogonadal men has not been fully evaluated and remains an area of active interest.

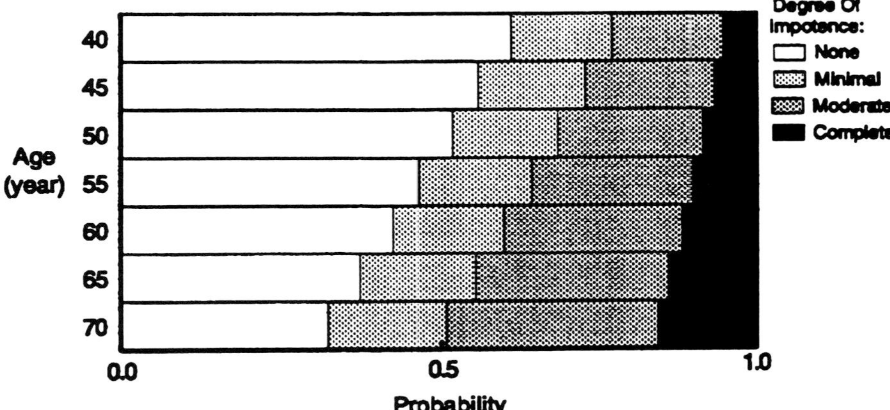

Fig. 3.2. Probability and degree of impotence in aging men. From Feldman et al,[3] with permission.

Acquired Hypogonadism

Gonadal insults from environmental factors, such as trauma, extreme heat, viruses, or radiation usually affect the more sensitive seminiferous tubules. However, those with severe bilateral testicular trauma, torsion, or surgical orchiectomy may also present with hypoandrogenism.[19]

Systemic Disorders

Sexual dysfunction is associated with some chronic illnesses. Decreased libido, hypotestosteronism, and primary or secondary hypogonadism, with or without hyperprolactinemia, have been found in debilitated patients. Although the exact cause and effect mechanism between illness and sexual function is unclear, treatment of these men involves correction of the underlying condition. If successful, libido and erectile function are usually restored.

Acute Illness

Patients with myocardial infarction, sepsis, or respiratory failure can have temporarily reduced androgen production and subsequent sexual dysfunction.[20] A hypothalamic–pituitary abnormality is usually suspected. In select patients, the hypogonadism is very severe, aggravating the catabolic state. Steroid supplementation in such circumstances may be beneficial.

Acquired Immunodeficiency Syndrome (AIDS)

AIDS has multiple effects on the endocrine system. As the disease progresses, many men infected with the human immunodeficiency virus (HIV) complain of decreased libido. Serum testosterone falls in parallel with the CD4$^+$ count.[21] Serum prolactin usually remains normal. A defect in the hypothalamic–pituitary axis is thought to be the cause of the hypogonadotropic hypogonadism found in the majority of the men. Some investigators have suggested that there is altered paracrine regulation of Leydig cells secondary to cytokine cascade activation in AIDS patients. This may contribute to the hypotestosteronism seen in these individuals.[22] Additionally, AIDS treatment drugs, such as ketoconazole, can reduce androgen production by interfering with key enzymes in steroidogenesis.

Liver Disease

Sexual dysfunction and gynecomastia are commonly seen in men with chronic liver disease. The exact cause of the impotence is not known. However, elevated SHBG levels associated with chronic liver disease reduce the amount of bioavailable testosterone. A hypothalamic–pituitary abnormality is suspected secondary to inappropriately low LH levels. Elevated estrogens, secondary to decreased hepatic degradation, in those with liver disease may further inhibit LH secretion. The resultant hyperestrogenic state is an important factor in the frequently observed gynecomastia and testicular atrophy. Alcoholic cirrhosis is the most common cause of liver failure, and alcohol itself may be directly toxic to the hypothalamic–pituitary axis and testes.

The degree of gynecomastia is related to the increased estrogen-to-testosterone ratio. Gynecomastia may actually become more pronounced with testosterone replacement as the exogenous androgen is aromatized to estrogen.

Renal Failure

Many men with end-stage renal disease complain of decreased libido and erectile ability. Hypogonadotropic hypogonadism is detected in the majority of cases. Abnormalities exist throughout the hypothalamic–pituitary–gonadal axis. Serum testosterone levels fail to rise appropriately after the exogenous administration of human chorionic gonadotropin (hCG), suggesting an abnormality of intrinsic testicular function. Increased production and decreased renal clearance of prolactin in renal failure patients likely contributes to the sexual dysfunction. Renal transplantation often corrects the hormonal derangements, whereas dialysis does not.

Sickle Cell Disease

Sickle cell disease causes testicular injury and hypoandrogenism with elevated LH levels. Testosterone replacement is effective in reversing the associated erectile dysfunction.

Nutritional Disorders

Hypogonadotropic hypogonadism may be related to both malnutrition and severe obesity. Correction of nutritional deficiencies and weight reduction may restore normal androgen production.

Medications

Adverse side effects of some medications include hypoandrogenism, hyperestrogenism, hyperprolactinemia, decreased libido, and erectile dysfunction. Spironolactone blocks testosterone synthesis and competitively binds to the same receptor. Antiulcer agents, such as cimetidine and other H_2-blockers, block androgen receptor binding. Phenothiazines and verapamil, among others, can cause hyperprolactinemia. Digitalis can decrease serum testosterone and increase serum estradiol levels. Ketaconazole blocks androgen synthesis. A number of cytotoxic, alkylating, and other chemotherapeutic agents have multiple adverse effects on the hypothalamic–pituitary–gonadal axis at one or more levels (Table 3.2).

Specific Endocrinopathies

Libido and erectile function are dependant upon androgen availability. Hypoandrogenism is the most common endocrinopathy associated with male sexual dysfunction. With milder states of hypogonadism, erectile function may be relatively preserved, but libido decreased. Causes of hypoandrogenism are hypothalamic–pituitary lessons (secondary or hypogonadotropic hypogonadism), gonadal disorders (primary or hypergonadotropic hypogonadism), and hyperprolactinemia.

Hyperprolactinemia

Hyperprolactinemia can be found in about 1% to 16% of men with impotence.[22] Nearly half of all patients with elevated prolactin have no demonstrable pituitary abnormality and are termed idiopathic. One-third have a documented pituitary tumor (prolactinoma), and a substantial number may have small microadenomas not demonstrable by imaging techniques. The remainder have hyperprolactinemia

TABLE 3.2. Drugs Associated with Impotence

Central nervous system	α-Methyldopa, barbiturates, benzodiazepines, butyrophenones, carbamazepine, clonidine, ethanol, fluoxetine, heroin, methadone, morphine, phenothiazines, phenytoin, primidone, reserpine
Anticholinergic	Atropine, butyrophenones, disopyramide, ganglionic blocking agents, phenothiazines, tricyclic antidepressants
Antiadrenergic	Benzhexol, benztropine, bethanidine, debrisoquin, propranolol, prazosin, phenoxybenzamine, phentolamine, thioridazine
Antiandrogen	Cimetidine, cyproterone acetate, estrogens, finasteride, ketoconazole, progestins, spironolactone
Others	Amphetamines, cocaine, monoamine oxidase inhibitors, thiazides

With permission from Mulcahy JJ: Hormonal evaluation and treatment of the patient with sexual dysfunction. In Chapter 116. Impotence. Part VIII: Endocrinology of the male Excerpted from *Principles and Practice of Endocrinology and Metabolism*, ed 2. Philadelphia; Lippincott, 1995, p 1091.)

due to medication effects, hypothyroidism, or other systemic illnesses, such as renal or liver failure. Plasma prolactin levels may vary from mildly elevated (15 to 25 ng/ml) to values in the thousands. The highest prolactin levels are seen in those with prolactinomas. In patients with a prolactin level of 100 ng/ml, 50% will have a pituitary tumor.[23] Levels above 200 ng/ml are almost always associated with a tumor.

Although most men with hyperprolactinemia present with decreased libido and erectile dysfunction, occasionally the mass effects of an enlarging pituitary tumor will cause visual field defects, headaches, or other endocrinopathies. Often serum testosterone is low, but testosterone replacement does not always correct the sexual dysfunction because the elevated prolactin interferes with end-organ responsiveness.[23]

Diagnostic imaging of the pituitary gland is necessary in all patients with elevated prolactin in an attempt to document a pituitary tumor. Those cases where no tumor is demonstrable and no other cause for hyperprolactinemia is evident are classified as idiopathic hyperprolactinemia. A substantial number of these cases are now thought to represent microadenomas.

Treatment is based on the underlying cause. In those with hypothyroidism, thyroid replacement usually restores prolactin levels to normal. If medications are the cause, they should be discontinued when possible or altered under medical council. Medications known to cause hyperprolactinemia include verapamil, amoxepin, cocaine, metoclopramide, dopamine receptor antagonists (phenothiazine), monoamine inhibitors (α-methyldopa), and monoamine depleters (reserpine). Patients with large, functioning pituitary tumors (macroprolactinomas) require surgical intervention. Medical therapy with the dopaminergic agonist bromocriptine or pergolide is considered in those with idiopathic hyperprolactinemia or small prolactinomas, less than 1.0 cm in diameter (microprolactinoma). Gradual administration of bromocriptine at 2.5 to 7.5 mg/day will restore serum prolactin levels to normal and minimize common side effects, such as gastrointestinal discomfort, sinus congestion, and orthostatic hypotension.

Pituitary and Hypothalamic Diseases

A low serum testosterone level without elevated gonadotropins suggests pituitary or hypothalamic dysfunction. Men with secondary testicular failure will have atrophic testicles and prostate atrophy initially, then loss of other androgenic effects. Klyde[23] reported that the most frequent cause of secondary hypogonadism in an impotent male population is an idiopathic, isolated LH deficiency probably resulting from hypothalamic dysfunction. A hypothalamic versus pituitary cause is suggested after observing an LH rise after GnRH stimulation.

LH deficiency may also be caused by pituitary tumors that may be functioning or nonfunctioning. Nonfunctioning tumors or glycoprotein-secreting tumors (previously termed *chromophobe adenomas*) are the most common cause of panhypopituitarism. Patients may complain of headaches and visual problems, or they may have other clinical features related to the deficient hormones. The hypogonadal state may be a result of damage to the gonadotropic-producing cells by the pituitary tumor. Other nonfunctioning tumors include craniopharyngioma, meningioma, optic glioma, astrocytoma, lymphoma, and metastatic carcinoma. These tumors' destructive effects cause diminished gonadotropin secretion, initially. A fall in hGH, thyrotropic hormone (TSH), and finally adrenocorticotropic hormone (ACTH) is then seen. Although sexual dysfunction is an early clinical manifestation of this panhypopituitarism, most men delay medical care until they exhibit features of hypothyroidism or adrenal insufficiency.

Functioning pituitary tumors associated with sexual dysfunction include gonadotropin-producing adenomas, growth hormone-producing tumors, ACTH-producing tumors, TSH-producing tumors, and prolactinomas. Gonadotropin-producing tumors are usually recognized by symptoms caused by tumor growth. Gonadotroph cell hormonal hypersecretion has little clinical effect. Hence, sexual dysfunction is an uncommon complaint in those with gonadotropin-producing tumors. Treatment usually involves surgery and irradiation.

TSH-producing pituitary tumors are rare and occasionally may be associated with hypogonadism. Laboratory findings include an elevated (thyroxine) T_4 and normal-to-high TSH in those suspected of having hyperthyroidism. Radiographic findings suggest a pituitary adenoma.

hGH-producing tumors are the most common cause of acromegaly. The expanding pituitary tumor may cause pituitary failure and hypogonadism. Hyperprolactinemia, found in 20% to 40% of these cases, is caused by secretion by the hGH-producing cells or via disruption of the portal blood flow by the expanding tumor, thereby interrupting prolactin inhibiting factor.[24] Clinical findings suggest the diagnosis.

Treatment of pituitary adenomas can be surgical, irradiational, medical, or a combination of approaches for larger tumors. The goal of treatment should be to normalize endocrine function and address the expanding tumor, if present and symptomatic. Success from surgical therapy is inversely proportional to the tumor size. Hence, surgery is most curative for microadenomas. Irradiation is now reserved for surgical failures. Bromocriptine, or pergolide, is sometimes useful in prolactin-secreting acromegalic tumors.

Thyroid Disease

Erectile dysfunction is a common complaint in men with hyperthyroidism or hypothyroidism. The mechanism by which thyroid hormone excess and deficiency cause sexual dysfunction differs.

Hyperthyroidism or toxicosis results from chronic exposure to elevated thyroid hormone. Clinical manifestations include weight loss, palpitations, heat intolerance, diaphoresis, and weakness. Commonly, only tachycardia or atrial fibrillation is seen in the elderly. Physical exam often reveals a nervous, tachycardic individual. Most patients with hyperthyroidism will have elevated T_4 and (triiodothyronine) T_3 levels and totally suppressed TSH. Although prolactin secretion is elevated in hyperthyroidism, so is the metabolic clearance rate. Accordingly, serum prolactin levels may be normal or subnormal. SHBG is increased and results in an elevated total testosterone; however, the amount of bioavailable testosterone is decreased.[25] Increased peripheral aromatization of androgens to estrogens may partially suppress gonadotropin secretion. The hyperestrogenism of hyperthyroidism may also adversely affect libido and is the cause of the associated gynecomastia. Testosterone replacement will not improve libido and may augment the gynecomastia. Restoration to the euthyroid state with current medical and/or surgical methods will reverse the associated sexual dysfunction.

Hypothyroidism or myxedema is a clinical condition in which there is generalized metabolic slowing due to decreased production of T_4. These patients will typically demonstrate weight gain, skin dryness, deepening of the voice, cold intolerance, lethargy, and constipation. Bradycardia, dry hair and skin, dull expression, and delayed deep tendon reflexes are common findings on physical exam. A goiter may also be present. Low T_4 and elevated TSH confirm the diagnosis. Hyperprolactinemia, resulting from the stimulatory effect of thyrotropin-releasing hormone (TRH) on pituitary prolactin secretion, is common and probably contributes to the hypogonadism and decreased libido. Thyroid hormone replacement with L-thyroxine is effective in restoring sexual potency; however, it may take months for full recovery.

Adrenal Disease

Excess adrenal corticosteroids in patients with Cushing's syndrome can produce a hypogonadal state resulting in decreased libido and erections. Most commonly, this is iatrogenic secondary to glucocorticoid therapy for nonendocrine disorders. Cushing's disease is caused by a pituitary tumor and is the most frequent cause (approximately 70%) of endogenous hypercortisolism. Central obesity, protuberant abdomen, full plethoric faces, and increased supraclavicular fat deposits are classic physical findings. Urinary-free cortisols will be elevated. Correction of the hypercortisolism will usually reverse the sexual dysfunction.

Adrenal insufficiency causes a generalized debilitated state that interferes with normal sexual function. The marked decrease in cortisol commonly results in an insidious presentation characterized by weight loss, fatigue, malaise, hypotension, and prominent gastrointestinal symptoms. Libido and erectile potency can be maintained in properly treated patients.

Autoimmune Disease

Polyglandular autoimmune disease is an autosomal dominant disorder that results in multiple endocrine failure. In addition to testicular failure, these patients may have thyroid, adrenal, or β-cell pancreatic islet deficiency (Type I diabetes). Associated autoimmune disorders include myasthenia gravis, pernicious anemia, and vitiligo. Distinction between these multiple endocrine failure patients and those with hypopituitarism is vital for proper treatment.

Estrogen Excess

Hyperestrogenism causes LH suppression, and later, diminished testosterone production. This is most commonly seen in obese men. The mechanism probably involves increased conversion of testosterone to estrogen in the excess adipose tissue.[26] Patients with chronic hepatitis, cirrhosis or other chronic liver diseases may have hyperestrogenism secondary to hepatic aromatization of testosterone to estrogen.[27] In addition, elevated SHBG levels result in a reduction in bioavailable or active testosterone.

Hyperestrogenism can also be caused by excess production of dehydroepiandrosterone (DHEA) in patients with congenital adrenal hyperplasia (CAH). In the more common forms, adrenal hydroxylase enzyme is deficient in these patients and, therefore, cortisol secretion is decreased. The resulting increase in pituitary ACTH secretion leads to increased DHEA production.[28] This adrenal androgen can then be converted to estrogen in the liver and adipose tissue. Although rare, gynecomastia and a female fat distribution pattern may appear in some men. Laboratory evaluation will reveal low testosterone and LH with an elevated total estrogen (estrone + estradiol). Measurement of estradiol alone is inadequate because much of the estrogen in men is estrone.

Weight loss and suppression of DHEA production with supplemental glucocorticoids can be effective in restoring sexual potency. If estrogen–testosterone imbalance is the only cause of sexual dysfunction, testosterone replacement can be helpful.

Diabetes Mellitus

Diabetes is the most common endocrine abnormality associated with erectile failure. Diabetes-related sexual dysfunction is present in 35% to 75% of patients, increases with age, and is present in all men suffering from autonomic diabetic neuropathy.[29] A commonly quoted overall statistic is that 50% of men with diabetes for 15 yr or more will be impotent. An acute onset of impotence may result from the metabolic derangements of poorly controlled diabetes and may improve with better glucose control. However, most men with diabetes experience a gradual loss of erectile ability, which is often associated with related complications, such as neuropathy, vascular disease, nephropathy, and retinopathy. Men with a strong family history of adult onset or Type II diabetes, and who have not had a recent physical examination, can present with erectile difficulties as the initial presentation of their diabetes.

Impotence in diabetic men may result from either neuropathy, vascular disease, or a combination. Recent studies have documented that the corpus cavernosum tissue from diabetic men has impairment of both endothelium-derived relaxing factor (EDRF)-mediated smooth muscle relaxation and autonomic nerve-mediated relaxation.[30]

For the most part, hormonal factors per se do not appear to be directly related to the sexual dysfunction. LH and testosterone levels are usually normal, and testosterone replacement in these situations will not improve potency.

Recent studies of patients with insulin-dependant diabetes mellitus have clearly demonstrated a marked decrease in the incidence and progression of microvascular disease and neuropathy with tighter glycemic control.[31] Based on similar findings in both American and European studies relating glycemic control to target organ complications, it is highly likely that improved glycemic control will be of benefit in preventing or delaying irreversible erectile dysfunction.

EVALUATION OF HORMONAL-RELATED SEXUAL DYSFUNCTION

History and Physical Exam

Proper evaluation of men with sexual dysfunction should always start with a complete history and physical exam. Organic and psychogenic causes of impotence should be identified. Organic causes are usually characterized by an insidious change in the rigidity or ability to sustain morning, coital, or masturbation-related erections. Libido must be accurately assessed. Indeed, decreased libido and impotence are the earliest signs of low serum testosterone. The clinician should search for relevant comorbid risk factors, such as diabetes mellitus, hypertension, coronary artery disease, peripheral vascular disease, alcoholism, smoking, and neurologic or endocrine disorders. A complete drug history is equally important, as 16 of the 200 most commonly prescribed drugs in the United States can cause impotence.

The physical exam should include a careful evaluation of hair and fat distribution, skin texture, thyroid size and consistency, gynecomastia, central and distal pulses, deep tendon reflexes and vibratory sensation, penis and testicles, and a rectal exam focusing on prostate size and consistency.

Routine Laboratory Evaluation

Routine laboratory tests (complete blood count and chemistries) can be helpful to confirm a disease process suspected by history and physical exam. Screening for diabetes mellitus, hyperlipidemia, and other systemic disorders, such as liver and renal disease, is valid in select patients. Impotence from diabetes is related to the duration and severity of the disease. Therefore, testing for glycosylated hemoglobin (a measure of the average glucose for the prior 2 to 3 months) may be more informative than a random glucose level.

Hormonal Screening

The purpose of hormonal screening is to identify a significant endocrinopathy and to identify impotent patients who might respond to endocrine therapy. Unfortunately, no aspect of the evaluation of male sexual dysfunction is as controversial as hormonal screening. Recommended baseline screening ranges from thyroid function tests, LH, FSH, prolactin, and testosterone to a single total testosterone determination. In an era of ever-increasing cost containment, disagreement mounts as to what constitutes a minimum hormonal evaluation for sexual dysfunction.

Thyroid function tests are touted by some to be particularly important in the elderly, where there is a high prevalence of subclinical thyroid dysfunction.

Because testosterone is secreted episodically in response to LH, some investigators argue that a single testosterone determination could be normal in a patient with an underlying endocrinopathy, and no further endocrine evaluation would have been performed.[32] Alternatively, a single mild-to-moderately low testosterone level may not necessarily indicate true deficiency. Accordingly, some recommend serial or pooled blood collections for LH and total testosterone.[33] Studies have shown free testosterone levels to be more predictive of a potential positive response to androgen replacement therapy versus total testosterone, especially in patients who have only partial erectile dysfunction.[34] However, free testosterone cannot detect significant endocrinopathies, such as pituitary tumors, any better than total testosterone. Others argue that the age-related increase in SHBG produces a reduction in unbound (free) testosterone. Because they believe that non-SHBG-bound testosterone is the only biologically active form, measurement of free testosterone in men older than 60 yr or who have altered levels of SHBG is recommended.[35] Conversely, other studies have demonstrated that protein-bound testosterone may be as important as unbound testosterone in regulating male sexual function.

Some investigators believe that even modest elevations in prolactin, in the presence of normal testosterone, can cause impotence. Therefore, they recommend prolactin and testosterone determinations as initial hormone screening.[36] Others emphasize that the yield of routine prolactin screening is low and highly questionable on the basis of contemporary health economics.[37] These investigators believe that modest increases in serum prolactin, in the presence of normal testosterone, require a vigorous search for other causes before a hasty diagnosis and treatment plan is instituted.[38–40] Akpunonu et al.[41] reported the prevalence of hyperprolactinemia in 299 men with impotence to be 1.4%. They concluded that because the prevalence of hyperprolactinemia is low, routine measurement of prolactin levels is not indicated. In fact, selective prolactin determination only in patients with low testosterone saved $2,574 per case detected.[41] In another study by Lehmann et al.,[42] 107 impotent men underwent a full endocrine evaluation. Approximately 16% had low testosterone and 3% had hyperprolactinemia. Lehmann and colleagues concluded that a single total testosterone measurement was adequate. If low, repeated measurements, combined with LH, FSH, and prolactin will identify patients with endocrine-related erectile dysfunction.[42] Lewis and Barrett[43] also recommend that a serum prolactin level be obtained only as a secondary hormonal test if the testosterone level is low, unless the patient reports a significantly decreased libido, a visual field defect, or extreme headaches.

Preferred Evaluation Of Testosterone Deficiency

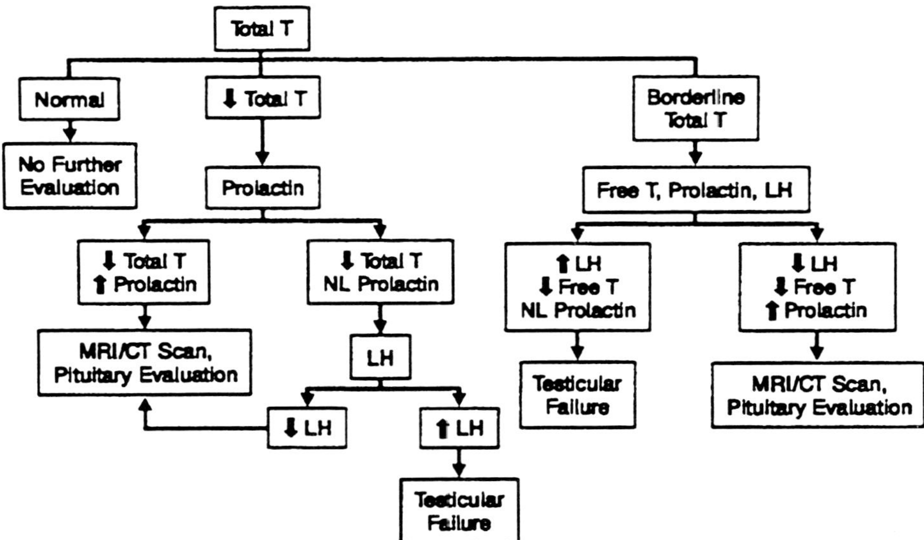

Fig. 3.3. Proposed preferred evaluation of testosterone deficiency. Reproduced with permission from Murdock MI: Urologist's approaches to diagnosis and treatment of male hormone deficience states. In Perspectives of Male Hormone Replacement Therapy (symposium program workbook, Aventura, FL, January 12–13, 1996). Philadelphia, SmithKline Beecham Pharmaceuticals, 1996.

Although there is no universally agreed upon protocol, the preponderance of current opinion suggests obtaining a total testosterone level (preferably in the early morning, when testosterone and prolactin levels are high), initially. If the total testosterone is low, then a serum prolactin determination is warranted. Further laboratory and endocrine testing, such as glycosylated hemoglobin, FSH and LH, thyroid function, and a total estrogen level, may be needed based on the patient's clinical presentation and degree of testosterone deficiency (Fig. 3.3).

Additional Assessments

Initial impressions may need to be corroborated, when necessary, by a series of additional examinations including NPT, psychologic, neurologic, and vascular testing (i.e., duplex Doppler imaging in combination with intracavernosal vasodilator injection).

Radiographic Studies

MRI can be helpful in diagnosing hemochromatosis. When hypothalamic pituitary abnormalities are suspected, a computed tomographic (CT) scan or MRI of the skull will reveal a prolactin-secreting tumor if the serum prolactin is elevated or a nonprolactin-secreting tumor in cases of hypogonadotropic hypogonadism (Fig. 3.4).

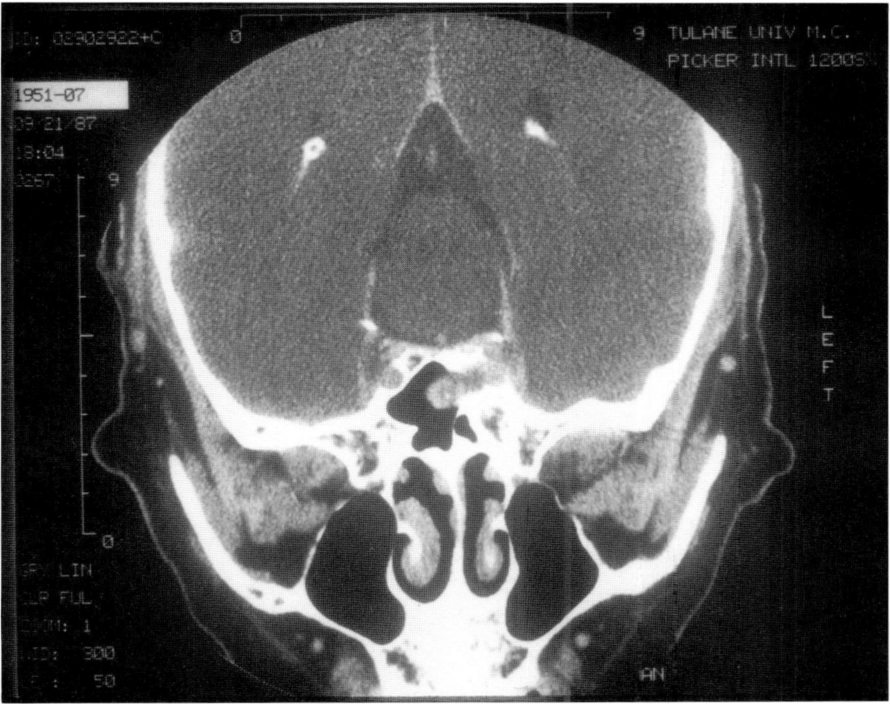

Fig. 3.4. MRI of brain demonstrating pituitary prolactinoma.

TREATMENT SUMMARY

Androgen Replacement

Ideally, in the presence of testosterone deficiency, androgen replacement therapy should restore the normal endocrine milieu and restore all androgen-dependent physiologic functions. Many times, however, this is a difficult or impossible task. The main goal, then, is to return and maintain normal sexual function in hypogonadal men.

Testosterone replacement is used in both primary and secondary hypogonadism because it is easier and less expensive than pulsatile parenteral gonadotropin stimulation. Presently, the most commonly used forms of androgen replacement are the depot formulations of the long-acting esters of testosterone, enanthate and cypionate. These esters are converted to free testosterone in the circulation. The esterified forms of testosterone have greater lipid solubility and duration of action. The doses should be individualized, but administration of 200 to 300 mg every 2 or 3 wk is customary. Unfortunately, this method is far from ideal physiologic replacement. Supraphysiologic, followed by subnormal plasma testosterone levels, have been reported using the above dosing schedule.

Oral testosterone derivatives (17α-alkylated forms) have been associated with severe hepatotoxicity in some patients. Although these androgens are metabolized more slowly than testosterone, their short physical half-life (3 hr) requires multiple daily dosing. Another shortcoming to this form of therapy is that plasma levels cannot be readily determined by most currently used testosterone assays. A final disadvantage of this mode of therapy is that bioconversion of alkylated testosterone to estradiol does not occur. Therefore, patients on oral testosterone therapy may be at higher risk for cardiovascular disease. In the rare patient who cannot tolerate parenteral androgens, methyltestosterone 25 to 50 mg orally per day, or fluoxymestrone 5 to 10 mg orally per day may be used with careful monitoring of hepatic function.

Transdermal testosterone preparations (TTS-T) are the newest and are rapidly becoming a very popular form of androgen replacement. TTS-T is convenient, reliable, and more closely mimics normal physiologic testosterone secretion while avoiding the undesirably high testosterone levels that may be seen with depot preparations. This route avoids passage of high drug concentrations through the liver. Knowledge that scrotal skin is much more permeable to testosterone than other skin sites led to the development of transscrotal testosterone preparations (e.g., Testoderm; Alza Co., Palo Alto, CA). Serum testosterone levels peak between 2 and 6 hr after patch application, followed by a gradual fall into the hypogonadal range within 24 hr. Accordingly, the patches must be applied to the scrotal skin every day. Another potential benefit is that, with early morning application of the patch, the normal diurnal pattern of testosterone secretion is mimicked. On the negative side, some are concerned over possible undesirable long-term effects. The scrotal skin has significant 5α-reductase activity. Therefore, a large proportion of the testosterone absorbed through the scrotal skin is converted to DHT, resulting in supraphysiologic levels. It is possible that these supranormal DHT levels may increase the risk for benign prostatic hypertrophy (BPH) and prostate cancer.

A transdermal testosterone delivery system for nongenital skin has recently been developed (i.e., Androderm; SKB, Philadelphia, PA). It uses a permeation-enhancing vehicle to allow for efficient testosterone absorption through nonscrotal skin. Two patches daily applied to the abdomen, back, thighs, or upper arms produced normal plasma testosterone levels. The normal diurnal pattern can be mimicked by applying two patches nightly. The excess DHT levels associated with the transscrotal testosterone delivery approach do not occur with this method. Adverse skin reactions were noted in 9%, similar to other transdermal preparations. Changes in prostate volume, mean prostate specific antigen (PSA), and plasma lipids were not significantly different from appropriate comparison groups. Future studies are planned to evaluate the effect of this form of testosterone delivery on erectile function and in elderly men with low serum testosterone levels.[44]

Before the administration of any androgen, a serum PSA should be obtained, and men older than 50 yr must be evaluated for BPH and prostate cancer. Sleep apnea or polycythemia may worsen with androgen replacement. Liver function should be assessed before and periodically (e.g., annually) during testosterone therapy. Gynecomastia is rarely a problem, except in men with hepatic cirrhosis. Priapism can occur in chronically androgen-deficient patients on high replacement doses.

Other Therapies

Several new dopamine agonists have been developed for the treatment of some prolactin-secreting pituitary tumors. These include pergolide, carbegoline, and octreotide. However, most believe that these patients should promptly be referred to an appropriate specialist for treatment.

Occasionally, some men with erectile dysfunction and hypogonadotropic hypogonadism may have a better clinical response to GnRH or clomiphene stimulation, with an increase in serum testosterone. Therefore, clomiphene administered in doses of 12.5 to 50 mg per day continuously or on a 25-day cycle with a 5-day "rest period" can be effective in this group of patients.

SUMMARY

Sexual dysfunction is common among men, and its incidence increases with age and various medical disorders. More and more men are seeking the help of physicians because of an increasingly liberal attitude towards sexuality, greater emphasis on quality of life, recognition that impotence is most commonly organic and not psychogenic, and improved diagnostic and therapeutic techniques. Because of the complex nature of hormonal-related sexual dysfunction, a scientific and systematic approach is required to detect and treat the underlying condition. Ultimately, this must be accomplished in the confines of present day medical economics. Only with a complete understanding of the principles of male sexual endocrinology and related abnormalities can an accurate, practical, and effective treatment plan be instituted.

REFERENCES

 1. Kinsey AL, Pomeroy WB, Martin CE: *Sexual Behavior in the Human Male*. Philadelphia, Saunders, 1948.

2. Diokno AL, Brown MB, Herzog AR: Sexual function in the elderly. *Arch Intern Med* 150:197–200, 1990.

3. Feldman HA, Goldstein I, Hatzichristou DG, et al: Impotence and its medical and psychosocial correlates: results of the Massachusetts Male Aging Study. *J Urol* 151:54–61, 1994.

4. Vermulen A: Androgens and the aging male. *J Clin Endocrinol Metab* 73:221–224, 1991.

5. Bardin CW, Paulsen CA: The testes. In Williams RH (ed): *Textbook of Endocrinology*, ed 6. Philadelphia, Saunders, 1981.

6. Griffin JE, Wilson JD: Disorders of the testes and male reproductive tract. In Wilson JD, Foster DW (eds): *Textbook of Endocrinology*, ed 7. Philadelphia, Saunders, 1986.

7. Carmel PW, Araki S, Ferin M: Pituitary stalk portal blood collection in rhesus monkeys: evidence for pulsatile release of gonadotropin-releasing hormone (GnRH). *Endocrinology* 99:243–248, 1976.

8. Decker MH, Loriaux DL, Cutler GB, Jr: A seminiferous tubular factor is not obligatory for regulation of plasma follicle-stimulating hormone in the rat. *Endocrinology* 108:1035–1039, 1981.

9. Sarten RJ: Independent effects of testosterone and estradiol on the secretion of gonadotrophins in man. In Troen P, Nankin HR (eds): *The Testis in Normal and Infertile Men.* New York, Raven Press, 1977.

10. Rosen SN, Weintraub BD: Monotropic increase of serum FSH correlated with low sperm count in young men with oligospermia and aspermia. *J Clin Endocrinol Metab* 32:410–416, 1971.

11. Saez JM, Forest MG: Kinetics of human chorionic gonadotropin-induced steroidogenic response of the human testis. I. Plasma testosterone: implication for human chorionic gonadotropin stimulation test. *J Clin Endocrin Metab* 49:278–283, 1979.

12. Labrie F, Belanger A, Cusan L, et al: Antifertility effects of LH-RH agonists in the male. *J Androl* 1:209–212, 1980.

13. Kalla NR, Nisula BC, Menard R, et al: The effect of estradiol on testicular testosterone biosynthesis. *Endocrinology* 106:35–39, 1980.

14. Darney KJ, Ewing L: Autoregulation of testosterone secretion in perfused rat testes. *Endocrinology* 109:993–995, 1981.

15. Cunningham GR, Karacan I, Ware JC, et al: The relationship between serum testosterone and prolactin levels and nocturnal penile tumescence (NPT) in impotent men. *J Androl* 3:241–245, 1982.

16. Kwan M, Greenleaf WJ, Mann J, et al: The nature of androgen action on male sexuality: a combined laboratory self-report study on hypogonadal men. *J Clin Endocrinol Metab* 57:557–562, 1983.

17. Davidson JM: Hormones and sexual behavior in the male. *Hosp Pract* 10:126–132, 1975.

18. Carter JN, Tyson JE, Tolis G, et al: Prolactin-secreting tumors and hypogonadism in 22 men. *N Engl J Med* 299:847–852, 1978.

19. Zonsein J: Diagnosis and management of endocrine disorders. *Urol Clin North Am* 22:789–802, 1995.

20. Spratt DI, Bigos ST, Beitins I, et al: Both hyper- and hypogonadotropic hypogonadism occur transiently in acute illness: bio- and immunoactive gonadotropins. *J Clin Endocrinol Metab* 75:152–157, 1992.

21. Croxson TS, Chapman WE, Miller LK, et al: Changes in the hypothalamic-pituitary-gonadal axis in human immunodeficiency virus-infected homosexual men. *J Clin Endocrinol Metab* 68:317–321, 1989.

22. Villette JN, Bourin P, Noinel, et al: Circadian variations in plasma levels of hypophyseal, adrenocortical and testicular hormones in men infected with human immunodeficiency virus. *J Clin Endocrinol Metab* 70:572–577, 1990.

23. Klyde BJ: Hormonal causes of male sexual dysfunction. In Whitehead D, Nagler H (ed): *Management of Impotence and Infertility.* Philadelphia, Lippincott, 1994.

24. Melmed S: Acromegaly. *N Engl J Med* 322:966–976, 1990.

25. Rosner W: The function of corticosteroid-binding globulin and sex hormone-binding globulin: recent advances. *Endocrin Rev* 11:80–91, 1990.

26. Roncari DAK, Van RLR: Promotion of human adipocyte precursor replaction by estradiol in culture. *J Clin Invest* 62:503–568, 1977.

27. Aldercreutz H: Hepatic metabolism of estrogens in health and disease. *N Engl J Med* 290:1081–1083, 1974.

28. Marynick SP, Chakmakjian ZH, McCaffree DL, et al: Androgen excess in cystic acne. *N Engl J Med* 308:981–986, 1983.

29. Ellenberg M: Impotence in diabetes: the neurologic factor. *Ann Intern Med* 75:213–219, 1971.

30. Saenz de Tejada I, Goldstein I, Azadzoi K, et al: Impaired neurogenic endothelium-mediated relaxation of penile smooth muscle from diabetic men with impotence. *N Engl J Med* 320:1025–1030, 1989.

31. The Diabetes Control and Complications Trial Research Group: The effect of intensive treatment of diabetes on the development and progression of long-term complications in insulin-dependent diabetes mellitus. *N Engl J Med* 329:977–1036, 1993.

32. Pryor JL: Editorial comment. Johnson AR, Jarow JP. Is routine endocrine testing of impotent men necessary? *J Urol* 147:1542–1544, 1992.

33. McClure RD: Endocrine investigation and therapy. *Urol Clin North Am* 14:471–488, 1987.

34. Carani C, Zini D, Baldini A, et al: Effects of androgen treatment in impotent men with normal and low levels of free testosterone. *Arch Sex Behav* 19:223–234, 1990.

35. Cunningham GR, Hirshkowitz M: Impotence. In Becker KL, Brenner WJ (eds): Endocrinology of the male. Excerpted from *Principles and Practice of Endocrinology and Metabolism.* Philadelphia, Lippincott, 1995.

36. Leonard MP, Nickel CJ, Morales A: Hyperprolactinemia and impotence: why, when, and how to investigate. *J Urol* 142:992–994, 1989.

37. Sigman M, Jarow J: Endocrine testing of infertile men: indications and results. *Fertil Steril* 64:549, 1995.

38. Nickel JC, Morales A, Condra M, et al: Endocrine dysfunction in impotence: incidence, and significance and cost-effective screening. *J Urol* 132:40–43, 1984.

39. Miller JB, Howards SS, McLeod RM: Serum prolactin in organic and psychogenic impotence. *J Urol* 124:862–864, 1980.

40. Benson GS: The clinical evaluation of the patient presenting with erectile dysfunction: what is reasonable? *Semin Urol* 8:94–99, 1990.

41. Akpunonu BE, Mutgi AB, Federman DJ, et al: Routine prolactin measurement is not necessary in the initial evaluation of impotence. *J Gen Intern Med* 9:336–338, 1994.

42. Lehmann K, Schopke W, Brutsch HP, et al: [Which hormone determinations are necessary in the initial assessment of erectile dysfunction?] [German] *Schweiz Rundsch Med Prax* 83:1030–1033, 1994.

43. Lewis RW, Barrett DM: Modern management of male erectile dysfunction. *AUA Update* series 14(20), 1995.

44. Winters SJ: Pharmacology of testosterone and current androgen replacement therapies. In *Perspectives on Male Hormone Replacement Therapy* (symposium program workbook, Aventura, FL, Jan 12–13, 1996). Springfield, NJ, Scientific Therapeutics Information, 1996.

4

Nocturnal Penile Tumescence Monitoring

James A. Daitch
Milton M. Lakin
Drogo K. Montague

Erectile dysfunction (ED), the inability to achieve or maintain an erection of sufficient rigidity to perform sexual intercourse in greater than 25% of attempts, affects an estimated 18 million Americans.[1,2] Normal erectile function involves complex interactions between psychologic, neurologic, hormonal, and vascular systems. Failure in any one of these systems may lead to ED. With many treatment options available, an accurate assessment of each patient's ED etiology is crucial. This is particularly important with regard to distinguishing psychogenic from organogenic ED, as surgical intervention for psychogenic ED is inappropriate, and psychotherapy for organic ED is ineffective.

In 1940, Halverson first described nocturnal penile tumescence (NPT), or sleep erections, in infants.[3] Four years later, Ohlmeyer and associates described periodic sleep erections in men 20 to 40 yr old.[4] Approximately 10 yr later, Aserinsky and Kleitman reported the existence of rapid eye movement (REM) sleep described as regularly occurring periods of bilateral synchronous eye movements during stage 1 EEG activity.[5] Aserinsky also noted a distinct association between REM sleep and the erectile episodes previously described by Ohlmeyer.[6] Systematic efforts to associate NPT and REM sleep began, and by the mid 1960s two separate groups led by Fisher[7] and Karacan[8] reported NPT episodes associated with 80% to 90% of REM periods in healthy young adults. By 1976, through a series of studies involving over 2,000 healthy boys and men, Karacan and associates had documented the existence of sleep-related erections in all healthy males 3 to 79 yr old.[9–14] Although he noted both quantitative and qualitative changes in NPT with increasing age, the overwhelming consistency of this phenomenon led Karacan to hypothesize that monitoring sleep erections could have diagnostic and prognostic significance in the differentiation of psychogenic from organogenic ED.[15] This would be the first objective test of erectile function. The working assumption is that during sleep emotional factors such as fear and anxiety are neutralized, and subjects suffering from psychogenic ED therefore have normal NPT. However, for patients with organic ED, the underlying cause (vascular, hormonal, or neurologic) does not change with sleep, and abnormal sleep erections persist. As other investigators began testing NPT monitoring, a second assumption of NPT became apparent; for NPT to be accurate, the mechanisms involved in sleep erections must be the same as those responsible for sexually stimulated erections. Although there is some question as to the validity of the two aforementioned assumptions, NPT has emerged as a time-tested reliable technique to aid in the evaluation of ED.

NPT METHODOLOGY

Formal NPT testing takes place over two to three consecutive nights in a sleep laboratory. Subjects are to abstain from alcohol, caffeine, and medications that may affect erections or sleep for at least 6 to 8 hr prior to the test. Patients must sleep normally to permit a valid test, as sleep erections occur primarily during REM sleep. In order to adequately assess REM sleep, electroencephalographic (EEG), electro-oculographic (EOG), and submental electromyographic (EMG) measures are recorded during NPT testing. Numerous studies have demonstrated that subtle sleep disorders such as sleep apnea or hypopnea and nocturnal myoclonus (periodic leg movements) may disrupt NPT without apparent EEG changes.[16–18] Hence, nasal and oral thermistors (airflow), pulse oximetry, and anterior tibialis EMG measurements are also recommended.

Penile tumescence is measured by using two mercury-in-rubber strain gauges, one placed at the penile base and the other just behind the glans penis. The strain gauges are expandable rubber loops containing a thin column of mercury. When the loop circumference increases, the mercury column is thinned and electrical resistance through the mercury is increased. This is translated into pen deflection on a recording device. The strain gauges are calibrated using three cylinders of increasing circumferences (70, 80, and 90 mm), so that an increase in circumference of 1 mm corresponds to a 1-mm pen deflection on the recording paper. Discrepancies between base and tip tumescence are noted. Simultaneous recorded changes in penile circumference and sleep parameters permit the differentiation of REM from non-REM (NREM) sleep erections, and assure the quality of sleep during the study.

NPT INTERPRETATION

The analysis of NPT test results has evolved over the past 30 yr, with most studies employing different decision rules to classify sleep erections as normal or abnormal. In general, a combination of the following parameters is used to assess sleep erections:

Degree: an increase in penile circumference over the flaccid state, measured in millimeters at the base. During the three nights of testing, the greatest penile circumference is noted on the recorded data. If this circumference is estimated to be a full erection by direct observation, then any episode with a circumference between 81% and 100% of this greatest circumference is considered to be a maximum episode. Episodes with a circumference of 25% to 80% of the greatest penile circumference are considered partial episodes. Increases less than 25% are not considered erection episodes. If direct observation of the greatest penile circumference is estimated to represent less than a full erection, then the trained observer extrapolates the circumference at which a full erection would occur, and uses this number to categorize tumescent episodes.[19,20]

Frequency: mean number of total and maximum episodes per night.

Duration: mean time per night spent in all erectile episodes, maximum episodes, and episodes with simultaneous REM sleep.

By comparing the above factors with norms established primarily through Karacan's work,[19-14] patients were successfully classified as suffering from psychogenic or organic ED in approximately 80% to 95% of cases.[21] It soon became evident, however, that there were large interindividual differences in circumferential changes related primarily to anatomic variations among subjects. For example, a 16-mm circumferential increase may represent a full erection in one man, but correspond to a flaccid state in another. In addition, Wein and associates reported significant penile tumescence without sufficient rigidity for vaginal penetration in 17% of 134 patients with ED.[22] Subsequent studies corroborated these findings; maximum tumescence can be reached prior to achieving significant rigidity.[23,24] Since rigidity is the most important factor involved in successful intromission, NPT testing and results interpretation have been modified.

Rigidity measurements are taken usually on the third night of testing by awaking the patient during a tumescent episode equal to the greatest degree of tumescence observed on the previous nights of testing. This erection is rated on a scale of 0–100% rigidity by both the patient and a trained observer, and a photograph is taken. In addition, a tonometer device is used to objectively measure the axial rigidity of the erection. This device is basically a syringe with a rubber cap on one end, and a sphygmomanometer on the other end. The cap is placed over the tip of the penis and pressure is applied until the penis buckles. Based on Karacan's observations, a buckling pressure of 100 mm Hg represents sufficient rigidity for vaginal penetration. Buckling pressures between 60 and 100 mm Hg are of questionably sufficient rigidity, and buckling pressures < 60 mm Hg are of insufficient rigidity for intromission.[19]

Unfortunately, few studies have examined the accuracy of NPT testing in patients diagnosed with organic or psychogenic ED based on information independent of NPT results.

Marshall and associates assigned patients with ED to one of four diagnostic groups on the basis of clinical history alone: organic ED, psychogenic ED, mixed etiology, and uncertain etiology.[21] NPT results correlated with the clinical categorization of psychogenic and organic ED in 95% of cases. Schiavi and colleagues studied four age-matched groups formed on the basis of clinical evidence independent of NPT information.[20] Analysis of NPT testing results demonstrated that specific NPT parameters could discriminate diabetic men with organic ED from diabetics with normal erectile function, men with psychogenic ED, and normal controls with 77.8% to 88.9% accuracy. Still, questions about the accuracy of sleep erections in predicting the quality of sexually stimulated erections remain.

False-positive NPT

One concern is that the quality of sleep erections may overestimate the quality of sexually induced erections. In these patients the NPT result is positive (i.e., adequate sleep erection), but the patient truly has organic ED. A few studies have demonstrated this to be the case, particularly in patients with neurogenic ED.

Neurogenic ED

Ghezzi and associates performed pudendal evoked potential (PEP), bulbocavernosus muscle motor evoked potential, and bulbocavernosus reflex (BCR) examinations in a total of 14 multiple sclerosis (MS) patients with or without ED.[25] When the results were compared to NPT results and clinical evaluations, neither NPT nor neurologic testing could distinguish MS patients with normal erectile function from MS patients with ED. Kirkeby and associates evaluated 26 MS patients with ED.[26] They found a 36% false-positive rate in NPT results. While these studies are small and lack sufficient controls, they do illustrate the need to carefully interpret NPT results among patients with neurologic disorders.

Pelvic Steal Syndrome

Another source of false-positive NPT results, termed the "pelvic steal syndrome," has been described. Case reports have demonstrated that patients with compromised penile vascular supply may obtain adequate erections, but rapidly lose rigidity with movement of lower extremities or pelvic thrusting.[27] This is thought to be due to the shunting of blood away from the penis and toward the buttocks muscles. The prevalence of this phenomenon among patients with ED is unclear.

False-negative NPT

Several concerns regarding false-negative NPT results have been raised. In these patients the NPT result is negative (i.e., inadequate sleep erections), but the patients do not have organic ED.

NPT and Age

Since the early work of Karacan and associates, NPT has been shown to change with increasing patient age.[9–14] For example, the total tumescence time relative to the sleep time peaks at 3–5 yr and again between 10 and 19 yr; after age 19 this declines slightly but steadily as the healthy patient ages. In addition, the number of REM-related NPT episodes per night also steadily decreases, as does the average length of these episodes. Perhaps most important, the number of full erections decreases and the number of partial erections increases in normal males as they age. During puberty >6 erections occur per night, with over 2.5 hr (40%) of sleep time spent with erections. By age 60, this decreases to 3–4 erections per night, with duration approaching 20% of total sleep time. Schiavi and colleagues examined 40 healthy subjects 23–73 yr old and also found decreased number and duration of erectile episodes with increased age.[28] In addition, they noted a significant decrease in maximum rigidity during NPT in older men, despite clinical potency. A subsequent study by Burris and associates demonstrated decreased duration of erectile episodes with increased age, but the number of erectile episodes and rigidity did not change significantly among subjects 21–75 yr old.[29]

Hence, NPT changes with age. Although the parameters used to interpret NPT results are currently equivalent for all patients, consideration should be given to patient age when drawing conclusions about the etiology of ED based on NPT.

NPT and Sleep Disorders

As previously mentioned, patients must sleep normally to allow valid NPT testing, since subtle sleep disorders such as sleep apnea, hypopnea, or nocturnal myoclonus may disrupt NPT.[16–18] In addition to affecting NPT, sleep apnea may be associated with ED itself.[30] Schiavi and associates, however, did not find sleep disorders to be involved in ED among 70 healthy older men when the data was controlled for age.[31] It is clear, however, that the quality of sleep must be assessed in all patients undergoing NPT to avoid potential false-negative results.

NPT and Depression

Depressed patients often report decreased libido and changes in erectile function. Roose and colleagues first reported impaired NPT in two severely depressed patients.[32] Interestingly, NPT results improved after clinical recovery from depression. Thase and associates subsequently concurred with these findings.[33–35] They found that approximately 20% of all depressed men had severely impaired NPT which normalized after the depression was treated. In addition, they described an uncoupling of REM sleep and NPT among depressed patients. The impaired NPT was thought to be a neurophysiologic correlate of depression. Although some studies identify no significant change in NPT during the acute phases of depression,[36,37] patients with ED should be carefully screened for signs of depression, and if indicated, treated before further workup of their ED.

NPT and Anxiety

In addition to depression, other psychological factors may influence NPT. A number of studies suggest that anxiety may affect NPT. Although he noted more pronounced abnormalities in patients with organic ED, Johanović reported marked NPT impairment in both acute and chronic psychogenic ED.[38] In addition, he described impaired NPT on the first night of sleep laboratory testing.[39] This is thought to be due to anxiety associated with unfamiliar sleep surroundings and NPT equipment. Although others have subsequently described this "first night effect" of NPT monitoring, several groups have not found any evidence of a "first night effect."[37,40–41]

Karacan and associates noted that dream anxiety interfered with the erection cycle among 16 young men examined over a 6-wk period.[42] Fisher's group also noted impaired sleep erections associated with high anxiety dreams.[43] Hence, despite its ability to distinguish psychogenic from organogenic ED, NPT can be affected by psychological factors.

NPT and Drugs

Various studies have demonstrated a tendency for drugs to impair NPT.[44-49] Among the most common culprits are antihypertensives, anticholinergics, anxiolytics, antidepressants, alcohol, and tobacco (Table 4.1) Despite the known detrimental effects of alcohol on NPT, Schiavi and colleagues noted no significant difference in NPT results between healthy chronic alcoholics who had achieved sobriety for ≥ 2 months and nonalcoholic volunteers.[47] Based on their results and those of previous studies, they concluded that the abnormal NPT associated with alcoholism can reverse itself after alcohol abstention. Similarly, Elist and associates demonstrated that impaired NPT normalized in 7 of 20 (35%) cigarette smokers 6 wk after smoking cessation.[49] While the effects of drugs on NPT may be temporary, it is crucial to limit their use in the proximity of NPT testing.

NPT and Hypogonadism

While hypogonadal men clearly have ED and typically have abnormal NPT, several studies confirm that hypogonadal men do achieve erections in response to erotic stimuli.[50-53] These authors have demonstrated that sleep erections are androgen-dependent, whereas erotic erections are not. This has led to speculation that sleep erections and erotic erections are mediated through different neurophysiologic pathways.[54-56]

Results in patients with neurologic lesions support this view. Based on the observation that psychogenic erections can occur in men with a complete lesion below T12-L2, while reflex erections can occur in some men with complete chronic spinal cord injuries if the conus, sacral anterior roots, and posterior roots are intact, some have concluded that psychogenic erections are mediated by T12-L2 segments, and reflex erections by S2-S4 segments.[57,58] This lends further credence to the caveat mentioned above, that NPT must be interpreted carefully in men with neurologic disorders.

In summary, NPT testing is estimated to have a false-negative rate of approximately 10–20%.[40,59] Given the pitfalls of NPT mentioned previously, NPT test

Table 4.1. Drugs Impairing NPT

Alcohol
Antiandrogens
Anticholinergics
Anticonvulsants
Antidepressants
Anxiolytics
Barbiturates
Benzodiazepines
Cocaine
Diuretics (hydrochlorothiazide in doses > 50 mg/d, spironolactone)
Marijuana
Narcotics
Sympatholytics (α-methyldopa, beta-blockers, clonidine, guanethidine, reserpine)
Tobacco

Table 4.2. Factors Affecting NPT Results

False-positive NPT Result	*False-negative NPT Result*
Neurogenic erectile dysfunction	Anxiety
Pelvic steal syndrome	Drug/medication usage
	Elderly healthy patient
	Hypogonadism
	Major depression episode
	Sleep disorders

results must be interpreted cautiously (Table 4.2). Compared to other objective diagnostic tests that attempt to distinguish psychogenic from organic ED, however, NPT testing appears to be the most accurate.[59–62] In addition, NPT testing is noninvasive.

ALTERNATIVE NPT MONITORING TECHNIQUES

While formal NPT testing is considered the gold standard for differentiating psychogenic from organic ED, test administration is very difficult, logistically cumbersome, time-consuming, and expensive. As a result, simpler, less expensive tests were developed in an effort to maximize the diagnostic benefits of NPT while minimizing the costs.

Portable NPT

Portable NPT monitoring consists of the mercury-in-rubber strain gauges described earlier, connected to a portable device which records penile tumescence. The patient is instructed to connect the strain gauges at home before sleeping, disconnecting them in the morning upon awakening. Administering the test at home is much more convenient for the patient, and reduces the overall test cost by limiting the number of trained observers necessary to administer the test. However, due to the lack of simultaneous EMG data, significant motion artifact often results in difficult test interpretation.[63] In addition, no rigidity data is obtained, and without simultaneous EEG data, the quality of sleep and therefore test validity cannot be assured. The use of home NPT monitoring with strain gauges has been largely abandoned.

Stamp Test

In 1980, Barry and associates described a technique using stamps to measure NPT.[64] Just prior to sleep, a strip of four stamps are wrapped snugly around the penis and the overlapping stamp is moistened to provide a $\frac{1}{2}$ to 1 stamp overlapping seal. In the morning the patient inspects the ring to determine if it has broken at the perforations. The test is repeated for three consecutive nights. If the ring remains unbroken, no significant NPT has occurred, and the patient has organic ED, however if breakage occurs, the patient has psychogenic ED. Of 22 men with normal erectile function, only four (18%) had a false-negative stamp test. Similarly, only one of 11 men with ED (9%) had a false-positive stamp test. Marshall and associates validated these findings by assessing stamp breakage in 15 healthy men watching erotic videos.[65] They found stamp breakage at 80–100% of full erection, however, this data provided no insight into the accuracy of the stamp test in a clinical setting. In a subsequent study, Marshall's group simultaneously performed formal NPT monitoring and the stamp test in 25 patients with ED.[66] In 16 of 20 patients with stamp breakage, NPT results were negative (80% false-positive rate). However, when stamp breakage did not occur, all patients had abnormal NPT. The large false-positive rate is thought to be due to patient movement breaking the stamps, progressive weakening of the perforations due to repeated partial erections, and/or moistening of the stamps during sleep. Hence, the stamp test is considered valid in only the small proportion of patients in whom the test is negative.

Snap-Gauge*

In an effort to improve on the stamp test, Ek and associates introduced the Snap-Gauge band.[67] This is a Velcro band fitted around the penis with three colored plastic film elements arranged in parallel (Fig. 4.1). Each film ruptures at a radial force selected to correspond to intracavernosal pressures found in erections (90–180 mm Hg). Ten ounces of radial force ruptures the blue film, 15 oz ruptures the red film, and 20 oz ruptures the clear film. The Snap-Gauge is worn for three consecutive nights. In their study of 66 patients with ED, Ek's group demonstrated that

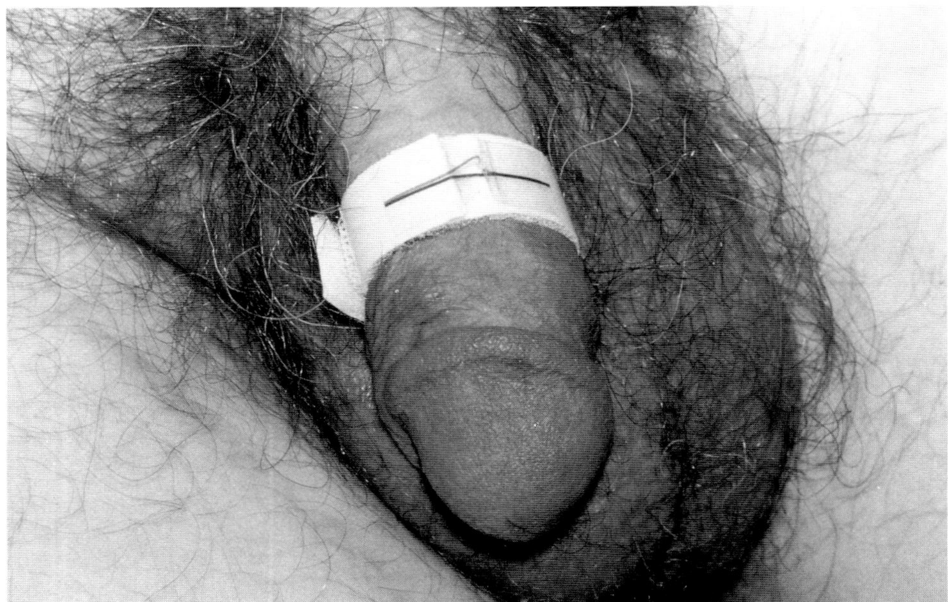

Fig. 4.1. Snap-Gauge device.

* Dacomed Corp., Minneapolis, MN

Snap-Gauge results correlated well with NPT test results. Similarly, Condra and associates reported a correlation between increased degree of tumescence and increased number of Snap-Gauge films broken.[68] However, neither of these studies measured rigidity independent of the Snap-Gauge. In 1988, Ellis and associates compared Snap-Gauge results to visual assessments of erectile rigidity during simultaneous formal NPT monitoring.[69] Their criteria for absent rigidity was zero to one Snap-Gauge film broken. Patients breaking two to three films were categorized as having rigid erections. Using this criteria, the Snap-Gauge performed with 70% sensitivity and 80% specificity. However, when carefully analyzing the data, among patients who broke two to three films, 46% had nonrigid erections by visual inspection. Only 11% of patients with Snap-Gauge determined nonrigid erections actually had rigidity by visual inspection. Allen and colleagues reported similar results in their study of 100 patients with ED; when no films were broken the Snap-Gauge was accurate, however, if even one element broke, the test was very inaccurate.[70] In a subsequent study, Allen and Brendler found Snap-Gauge results to misclassify approximately one-third of all patients with ED.[71] The Snap-Gauge is more accurate than the stamp test, however, it suffers the same shortcomings with regard to lack of information concerning partial rigidity, number of erections, and duration of erectile episodes. A device was needed that could measure rigidity continuously.

RigiScan*

Formal NPT testing provides continuous tumescence monitoring, but furnishes rigidity information only at discrete times when the patient is awakened. Erections in older patients tend to rapidly detumesce upon patient awakening, and these rigidity measurements are subject to observer error.[72] In 1985, Bradley and colleagues described a device which provided continuous measurement of both penile rigidity and tumescence.[73] This apparatus was modified and made commercially available as the RigiScan device (Dacomed Corp., Minneapolis, MN). The RigiScan consists of a portable battery-powered unit which is strapped around the thigh (Fig. 4.2). It has two loops connected to a DC torque motor. One loop is placed at the penile base, the other just behind the corona.

To measure tumescence, the loops tighten around the penis every 30 sec with a force of 1.7 newtons and the penile circumference (loop length) is recorded. A second circumference measurement is taken 15 sec later without active tightening of the loops. If tumescence increases 10 mm or more from baseline, rigidity measurements are initiated.

Rigidity is measured every 30 sec by the loops tightening with a force of 2.8 newtons. Rigidity is expressed as a percentage, with 100% equaling the rigidity of a noncompressible rubber shaft. When tumescence decreases to within 10 mm of baseline, rigidity measurements are discontinued until the next episode of adequate tumescence.

The RigiScan allows for the recording of three uninterrupted 10-hr sessions. Data can then be downloaded into a microprocessor where the nocturnal penile tumescence and rigidity (NPTR) information can be analyzed, displayed, and printed.

---

* Dacomed Corp., Minneapolis, MN.

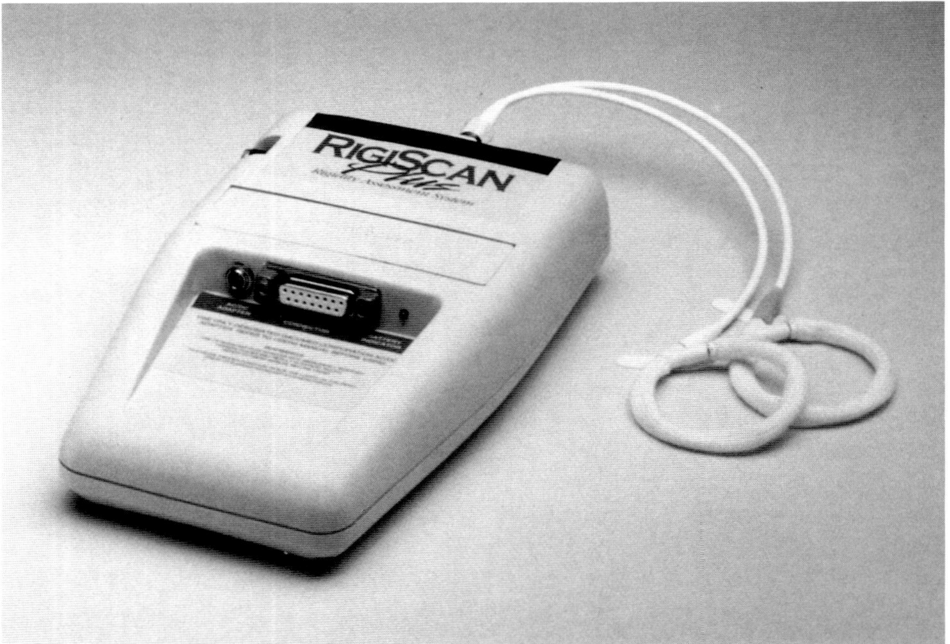

Fig. 4.2. RigiScan device.

Like the stamp test and Snap-Gauge, the RigiScan measures radial rigidity. Although axial rigidity is the most crucial measurement predicting vaginal penetration, there is a linear relationship between axial and radial rigidity.[24,73] In addition, radial rigidity is functionally related to intracavernous pressure, the true measure of rigidity.[24]

In Bradley's initial study, NPTR results were compared between 11 healthy controls and 11 patients presenting with ED. Healthy subjects averaged 4 erectile episodes per night, with a mean maximum rigidity of 74.7%. Men with ED averaged 3.3 episodes per night, with a mean maximum rigidity of 51.8%.[73] Subsequent normative data supplied by the Dacomed Corporation on over 500 patients defined a normal RigiScan study as containing 3–6 erection episodes each lasting 10–15 min per 8 hr of sleep. In addition, at least one nocturnal erection must contain a circumference increase of ≥ 3 cm at the penile base and ≥ 2 cm at the tip sustained for at least 10 min at a rigidity $\geq 70\%$ (Fig. 4.3). Rigidity between 40% and 70% is borderline, and rigidity $< 40\%$ is insufficient for vaginal penetration[74] (Fig. 4.4). Finally, there should be no evidence of dissociation or uncoupling. Dissociation describes normal penile base rigidity with concurrent abnormal tip rigidity (Fig. 4.5). Uncoupling refers to normal tumescence with significantly reduced or absent rigidity (Fig. 4.6). A number of studies have examined the accuracy of these parameters.

Bain and Guay examined the reproducibility of the RigiScan by testing 17 men presenting with ED, and repeating the test 39 days later.[75] Repeated test results were identical in all but two patients; one had ingested alcohol in close proximity to the repeat test and the other suffered a febrile illness during repeat testing. Hence,

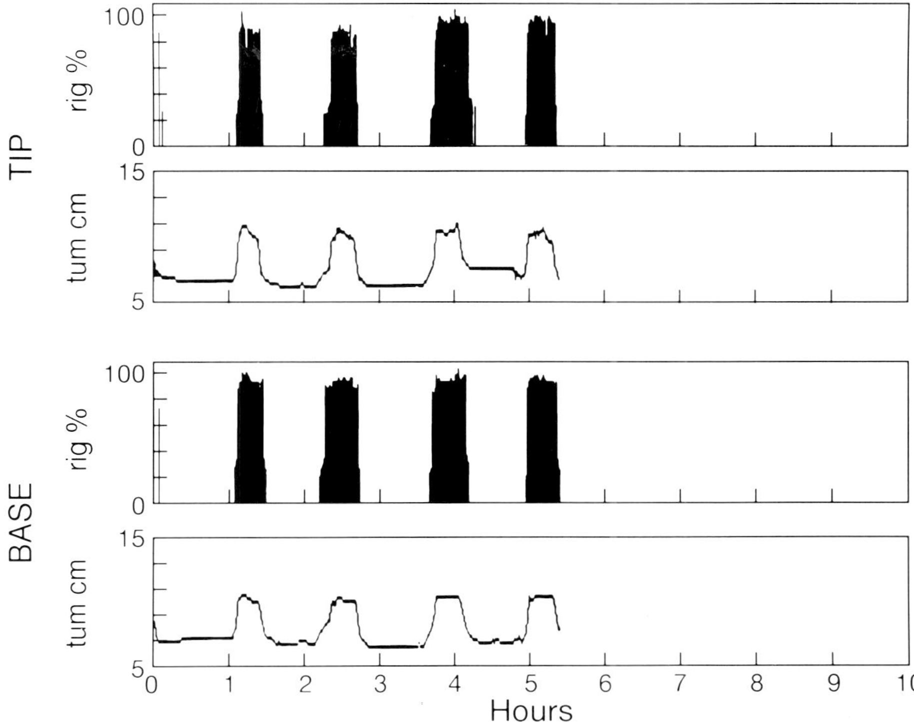

Fig. 4.3. Normal RigiScan demonstrating four erectile episodes each lasting >15 min with base and tip rigidity near 90%.

RigiScan results are reproducible, but also are sensitive to factors affecting any NPT test.

To evaluate the accuracy of NPTR, Kaneko and Bradley classified 105 patients as having psychogenic or organic ED based on data independent of NPT results. Subsequent NPTR testing confirmed or enabled the correction of the initial classification in all but one patient.[76] In addition, they also noted dissociation and uncoupling among the RigiScans of several patients with ED. This provided further support to the parameters outlined in previous studies.

Van Nueten and colleagues compared NPTR results in 100 patients with ED to results obtained through endocrinologic, neurologic, and vascular testing.[77] This group redefined normal base rigidity as 65%, and normal tip rigidity as 60%. Using these criteria, among 51 patients with normal NPTR, only five (9.8%) were misclassified as having psychogenic ED. All five patients were subsequently found to have neurogenic ED. Among 37 patients with abnormal NPTR, no patients were subsequently found to be misclassified. Of the remaining 12 patients with borderline NPTR results, five (42%) were found to have psychogenic ED, and seven (58%) had organic ED.

To examine if NPTR testing could delineate subtypes of organic ED, Sohn and associates classified 73 patients with organic ED into one of four groups on the basis of invasive testing independent of NPTR results: (1) neurogenic ED, (2)

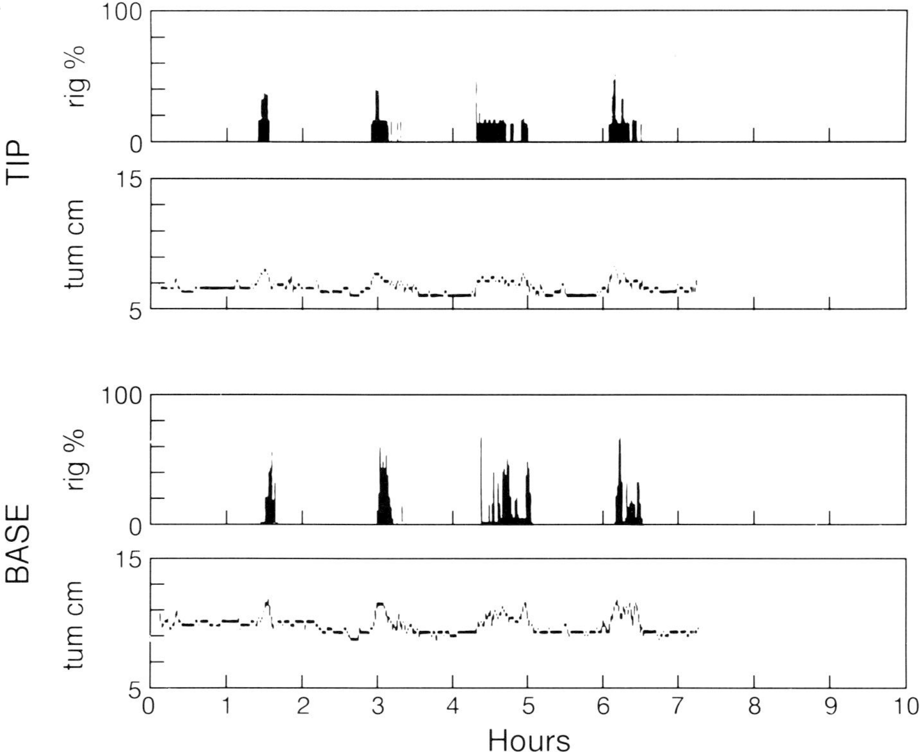

Fig. 4.4. Abnormal RigiScan of a patient with organic erectile dysfunction. Note inadequate tumescence at base and tip, as well as rigidity ranging from only 20% to 40%.

arteriogenic ED, (3) venogenic ED, and (4) combined arteriovenogenic ED.[78] When compared to subsequent NPTR results, they found a reduction in number of erectile events and degree of rigidity in men with neurogenic ED. Among vascular etiologies, there was no change in the number of erectile episodes, however, arteriogenic and venogenic ED patients had significantly reduced rigidity, and combined arteriovenogenic patients displayed even further reduced rigidity. Despite these differences, no pathognomonic pattern of neurogenic or vasculogenic ED could be derived from this study. Similar to Van Nueten's group, Sohn's group found that among patients with organic ED, NPTR testing misclassified 12.3% of patients as having psychogenic ED.

Allen and associates compared the evaluation of rigidity by NPTR to formal NPT testing.[79] Ten impotent patients underwent axial measurements of NPT rigidity with a tonometer during simultaneous RigiScan. Overall, radial rigidity correlated well with axial rigidity measurements. However, in the subset of measurements when radial rigidity was >60%, the RigiScan could not differentiate axial rigidities between 450 and 900 gm. Hence, this group concurred with those above, that positive NPTR results (i.e., normal NPTR) must be interpreted cautiously.

Licht and colleagues also compared RigiScan radial rigidity measurements to axial rigidity determined during simultaneous formal NPT.[80] Among 28 patients

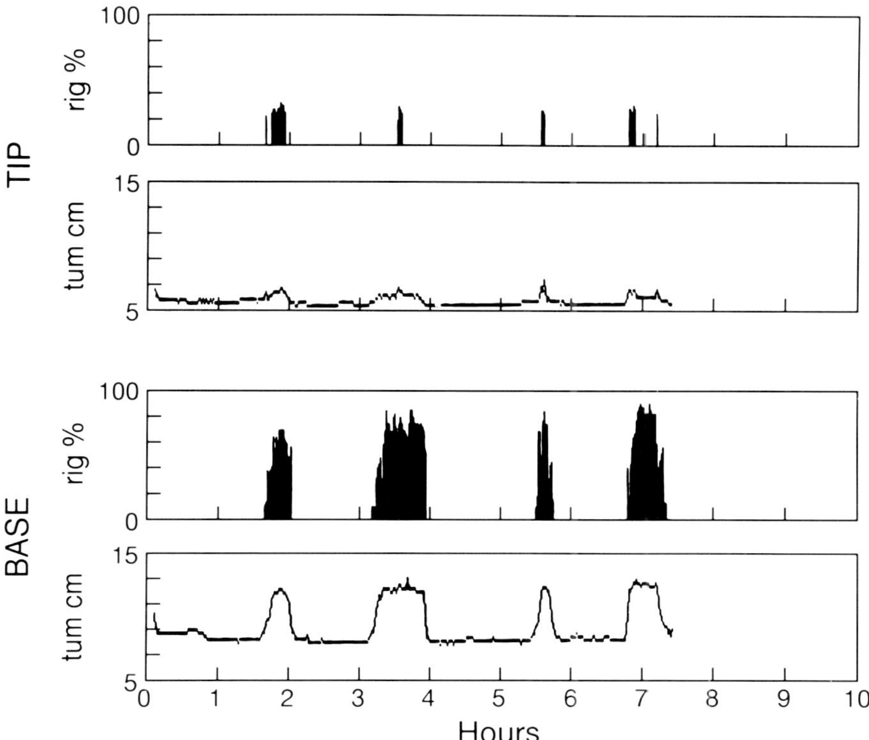

Fig. 4.5. Dissociation. RigiScan of a patient with Peyronie's disease demonstrates good base rigidity, but poor tip rigidity.

with ED and measurable NPT, RigiScan tip rigidity correlated poorly with axial buckling pressure measurements. However, RigiScan base rigidity measurements agreed with axial buckling pressure determinations in 90% of all cases. Using trained observer assessment of a functional erection as the gold standard, a Rigi-Scan base rigidity of ≥55% had an 85% sensitivity and 91% specificity in determining adequate erections. The previously established normal value of 70% was found to have a specificity of 97%, but a sensitivity of only 42%. Hence, in contrast to previous studies which demonstrated that NPTR tended to overestimate psychogenic ED, they concluded that NPTR tended to overestimate organic ED. Highly accurate results could be obtained by modifying NPTR test interpretation.

In an effort to further improve the precision of NPTR, Levine and Carroll analyzed new software which aids in accurate interpretation of RigiScan results.[41] This software summarizes an entire night of tumescence and rigidity data into single values in order to provide easier comparisons between NPTR results. This is accomplished by using time-intensity area measures. For example, rigidity is calculated by multiplying the minutes spent at a given rigidity level by that rigidity value itself. This product is summed across the entire event and termed the rigidity activity unit (RAU). Similarly, tumescence activity units (TAU) represent the product of the duration of each erectile episode by the percentage increase in tumescence for that episode. Based on data from 44 men with normal sexual functioning, nomograms

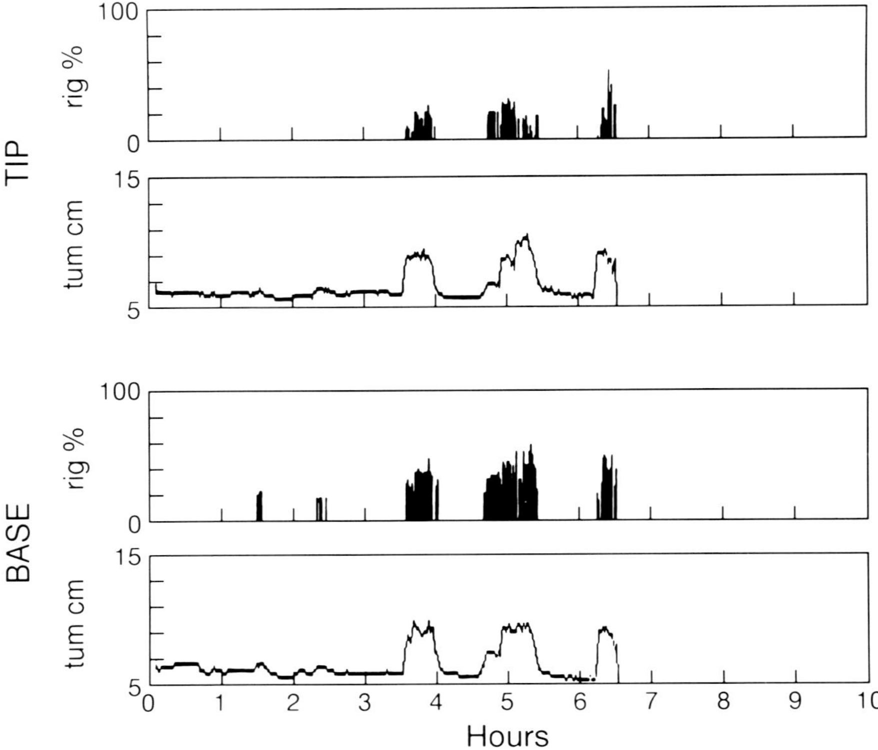

Fig. 4.6. Uncoupling. RigiScan with adequate tumescence at base and tip, but poor base and tip rigidity.

for RAU and TAU were generated. Hence, by plotting an individual's RAU and TAU values on the nomogram, the percentile ranking of his NPTR results (compared to this group of normals) can be calculated. Additional normative data is needed to provide more accurate RAU and TAU population distribution curves, however, this approach to NPTR interpretation will help to objectify NPTR test results.

Overall, then, the RigiScan device can distinguish functional from inadequate erections in the vast majority of cases. Although it suffers many of the same shortcomings of any NPT test, the RigiScan is a reasonable alternative to more expensive and cumbersome formal NPT testing.

FUTURE USE OF NPTR

In an effort to further reduce the cost of NPTR while improving its accuracy, recent studies have addressed monitoring erections during monitoring naps (diurnal penile tumescence or DPT). Gordon and Carey first described adequate sleep erections in seven healthy subjects during morning naps.[81] To assure adequate naps, subject sleep was intentionally abbreviated on the night before testing. All subjects manifested normal erections and REM sleep during their 3-hr naps. Similar results were obtained in a subsequent study examining 30 sexually functional males.[82] Morales and associates demonstrated excellent internal consistency between NPT results and DPT results among individual patients.[83] Although additional normative data is needed, DPTR testing does provide the potential advantages of reducing the cost and inconvenience of formal NPT, while supplying the EEG, EOG, and EMG data necessary to ensure adequate sleep during testing.

Other groups have used the RigiScan device to permit objective quantification of erectile rigidity associated with visual erotic stimulation (VES) or intracavernous injection of vasoactive medications (ICI). Djamilian and associates demonstrated RigiScan monitoring to be highly accurate in objectively evaluating the erectile response to ICI.[84] Ogrinc and Linet used modified RigiScan software to allow real-time analysis of erectile episodes.[85] RigiScan readings and simultaneous trained observer assessments were recorded every 5 min after patients with ED were injected with intracavernous prostaglandin E_1. Based on 521 injections, the established criteria of $\geq 70\%$ as adequate rigidity had a sensitivity of 47.6% and a specificity of 95.8% for determining functional erections. When altering this to consider a rigidity of $\geq 60\%$ as adequate, sensitivity improved to 70.8%, with a specificity of 85.0%.

No single test can distinguish psychogenic from organic ED. NPT monitoring, however, is the only objective test of erectile function that has been evaluated across all age groups in both healthy patients and in those with ED. When interpreted carefully, with attention to patient history, physical examination, and the previously mentioned caveats, NPT results are highly accurate. Hence, NPT monitoring remains an essential component in the evaluation of ED.

REFERENCES

1. Masters WH, Johnson VE: *Human Sexual Inadequacy*. Boston, Little, Brown & Co, 1970, p 157.
2. Goldstein I: Editorial: Impotence. *J Urol* 152:1119–1120, 1994.
3. Halverson HM: Genital and sphincter behavior of the male infant. *J Gen Psychol* 56:95–136, 1940.
4. Ohlmeyer P, Brilmayer H, Hullstrung H: Periodische Vorgange im Schlaf. *Pflugers Arch* 248:559, 1944.
5. Aserinsky E, Kleitman NA: A motility cycle in sleeping infants as manifested by ocular and gross bodily activity. *J. Appl Physiol* 8:11–18, 1955.
6. Aserinsky E: Ocular motility during sleep and its application to the study of rest-activity cycles and dreaming. Doctoral dissertation, University of Chicago, 1953.
7. Fisher C, Gross J, Zuch J: Cycle of penile erections synchronous with dreaming (REM) sleep. *Arch Gen Psychiatry* 12:29–45, 1965.
8. Karacan I: The developmental aspect and the effect of certain clinical conditions upon penile erection during sleep. International Congress. Series, Princeton, NJ, *Excerpta Medica* 1966, 150:2356–2359.
9. Hursch CJ, Karacan I, Williams RL: Some characteristics of nocturnal penile tumescence in early middle-aged males. *Compr Psychiatry* 13:539–548, 1972.

10. Karacan I, Hursch CJ, Williams RL: Some characteristics of nocturnal penile tumescence in elderly males. *J Gerontol* 27:39–45, 1972.

11. Karacan I, Hursch CJ, Williams RL, et al: Some characteristics of nocturnal penile tumescence during puberty. *Pediatr Res* 6:529–537, 1972.

12. Karacan I, Hursch CJ, Williams RL, et al: Some characteristics of nocturnal penile tumescence in young adults. *Arch Gen Psychiatry* 26:351–356, 1972.

13. Karacan I, Salis PJ, Thornby JI, et al: The ontogeny of nocturnal penile tumescence. *Waking Sleeping* 1:27–44, 1976.

14. Karacan I, Williams RL, Thornby JI, et al: Sleep-related penile tumescence as a function of age. *Am J Psychiatry* 132:932–937, 1975.

15. Karacan I: Clinical value of nocturnal erection in the prognosis and diagnosis of impotence. *Med Aspects Hum Sex* 4:27, 1970.

16. Pressman MR, DePhillipo MA, Kendrick JI, et al: Problems in the interpretation of nocturnal penile tumescence studies: disruption of sleep by occult sleep disorders. *J Urol* 136:595–598, 1986.

17. Hirshkowitz M, Karacan I, Gurakar A, et al: Hypertension, erectile dysfunction, and occult sleep apnea. *Sleep* 12:223–232, 1989.

18. Hirshkowitz M, Karacan I, Arcasoy MD, et al: The prevalence of periodic limb movements during sleep in men with erectile dysfunction. *Biol Psychiatry* 26:541–544, 1989.

19. Karacan I, Salis PJ, Williams RL: The role of the sleep laboratory in diagnosis and treatment of impotence. In Williams RL, Karacan I, Frazier SH (eds): *Sleep Disorders, Diagnosis and Treatment*. New York, John Wiley and Sons, 1978, pp 353–382.

20. Schiavi RC, Fisher C, Quadland M, et al: Nocturnal penile tumescent evaluation of erectile function in insulin-dependent diabetic men. *Diabetologia* 28:90–94, 1985.

21. Marshall P, Surridge D, Delva N: The role of nocturnal penile tumescence in differentiating between organic and psychogenic impotence: the first stage of validation. *Arch Sex Behav* 10:1–10, 1981.

22. Wein AJ, Fishkin R, Carpiniello VL, et al: Expansion without significant rigidity during nocturnal penile tumescence testing: a potential source of misinterpretation. *J Urol* 126:343–344, 1981.

23. Metz P, Wagner G: Penile circumference and erection. *Urology* 18:268–270, 1981.

24. Frohrib DA, Goldstein I, Payton TR, et al: Characterization of penile erectile states using external computer-based monitoring. *J Biomech Engin* 109:110–114, 1987.

25. Ghezzi A, Malvestiti GM, Baldini S, et al: Erectile impotence in mutiple sclerosis: a neurophysiological study. *J Neurol* 242:123–126, 1995.

26. Kirkeby HJ, Poulsen EU, Petersen T, et al: Erectile dysfunction in multiple sclerosis. *Neurology* 38:1366–1371, 1988.

27. Goldstein I, Siroky MB, Nath RL, et al: Vasculogenic impotence: role of the pelvic steal test. *J Urol* 128:300–306, 1982.

28. Schiavi RC, Schreiner-Engel P: Nocturnal penile tumescence in healthy aging men. *J Gerontol* 43:M146–M150, 1988.

29. Burris AS, Banks SM, Sherins RJ: Quantitative assessment of nocturnal penile tumescence and rigidity in normal men using a home monitor. *J Androl* 10:492–497, 1989.

30. Guilleminault C, Eldridge FL, Tilkian A, et al: Sleep apnea syndrome due to upper airway obstruction. a review of 25 cases. *Arch Intern Med* 137:296–300, 1977.

31. Schiavi RC, Mandeli J, Schreiner-Engel P, et al: Aging, sleep disorders, and male sexual function. *Biol Psychiatry* 30:15–24, 1991.

32. Roose SP, Glassman AH, Walsh BT, et al: Reversible loss of nocturnal penile tumescence during depression: a preliminary report. *Neuropsychobiology* 8:284–288, 1982.

33. Thase ME, Reynolds III CF, Glanz LM, et al: Nocturnal penile tumescence in depressed men. *Am J Psychiatry* 144:88–92, 1987.

34. Thase ME, Reynolds III CF, Jennings JR, et al: Nocturnal penile tumescence is diminished in depressed men. *Biol Psychiatry* 24:33–46, 1988.

35. Thase ME, Reynolds II CF, Jennings JR, et al: Diminished nocturnal penile tumescence in depression: a replication study. *Biol Psychiatry* 31:1136–1142, 1992.

36. Steiger A, Holsboer F, Benkert O: Studies of nocturnal penile tumescence and sleep electroencephalogram in patients with major depression and in normal controls. *Acta Psychiatr Scand* 87:358–363, 1993.

37. Nofzinger EA, Thase ME, Reynolds III CF, et al: Sexual function in depressed men. *Arch Gen Psychiatry* 50:24–30, 1993.

38. Johanović UJ: Sexuelle Reaktionen und Schlafperiodik bei Menschen. Ergebnisse experimenteller Untersuchungen. *Beitr Sexualforsch* 51:1, 1972.

39. Johanović UJ: Der Effekt der ersten Untersuchungsnacht auf die Erektionen im Schlaf. *Psychother Psychosom* 17:295, 1969.

40. Fisher C, Schiavi RC, Edwards A, et al: Evaluation of nocturnal penile tumescence in the differential diagnosis of sexual impotence. *Arch Gen Psychiatry* 36:431–437, 1979.

41. Levine LA, Carroll RA: Nocturnal penile tumescence and rigidity in men without complaints of erectile dysfunction using a new quantitative analysis software. *J Urol* 152:1103–1107, 1994.

42. Karacan I, Goodenough DR, Shapiro A, et al: Erection cycle during sleep in relation to dream anxiety. *Arch Gen Psychiatry* 15:183–189, 1966.

43. Fisher C, Schiavi R, Lear H, et al: The assessment of nocturnal REM erection in the differential diagnosis of sexual impotence. *J Sex Marital Therapy* 1:277–289, 1975.

44. Kowalski A, Stanley RO, Dennerstien L: The sexual side-effects of antidepressant medication: a double-blind comparison of two antidepressants in a non-psychiatric population. *Br J Psychiatry* 147:413–418, 1985.

45. Rosen RC, Kostis JB, Jekelis A, et al: Sexual sequelae of antihypertensive drugs: treatment effects on self-report and physiological measures in middle-aged male hypertensives. *Arch Sex Behav* 23:135–152, 1994.

46. Karacan I, Hirshkowitz M, Howell J, et al: Smoking more than a pack-per-day has a worsening effect on impotence. *Sleep Res* 17:287, 1988.

47. Schiavi RC, Stimmel BB, Mandeli J, et al: Chronic alcoholism and male sexual function. *Am J Psychiatry* 152:1045–1051, 1995.

48. Hirshkowitz M, Karacan I, Howell JW, et al: Nocturnal penile tumescence in cigarette smokers with erectile dysfunction. *Urology* 39:101–107, 1992.

49. Elist J, Jarman WD, Edson M: Evaluating medical treatment of impotence. *Urology* 23:374–375, 1984.

50. Kwan M, Greenleaf WJ, Mann J, et al: The nature of androgen action on male sexuality: a combined laboratory-self-report study on hypogonadal men. *J Clin Endocrinol Metab* 57:557–562, 1983.

51. O'Carroll RE, Shapiro C, Bancroft J: Androgens, behaviour and nocturnal erection in hypogonadal men: the effects of varying the replacement dose. *Clin Endocrinol* 23:527–538, 1985.

52. Burris AS, Banks SM, Carter S, et al: A long-term, prospective study of the physiologic

and behavioral effects of hormone replacement in untreated hypogonadal men. *J Androl* 13:297–304, 1992.

53. Carani C, Bancroft J, Granata A, et al: Testosterone and erectile function, nocturnal penile tumescence and rigidity, and erectile response to visual erotic stimuli in hypogonadal and eugonadal men. *Psychoneuroend* 17:647–654, 1992.

54. Weiss HD: The physiology of human penile erection. *Ann Intern Med* 76:793, 1972.

55. Condra M, Morales A, Surridge DH, et al: The unreliability of nocturnal penile tumescence recording as an outcome measurement in the treatment of organic impotence. *J Urol* 135:280–282, 1986.

56. Wincze JP, Bansal S, Malhotra C, et al: A comparison of nocturnal penile tumescence and penile response to erotic stimulation during waking states in comprehensively diagnosed groups of males experiencing erectile difficulties. *Arch Sex Behav* 17:333–348, 1988.

57. Brindley GS, Polkey CE, Rushton DN, et al: Sacral anterior root stimulators for bladder control in paraplegia: the first 50 cases. *J Neurol Neurosurg Psychiatry* 49:1104–1114, 1986.

58. Rushton DN: Sexual and sphincter dysfunction. In Bradley WG, Daroff RB, Fenichel GM, et al (eds): *Neurology in Clinical Practice*. Boston, Butterworth-Heinemann, 1991, pp 389–390.

59. Shvartzman P: The role of nocturnal penile tumescence and rigidity monitoring in the evaluation of impotence. *J Fam Pract* 39:279–282, 1994.

60. Allen RP, Brendler CB: Nocturnal penile tumescence prediction response to intracorporeal pharmacological erection testing. *J Urol* 140:518–522, 1988.

61. Buvat J, Buvat-Herbaut M, Lemaire A, et al: Recent developments in the clinical assessment and diagnosis of erectile dysfunction. *Ann Rev Sex Res* 1:265–308, 1990.

62. Allen RP, Engel RM, Smolev JK, et al: Comparison of duplex ultrasonography and nocturnal penile tumescence in evaluation of impotence. *J Urol* 151:1525–1529, 1994.

63. Marshall P, McGrath P, Schillinger J: Importance of electromyographic data in interpreting nocturnal penile tumescence. *Urology* 22:153–156, 1983.

64. Barry JM, Blank B, Boileau M: Nocturnal penile tumescence monitoring with stamps. *Urology* 15:171–172, 1980.

65. Marshall P, Earls C, Morales A, et al: Nocturnal penile tumescence recording with stamps: a validity study. *J Urol* 128:946–947, 1982.

66. Marshall P, Morales A, Phillips P, et al: Nocturnal penile tumescence with stamps: a comparative study under sleep laboratory conditions. *J Urol* 130:83–89, 1983.

67. Ek A, Bradley WE, Krane RJ: Nocturnal penile rigidity measured by the Snap-Gauge band. *J Urol* 129:964–966, 1983.

68. Condra M, Fenemore J, Reis K, et al: Screening assessment of penile tumescence and rigidity. *Urology* 29:254–257, 1987.

69. Ellis DF, Doghramji K, Bagley D: Snap-gauge band versus penile rigidity in impotence assessment. *J Urol* 140:61–63, 1988.

70. Allen J, Ellis DL, Carroll JL, et al: Snap-gauge band versus multidisciplinary evaluation in impotence assessment. *Urology* 34:197–199, 1989.

71. Allen R, Brendler CB: Snap-gauge compared to a full nocturnal penile tumescence study for evaluation of patients with erectile impotence. *J Urol* 143:51–54, 1990.

72. Bradley WE: New techniques in evaluation of impotence. *Urology* 29:383–388, 1987.

73. Bradley WE, Timm GW, Gallagher JM, et al: New method for continuous measurement of nocturnal penile tumescence and rigidity. *Urology* 26:4–9, 1985.

74. RigiScan ambulatory rigidity and tumescence system. Document no. 750-156-0486, Dacomed Corporation, Minneapolis, Minnesota, 1986.

75. Bain CL, Guay AT: Reproducibility in monitoring nocturnal penile tumescence and rigidity. *J Urol* 148:811–814, 1992.

76. Kaneko S, Bradley W: Evaluation of erectile dysfunction with continuous monitoring of penile rigidity. *J Urol* 136:1026–1029, 1986.

77. Van Nueten J, Verheyden B, Van Camp K: Role of penile nocturnal tumescence and rigidity measurement in the diagnosis of erectile impotence. *Eur Urol* 22:119–122, 1992.

78. Sohn MH, Seeger U, Sikora R, et al: Criteria for examiner-independent nocturnal penile tumescence and rigidity monitoring (NPTR): correlations to invasive diagnostic methods. *Int J Impot Res* 5:59–68, 1993.

79. Allen RP, Smolev JK, Engel RM, et al: Comparison of RigiScan and formal nocturnal penile tumescence testing in the evaluation of erectile rigidity. *J Urol* 149:1265–1268, 1993.

80. Licht MR, Lewis RW, Wollan PC, et al: Comparison of RigiScan and sleep laboratory nocturnal penile tumescence in the diagnosis of organic impotence. *J Urol* 154:1740–1743, 1995.

81. Gordon CM, Carey MP: Penile tumescence monitoring during morning naps: a pilot investigation of a cost-effective alternative to full night sleep studies in the assessment of male erectile disorder. *Behav Res Ther* 31:503–506, 1993.

82. Gordon CM, Carey MP: Penile tumescence monitoring during morning naps to assess male erectile functioning: an initial study of healthy men of varied ages. *Arch Sex Behav* 24:291–307, 1995.

83. Morales A, Condra M, Heaton JPW, et al: Diurnal penile tumescence recording in the etiological diagnosis of erectile dysfunction. *J Urol* 152:1111–1114, 1994

84. Djamilian M, Stief CG, Hartmann U, et al: Predictive value of real-time RigiScan monitoring for the etiology of organogenic impotence. *J Urol* 149:1269–1271, 1993.

85. Ogrinc FG, Linet OI: Evaluation of real-time RigiScan monitoring in pharmacological erection. *J Urol* 154:1356–1359, 1995.

5

Psychological Evaluation and Sex Therapy

Stephen B. Levine
Stanley E. Althof

When urologists evaluate and manage erectile dysfunction, they are inescapably thrust into the domain usually occupied by the mental health professional. This domain is filled with a type of complexity—emotion, meaning, secrets, conflicting motivation, and paradox—for which well-trained urologists are unprepared. The urologist's situation is similar to that of mental health professionals who deal with impotence (the traditional, but currently out-of-favor term for erectile dysfunction).[1] These psychiatrists and psychologists are not well prepared to grasp the content of the other 13 chapters of this book. In the past, each specialty has avoided the uncertainties of the other's realm by declaring "Ninety percent of erectile dysfunction is a disease of the penis . . . or in the head!" Each declaration was based on the fundamentally erroneous either organic/or psychogenic assumption.[2]

This chapter presents five topics: (*1*) the mental health professional's evaluation; (*2*) the pathogenesis of acquired and lifelong psychogenic erectile dysfunction; (*3*) how to refer for psychological evaluation and therapy; (*4*) psychology of treating organic dysfunction; (*5*) the factors that mitigate against urologic solutions.

THE MENTAL HEALTH PROFESSIONAL'S EVALUATION

After the psychological and urologic evaluation, the patient's erectile problem should be classifiable into either an organic, psychogenic, mixed, or idiopathic category and the specific etiologic factors should be enumerated. This is accomplished by integrating three groups of data: the pattern of the erections; the social and psychological events preceding the onset of the symptom; the urologic and laboratory findings. The steps of the clinical process—evaluation, diagnostic grouping, etiologic specification, and treatment—are taken in that order. Both the urologist and the mental health professional are necessary to fully appreciate a particular man's clinical complexity.

74

Diagnosis of Psychogenic Erectile Dysfunction

Erectile Pattern

The patient is placed in the psychogenic category when the clinician recognizes that the man's neural, vascular, and endocrine capacities to generate adequate erections are intact. Selective erectile dysfunction is its diagnostic hallmark. Despite the fact that the man cannot initiate or maintain reliable erections with a partner, he consistently does so under other circumstances. Stand-up, rigid, lasting erections when intercourse is not being attempted usually alert clinicians that the patient belongs in this generic category. These adequate erections occur during the night or early mornings, during kissing or petting behaviors, during masturbation, with certain partners, in response to magazines or videos, or spontaneously. To prevent a miscategorization, the clinician looks for an inconstant physical factor, such as intermittent substance abuse or medication use, that might explain the selective pattern. Lacking this, the diagnosis of psychogenic erectile dysfunction typically jumps out at the doctor.

The diagnosis is easiest to make in young men because their drive, ease of arousal, and degree of responsiveness to erotic stimuli are great. Its recognition becomes more difficult during mid-life because sexual neurophysiology becomes less efficient. Erections are more easily suppressed in mid-life by the emotional states that accompany relationship problems, vocational stresses and disappointments, concerns over children, and financial dangers.

The frequency, duration, and fullness of nocturnal erections are significantly impaired by depression.[3] Therefore, the clinician must be careful not to use erection patterns alone when making this diagnosis in a middle-aged man who is experiencing social and psychological misery. The clinician judiciously weighs the infrequently adequate erection against the man's emotional state.

Considerations of men's emotional circumstances are even more important in patients over 55 yr of age. In this age group, psychogenic erectile dysfunction may be present despite the fact that no adequate erections have been detected for many months. Pure organic cavernosal insufficiency is the most common misdiagnosis in men over 60. When much has changed in the man's life before the onset of the erectile problem, the mental health professional does not readily rule out an important psychogenic factor.

Social History

The *Diagnostic and Statistical Manual-IV (DSM-IV)*, the official psychiatric nosology, asks the clinician to make a vital distinction between acquired and lifelong forms of the disorder.[4] Acquired erectile dysfunction—that is, impotence that occurs after a long period of successful intercourse—is the far more prevalent variety.[5] The social changes that typically precede acquired impotence involve: relationship alienation; divorce; death of a spouse; vocational or financial failure; loss of personal or spousal health. Each of these set of circumstances triggers impotence by eliciting feelings and conflicts that resurface when intercourse is attempted.

Men with lifelong erectile dysfunction usually have social histories that lack such antecedent life events. Since potency has never been securely present and the patient is often younger, the mental health of professional's attention is drawn to developmental matters such as sexual identity, general personality functioning, and psychiatric diagnoses. Occasionally a young man who has failed on his first several intercourse attempts is seen in consultation. Although strictly speaking he has lifelong erectile dysfunction, what follows about lifelong erectile dysfunction does *not* apply to him. In contrast, those who have been unable to erect with a partner for many years and whose potency was only briefly intact are basically similar to men with lifelong erectile dysfunction.

Specifying the Psychological Disorder

After making the lifelong versus acquired distinction, the mental health professional seeks to further explain the symptom. The doctor reaches a tentative history-based hypothesis about the psychological dilemma the patient is struggling with — widower's impotence, marital discord, homosexuality, depression, pedophilia, transvestism, etc.

Medical History and Laboratory Findings

The urologist quickly becomes aware of the man's medical history, his physical examination findings, and the results of routine and selected laboratory evaluation. The absence of findings in this realm can be helpful in recognizing psychogenic erectile dysfunction when the pattern of erections is ambiguous, the antecedent evidents are not striking, and the patient and the therapist need to know the etiology within a short time period. When other elements in the evaluation, however, strongly point to a psychogenic diagnosis, expensive or invasive tests should be undertaken with caution, since the interpretation of their results is often uncertain. Ideally, the laboratory tests are entirely normal.

Diagnosis of Organic Erectile Dysfunction

Erectile Pattern

The mental health professional's suspicion of organic impotence is raised by a history of a consistent erection deficit. Variations in erection attainment in terms of the degree of enlargement, capacity to be upright, duration, and rigidity are common within this deficit. Despite the variation, the penis may never be full, rigid, erect, or last more than a brief time. The best erections tend to occur upon awakening. Adequacy of erections tends to decrease in this order: middle of night or morning; masturbation; foreplay; intercourse. However, in a classic or extreme organic impotence, the erection deficit is the same under all circumstances. The patterns are often obtained by asking the patient to numerically rate his erections. For instance, if a full, lasting, stand-up erection is designated 10, a typical organic pattern may look like this: mornings—6; masturbation—4 to 6; foreplay—3 to 4; intercourse—0 to 3. The variations probably in part reflect the influence of anxiety about obtaining and maintaining the erection.

Performance Anxiety

Performance anxiety is observable among all men regardless of etiologic categories. It has two faces: the anticipation of erectile failure before sex begins and the vigilant preoccupation with monitoring the state of tumescence during it.[6] Rather than giving himself over to the pleasures of touching and being touched, he thinks about how adequate his erection is or will be.

The anticipation and dread of the loss of erection is highly destructive; it precludes arousal by substituting anxiety and inattention to sensation. In men with organic impotence, this almost inescapable mental process adds another deficit to the one brought about by the erection-impairing disease. Performance anxiety causes men to go through the motions of lovemaking, instead of participating in a relaxed sensual manner. This is the basis of the statements: all organic impotence has at least some psychologic causation, and performance anxiety is the final common pathway of all erectile dysfunction.

Several mysteries about organic erectile patterns merit emphasis. Many men with organic deficit patterns for long periods of time occasionally have a firm lasting morning erection. This leaves the clinician wondering whether the patient has psychogenic erectile dysfunction. The limitations of our understanding of pathophysiology of erection come into play. It is not known whether the neural pathways for the noctural erections are physiologically distinct from that which mediates erections during sexual behavior. If it is possible that organic pathophysiology in early and moderate stages is overridden by nocturnal psychic stimulation, the absence of a nocturnal erection may signify the most severe or advanced organic pathology.

The variations in the pattern of erections found among the organically impaired may be accounted for by three medical facts: (1) Organic impotence is caused by a large number of diseases with pathophysiologies that are distinct from one another—for example, multiple sclerosis subverts erections in the spinal cord by blocking neurotransmission, whereas antihypertensive agents interfere with brain and peripheral neural mechanisms. (2) The same diseases vary in severity from patient to patient—for example atherosclerosis can cause erections to hover between 0 and 2 if there are extensive blockages of aortoiliac-hypogastric arterial flow, or it can account for erections of 7 or 8 if fewer less extensive lesions are present. (3) The same disease may impair potency through multiple mechanisms. Diabetes, for instance, may lead to the loss of nerve fibers in the penis, the loss of neurotransmitter mechanisms for vasodilation of the sinusoids, and a decrement of desire and arousal from poor metabolic control and renal disease.

Social History

In easy-to-diagnose organic impotence, nothing dramatic has changed prior to or along with the decrements in erectile functioning. A wife's affair, a job loss, a child's drug abuse, an unhappy relationship affair, depression—the types of histories that are often obtained from men with acquired psychogenic erectile dysfunction are *not* obtained among these men. The patient *and* his partner testify that life is fine but his erections are not.

Diagnosis of Idiopathic Erectile Dysfunction

When the clinician cannot identify the cause of a patient's erectile problem with reasonable certainty, the case is classified as idiopathic. Time often reveals the true diagnosis, e.g., a pelvic malignancy, marital deterioration, secreted homosexuality. Some idiopathic impotence is simply an artifact of not including the partner in the evaluation process. Wives can provide clinicians with clarifying information about their husband's social and psychological state so that the correct diagnosis can be made. Even after thorough evaluations, however, there are cases in which the clinician does not know the cause.

Progress has been made in clarifying some previously enigmatic cases—so-called impotence of aging. The original observations that aging men's erections are slower to form, not as rigid, and shorter lasting have been epidemiologically confirmed and described in terms of degrees of impotence.[7] Using the sleep laboratory, psychometric, and clinical evaluations of happily married, extremely physically healthy men, Masters and Johnson's 1970 observations about the gradual decline in physiologic capacities between 55 and 74 yr of age were confirmed.

A crucial observation was made during this work: men with the same physiologic decrements were found among the impotent and the potent. This directs clinicians to the complexities of the sexual equilibrium, the interaction of sexual characteristics and attitudes that are hypothesized to determine the quality of sexual behaviors.[8] It is possible that some idiopathically impotent men develop sufficient performance anxiety to undermine their potency in response to their own perception of erectile decline or their partner's comments about their erections. The partner may respond to the man's worries by avoiding lovemaking and quietly retiring from sex. She may do this to prevent his humiliation or because she is happy to stop having sex with him. The woman at this phase of life often has her own arousal difficulties which adds to the man's inability to obtain and maintain arousal—the emotional key to any waking erection.

Erectile dysfunction is further generated by the decline in sexual drive that is usually conspicuously apparent by the late fifties. Because the man is not as often and as intensely aroused spontaneously or in response to lovemaking, he can comfortably refrain from sexual behavior for longer periods of time than earlier in his life. The decline in drive and erectability summate. These decrements are biogenic, although not necessarily the result of disease other than aging. The decline in drive is thought to be brain-based, the decline in potency penile-based, but changes in the mediators between the brain and penis are also likely to be contributory.

These nuances are difficult to perceive during the initial evaluation. Even after the couple is seen over an extended period of time, the situation may be missed. Clinicians need to guard against the mistake of assuming a case is organic when it is, in fact, idiopathic.

When idiopathic impotence occurs in a man younger than early fifties, the clinician needs to worry about hidden organic and psychogenic factors. Much idiopathic impotence may turn out to be mixed impotence because it combines a definite, though inconstant physiologic decline with a subtle, fluctuating psychological factor, which at different times derives from performance anxiety, female arousal inefficiencies, and emotions about social changes.

PATHOGENESIS OF PSYCHOGENIC ERECTILE DYSFUNCTION

A Metaphor

Urologists consider psychogenic erectile dysfunction to be one disease. Mental health professionals do not have the luxury of this illusion. Pure psychogenic erectile dysfunction is merely a symptom of some underlying enigma. Although the enigmas vary, the essence of most cases can be captured by a metaphor. The symptom is a message from his brain to his body not to cooperate with intercourse for some good reason. The reason is a partial mystery to the man because he cannot allow himself to believe that his dilemma affects his potency.

Etiologic Contributions from Three Time Periods

Psychogenic erectile dysfunction is usually generated by the resonating interaction of emotional forces from three time periods: the *present*, the *recent past*, and *childhood*. Performance anxiety, the factor in the *present*, distracts the man from other feelings he may be having about making love in general or to his particular partner. The recently impotent man typically does not appreciate the significance of the life changes from the *recent past*. He is either unsure of the personal meaning of these changes, denies the meaning, or can not link the meaning to his potency problem. Rather, he emphasizes his new lack of sexual confidence (a frequent phase for performance anxiety) as the cause of his problem; he remains befuddled about how he fell into its pernicious trap. The trap, however, diminishes the frequency of lovemaking to protect him and his partner from disappointment and the reexperiencing of performance anxiety.

Demystifying the psychogenic problem often requires understanding that intercourse acquires meanings from nonsexual experiences during earlier life. Therapists tend to describe these meanings in varying jargoned ways: failed tasks of psychological development, impairments in sexual identity, vulnerabilities of the self-system, oedipal issues, abuse, social learning difficulties, pregenital fixations, and transference. Whatever jargon therapists prefer, the words refer to *childhood developmental processes*.

The etiologic concept of resonation of forces from three time spheres provides a scheme for understanding both generic varieties of psychogenic erectile dysfunction.[9] A scheme is only a skeletal outline of the process of symptom generation and maintenance. The mental health professional's work is to add the flesh by noting the extent of performance anxiety, pinpointing the precipitating events, and defining their emotional meanings. This is also how therapy is done.

The Usual Precipitants of Acquired Psychogenic Erectile Dysfunction

New erectile dysfunction arises under diverse social and psychological circumstances, but these seem irrelevant because all the afflicted men clearly suffer from performance anxiety. This anxiety, which usually begins after one or two erectile failures, obscures from their view the fact that they have other thoughts and feelings that interfere with arousal. These reactions stem from the recent changes in his social situation and their reverberation with past developmental experiences. Making love creates a confrontation with his private emotional truths and performance anxiety helps him avoid focusing on them. Men are vulnerable to psychogenic impotence to the degree to which: they expect to be able to perform sexually regardless of social circumstances; they are unable to quickly experience and understand their emotions. The recurring precipitants of acquired psychogenic erection dysfunction will now be discussed.

Relationship Deterioration

The self-declaration of impotence in the face of alienation, mutual hostility, lack of psychological intimacy, and partner unreceptivity is a testimony to the man's expectation that his penis ought to be able to function under any conditions. Such optimism is not warranted even though the shocked man may emphasize that in his last marriage he was able to have intercourse when divorcing. It is reasonable for the clinician to presume that such a man's impotence involves some of the following: resentment; loneliness; confusion about who is correct about the couple's unresolved differences; guilt over his role in their troubles; reaction to his partner's unreceptivity and anger; fear of abandonment; helplessness to end their downward spiral.

Divorce

Many divorcing and divorced men are surprised by their unreliable erections. Initially, they cannot relate their bitterness, guilt, or fear of future attachment to their erection problem. They, too, expect their penises to operate autonomously. It is reasonable for the clinician to presume that such a man's impotence involves some of the following: love for his wife; fear of his rage at women; doubt about his lovability; doubt about his ability to love; despair over his children's pain and alienation; wariness that the new partner will eventually turn into an impossible person as his wife did; guilt over his dishonesty with new partners.

Death of Spouse

Most widowers are at least in their 50s. Their feelings about resuming a sexual life with a new partner are influenced by many factors, such as the duration and quality of the marriage, the cause of their wives' deaths, their own health. Many of these men have been through slow deaths from cancer, and began mourning well before the actual event. Because there are many partners available to physically healthy widowers, many men use dating as a distraction from being home alone and other inevitably difficult aspects of grief. It is reasonable for the clinician to presume that the impotence of recent widowers involves some of the following: unresolved grief; guilt about impulses to have multiple partners; sense that he belongs only to his wife; confusion about his new freedom; discomfort about his children's and friends' reactions to his dating and the specific women he dates.

Vocational Failure

Vocational adequacy is central to most men's identity and self-esteem. Vocational failure or threatened vocational failure creates feelings of despair, uncertainty, anxiety, unworthiness, and guilt, which may be most apparent when he attempts to make love. "I don't feel worthy of her any longer," may lurk behind the recent impotence of men with employment problems.

Loss of Personal or Spousal Health

Psychogenic potency problems are common after major health events, such as myocardial infarction, open heart surgery, stroke, or cancer. Fear of death during sexual activity or a heightened awareness of the recent close call may be most apparent to the man during lovemaking. The partner's reactions to the man's illness and new health status may not be completely worked through, and can create a subtle sexual unreceptivity that triggers erectile failure and performance anxiety. This is a two-way system: the deterioration of the partner's health may also lead to erectile impairment because of his new perceptions of his partner.

Usual Causes of Lifelong Psychogenic Erectile Dysfunction

Probably between 95% and 99% of men who desire to have intercourse do so by the time they are 30 yr old. Among those who repeatedly fail, immediate antecedent life events do not seem to play a major role in the pathogenesis. While performance anxiety is usually very much in evidence, the key elements of pathogenesis derive from remote developmental processes that leave the male intensely frightened of, or genuinely uninterested in, intercourse. The causes of the problem are related to those factors that explain the man's private sense of inadequacy and his strong, inarticulate fears of closeness to a woman. These powerful issues generate an emotional state that either precludes arousal entirely or overwhelms the physiologic impact of arousal.

Among some men with lifelong erectile dysfunction, intercourse is possible when certain unusual conditions of fantasy or behavior are met. These conditions typically involve meeting unconventional sexual identity needs, such as being partially dressed in women's attire or having a fantasy of being with a man. When conducting an evaluation of a man with (nearly) lifelong impotence, the mental health profession will give careful consideration to each of the three components of sexual identity—gender identity, orientation, and intention. Clinicians will not be surprised when, after initial denials, the patient reveals an unconventional eroticism involving his sense of inadequate masculinity and/or femininity, homosexuality or bisexuality, or unconventional behavioral requirements such as exhibitionism, voyeurism, pedophilia, or sadomasochism. Some of these men present themselves as having no sexual desire. Careful history taking reveals that most have adequate sexual drive since they masturbate regularly; they simply possess a strong motivation to avoid sexual behavior with a partner.

Unlike acquired erectile dysfunction in which there is no necessary relationship between a *DSM-IV* diagnosis and the problem, lifelong erectile dysfunction is often associated with a diagnosable major condition. Most of these conditions are Axis II diagnoses, such as obsessive-compulsive, schizoid, or borderline personality; some, however, have a significant Axis I problem, such as depression, psychosis, or anxiety disorder. The recurring associated mental situations among those with lifelong psychogenic erection dysfunction will now be discussed.

Gender Identity Problems

This is the least common of the sexual identity difficulties that lurk behind lifelong inability to have intercourse. Most of these men are transvestites. They acknowledge having recurrent fantasies of being a woman, cross-dressing in private, discovering that their potency is assured by wearing a female garment during lovemaking, or thinking that their partner's breasts and vagina are their own.

Homoeroticism

This is the most common source of lifelong impotence in many settings. Many men who have responded with arousal to male bodies and repeatedly masturbated to male images cannot calmly make the transition from their homoeroticism to a heterosexual identity and life style. Some of them attempt a heterosexual relationship and fail at intercourse, seemingly because the motivational aspects of their sexual desire are lacking. They may never have revealed their homoeroticism to their partners and often will not spontaneously reveal it to the clinician. Their performance anxiety seems to grow when they cannot sustain arousal during lovemaking. Homosexual men can also have psychogenic impotence with male partners if their conflicts about sexual expression with males are largely unresolved, but this is far less frequently encountered than homoerotic men trying to participate in marital sexual behavior.

Paraphilia

Men with longstanding, highly arousing, unusual erotic fantasies that are associated with a compulsion to masturbate or act out with a partner usually have some impairment of conventional heterosexual function as well.[10] This impairment is most often manifested as an avoidance of lovemaking, but is also commonly involves impotence or inability to ejaculate in the vagina. The presence of the paraphilia usually must be elicited from the patient by careful questioning.

Abuse History

Heterosexual potency requires two capacities: to be aroused by a woman and to be able to neutralize the ordinary fear and nervousness about entering her body. Sexual identity problems limit the capacity to respond to women with arousal. When those with serious sexual identity problems are excluded, however, a large group of men who cannot neutralize their anxiety about lovemaking remain. These young men transfer feelings toward their parents or other earlier significant attachments to their partner because of the unconscious assumption that she will hurt him just as "they" did. The hurt may have been the result of egregious psychological abandonment, beatings, sexual abuse, or prolonged overly close relationships with their mothers. The patient's problem indicates that he is pessimistic about finding anyone who is trustworthy enough to share his bodily experience with him.

HOW TO REFER FOR PSYCHOLOGICAL EVALUATION AND THERAPY

Patients with psychogenic and mixed erectile dysfunction are the usual ones who should be considered for referral. The doctor's diagnosis that his erectile dysfunction is significantly contributed to by psychological factors should be delivered as news that may carry a positive prognosis. To the patient, the diagnosis of psychogenic erectile dysfunction initially means that the problem is "just in my head, it is not physical." To the psychotherapist, the symptom usually means the man does not feel safe in emotionally attaching to another person. The therapist is safe in assuming that the symptom is the patient's way of resolving a hidden drama between his wishes for sexual intercourse and his fears about the consequences of emotional attachment. A man may not want a referral to a mental health professional because he is dimly aware of this complexity and he is embarrassed to acknowledge that he is unable to manage the complexity on his own. Therapy needs to provide the patient with dignity, understanding, the opportunity to feel, and the chance to become better acquainted with how his mind operates. Therapy gives the man a chance to find a less burdensome, more direct manner of expressing his private feelings about himself and his situation. Referrals to a mental health professional from a urologist or primary care physician are facilitated if the doctor has some understanding of the above, personally knows the mental health professional, and offers hope. Six months of regular therapy is a minimal duration before declaring it unsuccessful and moving to another intervention. A follow-up visit at this time with the referring physician, therefore, is useful. If, however, the recently psychogenic impotent patient does not want a referral to a mental health professional, the urologist may suggest sensate focus exercises to him. These are essentially the instruction to make love four consecutive times without trying, no matter what happens, to have intercourse.[11] This often removes performance anxiety and enables some recently impotent men to recover.

Once a referral is made, the patient will either be in an individual or conjoint format. Conjoint therapy can be efficient and effective for impotence that is heavily derived from recent interpersonal conflicts in faithful couples. Conjoint therapy can prevent symptom resolution, however, when the man needs to discuss his sexual identity, inadequate sense of self, persistent desires for other partners, or childhood experiences that have left him deceitful, distrusting, and wary of closeness. Conjoint therapy is also not wise when the clinician has reason to believe that honesty will not be possible. Currently or recently unfaithful husbands should not be seen in conjoint therapies unless the infidelity is discussed because keeping such a secret from the partner is another betrayal of her.

Results for Lifelong Erectile Dysfunction

There is no reason to be optimistic about the ability of psychotherapy to create potency among those with long established lifelong erectile dysfunction. While some men are helped to establish a capacity for regular intercourse, this is far more likely to occur in heterosexual men in their twenties than in older men with significant feminine preoccupations or whose private orientation is almost exclusively homoerotic. Despite this low rate of success for lifelong erection problems, psychotherapy may help in other ways such as coming to grips with one's sexual identity and living more honestly. In already established couples, it may lead to better nonsexual relationships and in those who persist in individual therapy, improvements may occur in life function at work and in nonsexual relationships. Despite the optimism of early sex therapists, lifelong erection problems during conventional sexual intercourse are far more likely to persist than to be cured. This is because therapy seems unable to increase the man's motivation for intercourse. And this is the same reason why injections, for example, often fail—because the man does not have the motivation to consistently use them.

Results for Acquired Erectile Dysfunction

Not only are there published data to suggest that psychotherapists can be successful in a large percentage of cases,[12-14] but also a large body of clinical experience. Here, too, however, success depends on the recognition of and skill in dealing with the antecedent life events and their childhood reverberations—for example, helping a widower with his grief *and* his memories of his mother's sudden death during his adolescence. Prognosis is poor when the patient can not generate sexual desire for the partner.[15] The therapist needs to distinguish between the patient's genuine deep personal motive to bring his body to his partner from more superficial statements that, "of course, I want to have intercourse." Removing performance anxiety, helping to resolve an interpersonal conflict or a personal dilemma sometimes dramatically allows a genuine motivation to take over. Therapists generally do not have the capacity to generate the motivation to make love when the man no longer wants to remain with his partner.

Psychology of the Organic Erectile Dysfunction

The degree of performance anxiety depends on men's age, the importance of intercourse to their relationships, and the personal meaning of intercourse to them. Some elderly happily married men who have lost their potency long after their sexual drives have diminished seek consultation. Their wives are not complaining about the loss of intercourse. The man is seeing the urologist because he would prefer to have intercourse. He knows that many of his age mates are unable. Intercourse capacity has been lost but the man no longer is bothered by internal urges that demand an orgasm and neither is his partner. He generally only is interested in a pill without harmful side effects.

Younger men rarely display such equanimity. They suffer from their own subjective sense of masculine inadequacy. If their partners are pressuring them to have intercourse or threaten to end the relationship without it, their performance anxiety is quite high. If they perceive that their supportive loving wives miss the opportunity for intercourse but will not say so, they may feel guilty about their avoidance even though they cannot bring themselves to try to have intercourse. The sense of disgrace may reach dramatic proportions. Single men who perceive a world of women waiting for them may be eager to take one of the treatment options. Urologists soon learn, however, that not every organically impaired men, even young or middle-aged ones, is eager to use one of the highly efficacious treatments. Thus, even when the diagnosis is clearly organic, the treatment of patients must take into account psychological and social factors.

By the time the patient is evaluated, he has already demonstrated to himself that he can survive his lack of potency. Although he may feel badly about his erectile insufficiency, this does not necessarily mean that he now has deep motivation to resume the act. Or, if this is true, it does not necessarily mean that he is willing to place this at a high enough priority to take the time and spend the money to resume intercourse. This is often initially shocking to the physician because the patient has taken the time to seek consultation, can be helped, and yet, enigmatically, does not accept any but the least likely to help options.

FACTORS THAT MITIGATE AGAINST UROLOGIC SOLUTIONS

The Ideal Candidate for a Urologic Intervention

The ideal candidate has three characteristics: (1) a long history of good erectile function; (2) relatively recent—approximately less than 2 yr—garden variety organic dysfunction due to increasing fibrosis of the corporal smooth musculature; (3) regularly making love with his partner using his hands, mouth, vibrator, or limp penis. This history indicates that the woman is receptive, the man actually highly values sexual behavior, and neither has significant sexual inhibitions. It is merely up to the doctor to explain the options and let them choose and then support them with technical training and information. While cavernosal fibrosis is likely to be the most common organic etiology, many men will not meet or demonstrate these characteristics.

Complicating Psychosocial Factors

Low Sexual Motivation

The following psychosocial complexities—patient deceit, self-deception, and partner deception—may manifest low sexual desire. Sexual drive may or may not be present, but what is consistently lacking is the man's willingness to bring his body to his partner for sexual behavior. Because he is unwilling, his erections falter. He focuses on the unreliable erection and not the underlying circumstance that prevents erections.

Patient Deceit

What men say they want—that is, intercourse with their wife—is not always correct. Some men want to tell their wives that they have been to the doctor and that the physician suggests a workup or a treatment that the wife and he agree is unreasonable. He may not tell the doctor that is potent with another partner, female or male, particularly if the doctor does not ask. And he may not tell the doctor that he is only potent when he dresses in woman's clothing or has a bizarre fantasy or can have his wife dress up in a special way. While a mental health professional is more likely to elicit such a history, we, too, do not always elicit the truth.

Self-deception

Some men will tell themselves that they avoid sex because erections are no longer dependable. They will not admit to themselves that they possess little motivation to make love with their partners. They may be visiting the urologist to be potent so that he can delay visiting a divorce lawyer or before they give up entirely on the aspiration to make love with their partner. All recommendations from the urologist are refused.

Partner Deception

Some wives blame the lack of sex on the man's impotence when it is their lack of motivation to have sex that has initially created the erectile dysfunction. The wife may be having an affair of which he is unaware or he may know it but is too ashamed to admit it to the doctor.

General Psychological Barriers to Urologic Treatments

Bodily Integrity

The urologist's behavior should indicate to the patient that he is aware of the ordinary human need to maintain bodily integrity. The penis is a beloved organ and the idea of injecting it, or incising it for a prosthesis is initially unthinkable to almost everyone. The doctor's initial reassurances are often insufficient to quell anxiety about penile damage. It has to be repeated over time.

Aesthetic Barrier

The urologist also needs to be sensitive to the fact that there is an aesthetic aspect to intercourse and that the idea of the treatments may take some getting used to for both partners. "I don't want to stick my penis in that cylinder!" Aesthetic repulsion is often mixed up with the more accessible fear of pain, injury, or long-term complication. Some men think or say, "Call me when you have an effective pill, doctor!" To counter these problems, the urologist and staff need to acknowledge them specifically so that the patient knows that the doctor knows what he is experiencing.

Barriers to Relating to Errors in the Doctor–Patient Relationship Physicians may inadvertently behave in ways that interfere with patients' trust:

Insensitivity to the Patient's Subjective Experience. Some of our errors involve inattention to the subjective experience of consulting a doctor about impotence. We are accused of not appreciating how difficult it is to tell us about the problem. We fail to indicate to the man that we are aware of the inherent "abnormality" and attendant embarrassment of attaining an injection-erection on the examination table, particularly if a nurse or another physician is in the room. Jokes are dangerous because when we joke about impotence or the future good erections, the man takes the clue and laughs, but may be offended.

Oversimplifying Sexual Complexity. Other errors relate to our remarks that indicate to patients that all we think is involved in sex is a hard erection. Many men by their late 50s have long been aware that sex is always imbedded in relationship complexities. When we quickly reassure them that they will be fine with this treatment, particularly without asking them about the wife's alienation and disinterest in being a sexual partner, we announce our naiveté to them.

Rushed consultation with incomplete discussion of the options. Some errors relate to our rush. We provide incomplete or unbalanced presentations of the therapy options. By now journalists have repeatedly brought information about the treatments to the public via newspapers, magazines, and television programs. When a urologist seems to favor one treatment, quickly dismisses another without explaining the reasons why it would not be best for him, fails to mention an option, or schedules the next step without suggesting that the man and his partner think about this to formulate questions, the polite patient may not return. Some men have heard exaggerated stories about the treatments—severe pain, reoperations, ineffective, nodule formation—so the urologist or the urologic nurse has to be able to calmly discuss the side effect profiles of each approach. Costs, initially and over time, also need to be brought to the patient's awareness. Some of this can be accomplished or reinforced by written or other media material, but the doctor must be able to speak about it and listen to the man and his partner's concerns. In most clinical situations, the doctor recommends, and the patient decides after deliberation. Impulsive decision making by the patient should alert the doctor to consider slowing down the process somewhat, particularly when an implant is the treatment the patient impulsively chooses. The urologist needs to protect himself from unsatisfied patients, some of whom may become litigious if their potency is not significantly improved and they experience physical or emotional hardship.

Of course, none of these barriers are insurmountable, even though no urologist will be able to overcome every man's private objections to proceeding with mechanical treatment of his erectile dysfunction. This clinical reality is a long way from the common marketing ploy, "virtually every man can be helped with this problem."

REFERENCES

1. NIH Consensus Conference: Impotence. *JAMA* 270(1):83–90, 1993.
2. Althof SE, Seftel AD: The evaluation and management of erectile dysfunction. *Psychiatr Clin North Am* 18(1):177–192, 1995.
3. Thase ME, Reynolds CF, Glanz LM, et al: Nocturnal penile tumescence in depressed men. *Am J Psych* 144:89–92, 1987.
4. American Psychiatric Association: *DSM-IV*. Washington, DC, American Psychiatric Press, 1994.
5. Feldman HA, Goldstein I, Hatzichristou DG, et al: Impotence and its medical and psychosocial correlates: results of the Massachusetts aging study. *J Urol* 151:54, 1994.
6. Masters WH, Johnson V: *Human Sexual Inadequacy*. Boston, Little Brown, 1970.
7. Schiavi R, Schreiner-Engel P, Mandeli J, et al: Healthy aging and male sexual function. *Am J Psychiatry* 147(6):766–771, 1990.
8. Levine SB: *Sexual Life: A Clinician's Guide*. New York, Plenum, 1992, Chapter 4, The Sexual Equilibrium.

9. Levine SB: *Sexual Life: A Clinician's Guide.* New York, Plenum, New York, 1992, Chapter 10, Erection Problems.

10. Levine SB, Risen CB, Althof SE: An essay on the diagnosis and nature of paraphilia. *J Sex Marital Ther* 6(2):89–102, 1990.

11. Hunter J: *Treatise on Venereal Disease.* London, Mr G Nicol and Mr J Johnson, 1788, pp 203–204.

12. Kilmann PR, Milan RJ, Boland JP, et al: Group treatment for secondary erectile dysfunction. *J Sex Marital Ther* 13(3):168–182, 1987.

13. Hawton K, Catalan J, Martin P, et al: Long-term outcome of sex therapy. *Behav Res Ther* 24(6):665–675, 1986.

14. Hawton, K, Catalan J, Fagg J: Sex therapy for erectile dysfunction: characteristics of couples, treatment outcome, and prognostic factors. *Arch Sex Behav* 21(2):161–175, 1992.

15. Mohr DC, Beutler LE: Erectile dysfunction: a review of diagnostic and treatment procedures. *Clin Psychol Rev* 10:123–150, 1990.

6

Noninvasive Arterial Evaluation of the Patient Complaining of Erectile Dysfunction with Color Duplex Doppler Ultrasound

Gregory A. Broderick

INTRODUCTION: ERECTILE DYSFUNCTION, PREVALENCE, AND ASSOCIATION WITH AGING

A conservative estimate of the number of men in the United States suffering with complete erectile dysfunction is 10–20 million; when partial erectile dysfunction is included, the estimate jumps to 30 million.[1] Long before current appreciation of medical risk factors, clinical studies documented a relationship with age and male sexual dysfunction. Age-specific prevalence of erectile dysfunction is estimated to be 5% at age 40 increasing to 15–25% by age 65. The ratio of organic to psychological dysfunction also varies with age: 70% of patients under 35 yr of age having a psychogenic etiology, and 85% of men over 50 yr of age having organic impotence.[2] Patient accounts of coital frequency reveal a similar age trend: 75% of men in their seventh decade reporting coitus once monthly and 37% of patients 61–65 yr old describing weekly coitus. Only recently has normative community-based data become available.[3] The Massachusetts Male Aging Study (MMAS) assessed the prevalence of impotence among 1,290 men ranging in age from 40 to 70 yr. Men rated their potency on a four-point scale: not impotent, minimally impotent, moderately impotent, and completely impotent. A complaint of impotence was offered by 51% of men. Diabetes, hypertension, and coronary artery disease were each associated with increased probability of impotence complaints; these risks were amplified by concurrent smoking. Complete impotence was most prevalent among men taking medications: hypoglycemics, antihypertensives, vasodilators, and cardiac drugs.

Urologists can usually direct patients toward therapy with the information from a good sexual history, medical history, physical examination, and basic blood tests.

When diagnostic testing is indicated or desired, the penile blood flow study (PBFS) which consists of an intracavernous challenge of a vasoactive agent and assessment by color duplex Doppler ultrasound (CDDU) is the most reliable and least invasive means of specifying vascular erectile dysfunction. Furthermore, PBFS/CDDU efficiently selects patients who are candidates for more invasive testing.[4–7] The history, principles, and techniques of CDDU are reviewed as are the most recent criteria for distinguishing arterial insufficiency from cavernous venous occlusive disease, high-flow from low-flow priapism, and for preoperative staging of Peyronie's disease. CDDU provides a detailed examination of the vascular anatomy of the penis and elucidates the dynamics of erection.

INVESTIGATING PENILE BLOOD FLOW

Numerous diagnostic tests have been employed to evaluate penile hemodynamics: penile plethysmography, penile blood pressures, penile brachial index, duplex Doppler sonography, dynamic infusion cavernosometry/cavernosography, nuclear washout radiography, and color duplex Doppler ultrasound. In 1971 Gaskell devised one of the first noninvasive assessments of penile arterial inflow. He used a photometer to quantify the absorption of light by the pigment oxyhemoglobin in the glans penis. An occlusive cuff at the base of the penis was slowly loosened; the pressure at which oxyhemoglobin became measurable in the glans was assumed to reflect the penile systolic blood pressure.[8] Unfortunately flow to the glans is primarily supplied by the dorsal arteries, which may not share the same degree of pathology as the cavernous arteries. Abelson used the Doppler stethoscope to measure penile blood pressure in flaccidity, comparing this value to systolic brachial pressure: the penile-brachial index (maximal systolic penile pressure divided by systolic brachial artery pressure = PBI).[9] Michal and Goldstein modified the PBI test with a dynamic component by adding lower extremity and pelvic musculature exercises, with Doppler stethoscope auscultation made before and after exercise.[10,11] A decrease in the ratio of penile systolic pressure (<0.15) was indicative of pelvic steal, or significant penile inflow disease. Subsequent reviews comparing the PBI to pharmaco-penileangiography found PBI values from normal patients overlapped with those from impotent patients. Technically the PBI was subject to the same source of error as Gaskell's photometer: pressures were inadvertently obtained from the dorsal artery not reflecting the central cavernous inflows.[12]

Arteriography has been the gold standard of vascular investigations. Accurate penile angiography requires pharmacologically induced erection as the vessels of the flaccid shaft are contracted and tortuous. High-osmolality contrast agents are painful, may induce anaphylaxis, and may require intravenous sedative-anesthesia. Some centers use epidural or spinal anesthesia to reduce vasospasm.[13,14] Low-osmolality contrast agents limit angiographic morbidity (pain and allergy) but are more expensive.

Indisputably arteriography provides the best anatomic information about the origin of the common penile arteries, but this data has been difficult to correlate with patient complaints and with erection dynamics.[15] The common penile artery typically arises from the third segment of the internal pudendal artery (IPA) as it passes through the urogenital diaphragm. The paired common penile arteries generally arise from the ipsilateral IPA but may originate from one internal pudendal artery, or from an accessory internal pudendal artery. The accessory IPA may take origin from the hypogastric artery, remnant of the umbilical, ischial, or obturator arteries. An accessory IPA is more common on the right, but prevalence has been variably described from 4% to 70%. Performing selective internal pudendal arteriography (missing an accessory IPA) has an inherent false-positive rate for diagnosing penile inflow disease.[14,16–19] More importantly, deviations from paired common penile arteries have been documented in 50% of normally potent volunteers; unilateral absence or hypoplasia of a dorsal artery has been shown in up to 30% of volunteers.[13] Anatomic variation of penile arterial anatomy appears to be the rule rather than the exception: with unilateral or bilateral origin of the cavernous arteries, distal shaft communications between the dorsal and central cavernous arteries, and anastomosis between the corpus spongiosum and cavernous body.[20] The problem for the arteriographer has been twofold: differentiating congenital variations in penile arterial anatomy from acquired abnormalities and correlating anatomic alterations in the pattern of vascular inflow with the complaints of impotence. For the patient there remains the discomfort of the intra-arterial contrast, exposure to ionizing radiation, risk of minor or severe dye reaction, and potential for endothelial cell and smooth muscle damage following ionic contrast agents. As screening test phalloarteriography is overly invasive and unfortunately nonspecific of penile hemodynamics.[21]

PENILE BLOOD FLOW STUDY

In 1982, during the course of vascular reconstructive surgery Ronald Virag noted that infusion of papaverine into the hypogastric artery produced erection.[22] In 1983 a dramatic demonstration of the efficacy of penile self-injection was offered by Charles Brindley, who subsequently popularized the use of alpha-blockers (phenoxybenzamine and phentolamine) and intracorporal injection.[23,24] Zorgniotti and Lefleur promoted penile injection therapy with the drug combination: papaverine/phentolamine.[25] In 1986 Ishi published the first clinical series of prostaglandin E_1 (PGE_1) treated patients.[26,27] Many clinicians have subsequently turned to the benefits of combination therapy: exploiting the individual pharmaco-relaxing properties of different agents, reducing the pain associated with PGE_1 reducing the risk of corporal fibrosis and hepatic dysfunction associated with papaverine, and minimizing the cost and volume of penile injections. Bennett et al in 1991 first described the clinical efficacy of trimix: papaverine, phentolamine, and PGE_1[28] in July 1995 Upjohn Company (Kalamazoo, Michigan) received Food and Drug Administration approval to market injectable PGE_1 (Caverject) specifically for the diagnosis and treatment of male impotence. The demonstration that vasoactive injections could produce penile erection without benefit of psychic or tactile stimuli revolutionized the diagnosis and treatment of erectile dysfunction by providing a direct test of end organ integrity and therapy specifically for vascular deficiency.

A penile blood flow study (PBFS) consists of an intracavernous injection and an observer's visual rating of the consequent erection; the test is the most commonly used diagnostic procedure for impotence. PBFS is simple, minimally invasive, and performed without monitoring equipment. A positive injection test in a neurologically normal patient implies psychogenic impotence, presumably excluding significant venous or arterial insufficiency.[29,30] All too often the penile response is suboptimal, leaving the clinician questioning: "Does my patient have severe arterial insufficiency, venous leakage, or high anxiety?" A standard intracavernous test dosage has never been established for any agent. Furthermore, a contemporary hemodynamic investigation suggests that a positive injection test is associated with normal veno-occlusion (low flow to maintain erection values of 0.5 to 3 ml per minute during cavernosometry and minimal contrast or no contrast leakage during cavernosography), but not necessarily with normal arterial function. In as many as 19% of patients the test may be a false negative. Despite the presence of an erection there may be a significant disparity between the systemic and cavernous systolic arterial pressures. A normal PBFS then indicates meeting or exceeding a threshold response for intracavernous pressure (≥ 80 mm Hg) which may occur in the presence of a significant gradient between systemic systolic pressure and cavernous systolic pressure. A positive injection test only selects patients for home injection therapy; it does not rule out mild arterial insufficiency.[31] In 1985 Lue and Hricak introduced the technique of high-resolution sonography and quantitative Doppler spectrum analysis to document changes in cavernous arterial flow after intracorporal injection of papaverine.[32]

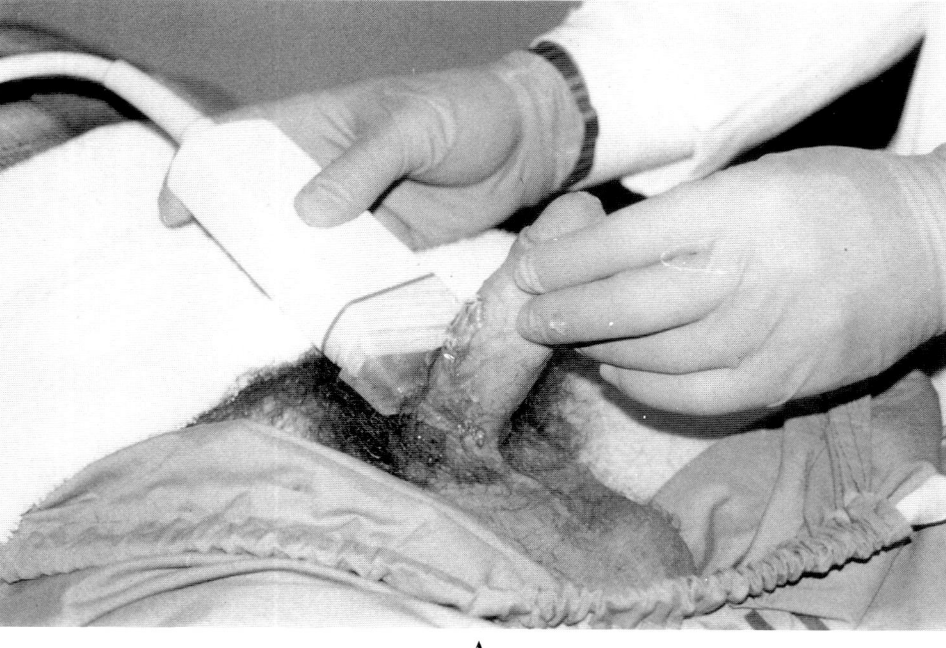

A

Fig. 6.1. A: The penis is held in the anatomic position of erection with the scanning probe in the transverse position. **B:** Transverse color Doppler image following a 6-µg injection of PGE_1 reveals the normal vascular anatomy. RCA = right cavernous artery; LCA = left cavernous artery; DDV = deep dorsal vein; LDA = left dorsal artery; CS = corpus spongiosum. **C:** Sagittal image 5 min after injection of dilator. Right dorsal artery (RDA), RCA, LCA. Central sinusoids beginning to fill (*arrows*). Note blood-distended sinusoids appear more hypoechoic than surrounding tissue.

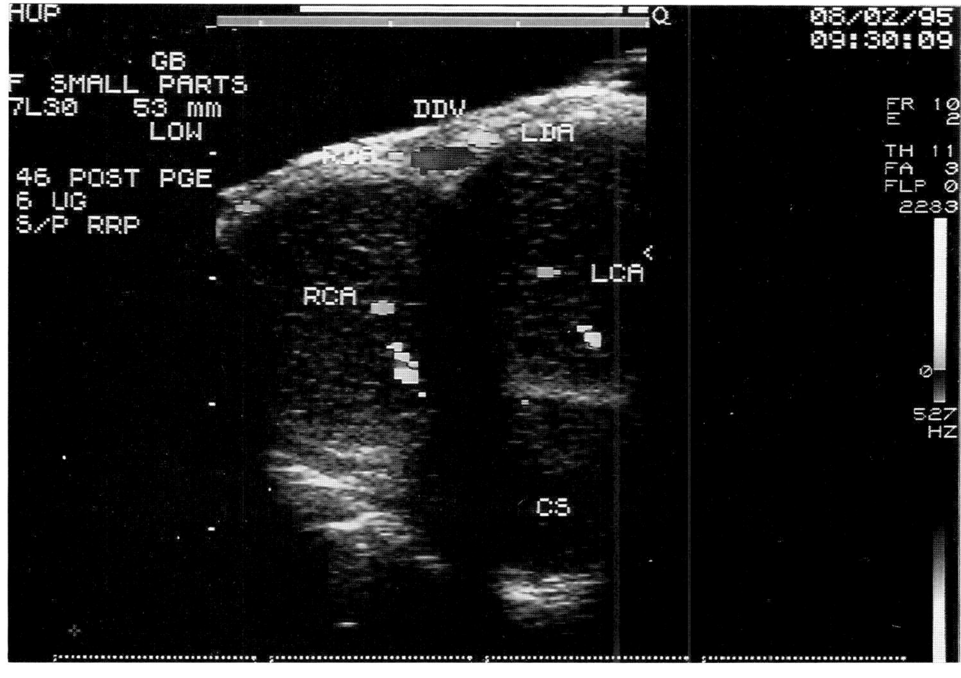

B

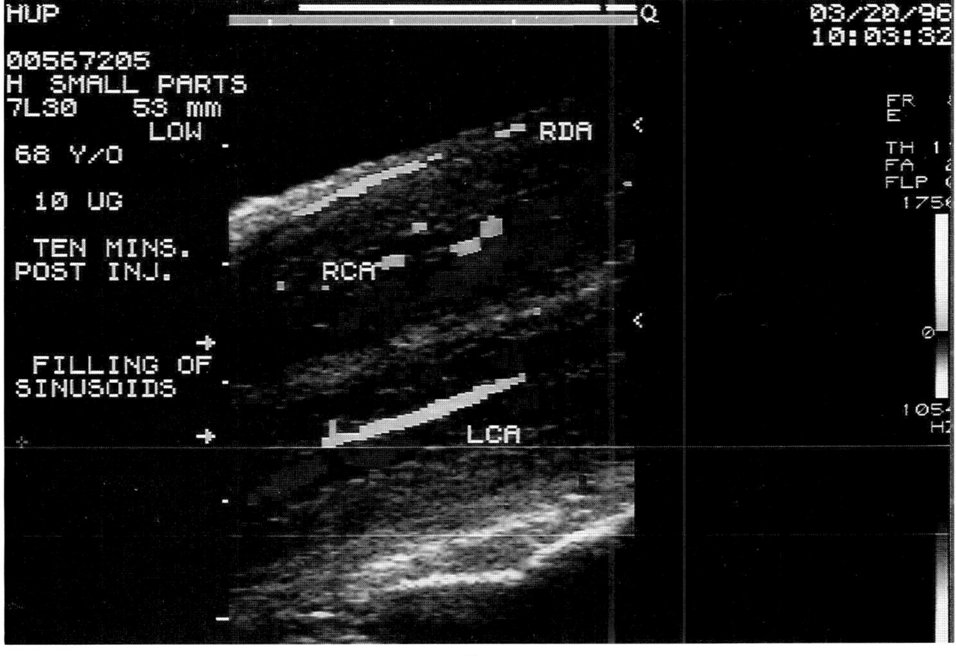

C

Fig. 6.1—Continued

CDDU ANATOMY

The human penis consists of three corpora: the paired corpora cavernosa and the ventral corpus spongiosum, which forms the glans penis distally. The cavernous bodies share a fenestrated septum, permitting them to neurophysiologically function or pharmacologically respond as a single unit. The tunica albuginea of the corpora cavernosa has a thickness of 2–3 mm in the flaccid state. The tunica albuginea of the corpus spongiosum is much thinner. Each of the corporeal bodies is surrounded by a dense fascial structure, Buck's fascia. With real-time ultrasound the corpus cavernosum and spongiosum have a homogeneous medium echogenicity which is distinguished from the hyperechoic tunica albuginea and septum (Fig. 6.1). The normal tunica albuginea has a uniform thickness and echogenicity; the subcutaneous tissues and Buck's fascia are not identifiable sonographically except by the location of the dorsal vascular bundle: paired dorsal arteries (DA) and deep dorsal vein complex (DDV) (Figs. 6.1B, 6.2B). The proximal penis (crural bodies) is anchored to inferior pubis. The penile bulb is surrounded by the bulbocavernosus (or bulbospongiosus) muscle. The crura and proximal part of the shaft are covered by the ischiocavernosus muscles. Whereas the pendulous penis is easily imaged from either the dorsal (Figs. 6.1 and 6.2) or ventral projection, the proximal third of the penis may be imaged in transverse or sagittal view but only by scanning from the ventral penis above or below the scrotum. The urethral lumen will be compressed, but can be imaged by retrograde filling with sterile gel or water.[33,34] The glans penis is covered with very thin and firmly adherent skin, has no fibrous sheath, and contains much connective tissue.

PENILE INFLOW

The penis is supplied mainly by the internal pudendal artery; after giving off the perineal artery in Alcock's canal, it becomes the common penile artery. Branches of the penile artery consist of the bulbar, urethral (spongiosal), dorsal, and cavernous arteries. The cavernous artery penetrates the tunica albuginea and enters the crura of the corpora cavernosa along with the cavernous veins and cavernous nerves. The cavernous arteries are easily identified by their echogenic walls; in the flaccid state the arteries are tortuous and ≤0.5 mm in diameter. Although with CDDU low blood flows of the flaccid penis are visible, cavernous flows preceding injection of vasodilator depend on the patient's sympathetic tone (anxiety) and are of no predictive value.[4,35] Cavernosal tissue is spongelike and composed of a meshwork of interconnected cavernosal spaces, which are lined by vascular endothelium and separated by trabeculae, containing bundles of smooth muscle in a framework of collagen, elastin, and fibroblasts. The terminal helicine arteries are multiple, muscular and corkscrew-shaped arteries (150–350 μm) that open directly into the cavernous spaces and act like resistance arteries (Fig. 6.3). The corporal tissue becomes more hypoechoic (darker) as the sinusoids distend with blood, making the echogenic walls of the cavernous arteries more obvious sonographically (Fig. 6.1C). The dorsal artery enters the penis and continues distally beneath Buck's fascia between the centrally located deep dorsal vein(s) and the paired dorsal nerves. The urethral

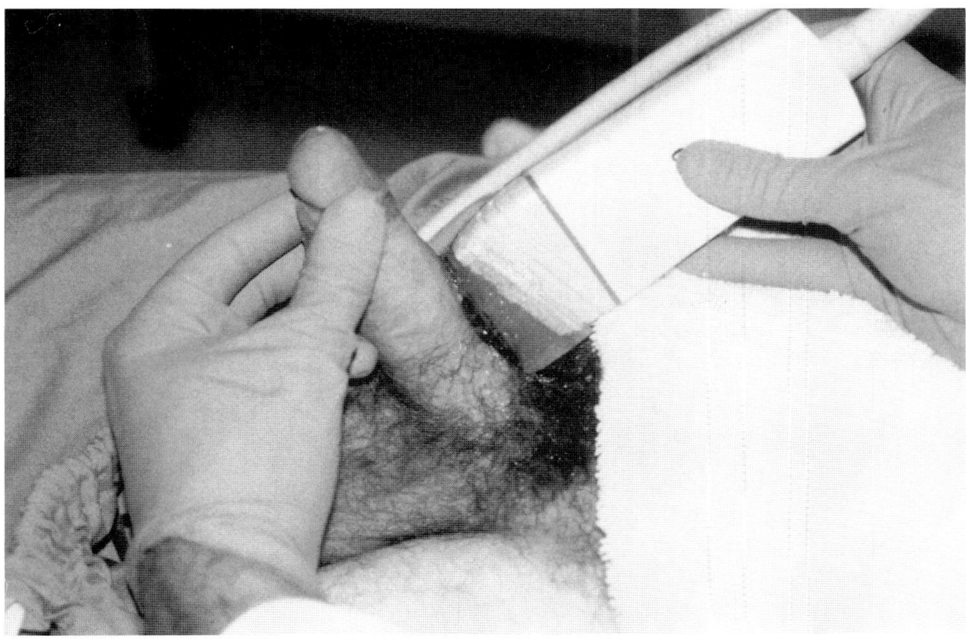

A

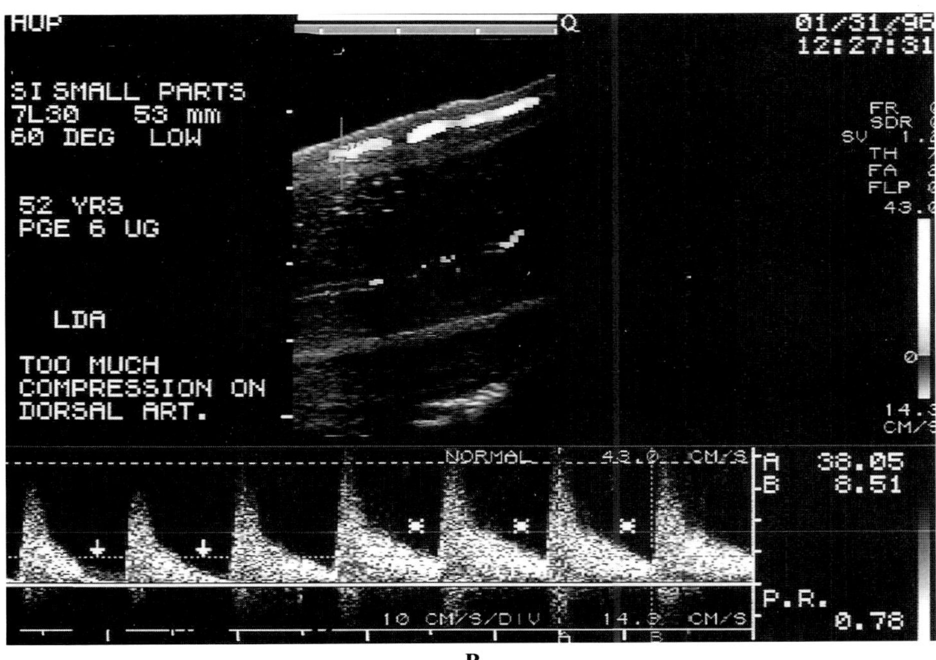

B

Fig. 6.2. A: Probe held in the sagittal position from the dorsum. Note cushion of ultrasound gel between stand-off wedge of transducer and penile shaft. **B**: Sagittal view of right dorsal artery (RDA); too much compression (*arrows*) dampens dorsal vascular flow and will alter both systolic and diastolic waveforms.

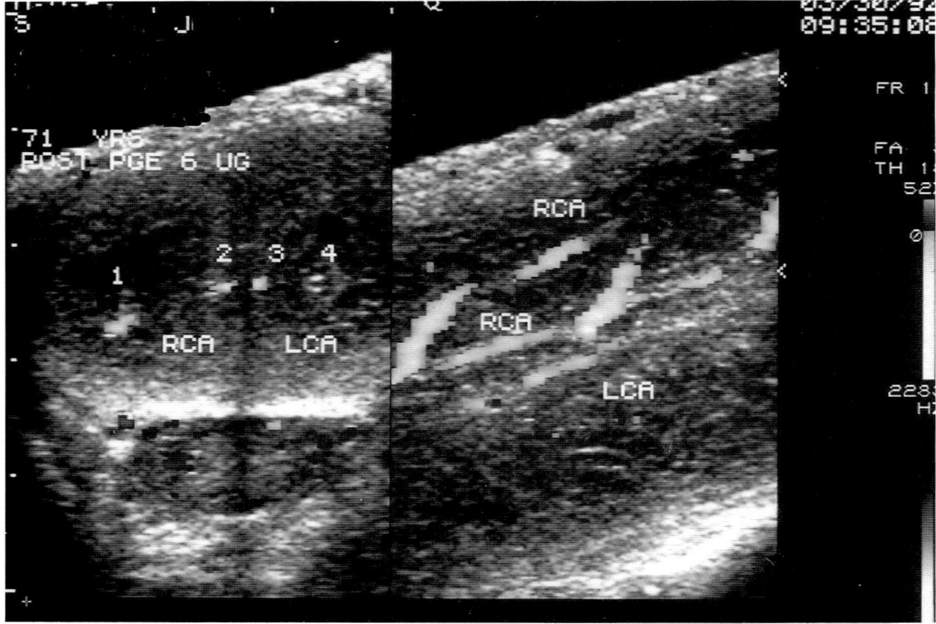

Fig. 6.3. Transverse and sagittal images of central cavernous arteries and branching helicine arterioles.

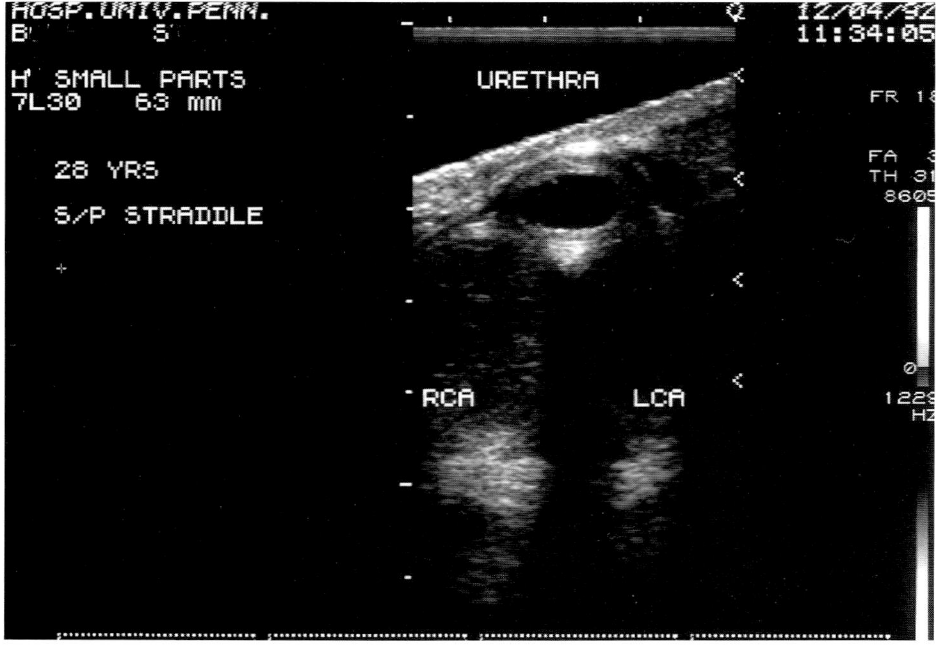

Fig. 6.4. The pendulous penis may be scanned from the ventral aspect. This transverse image shows the proximal bulb. Imaging of the urethral lumen is possible when the urethra is filled in a retrograde fashion with gel or water.

artery runs longitudinally through the corpus spongiosum lateral to the urethra (Fig. 6.4). This supplies corpus spongiosum, the urethral tissue, and the glans penis. The bulbar artery enters the bulb of the penis shortly after its origin. Recently described anatomic variations of penile arterial supply include dorsal to cavernous, cavernous to cavernous, and cavernous to urethral collaterals, duplication of the cavernous artery, and unilateral absence of a dorsal artery.[13]

PENILE OUTFLOW

Based on scanning electronic microscopy of vascular corrosion casts, Banya et al suggested two circulatory routes in the human corpora.[36] One route goes from the cavernous artery to capillary networks collected into the venular plexus just beneath the tunica albuginea; this is suggested to serve as a main circulatory pathway during the flaccid state. The other route is through the cavernous artery, to the helicine arteries to the cavernae (sinusoids), which are then emptied into the postcavernous venules. This ultrastructural detail is not visualized sonographically.

The deep venous system drains both the corpora cavernosa and the corpus spongiosum. The postcavernous venules coalesce to form larger emissary veins that pierce the tunica albuginea. The emissary veins of the middle and distal penis join to form the circumflex veins, which empty into the deep dorsal vein. Both the emissary and circumflex veins have valves. The short emissary veins of the proximal penis form the cavernous vein, which empties into the internal pudendal vein (Fig. 6.5).

The intermediate set of veins is deep to Buck's fascia. Veins from the glans penis form a retrocoronal plexus that drains into the deep dorsal vein. The deep dorsal vein courses proximal in the midline between the two corpora cavernosa and empties into the periprostatic plexus. The superficial dorsal vein drains the skin and the subcutaneous tissue superficial to Buck's fascia, draining into the superficial external pudendal vein.

ERECTION HEMODYNAMICS

Erection is a complex event regulated by the tone of smooth muscle composing the cavernous arterioles, venules, and sinusoids. Tumescence follows a decrease in corporal smooth muscle tension: decreasing arterial, arteriolar, and sinusoidal resistance. Decreasing resistance to arterial inflow bathes the cavernous tissues in highly oxygenated arterial blood. Venous outflow during erection is dynamically limited by distention of the sinusoids compressing the subtunical venular plexus against the inner layer of the tunica albuginea. The differential stretching of the two primary layers of the tunica albuginea during erection scissors closed the exiting emissary veins. The rigid penis is veno-occluded, in a low-outflow state, with distended sinusoids and elevated intracorporal pressure. During rigid erection, arterial inflows are paradoxically very low: by Doppler estimation 1.5–5.6 ml per minute, by phalloarteriography 4.7 ml per minute, by radioisotope study <5 ml per minute. Dynamic cavernosometry similarly reveals that with maximal smooth muscle relaxation rigid erection is associated with low flow to maintain values of 0.5–3 ml per

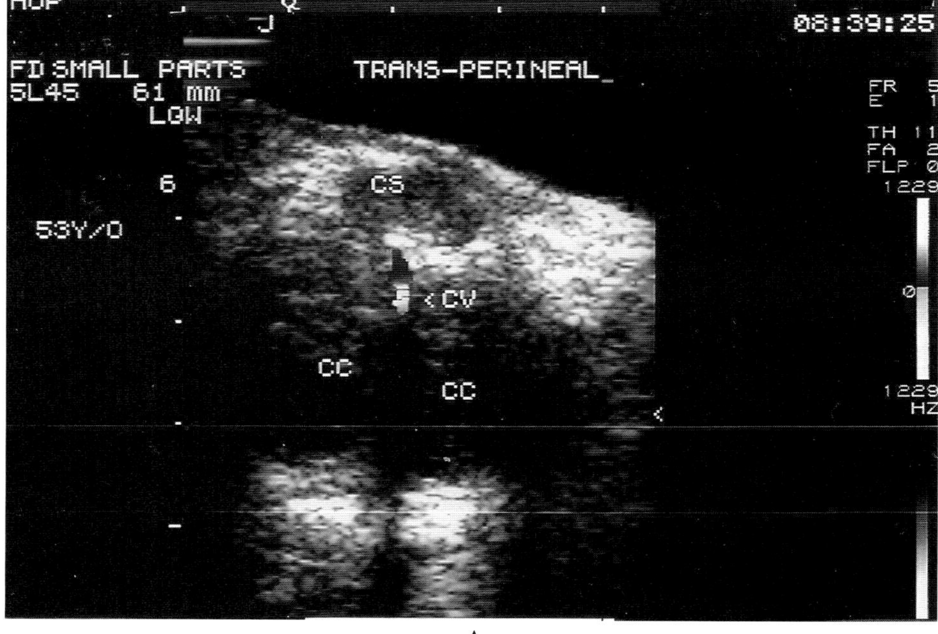

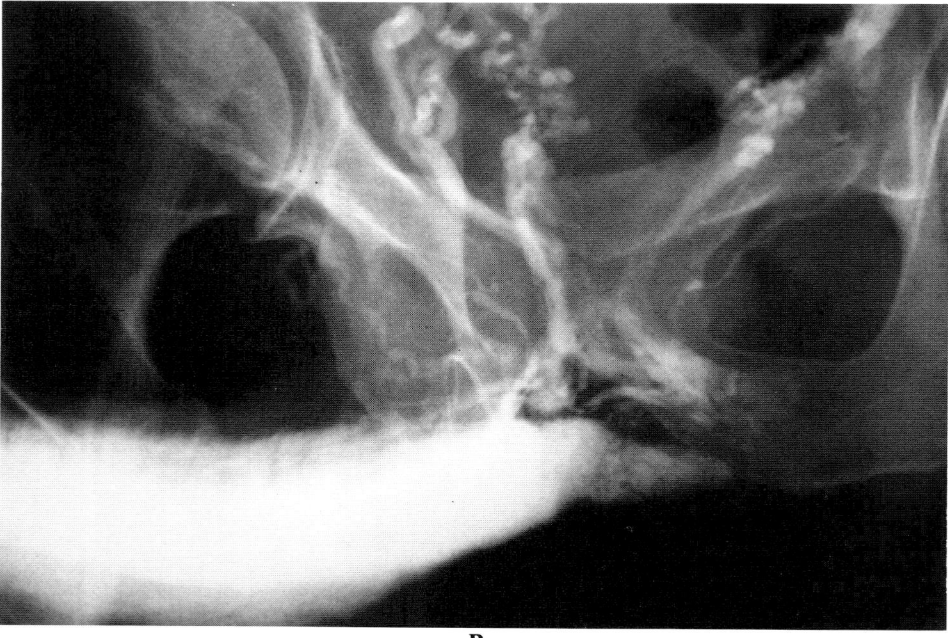

Fig. 6.5. A: Transverse sagittal scan of patient with severe veno-occlusive dysfunction revealing large cavernous vein. CS = corpus spongiosum; CV = cavernous vein; CC = corpus cavernosum. **B**: Dynamic cavernosogram of the same patient showing leakage via the cavernous and crural veins.

minute.[31,32,37] Detumescence and flaccidity are initiated and maintained by corporal smooth muscle contraction.

Lue and Wagner having studied the dynamics of erection in several species and have divided the progress from flaccidity to erection into distinct phases.[38,39] In the flaccid phase there is a dominant sympathetic influence. Electrical activity recorded from the smooth muscle of the corpus cavernosum indicates that the smooth muscle cells are contracting. In the latent or filling phase parasympathetic nervous activity dominates; there is increased blood flow through the internal pudendal and cavernous arteries. Peripheral resistance is decreased due to dilatation of the cavernosal and helicine arteries. The penis elongates. In the tumescence phase the intracavernous pressure increases rapidly. The compliance of the sinusoidal muscle is markedly enhanced, causing penile engorgement. In full erection the relaxed trabecular muscle expands and, together with the increased blood volume, compresses the plexus of subtunical venules, reducing venous outflow, increasing intracavernous pressure to within 10–20 mm Hg systemic systolic blood pressure. In the rigid erection phase cavernous pressure may increase well above the systolic pressure. As a consequence of voluntary or reflexogenic contraction of the ischiocavernosus and bulbocavernosus muscles suprasystolic pressures may be transiently achieved during pelvic thrusting.

These separate phases of erection documented in the laboratory in animals do have correlates with human erectile responses during PBFS (Fig. 6.6). There are many more variables in clinical testing, the first of which is the patient's pathology; arterial or venous insufficiency will preclude full erection. Secondly the threshold dosage for a single agent or multiple agents to reliably promote complete smooth muscle relaxation has never been established. Data on the minimal effective dosage of PGE_1 suggests 2 µg will produce erection in 38% of men with psychogenic impotence and 20% of men with vasculogenic erectile dysfunction.[40] In most diagnostic testing at least 10 µg of PGE_1 or 60 mg of papaverine is administered. Patterns of spectral waveform progression on CDDU have been correlated with a normal rigid response during PBFS.[4,41] Figure 6.6 is a composite of the phases of erection illustrated in the physiology laboratories of Lue and Wagner and the Doppler waveforms likely to be identified by the examiner during this idealized schema of progressive rigidity.[38,39,41] In the flaccid state arteriolar resistance is high; if flow is visualized only systolic flow will be evident and likely be < 15 cm/sec (phase 1, spectral waveform A). In the early filling phase arteriolar and sinusoidal resistance is decreasing (phase 2, spectral waveform B); both antegrade systolic and diastolic flow will be evident. When sinusoidal resistance is at its lowest (5–10 min) following penile injection the waveform is characterized by high forward flow during systole and diastole (phase 3, spectral waveform C). As intrapenile pressure increases, diastolic velocities decrease, with full erection the systolic waveforms will sharply peak and may be slightly less than during full tumescence; diastolic flow will be zero (phase 4, spectral waveform D). In rigid erection (phase 5, spectral waveform E) cavernous pressure will exceed systemic diastolic blood pressure and reversal of diastolic flow occurs. Similarly in the rigid erection phase the systolic waveform may be dampened. With climax sympathetic tone predominates, the arteriolar and sinusoidal muscles recoil. Because of falling intracavernous pressures pudendal arterial inflow transiently increases in the experimental model (phase 6), before intrinsic cavernous arterial resistance lowers cavernous inflow to basal flaccid levels. The

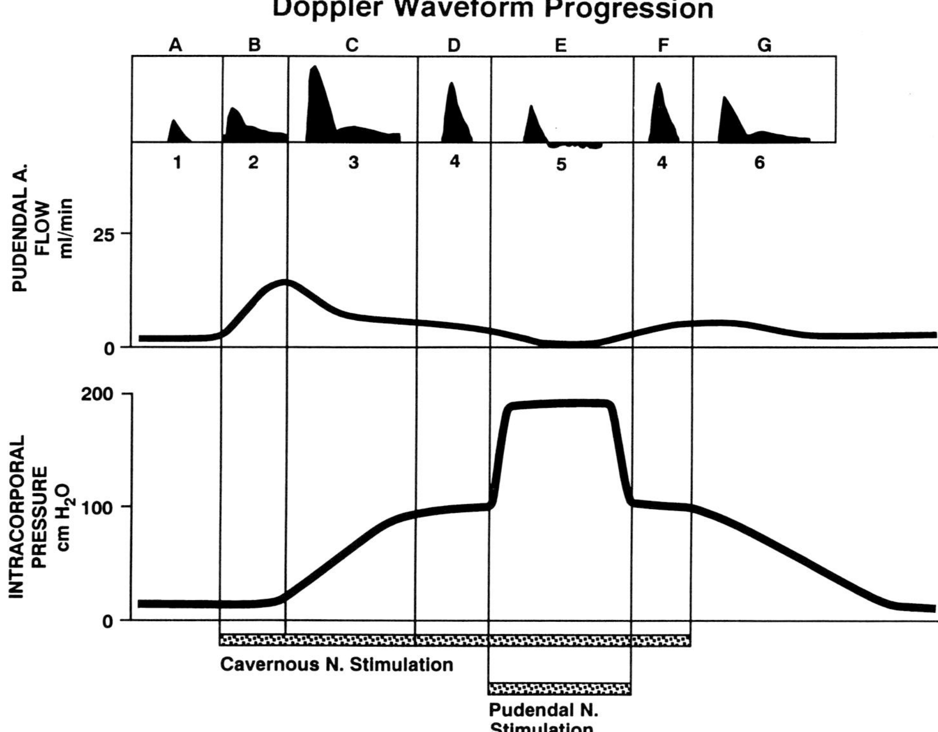

Fig. 6.6. Phases of Penile Erection. Modified and reproduced with permission from reference 38.

examiner should be familiar with each of these waveforms, and remember that in patients with arterial insufficiency progression may be arrested at waveform B (PSV < 25 cm/sec). Because of cavernous venous occlusive disease the progression may be arrested at waveform C or transiently advance through waveform D and then directly on to waveform G.

TECHNIQUE: INSTRUMENTS

Since its introduction by Lue in 1985, duplex Doppler penile sonography has proven to be an accurate and reproducible technique for evaluating erectile dysfunction. With the initial gray scale imaging of duplex sonography, study quality was highly dependent on the skill of the examiner. Vessel localization within the corporal tissue was difficult and dorsal vessel imaging all but impossible. The addition of color has facilitated consistent detection of dorsal, cavernous, and urethral vessels. CDDU permits the rapid acquisition and measurement of small vessels in low-flow states.[42–44] High-frequency linear array transducers (5 to 10 MHz) provide the best images of the penis; the higher the frequency the better the near field resolution. For this chapter all images were retrieved from a 7.0-MHz linear transducer with standoff wedge (Siemens/Quantum) or 7.5-MHz linear array transducer (Bruel & Kjaer); these permit continuous color encoded gray scale images during Doppler sampling. Others have reported adequate high-resolution penile imaging with (noncolor) gray scale 13.5-MHz probes.[45]

Color flow uses the imaging principles of pulsed Doppler: a pulse of ultrasound is emitted from the transducer, is reflected back and received. When the returning echo has a different frequency than the emitted frequency a Doppler shift has occurred; ultrasound reflecting back off a moving object (penile blood) causes a Doppler shift. Doppler frequency shift depends on several factors: frequency of the transducer, velocity of the moving object (penile blood), speed of sound through the medium (penile tissue), and angle between the Doppler beam and direction of blood flow. The blood flowing in a vessel which is approaching the transducer will produce echoes with a higher frequency than was emitted; blood flowing away produces a lower frequency. As blood flow velocities increase, Doppler shift increases. The Doppler shift is displayed on gray scale as spectrum (waveform) or in CDDU as two-dimensional color image. In CDDU the color display has an angle dependence just like the gray scale spectrum of the Doppler shift. If the vessel runs parallel to the skin surface, ultrasound scanning lines are perpendicular (90° Doppler angle); this will yield no Doppler shift and no color within the vessel. To correct this problem of physics, linear array transducers use phasing to steer the scan lines at a more appropriate angle or an angled standoff wedge on the end of the transducer to provide a nonperpendicular Doppler angle. The angled standoff wedge is acoustically neutral and is ideal for imaging penile vessels which are parallel to the skin. Arterial flow velocity determinations depend on the ultrasound beam–vessel angle; the optimal angle is 60°; the angle correction is set by the examiner. Since arterial flow velocities will be repeated several times after injecting vasodilator, particular attention should be made to maintaining the same angle of insonation. For example, arterial velocity in the same vessel will be calculated at 20 cm/sec, 25 cm/sec, 31 cm/sec, or 203 cm/sec as the probe–vessel angle is altered from 30° to 45° to 55° to 85° respectively![46–50]

EXAMINING PROTOCOL

The examination should be performed in a warm, darkened room. A warm, secure setting is essential to reduce anxiety and thus sympathetic cavernous smooth muscle tone. The patient should be assured that no one will come walking in during his testing. The patient should be supine. His attention should be directed at the ultrasound monitor with periodic explanation of images displayed: "You are going to see ultrasound views of your penile vessels; some of these run on the surface of the penis and two are central arteries providing the pressure to your erection. When the Doppler is activated, the sound you hear will be blood flowing into your penis with each heart beat."

The corporal bodies should be scanned in the transverse plane from base to tip to demonstrate normal anatomy (paired cavernous and dorsal arteries). The echotexture should be homogeneous; fibrotic processes are relatively hyperechoic in comparison. Peyronie's plaques will be denser than normal tunica; they may be

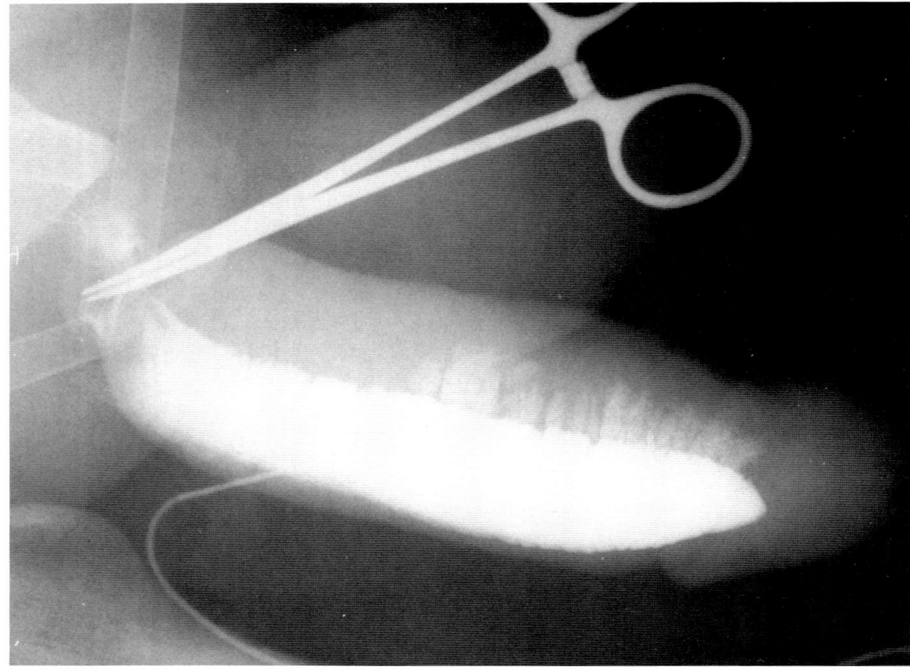

A

B

Fig. 6.7. A: The corporal septum is fenestrated; early phase cavernosogram with contrast initially crossing septum. **B**: Sagittal scan of right cavernous artery with collateral flow across the septum.

visible as linear echogenic thicknenings. If they cast an acoustic shadow, then calcification should be suspected and plain radiographs taken following PBFS/CDDU. The penile vessels and flow velocities are assessed in the sagittal plane (parallel to the long axis of the penis). Vessels may be scanned from dorsal or ventral aspects (Fig. 6.2). Lateral scanning will demonstrate both cavernous vessels in the same image, with the hyperechoic septum between both arteries (Fig. 6.7). Cavernous to cavernous collaterals are only imaged in the sagittal projection from the lateral penis. I have noted these vessels perforating the septum in more than 50% of men examined (Figs. 6.8 and 6.9). They are seen in patients with neurogenic and psychogenic impotence suggesting their origin is congenital. The dynamics of collateral flow are important; high-flow collaterals ≥ 25 cm/sec may supplement unilateral cavernous arterial insufficiency (Fig. 6.10). A dorsal projection is required to image the dorsal artery and ipsilateral cavernous artery (Fig. 6.11). Following vasodilator dorsal to cavernous collaterals were recently demonstrated in 59% of men; these were hemodynamically significant only in 15% of patients (≥ 25 cm/sec).[51] The dorsal arteries are not subjected to intracorporal pressure changes of progressive erection phases; therefore, even in well sustained rigidity antegrade diastolic flow persists. During peak erection, dorsal systolic flow is maximal. Copious acoustic gel on the surface of the penis and a light touch is needed not to alter flow dynamics of dorsal vessels by too much transducer compression (Fig. 6.2B).

All four penile arteries should be scanned at least from the level of the penoscrotal junction to glans. When there is asymmetry of cavernous flows (≥ 10 cm/sec) or when collaterals are seen, the crura should be examined to determine if proximal

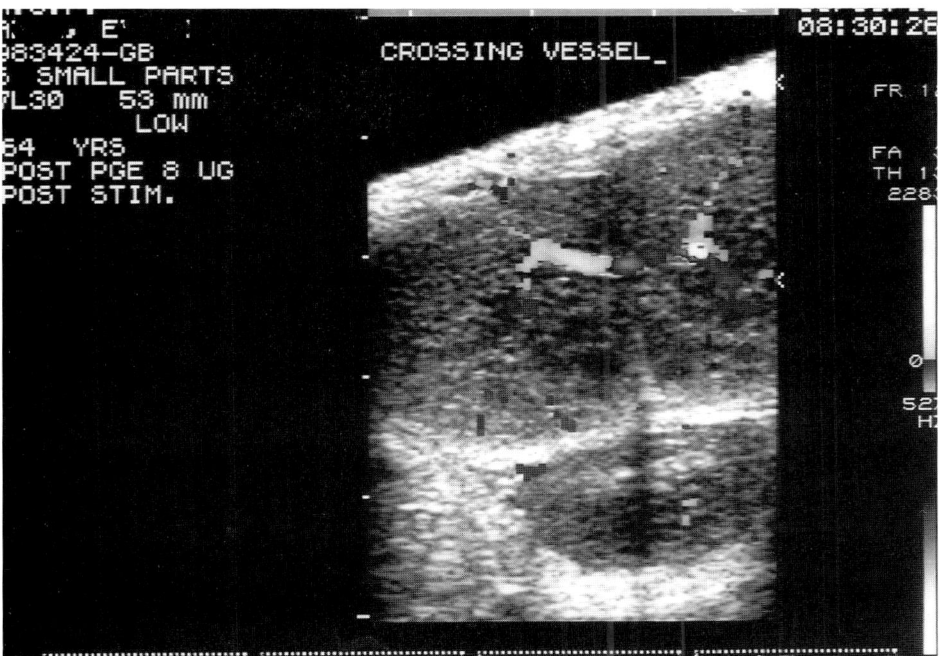

Fig. 6.8. Transverse image of cavernous arterial collateral crossing the septum.

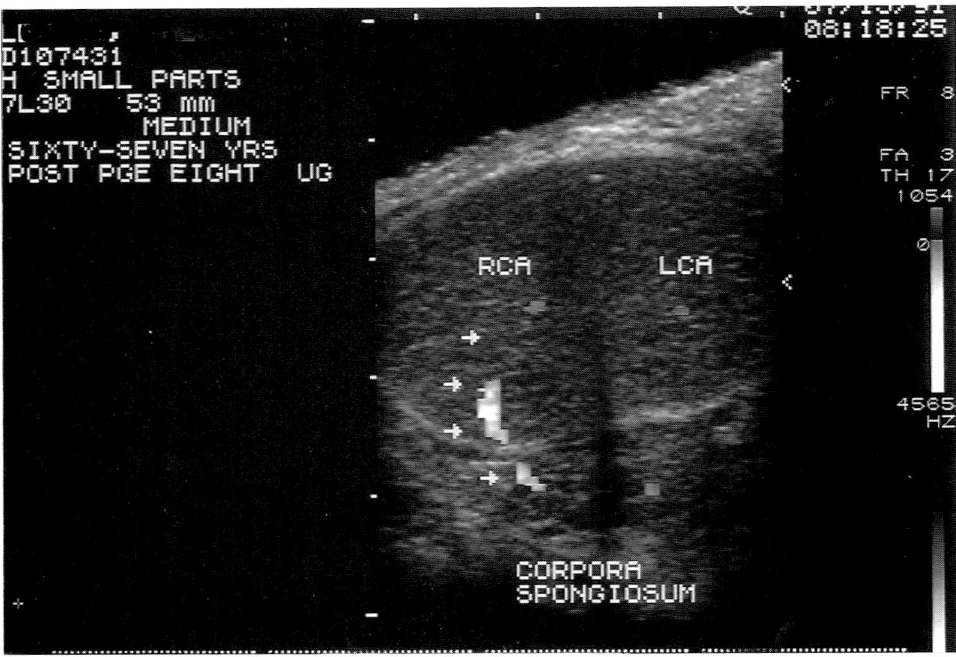

Fig. 6.9. Transverse image of right cavernous arterial (RCA) collateral to corpus spongiosum.

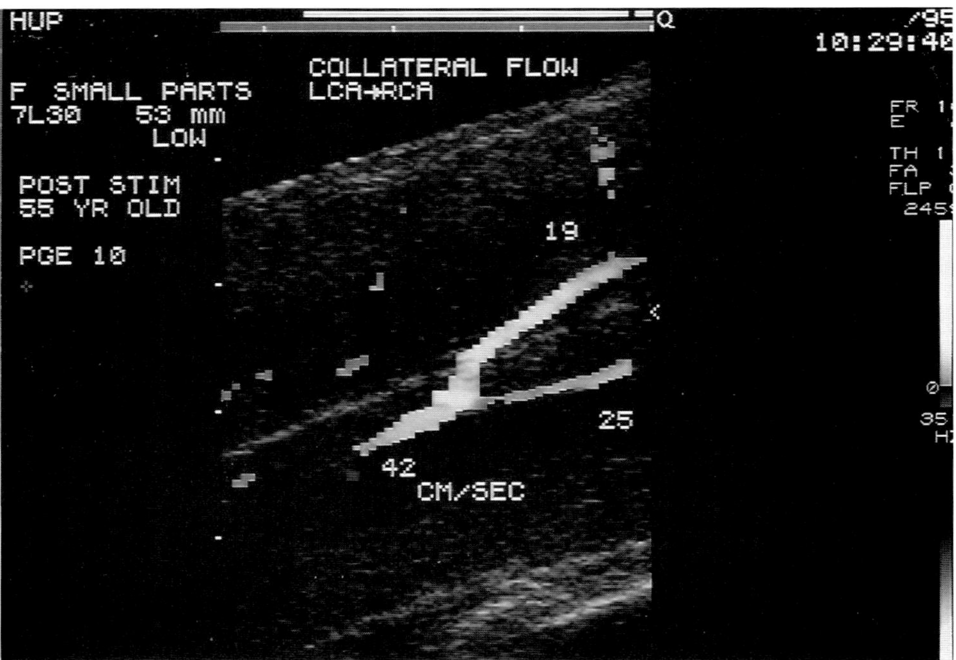

Fig. 6.10. Sagittal scan of cavernous artery collaterals, with 42 cm/sec flow in the proximal LCA, 25 cm/sec flow in distal LCA, and 19 cm/sec flow in the distal RCA.

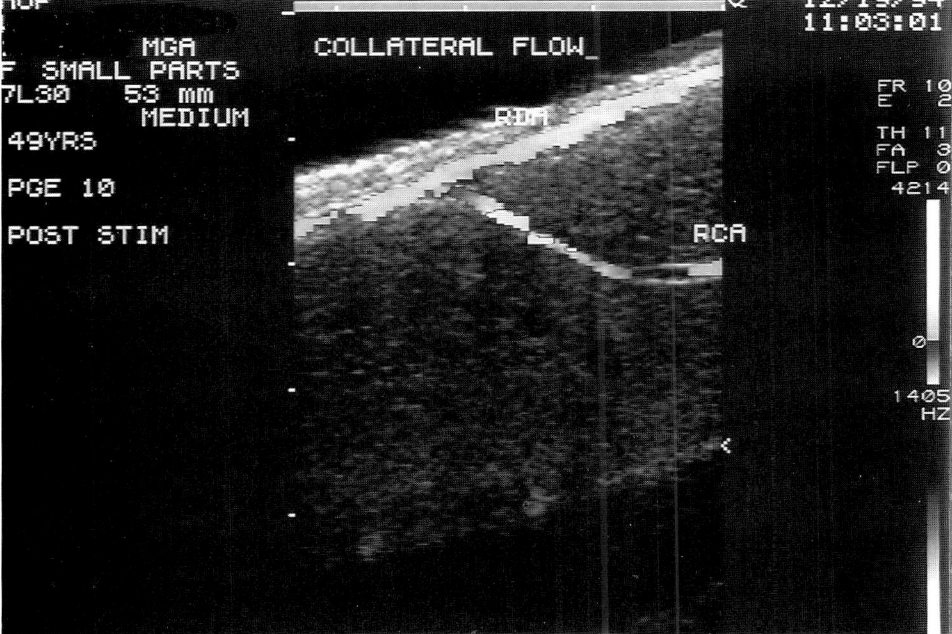

Fig. 6.11. Right dorsal artery (RDA) to right cavernous artery (RCA) collateral.

inflow disease exists (prepenile) or if intracorporal stenosis has resulted in decreased unilateral CDDU signal. If the patient's legs are abducted in a frog leg position, the perineum can be scanned, revealing the entry of the cavernous arteries into the penis. This view is especially helpful when searching for arterial sinusoidal malformations (fistula) causing high-flow priapism or if the patient develops a rapid rigidity. Cavernous flow velocities will be highest at the perineum and will segmentally diminish, distally. Several investigators have confirmed that systolic velocities of the cavernous arteries vary significantly as a function of sampling location.[52,53] Traditionally arterial velocities are measured at the penoscrotal junction (proximal pendulous shaft), from either the ventral or lateral–sagittal projections. If the penis has not assumed an erect posture, it should be held upright by the glans; this is the anatomic position of erection and serves to straighten the course of the cavernous and dorsal arteries. The principal source of error in flow velocity determinations is incorrectly assigned Doppler angle. Holding the shaft upright stretches the normally tortuous cavernous vessels and permits consistent measurements with the probe–vessel Doppler angle remaining set (60°).

Timing is important; arterial diameter and cavernous peak systolic velocities will maximize before rigid erection. Some investigators advocate continuous penile sampling for up to 30 min after penile injection.[54] Meuleman et al found peak velocities highest 5–10 min following vasodilator.[55] Fitzgerald et al found that 24% of patients tested did not reach maximum cavernous flow until 10–15 min after injection.[56] If initial measurements are made at 5–10 min after injection and thereafter full or rigid erection waveforms are not seen, a period of privacy and self-stimulation will enhance the penile response in $\geq 70\%$ of patients.[4] CDDU assessment is repeated immediately after self-stimulation, and notation is made of whether the response weakens or is sustained. Donatucci and Lue found that among 90 patients performing self-stimulation after PGE_1 challenge 74% improved; among those whose responses weakened within 5 min of stimulation 84% were noted to have moderate venous leakage on follow-up cavernosography.[57] Additionally it is very useful to visually rate the erectile quality during Doppler assessment: inadequate versus adequate versus unbending rigidity sustained for 20 min. Correlation of visual erection rating and Doppler parameters is an essential element in the diagnostic process: although the Doppler parameters are distinctly different, tumescence is characteristic of both severe veno-occlusive disease and arterial insufficiency; adequate erection suggests the patient will be a good candidate for home injection therapy, no matter what the final diagnosis. The patient should be questioned about whether the pharmacologic erection is similar, better or worse than those he gets at home.[4] Goldstein states the aim of PBFS/CDDU is to obtain hemodynamic data on the same quality of erection that the patient gets in the privacy of his own bedroom, "the best quality erection" (BQE).[45] If the answer to the BQE question is "no" then he recommends that the patient achieve maximal smooth muscle relaxation.[58] European investigators have recommended audiovisual sexual stimulation in lieu of or to supplement manual stimulation for PBFS.[59]

The initial duplex Doppler studies were performed after injection of 60 mg of papaverine.[15,60,61] Trimix has been used recently in efforts to achieve maximal smooth muscle relaxation: 0.2 ml of papaverine (6 mg), phentolamine (0.2 mg), and PGE_1 (2 µg).[45] Of the currently used agents PGE_1 is thought to have the greatest biocompatibility. PGE_1 is a corporal smooth muscle relaxant and has anti-adrenergic activity that may explain its efficacy in patients suffering high-anxiety, psychogenic erectile dysfunction.[27,62–64] PGE_1 (Caverject; Upjohn Co., Kalamazoo, MI) is the only FDA-approved injectable for the treatment of erectile dysfunction. In a recent dose-finding study, the median effective dosage was 5.0 µg in patients with vasculogenic dysfunction, producing a mean duration of erection of 37 min. Penile discomfort was noted in 34%, and prolonged erection (4–6 hr) in 5%.[40] In my experience with initial diagnostic intracavernous challenges, PGE_1 is highly effective with dosing of: 6 µg for patients 50–60 yr old and 10 µg for patients 60–70 yr old when coupled with privacy and self-stimulation. With this regimen of age-specific dosing, fewer than 4% of patients develop persistent rigidity of 2 hr. In my practice most patients with rigidity for 2 hr have been successfully managed with single injection of the α-adrenergic phenylephrine (100 µg/cc, using 1–2 cc); interestingly, reversal of partial erection or tumescence associated with pain resolves the penile ache as well.

CDDU AND PENILE INFLOW:
ARTERIAL ADEQUACY

The original parameter used to infer the integrity of penile circulation was cavernous peak systolic velocity (PSV). In efforts to further refine the diagnosis of cavernous inflow disease, Doppler parameters have been expanded: end diastolic arterial

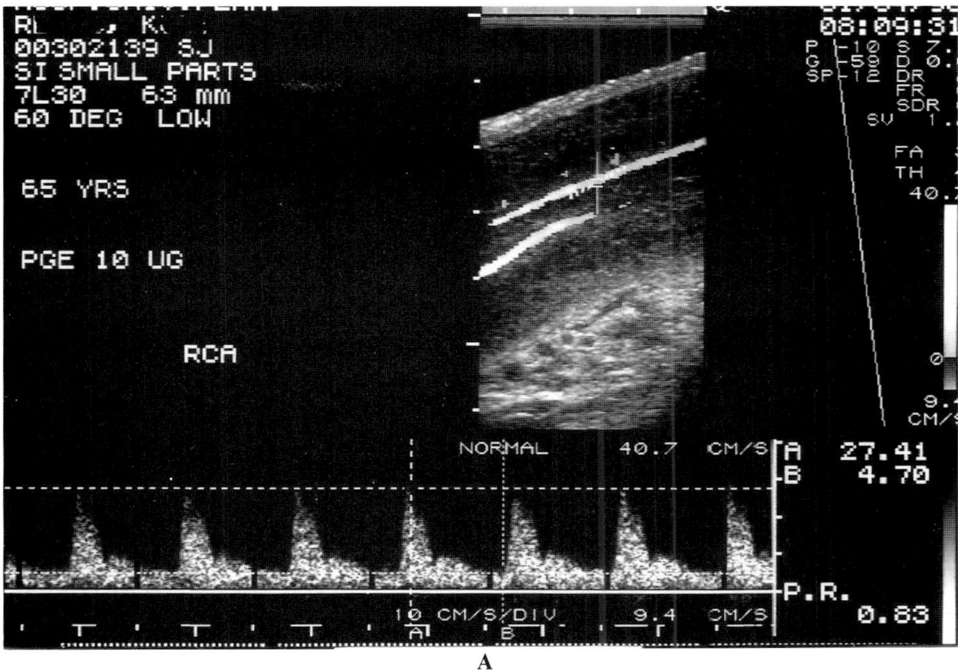

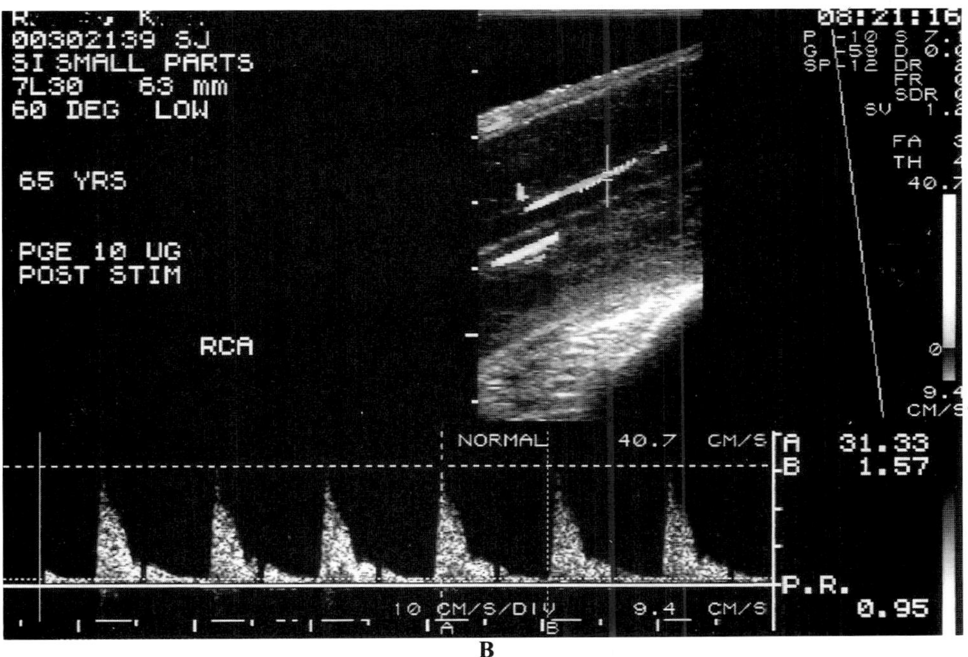

Fig. 6.12. A: Normal progression of Doppler waveform: response 5 min after penile injection of 10 μg PGE₁, RCA flow has a peak systolic of 27 cm/sec, end diastolic flow of 4.7 cm/sec, and resistive index 0.83. **B**: Following privacy and self-stimulation, peak systolic flow is 31 cm/sec, end diastolic flow is 1.57 cm/sec, and resistive index is 0.95.

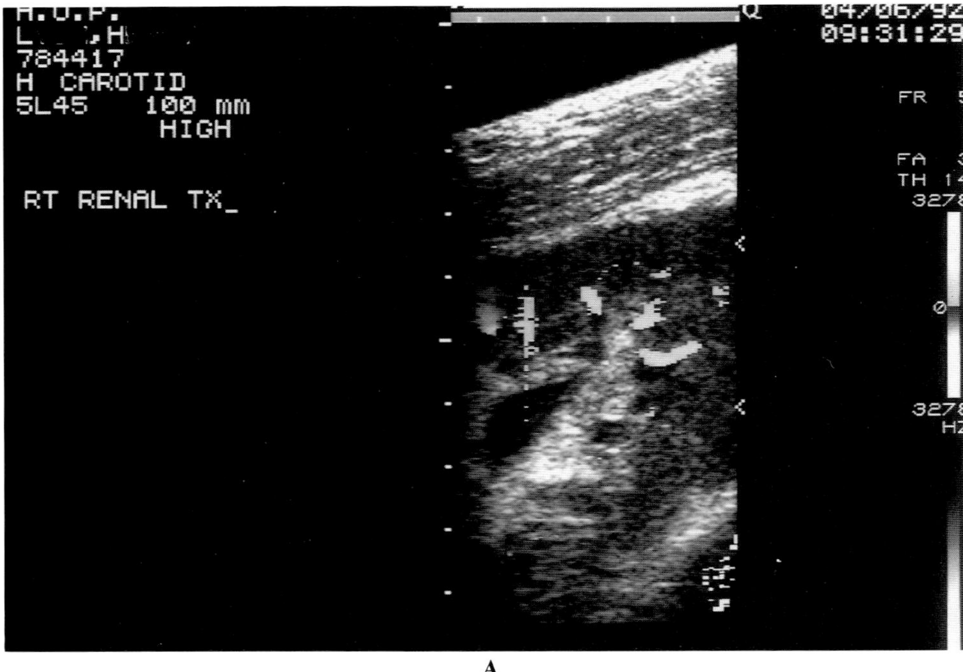

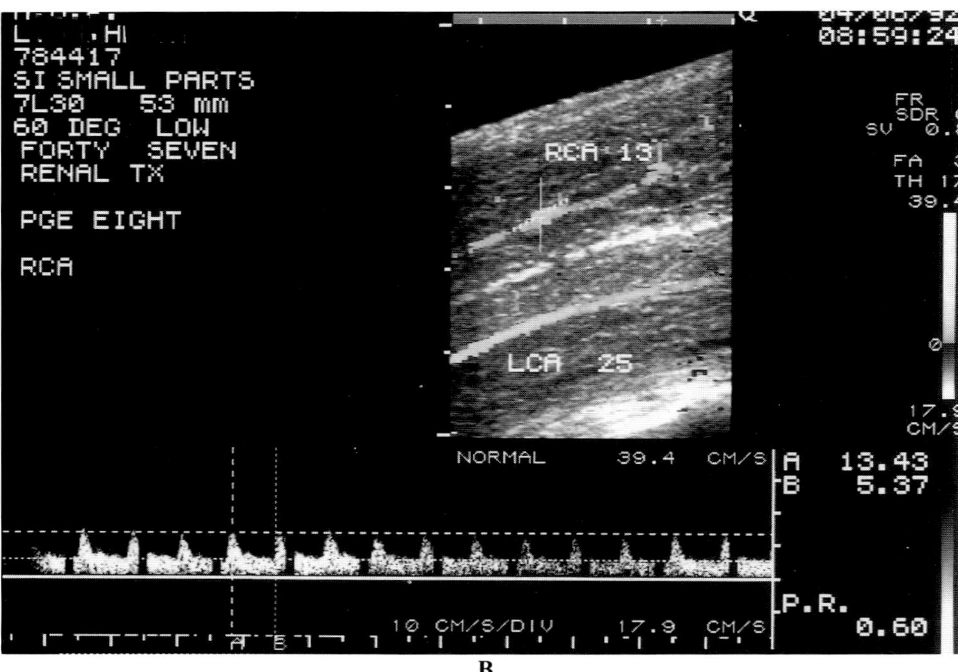

Fig. 6.13. A: Color Doppler of right renal transplant. **B**: Unilateral cavernous arterial insufficiency in right cavernous artery (RCA) with low peak systolic velocity in the right central artery, 13 cm/sec, suggesting a pelvic steal is occurring.

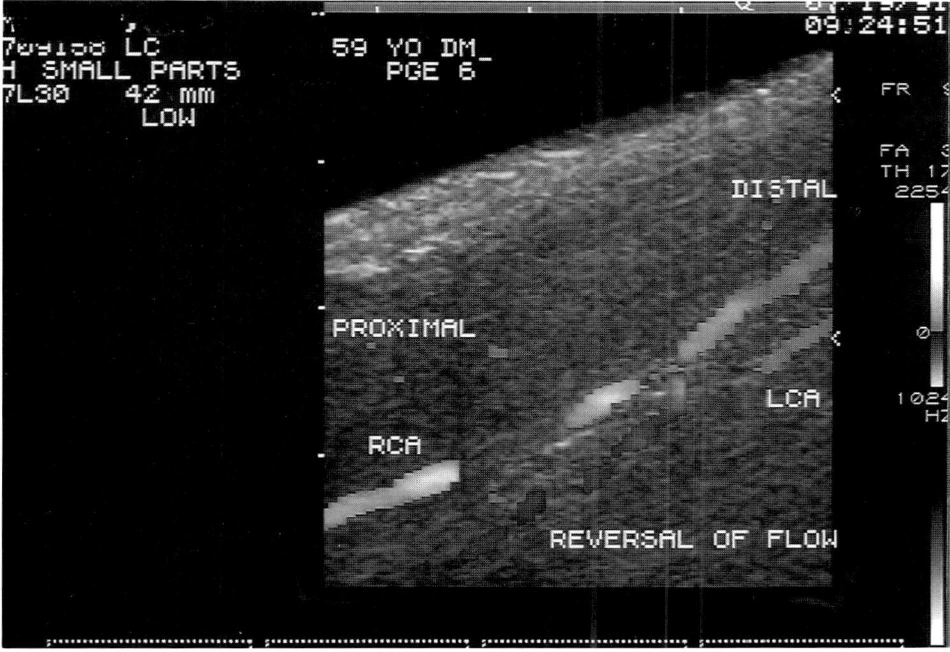

Fig. 6.14. Severe unilateral cavernous arterial insufficiency in 59-yr-old diabetic, with reversal of flow in the proximal left cavernous artery (LCA).

velocity (EDV, flow velocity measured during diastole immediately prior to take-off of the systolic waveform), systolic rise time (msec from the start of systolic velocity to the maximum value), and cavernous artery acceleration (peak flow velocity over systolic rise time).[35,65,66] Flow velocities should be measured 5 to 10 min after injection; a delay in response is typical in both the hypertensive and the anxious patient. A visual rating of erectile quality should be recorded each time a set of Doppler parameters is recorded.

Lue originally proposed that an adequate response in the cavernous arteries should produce a >0.7 mm postinjection arterial diameter and ≥ 25 cm/sec PSV. He found that if the cavernous arteries did not dilate by 75% there was a high likelihood of arterial disease.[67] Other investigators suggested increases of more than 100%, or could not confirm significant changes at all in pre- and postinjection cavernous arterial diameters.[44,68–70] The cavernous arterial diameters normally decrease from proximal to distal and measurement of cavernous arterial lumens actually exceeds ultrasound resolution of 7–10 MHz probes. In the University of California, San Francisco series, normal subjects had mean PSV of 34.8 cm/sec and mean arterial diameter 0.89 mm.[50] In a study from Baylor University normal volunteers had mean PSV of 40 cm/sec and mean arterial diameter of 1.0 mm.[71] Normal volunteers at the Harvard Medical School study had mean PSV of 47 cm/sec.[68] Each of these groups concurs that a peak systolic velocity <25 cm/sec signifies severe arterial disease. When penile angiography is compared to duplex Doppler examinations of the same patients, PSV < 25 cm/sec is consistently associated with

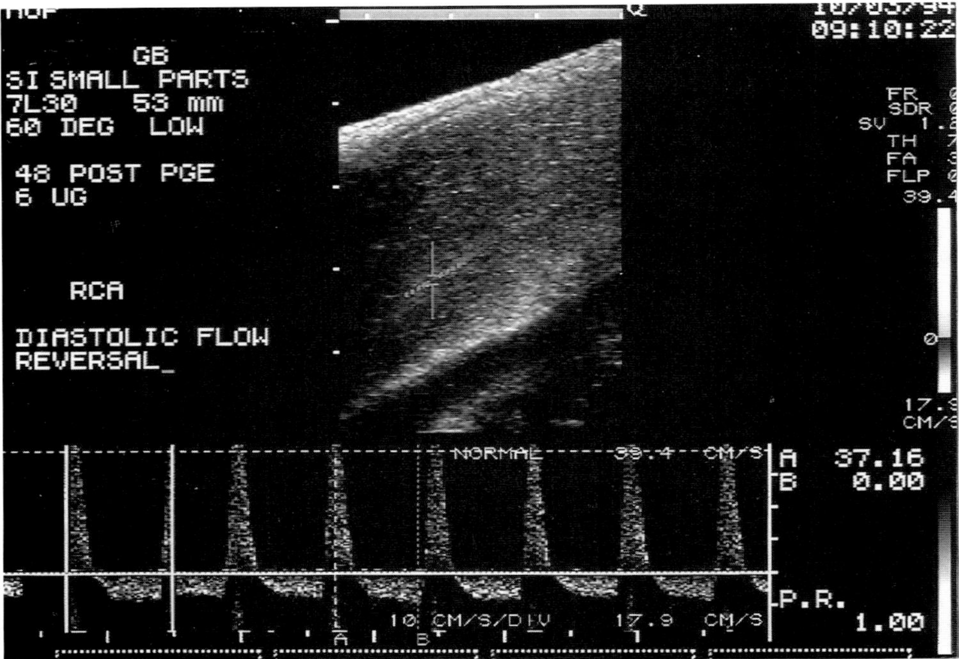

Fig. 6.15. Diastolic flow reversal is seen in the right cavernous artery (RCA), associated with rigid erection.

severe inflow disease. In the Mayo Clinic series PSV < 25 cm/sec had a sensitivity of 100% and specificity of 95% for selecting patients with abnormal pudendal arteriography (Fig. 6.12A, B).[72] A PSV of 35 cm/sec or more is generally associated with a normal penile arteriogram.[70] The Mayo Clinic group has recommended that in cases with a good clinical response to vasodilating injection and bilateral peak systolic velocities > 30 cm/sec with arterial dilation to 0.7 mm, arteriography should not be performed. When PSV is compared to cavernous arterial systolic occlusion pressures (CASOP) generated during dynamic infusion cavernosometry, a PSV ≥ 25 cm/sec predicts a normal CASOP with a sensitivity of 95% and specificity of 95%.[73] Asymmetry greater than 10 cm/sec between right and left cavernous inflows is abnormal; if cavernous inflows are asymmetric or absent at the perineum, suspect prepenile (pudendal) arterial disease. Intrapenile arterial disease is evident when crural inflows are adequate and symmetric but asymmetry of right versus left (R/L) PSVs is noted in the pendulous penis.[68,70] On CDDU severe unilateral cavernous arterial insufficiency may be associated with reversal of systolic flow proximal to the entry of a collateral (Figs. 6.13 and 6.14).

Schwartz correlated progressive changes in Doppler spectral waveform pattern with increasing intracorporal pressure in potent volunteers stimulated with papaverine/phentolamine.[41] Rigid erection was associated with intracorporal pressures ranging from 83 to 106 mm Hg. During tumescence both PSV and EDV increased, with corporal pressure ranging from 11 to 25 mm Hg. With rigidity EDV approached zero, and diastolic flow reversed when intracorporal pressures reached

63–83 mm Hg[74] (Fig. 6.15). In 1974 Planiol and Pourcelot derived the index of vascular resistance from the Doppler spectrum. The formula for resistive index is RI = PSV − EDV/PSV. RI calculation is not directly dependent on the probe vessel angle; it does not matter that the Doppler angle is not ideal (60°).[75] The value of RI depends on the resistance to arterial inflow, and in the context of corporal physiology this is a function of sympathetic tone in the flaccid state and of changing intra-corporal pressure during the various phases of erection following either natural or pharmacologic smooth muscle relaxation. As penile pressure equals or exceeds diastolic systemic pressure, diastolic flow in the corpora will approach zero and the value for RI approaches 1. During tumescence and until full rigidity, diastolic flow persists and the value for RI remains < 1.0. The RI correlates very well with visual rating of erectile responses as both are descriptions of penile rigidity/pressure. Both EDV and RI are useful parameters in predicting adequacy of veno-occlusion (see below).

PRESBYRECTIA: AGE-RELATED DECREASE IN ERECTION

As discussed above, age-related decreases in erectile function have long been evident in clinical series and have now been verified in normative community groups such as the Massachusetts Male Aging Study.[76] Wespes has observed an age-related decrease in smooth muscle content, using computerized morphometry to analyze penile biopsies. Comparing young patients with penile curvature but hemodynamically adequate erections to elderly patients with erectile dysfunction, he found: young patients have corpora composed of 40–52% smooth muscle, patients with corporal veno-occlusive dysfunction have 19–36% smooth muscle, and patients with arterial impotence have 10–25% smooth muscle with collagen content correspondingly increased.[77] Several observations support a link between the mechanism of corporal smooth muscle (CSM) relaxation and CSM degeneration.[78,79] At low oxygen tensions found in the flaccid penis, nitric oxide synthase activity is inhibited. As a consequence of cavernous artery relaxation, oxygenated blood is delivered to the corpus cavernosum. In the oxygen-enriched corpora the autonomic dilator nerves, and endothelium of the sinusoids increase synthesis and release of nitric oxide, the principal corporal dilator. PGE synthesis in rabbit corpus cavernosum is similarly regulated by oxygen tension. Under hypoxic conditions, endothelial cell cultures increase synthesis of endothelin-1 and transforming growth factor-β1 (TGF-β).[79] TGF-β is a cytokine that includes collagen synthesis and accumulation. Levin et al have demonstrated that under hypoxic conditions the physiology of sinusoidal muscle is severely altered; coupling between CSM contraction and intracellular increases in calcium is abolished under hypoxic conditions.[80] Bringing this basic research on molecular growth factors and physiology together the following is hypothesized: in the aging male decreasing number and duration of nocturnal erections may be related to corporal hypoxia secondary to arterial or arteriolar insufficiency.

CDDU hemodynamic parameters of a normal erection do seem to vary with age. In a retrospective review of over 600 cases, 106 instances where intracavernous challenge with PGE$_1$ produced excellent well-sustained rigidity of at least 20 min were

Table 6.1. PBFS/CDDU Age-specific Parameters of Excellent Erections

AGE	RI (pre)	PSV (pre)	RI (post-stim)	PSV (post-stim)
20–29	0.88	39.5	0.95	53.7
30–39	0.81	32.7	0.94	45.0
40–49	0.79	32.3	0.93	43.2
50–59	0.81	27.8	0.94	33.4
60–69	0.79	28.7	0.91	33.0
70–79	0.84	26.9	0.96	32.9

Adapted from Broderick and Arger.[81]

documented in patients of various ages (Table 6.1). CDDU parameters were recorded 5 to 10 min after PGE_1 injection and repeated following privacy and self-stimulation. Mean PGE_1 dosages producing excellent erections by age group were: 5 µg (20–49); 6 µg (50–59); 10 µg (60–79). Rigid erection following privacy and self-stimulation was consistently characterized by RI > 0.90, but occurred over a range of PSVs which decreased with advancing age. The data suggests that cavernous arterial flow decreases with age and the technique of privacy and self-stimulation should permit safe and effective diagnostic dosage for the typical impotence patient with 10 µg. Resistive index (RI) parameter did not vary with age; perhaps the dynamics of veno-occlusion are the critical factor in the aging erectile response.[81]

CDDU AND PENILE OUTFLOW: DOCUMENTING VENO-OCCLUSIVE ADEQUACY

Failure of the veno-occlusive mechanism is reflected in the Doppler spectral waveform of the cavernous artery. The suspicion of venous leakage is raised when the patient has an excellent arterial response to injected vasodilator (≥ 30 cm/sec, PSV), with well-maintained EDV (>3–5 cm/sec), accompanied by transient rigidity after self-stimulation.

Quam found EDVs ranging between 0 and 24 cm/sec after intracavernous papaverine (60 mg). Among patients with peak systolic velocities >25 cm/sec, venous leakage on cavernosometry was predicted with a sensitivity of 90% and specificity of 56% when end diastolic flow was >5 cm/sec.[42] Fitzgerald using criteria of cavernous arterial adequacy (>25 cm/sec, PSV) and venous leakage (>5 cm/sec, EDV), noted that only three-fourths of patients achieved maximal responses to papaverine (60 mg) at 5 min. Data acquisition for a total of 30 min yielded a sensitivity of 95% and specificity of 83% for prediction of venous leakage.[56] Merckx et al injected patients with PGE_1 (20 µg) followed by Doppler analysis at 5-min intervals. Doppler parameters among 26 psychogenically impotent men were statistically identical to eight potent volunteers: at 5 min maximum PSV 49 cm/sec, maximum EDV 11 cm/sec, RI 0.78; at 10 min PSV was 38.8 cm/sec, EDV 3.7 cm/sec, RI 0.91. The RI was the only parameter that statistically differentiated the venous incompetence. Using this 5- and 10-min scanning protocol they noted a 93% correlation between CDDU and cavernosometry.[82] In the Mayo Clinic series of 1994 Lewis noted that an EDV of >3 cm/sec measured 15–20 min postinjection yielded a specificity of 94% and sensitivity of 69% for detection of venous leakage when compared with dynamic cavernosometry.[72] McMahon found RI calculations 15 min after injection correlated well with maintenance flow rates (from dynamic infusion cavernosometry) and cavernosal decay rates.[83] In a study from Japan, Naroda found RI > 0.9 was associated with normal dynamic infusion cavernosometry in 90% and RI < 0.75 was associated with venous leakage in 95% of patients.[84]

Although the definitive criteria for CDDU-diagnosed venous leakage have not been agreed upon, the examiner should reliably be able to select patients for more invasive investigations (dynamic infusion cavernosometry and cavernosography) by observing waveform progression through each phase of erection. When the Doppler spectral waveform continues to exhibit forward diastolic flow despite peak systolic flow (>30 cm/sec), a low-resistance state persists in the sinusoids and the patient may have venogenic impotence (Fig. 6.16). The dorsal arteries are not subjected to the intracorporal pressure changes with each phase of erection and well-sustained rigidity is associated with antegrade diastolic flow (Table 6.2). Deep dorsal vein flow persists during rigid erection; DDV flows are a function of dorsal arterial flow to the glans and should not be interpreted as evidence of corporal venous leakage (Fig. 6.17). When DDV flows are high a pattern respiratory venous variation may be

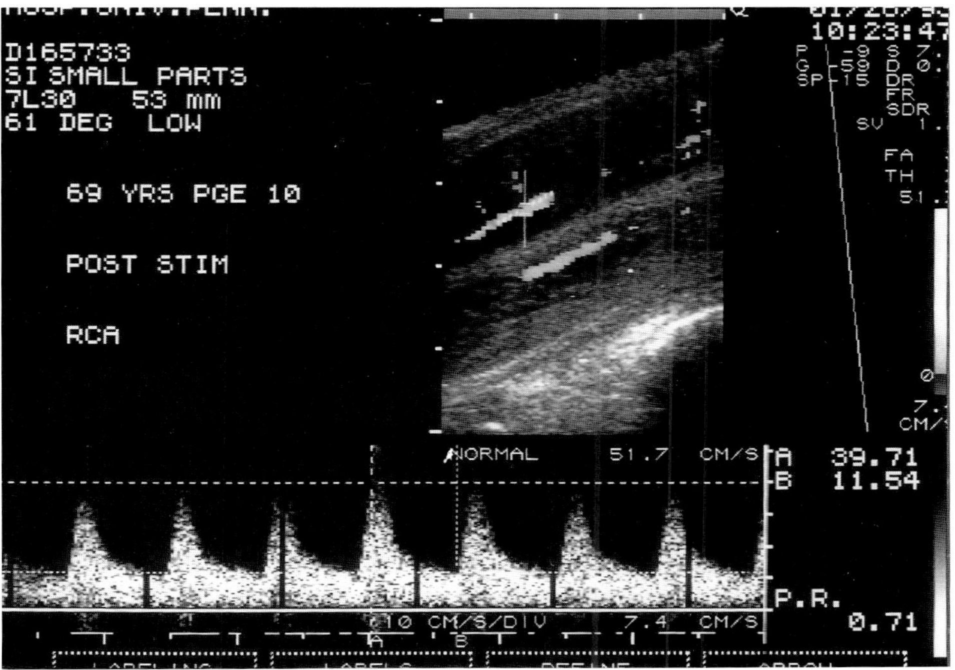

Fig. 6.16. An unequivocal diagnosis of cavernous venous occlusive disease based on ultrasound criteria can be given with cavernous arterial flows exceeding 35 cm/sec, end diastolic velocities remaining high (11 cm/sec), and resistive index low (0.71). Sagittal scan of 69-yr-old, following PGE$_1$ 10 µg and self-stimulation.

Table 6.2. Erectile Response Indicated by Doppler Flow

Doppler Flows (cm/sec)	Best Erectile Response		
	Inadequate	Adequate	Excellent
Deep dorsal vein	11.4	10.7	10.6
Cavernous artery (PSV)	24.1	28.1	40.9
Dorsal artery (PSV)	35.6	44.4	46.9
Cavernous artery (RI)	0.68	0.80	0.95

Adapted from Broderick.[4]

PSV = peak systolic velocity; RI = resistive index.

detected (Fig. 6.18). The primary veno-occlusive mechanism consists of passive compression of the subtunical venular plexus by the distended sinusoids. The secondary mechanism is the scissoring off of the emissary veins as they egress through the two layers of the tunica albuginea. Emissary veins unlike dorsal artery to cavernous artery collaterals are difficult to localize with CDDU presumably because of their low-flow state and easy compressibility (Fig. 6.19).

PRIAPISM: CDDU CHARACTERISTICS OF LOW FLOW AND HIGH FLOW

Priapism is a persistent erection that fails to subside after climax and is accompanied by penile pain and tenderness; it is an overfunction of a normal mechanism.[85] Traditionally priapism has been categorized as primary (spontaneous–idiopathic) or secondary to specific pathologies: sickle cell disease, leukemia, fat emboli, malignant infiltration, neurologic injury, alcohol, and psychotropic drugs. With the increasing popularity of pharmacologic erection programs, iatrogenic or therapeutically induced prolonged erection has become the most common cause of priapism.[86] Ischemic priapism is an obvious failure of the detumescence mechanism which may result from direct dysregulation of the cavernous–arterial–sinusoidal system through persistent stimulation of corporal relaxing factors, inhibition of neurotransmission normally terminating erection, or inactivation of the smooth muscle cellular cofactors that regulate corporal smooth muscle tone such as an altered metabolic environment (hypoxia, hypercarbia, and acidity).[87] We know that beyond a certain and as yet undefined time, the cavernous smooth muscle becomes refractory to recoiling. This condition is clinically well-recognized in emergency rooms and remains one of the few true urologic emergencies.

Histologic investigations reveal that after 24 h of ischemic priapism the corporal tissues become thickened and edematous. The natural history of untreated priapism is impotency with perhaps some erectile activity maintained in the proximal crura. Microscopy by Spycher and Hauri[88] demonstrates trabecular interstitial edema after 12 h followed by the destruction of sinusoidal endothelium, exposure of the basement membrane, and thrombocyte adherence by 24 hr. By 48 hr actual thrombus formation occurs in the sinusoidal spaces and the smooth muscle undergoes fibroblast-like cell transformation. CDDU is not needed to make the diagnosis of

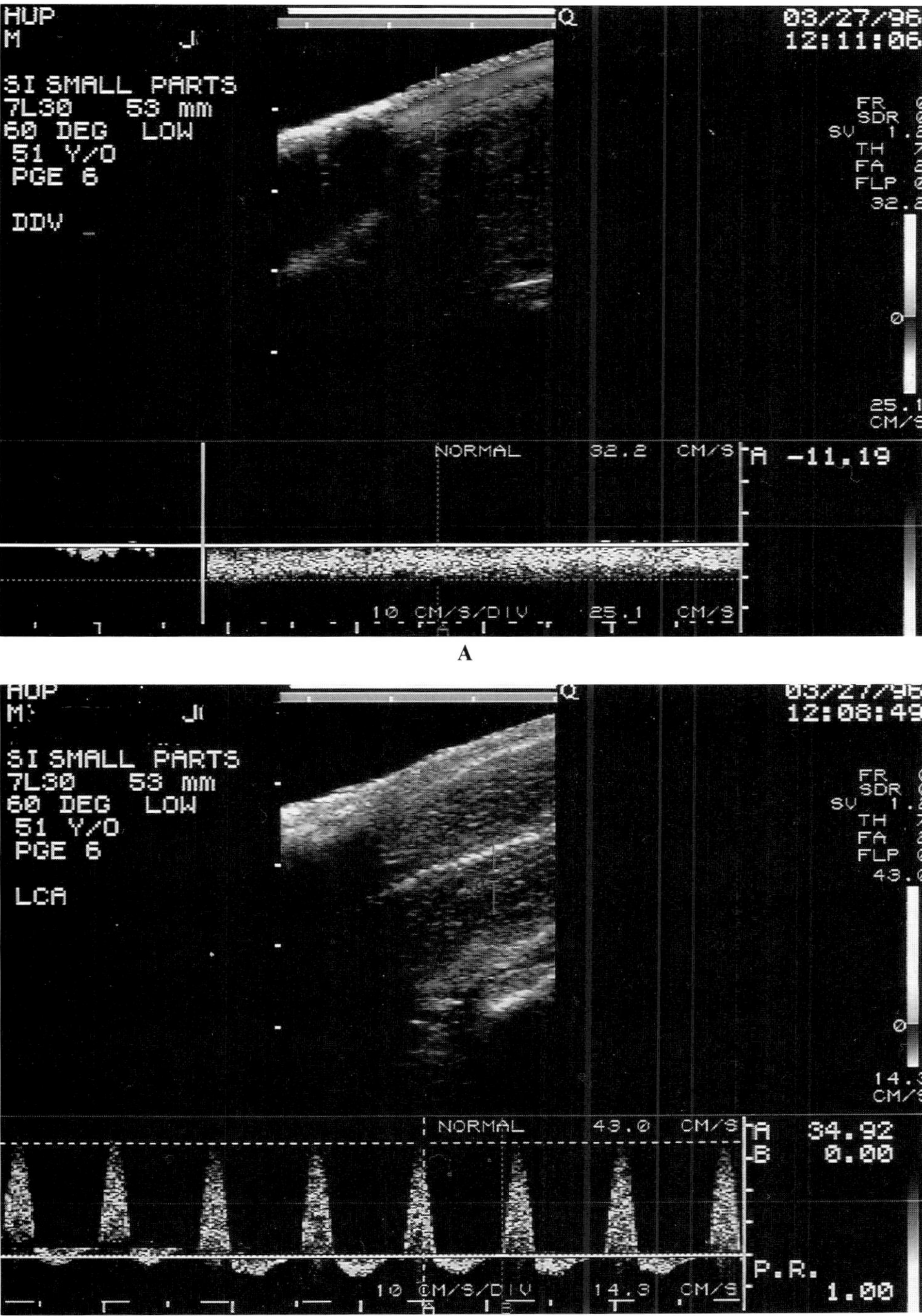

Fig. 6.17. A: Deep dorsal vein flow (DDV) persists during rigid erection, Patient MJ. **B**: Patient MJ; Doppler waveform of rigidity, with peak systolic velocity of 35 cm/sec and reversal of diastolic flow.

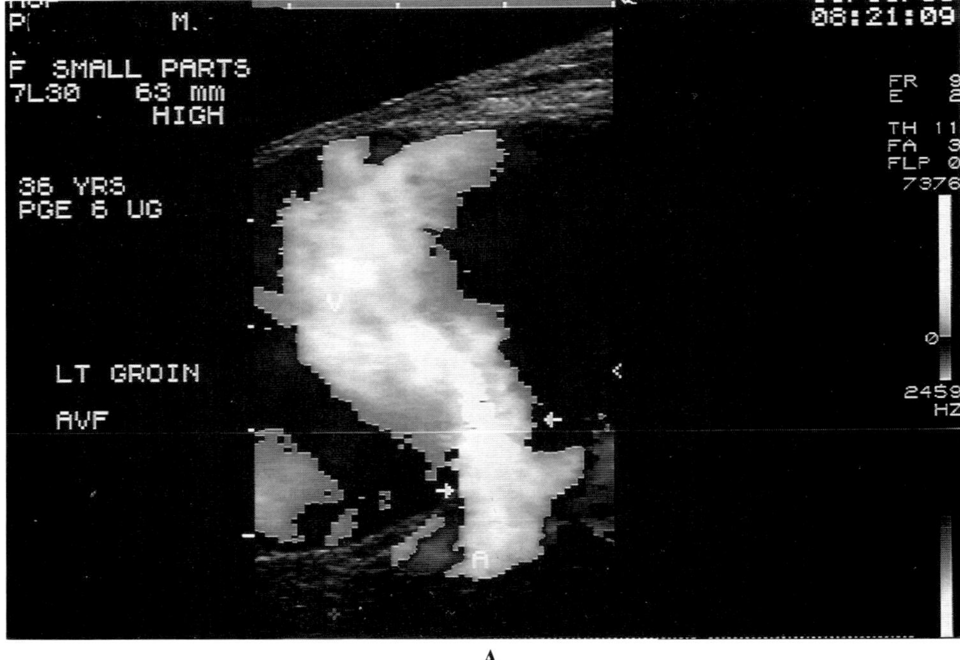

A

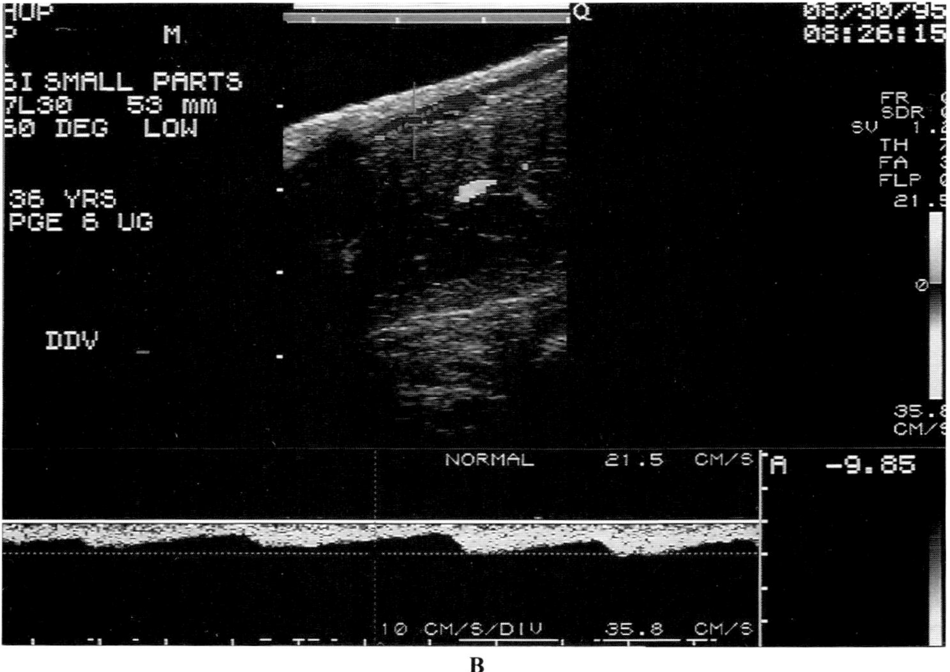

B

Fig. 6.18. A: Left groin arterial venous fistula (AVF), postoperative complication in Patient PM. **B**: Arterial waveform pattern in the deep dorsal vein (DDV) of Patient PM.

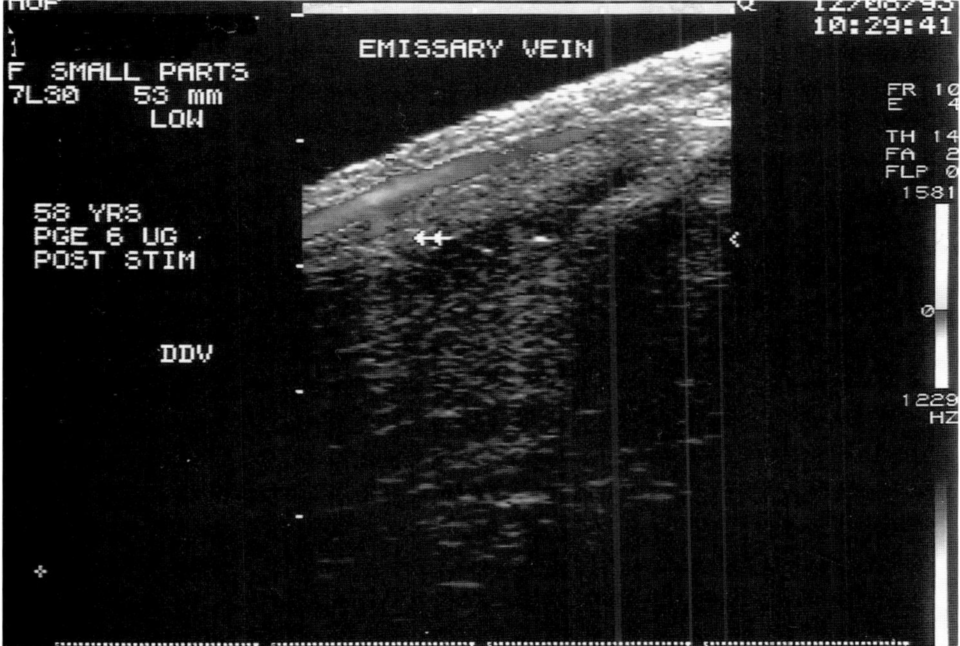

Fig. 6.19. Emissary veins perforating the tunica albuginea are rarely seen, because of their small size and low-flow state (*arrows*).

priapism; the diagnosis is established by history, examination, and penile blood gas. CDDU may be useful in follow-up of ischemic priapism to determine the extent of corporal fibrosis and the patency of the cavernous arteries (Fig. 6.20).

Our understanding of penile hemodynamics has led to classification of the prolonged erection as either ischemic–veno-occlusive or high flow–arterial. Of the various etiologies for priapism only one, trauma, has been attributed to "dysregulation" of inflow, producing high-flow priapism.[89,90] Hakim demonstrated the utility and accuracy of duplex Doppler in the diagnosis and management of high-flow priapism when compared to selective internal pudendal arteriography.[91] The investigators followed ten men with selective internal pudendal arteriography, duplex Doppler ultrasonography, and physical examinations. The duration of priapism was startling from 21 days to 36 yr; at the time of initial evaluation all patients gave history of blunt perineal or shaft trauma, and had bright red corporal aspirates. Six patients who were embolized had retrograde unilateral cavernous flows on CDDU follow-up suggesting permanent occlusion. The only consequence of expectant management was the "annoyance" of a turgid shaft. The authors conclude: duplex sonography is more accurate than physical examination and arteriography in predicting the existence and persistence of lacunar fistulae. Indeed all ten patients had delay in time to presentation from days to years during which they reported normal or improved sexual activity.

These cases are extremely rare; unlike low-flow veno-occlusive priapism there is no need for emergent intervention in high-flow priapism. It is essential to establish the correct classification of priapism by aspiration of bright red blood from the

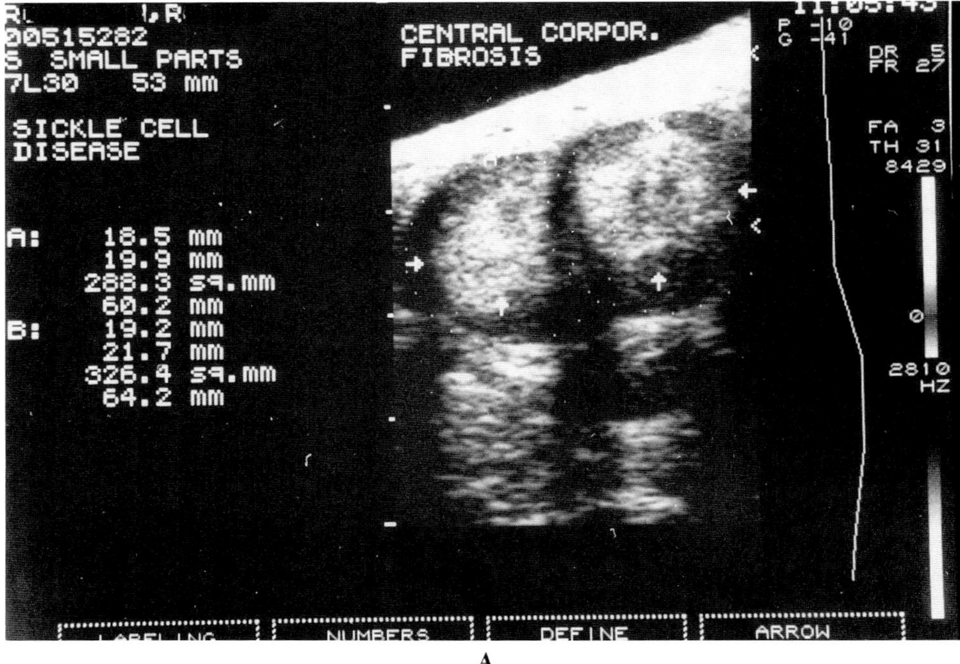

A

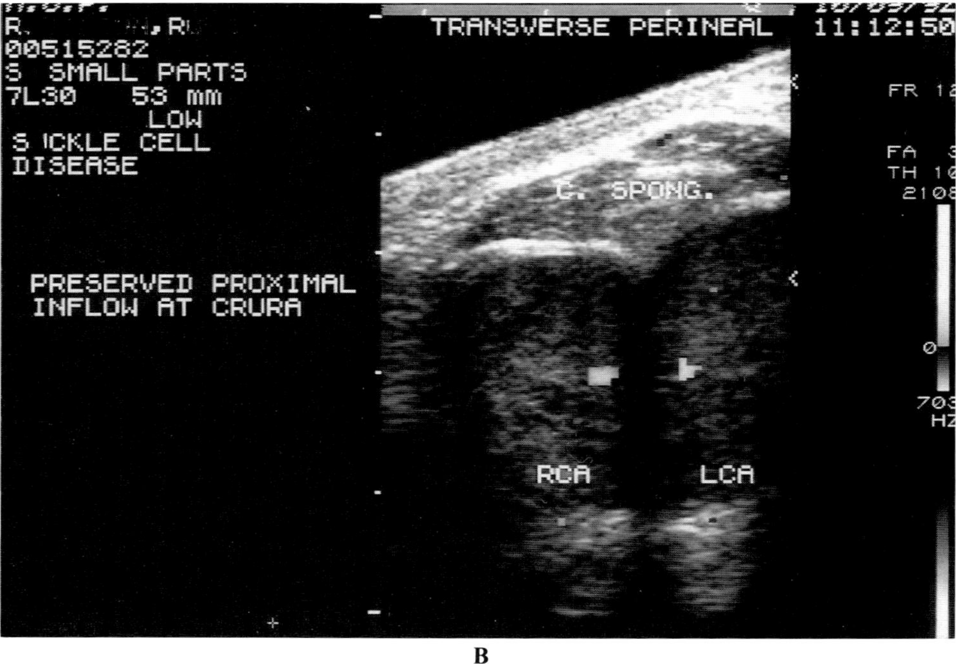

B

Fig. 6.20. **A**: Transverse scan from the dorsum in patient with recurrent sickle cell priapism; central corporal fibrosis appears hyperechoic (*arrows*). **B**: Proximal scan of same patient showing preservation of cavernous arterial inflow; note corporal tissue is more hypoechoic.

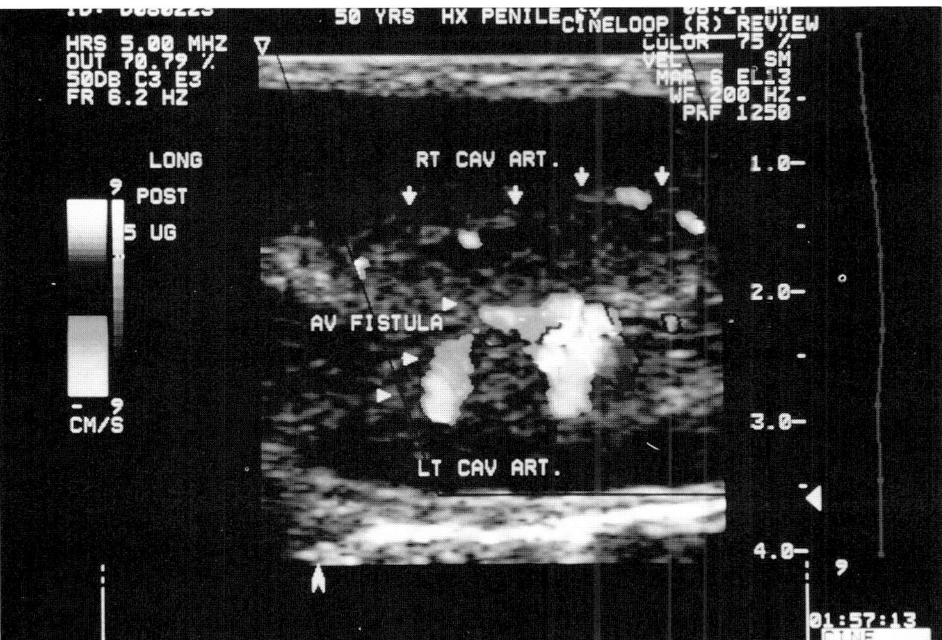

Fig. 6.21. Left cavernous sinusoidal fistula; note unregulated blood flow from disrupted left cavernous artery.

corpora, confirming high oxygen tension. Remote corporal injury may be evident on CDDU by hyperechoic changes within the corpora, a nonspecific finding consistent with scar formation. Disruption of the sinusoid architecture is evidenced by turbulent flow on CDDU, marking the site of arteriosinusoidal fistula (Fig. 6.21). In the acute phase on injury unregulated flow may be imaged without vascactive injection; in follow-up low-dosage vasoactive injection is needed. The crural bodies must be imaged from the ventrum (transperineum) by frog legging the patient and lifting the scrotum.

CDDU: STAGING OF PEYRONIE'S DISEASE

Surgical staging of Peyronie's disease must address both penile form and function. The tunica albuginea and dorsal vascular complex are well-imaged with CDDU. A standoff wedge increases near field resolution bringing into view dorsal plaques. The tunica albuginea is normally hyperechoic compared to the corpora proper. As the corporal bodies distend with blood the cavernous sinusoids become more hypoechoic increasing the contrast between the tunica and corpora. Penile plaques are hyperechoic thickenings of the tunica albuginea. The typical dorsal plaque underlies the dorsal vasculature. Denser plaques cast an acoustical shadow and are well-visualized in either the transverse or sagittal plains. Although most plaques localize to the proximal and middle third of the pendulous shaft, distal plaques can be identified (Fig. 6.22). Circumferential narrowing of the corporal bodies by plaque results in an hourglass shape to the erection; the patient complains of "hinging" with erection (Fig. 6.23). The sonographic correlate is a ring of thickened tunica. A similar but focal wedge is seen when penile deviation is lateral. Septal fibrosis is the most technically challenging abnormality to demonstrate. If increased tissue density is discrete, hyperechoic aggregates within the septum are seen. More diffuse septal fibrosis is identified by scanning in a sagittal plane parallel to the septum; from this vantage the denser septal fibers take on a veil-like appearance with posterior acoustical shadowing. In cases where acoustical shadowing is generated by dense plaques, plain radiographs should follow CDDU.

Potentially the most useful preoperative staging information is the demonstration of collaterals from the dorsal vascular bundle. Dorsal artery collaterals diving downward through the tunica to anastamose with the ipsilateral cavernous artery may be in close proximity to a plaque. Operative mobilization of the neurovascular bundle for plaque incision or excision in these cases would of necessity sacrifice the dorsal contribution to cavernous inflow. I have not been able to visualize plaque-associated vein leakage as some investigators have documented on dynamic cavernosography, but it is very difficult with current technology to image emissary veins despite their ubiquity.[92] My experience with CDDU suggests high-resolution sonography provides both a dynamic noninvasive vascular assessment of erectile function and can precisely localize penile plaques. Timing must take into account the dynamic phases of erection, the fact that penile pain may preempt complete smooth muscle relaxation, and the obstacle that severe penile deviations present to imaging.

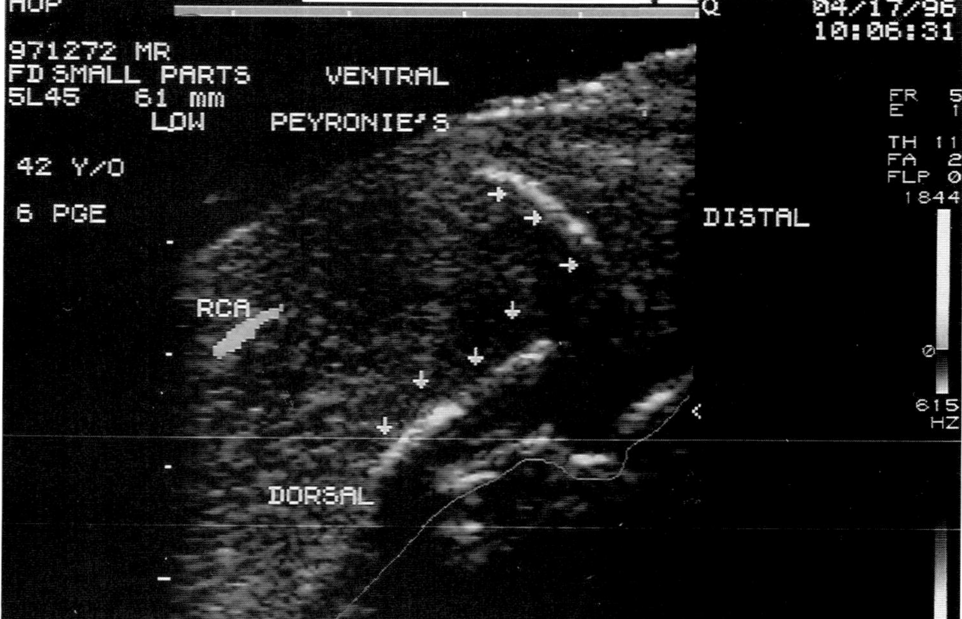

Fig. 6.22. Unusual Peyronie's plaque (*arrows*) of corporal tip; ventral sagittal scan shows corpora bodies ending within glans.

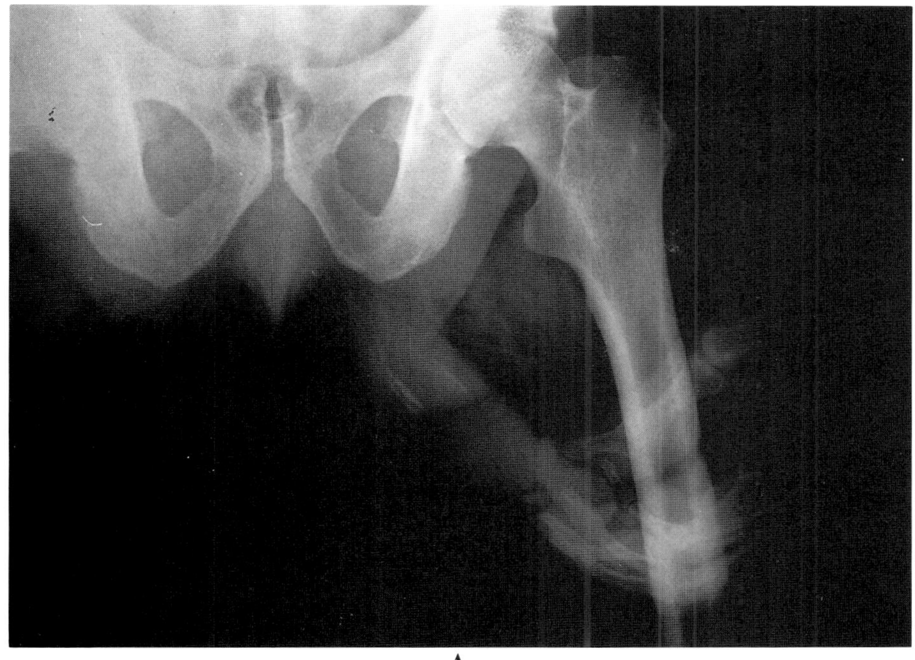

A

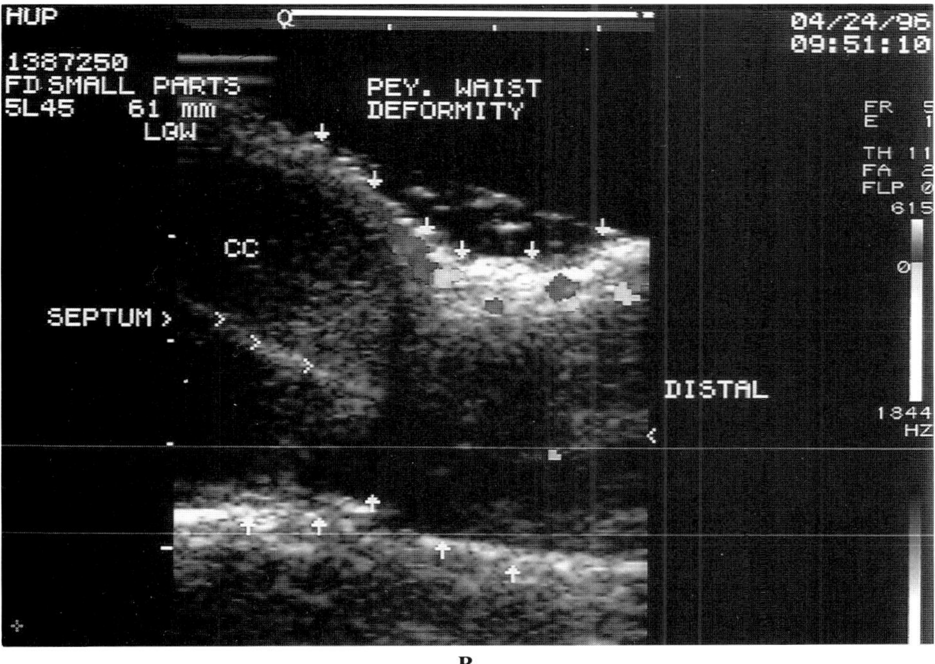

B

Fig. 6.23. A: Plain radiograph of calcified circumferential Peyronie's plaque. **B**: Sagittal CDDU image of same patients (*arrows*) highlights circumferential narrowing causing waist deformity.

The plaque should be imaged at 5–10 min in the latent/tumescent phase while the penis may still be straightened by the examiner, before the deformity associated with rigidity prevents imaging.

CONCLUSION

CDDU is minimally invasive and adds no additional risk to a diagnostic challenge of intracavernous vasoactive agent, the traditional penile blood flow study. CDDU/PBFS should be the first line of dynamic testing, when dynamic testing is performed. Doppler sonography is more accurate than physical examination alone following penile injection and exposes anatomic abnormalities as well as corporal hemodynamics unlike phalloarteriography. Important unanswered questions remain: What is an adequate first dosage in pharmacoerection testing? Should that dosage vary with age, or vasculogenic risk factors? False-positive evaluations can be avoided by either privacy and self-stimulation which enhance erectile responses with pharmacotesting in 70% of patients or redosing to achieve maximal smooth muscle relaxation.

REFERENCES

1. Consensus development conference statement: Impotence National Institutes of Health. *JAMA* 270(1):83–90, 1993.

2. Mellinger BC, Weiss J: Sexual dysfunction in the elderly male. *Am Urol Assoc Update Series* 11(19):146–152, 1992.

3. Feldman HA, Goldstein I, Hatzichristou DG, et al: Impotence and its medical and psychosocial correlates: results of the Massachusetts Male Aging Study. *Int J Impotence Res* 4(Suppl 2):A17, 1992.

4. Broderick GA, Arger PA: Duplex doppler ultrasonography: noninvasive assessment of penile anatomy and function. *Semin Roentgenol* 28(1):43–56, 1993.

5. Landwehr P: Penile vessels: erectile dysfunction. In Wolf K-J, Fobbe F (eds): *Color Duplex Sonography: Principles and Clinical Application.* Stuttgart, Thieme Medical Publishers, 1995, pp 204–215, .

6. Herbener TE, Seftel AD, Nehra A, et al: Penile ultrasound. *Semin Urol* 12(4):320–332, 1994.

7. King BF, Lewis RW, Mckusick MA: Radiologic evaluation of impotence. In Bennett AH (ed): *Impotence.* Philadelphia, WB Saunders, 1994, pp 52–91.

8. Gaskell P: The importance of penile blood pressure in cases of impotence. *Can Med Assoc J* 105:104, 1971.

9. Abelson D: Diagnostic value of the penile pulse and blood pressure: a Doppler study of impotence in diabetics. *J Urol* 113:636, 1975.

10. Michal V, Kramer R, Pospichal J: External iliac "steal syndrome". *J Cardiovasc Surg* 19:355, 1978.

11. Goldstein I, Siroky MB, North RI, et al: Vasculogenic impotence: role of the pelvic steal test. *J Urol* 128:300, 1982.

12. Schwartz AN, Lowe MA, Ireton R, et al: A comparison of penile brachial index and angiography: evaluation of corpora cavernosa arterial inflow. *J Urol* 143:510, 1990.

13. Bahren W, Gall H, Scherb W, et al: Arterial anatomy and arteriographic diagnosis of arteriogenic impotence. *Cardiovasc Intervent Radiol* 11:195–210, 1988.

14. Bookstein JJ, Lange EV: Penile magnification pharmacoarteric graphy: details of intrapenile arterial anatomy. *AJR* 148:883, 1987.

15. Rajfer J, Canan V, Dorey FJ, et al: Correlation between penile angiography and duplex scanning of cavernous arteries in impotent men. *J Urol* 143:1128–1130, 1990.

16. Breza J, Aboseif SR, Orivs BR, et al: Detailed anatomy of penile nerurovascular structures: surgical significance. *J Urol* 141:437–443, 1989.

17. Polascik TJ, Walsh PC: Radical retropubic prostatectomy: the influence of accessory pudendal arteries on the recovery of sexual function. *J Urol* 153:150–152, 1995.

18. Curet P, Grellet J, Perrin D, et al: Technical and anatomic factors in filling of distal portion of internal pudendal artery during arteriography. *Urology* 29:333, 1987.

19. Rosen MP, Greenfield AJ, Walker TG, et al: Arteriogenic impotence: findings in 195 impotent men examined with selective internal pudendal argiography. *Radiology* 174:1043, 1990.

20. Garibyan H, Lue TF: Anastomotic network between the dorsal and cavernous arteries in the penis. *J Urol* 143:221A, (1990).

21. Gall H, Bahren W, Scherb W, et al: Diagnostic accuracy of Doppler ultrasound technique of the penile arteries in correlation to selective arteriography. *Cardiovasc Intervent Radiol* 11:225, 1988.

22. Virag R: Intracavernous injection of papaverine for erectile failure. *Lancet* 2:398, 1982.

23. Brindley CS: Maintenance treatment of erectile impotence by cavernosal unstriated muscle relaxant injection. *Br J Psychiatry* 149:210, 1986.

24. Brindley CS: Cavernosal alpha-blockade: a new technique for investigating and treating erectile impotence. *Br J Psychiatry* 143:332, 1983.

25. Zorgniotti AW, Lefleur RS: Auto-injection of the corpus cavernosum with a vasoactive drug combination for vasculogenic impotence. *J Urol* 133:39, 1985.

26. Ishii N, Watanabe H, Irisawa C, et al: Studies on male sexual impotence report 18: therapeutic trial with prostaglandin E1 for organic impotence. *Jpn J Urol* 77:954–962, 1986.

27. Ishii N, Watanabe H, Irisawa C, et al: Intracavernous injection of prostaglandin E-1 for the treatment of erectile impotence. *J Urol* 141:323–325, 1989.

28. Bennett AH, Carpernter AJ, Barada JH: Improved vasoactive drug combination for pharmacloogical erection program. *J Urol* 146:1564, 1991.

29. Virag R, Frydman D, Legman M, et al: Intracavernous injection of papaverine as a diagnostic and therapeutic method in erectile failure. *Angiology* 35:79, 1984.

30. Lue TF: Impotence: a patient's goal directed approach to treatment. *World J Urol* 8:67, 1990.

31. Pescatori ES, Hatzichristou DG, Namburi S, et al: A positive intracavernous injection test implies normal veno-occlusive but not necessarily normal arterial function: a hemodynamic study. *J Urol* 151:1209–1216, 1994.

32. Lue TF, Hricak H, Marich KW, et al: Vasculogenic impotence evaluated by high resolution ultrasonography and pulsed Doppler spectrum analysis. *Radiology* 155:777, 1985.

33. McAninch JW, Laing FC, Jeffrey RB: Sonourethrography in the evaluation of urethral strictures. *J Urol* 139:294–297, 1988.

34. Benson CB, Doubilet PM, Richie JP: Sonography of the male genital tract. *AJR* 153:705–713, 1989.

35. Oates CP, Pickard PH, Powell PH, et al: The use of duplex ultrasound in the assessment of arterial supply to the penis in vasculogenic impotence. *J Urol* 153:354–357, 1995.

36. Banya Y, Ushiki T, Takagane H, et al: Two circulatory routes within the human corpus cavernosum penis: a scanning electron microscopic study of corrosion casts. *J Urol* 879:883, 1989.

37. Bookstein JJ: Cavernosal veno-occlusive insufficiency in male impotence: evaluation of degree and location. *Radiology* 164:175, 1987.

38. Aboseif SR, Lue TF: Hemodynamics of penile erection. *Urol Clin North Am* 15:1–7, 1988.

39. Andersson K-E, Wagner G: Physiology of penile erection. *Physiol Rev* 75(1):191–236, 1995.

40. Linet OI, Ogrinc FG: Efficacy and safety of intracavernosal asprostakil in men with erectile dysfunction. *N Engl J Med* 334(14):873–877, 1996.

41. Schwartz AN, Wang KY, Mack LA, et al: Evaluation of normal erectile function with color flow Doppler sonography. *AJR* 153:1155–1160, 1989.

42. Quam JP, King BF, James EM, et al: Duplex and color Doppler sonographic evaluation of vasculogenic impotence. *AJR* 153:1141–1147, 1989.

43. Paushter DM: Role of duplex sonography in the evaluation of sexual impotence. *AJR* 153:1161, 1989.

44. Collins JP, Lewandowski BJ: Experience with intracorporeal injection of papaverine and duplex ultrasound scanning for the assessment of arteriogenic impotence. *Baar J Urol* 59:84, 1987.

45. Herbner TE, Seftel AD, Nehra A, et al: Penile ultrasound. *Semin Urol* 12(4):320–332, 1994.

46. Burns PN: Hemodynamics and interpretation of Doppler signals. In Taylor KJW, Burns PN, Wells PNT: *Clinical Applications of Doppler Ultrasound*. New York, Raven Press, 1987.

47. Burns PN: Physical principles of Doppler ultrasound and spectral analysis. *J Clin Ultrasound* 15:567–590, 1987.

48. Foley WD, Erickson SJ: Color Doppler flow imaging. *AJR* 156:3–13, 1991.

49. Merritt CR: Doppler color flow imaging. *J Clin Ultrasound* 15:591–597, 1987.

50. Broderick GA, Lue TF: The penile blood flow study: evaluation of vasculogenic impotence. In Jonas U, Thon WF, Stief CG (eds): *Erectile Dysfunction*. Berlin, Heidelberg, New York, Springer-Verlag, 1991.

51. Wegner HEH, Andersen R, Knispel HH, et al: Evaluation of penile arteries with color coded duplex sonography: prevalence and possible therapeutic implications of connections between dorsal and cavernous arteries in impotent men. *J Urol* 153:1469–1471, 1995.

52. Paick JS, Won Lee S, Hyup Kim S: Doppler sonography of deep cavernosal artery of the penis: variation of peak systolic velocity according to sampling location. *Int J Impot Res* 6(1):A34, 1994.

53. Chung WS, Park YY, Back SY: The effect of measurement location of the blood flow parameters on their values during Duplex sonography. *Int J Impot Res* 6(1):A29, 1994.

54. Govier FE, Asase D, Hefty TR, et al: Timing of penile color flow duplex ultrasonography using a triple drug mixture. *J Urol* 153:1472–1475, 1995.

55. Meuleman EJH, Bemelmans BLH, Doesburg WH, et al: Penile pharmacological duplex ultrasonography: a dose effect study comparing papaverine, papaverine/phentolamine and PGE1. *J Urol* 148:63, 1992.

56. Fitzgerald SW, Erickson SJ, Foley WD, et al: Color Doppler sonography in the evaluation of erectile dysfunction: patterns of temporal response to papaverine. *AJR* 157:331–336, 1991.

57. Lue TF, Donatucci CF: The combined intracavernous injection and stimulation test: diagnostic accuracy. *J Urol* 148:61–62, 1992.

58. Nehra A, Hakim LS, Abokar RA, et al: A new method of performing duplex Doppler ultrasonography: effect of re-dosing of vasoactive agents on hemodynamic parameters. *J Urol* 153(4):415A, 1995.

59. Montorsi F, Guazzoni G, Barbieri L, et al: The effect of intracorporeal injection plus genital and audiovisual sexual stimulation versus second injection on penile color Doppler sonography parameters. *J Urol* 155:536–540, 1996.

60. Lue TF, Hricak H, Marich KW, et al: Evaluation of arteriogenic impotence with intracorporeal injection of papaverine and the duplex ultrasound scanner. *Semin Urol* 3:43–48, 1987.

61. Fitzgerald SW, Krysiewicz S, Mellinger C: The role of imaging in the evaluation of impotence. *AJR* 153:1133–1139, 1989.

62. Golub M, Zia P, Matsuno N, et al: Metabolism of prostaglandins A-1 and E-1 in men. *J Clin Invest* 59:1404, 1979.

63. Hamberg M: Biosynthesis of prostaglandin E-1 by human seminal vesicles. *Lipids* 11:249, 1976.

64. Hedquist P: PGE and prostaglandin and synthesis inhibitors of norepinephrine release from vascular tissue. In Robinson HJ, Vane ER (eds): *Prostaglandin Synthetase Inhibitors.* New York. Raven Press, 1973, p 303.

65. Meuleman EFJ, Bemelmans BLH, vanAsten W, et al: Assessment of penile blood flow by duplex ultrasonography in 44 men with normal erectile potency in different phases of erection. *J Urol* 147:51–56, 1992.

66. Mellinger BC, Fried JJ, Vaughan ED: Papaverine induced penile blood flow acceleration in impotent men measured by duplex scanning. *J Urol* 144:897, 1990.

67. Lue TF, Tanagho EA: Physiology of erection and pharmacological management of impotence. *J Urol* 137:829, 1987.

68. Benson CB, Vickers MA: Sexual impotence caused by vascular disease: diagnosis with duplex sonography. *AJR* 153:1149, 1989.

69. Shabsigh R, Fishman IF, Quesada ET, et al: Evaluation of vasculogenic erectile impotence using penile duplex ultrasonography. *J Urol* 142:1469, 1989.

70. Benson CB, Aruny JE, Vickers MA: Correlation of duplex sonography with arteriography in patients with erectile dysfunction. *AJR* 160:71–73, 1993

71. Shabisgh R, Fishman IJ, Shottland Y, et al: Comparison of penile duplex ultrasonography with nocturnal penile tumescence monitoring for the evaluation of erectile impotence. *J Urol* 143:924, 1990.

72. Lewis RW, King BF: Dynamic color doppler sonography in the evaluation of penile erectile disorders. *Int J Impot Res* 6(1):A30, 1994.

73. Rhee E, Osborn A, Witt M: The correlation of cavernous systolic occlusion pressure with peak velocity flow using color duplex doppler ultrasound. *J Urol* 153:358–360, 1995.

74. Schwartz AN, Lowe MA, Berger RE, et al: Assessment of normal and abnormal erectile

function; color doppler flow sonography versus conventional techniques. *Rad Sci North Am* 180:105–109, 1991.

75. Planiol T, Pourcelot L: Doppler effect study of the carotid circulation. In de Vlieger M, White DN, McCready VR (eds): *Ultrasonics in Medicine.* Amsterdam, Excerpta Medica, 1974, pp 104–111.

76. Kaplan HS: The concept of presbyrectia. *Int J Impot Res* 1:59, 1989.

77. Wespes E, deGoes PM, Schulman C: Vascular impotence: focal or diffuse penile disease. *J Urol* 1435:1436, 1992.

78. Kim N, Vardi Y, Padma-Nathan H, et al: Oxygen tension regulates the nitric oxide pathway. Physiological role in penile erection. *J Clin Invest* 91:3006–3012, 1993.

79. Saenz de Tejada I, Mooreland RB: Physiology of erection, pathophysiology of impotence, and implications of PGE₁ in the control of collagen synthesis in the corpus cavernosum. Proceedings of a Symposium, Kalamazoo, Michigan August 3–4, 1993. Excerpta Medica, pp 3–16.

80. Levin RM, Hypolite JA, Broderick GA: Dissociation of basal and stimulated tonic contraction of the corpus cavernosum with intracellular calcium during hypoxia. *J Urol* 153(4):A405, 1995.

81. Broderick GA, Arger PA: Penile blood flow study: age specific references ranges. *J Urol* 151(5):A371, 1994.

82. Merckx LA, De Bruyne RMG, Goes E, et al: The value of dynamic color duplex scanning in the diagnosis of venogenic impotence. *J Urol* 148:318–320, 1992.

83. McMahon CG, Daley J: Correlation of duplex ultrasonography, PBI, DICC and angiography in the diagnosis of impotence. *Int J Impot Res* 6(1):A32, 1994.

84. Naroda T, Yamanaka M, Matsushita K, et al: Evaluation of resistance index of the cavernous artery with color doppler ultrasonography for venogenic impotence. *Int J Impot Res* 6(1):D62, 1994.

85. Hinman F Jr: Priapism, reasons for failure of therapy. *J Urol* 83:420, 1960.

86. Broderick GA, Lue TF: Priapism and physiology of erection. *AUA Update Series* 7(29):225–232, 1988.

87. Broderick GA, Harkaway R: Pharmacological erection: time-dependent changes in the corporal environment. *Int J Impot Res* 6:9–16, 1994.

88. Spycher MA, Huuri D: The ultrastructure of the erectile tissue in priapirm. *J Urol* 135:142–147, 1986.

89. Witt MA, Goldstein I, Saenz de Tejada I, et al: Traumatic laceration of intracavernosal arteries: the pathophysiology of nonischemic, high flow arterial priapism. *J Urol* 143:129–132, 1990.

90. Walker TG, Gran PW, Goldstein I, et al: High-flow priapism: treatment with superselective transcatheter embolization. *Radiology* 174:1053–1054, 1990.

91. Hakim LS, Kulaksizoglu H, Mulligan R, et al: Evolving concepts in the diagnosis and treatment of arterial high flow priapism. *J Urol* 155:541–548, 1996.

92. Gasior BL, Levine FJ, Sowannesian A, et al: Plaque associated corporal veno-occlusive dysfunction in idiopathic Peyronie's disease: a pharmacavernosometric and pharmacocavernosographic study. *World J Urol* 8(2):90, 1990.

7

Penile Revascularization

Alexandru E. Benet
Jamil Rehman
Arnold Melman

The penis is a vascular organ and an erection is the result of a complex hemodynamic process. For an erection to occur, coordination of neural, vascular, and endocrine mechanisms, mediated by multiple neurotransmitters and complex hemodynamic processes are required.[1] Erectile dysfunction is a common problem that may affect as many as 30 million men in the United States.[2] Vasculogenic erectile dysfunction is believed to be the cause of 60 to 80% of men with organic erectile dysfunction.[3]

Vasculogenic erectile dysfunction may be treated by several treatment options. These include oral medications, vacuum devices, external splints, intracavernosal pharmacotherapy, penile implants, and vascular surgery. Of the options listed, intracavernosal pharmacotherapy is the most popular method.[4] Vascular surgery and specifically penile revascularization (inferior epigastric–penile bypass surgery) is the method expected to restore the patient's original erectile function without the need for additional treatment.

The fundamental technique of vascular surgery, named "three-stay suture technique,"[5] was first published by Carrel, who in 1912 was awarded the Nobel Prize for his development. After this revolutionary development, improved suturing materials, improved surgical techniques, the discovery of an anticoagulant substance by Howell which he named heparin,[6] and the introduction of the operating microscope[7] led to several improvements in medicine. During the last three decades the gold standard for vascular insufficiency is bypass surgery.[8,9]

This concept was adopted in the early 1970s by several urologists around the world, for the treatment of vasculogenic erectile dysfunction. In 1973 Michal et al.[10] first described the use of penile revascularization as a surgical treatment of erectile dysfunction. Initially they anastomosed the inferior epigastric artery directly to the corpus cavernosum[11] (Michal I) and subsequently end-to-side anastomosis of the inferior epigastric to the dorsal penile artery (Michal II).[12] With further refinements of microvascular surgery, additional techniques have evolved based on anastomoses of a donor arterial supply, usually the inferior epigastric artery to the dorsal arteries, deep dorsal vein, or the cavernosal arteries (Table 7.1).

TABLE 7.1. The History of Microvascular Penile Revascularization

1972	Michal I—Anastomosed inferior epigastric artery and corpus cavernosum
1977	Michal III—Anastomised inferior epigastric artery to dorsal penile artery
1980	Le-Veen Diaz—Arterialization of deep dorsal vein. He used saphenous vein graft to anastomose the femoral artery to the deep dorsal vein
1978 to 1988	Virag I—Inferior epigastric artery to deep dorsal vein end-to-side anastomosis, proximal vein open
	Virag II—Inferior or epigastric artery to deep dorsal vein end-to-side anastomosis, proximal vein tied
	Virag III—Interposition of Saphenous vein graft to deep dorsal vein end-to-side anastomosis, proximal vein tied
	Virag IV—Virag I plus veno-cavernous shunt
	Virag V—Virag II plus veno-cavernous shunt
	Virage VI—Virag III plus veno-cavernous shunt
1979	Crespo, Anastomised inferior epigastric artery to cavernosal artery
1979	Furlow-Fisher modification of Virag II with ligation of both proximal and distal ends of the deep dorsal vein
1982	McGregor & Konack, Direct anastomosis inferior epigastric artery to cavernosal artery
1983	McDougal and Jeffery modification of Michal II, anastomosed bilateral inferior epigastric arteries end to side to both dorsal arteries
1983	Hauri, Anastomosed Inferior epigastric artery to deep dorsal vein and dorsal artery joined together with creation arteriovenous fistula (Hauri fistula technique)
1984	Sharlip modification, Anastomosed inferior epigastric artery to proximal dorsal penile artery end to end fashion
1987	Carmignani Modification, Anastomosed inferior epigastric artery end to end to the proximal end of the transected dorsal artery and the distal stump of dorsal artery is anastomosed to the contralateral dorsal artery in an end-side fashion
1992	Lewis modification, Anastomosed inferior epigastric artery to an isolated segment of deep dorsal vein, end to end. Proximal and distant site of vein tied
1992	Junemann Modification of Hauri procedure. Three arterio-venous fistulae created instead of one to improve patency
1992	Austoni Modification, Anastomosed inferior epigastric artery to both the distal and proximal divided ends of the dorsal penile arteries
1995	Lund, Laproscopic retrieval of inferior epigastric artery

ETIOLOGY OF ARTERIOGENIC ERECTILE DYSFUNCTION

Erectile dysfunction develops if the arterial disease reduces the luminal diameter to such an extent that the blood supply to the penis decreases so that there is insufficient flow either to obtain or to maintain the erection. The best correlation with pudendal angiography was observed when the arterial occlusive disease occluded more than 50% of the luminal diameter of the penile artery.[13] Arteriogenic erectile dysfunction may be caused by generalized or localized blood vessel involvement.

The major risk factors for generalized vascular insufficiency include cigarette smoking, diabetes mellitus, hypertension, and hyperlipidemia.[14] Conditions affecting cardiac function and the major blood vessels will have an adverse effect on the blood flow to the penis during erection due to inadequate filling pressure.[15,16] Questioning a patient with vasculogenic erectile dysfunction may uncover overt signs of angina or intermittent claudication. These patients should be referred to the appropriate physician for investigation and management of these problems along with treatment of the erectile dysfunction.

Many conditions may affect the blood vessel function from aorta to end arterioles. Most conditions will lead to intimal plaque formation (atherosclerosis). As mentioned earlier, diabetes, hypertension, hyperlipidemia, and certain peripheral vasculopathies may lead to erectile dysfunction. Because the metabolic demands of the flaccid penis are low, only the most profound vascular occlusions (as sometimes observed in men with severe diabetes and hypertension) will result in gangrene of the penis. The usual event is that of impaired erection only.

The principal vascular supply to the penis is the internal pudendal artery and its branches. Injury to the internal pudendal artery usually does not produce ischemic damage to the penis unless collaterals are also damaged. The penis may get collateral supply from the external pudendal, obturator, and inferior gluteal arteries. These collaterals maintain tissue viability but are insufficient to meet the demands of increased blood flow needed to achieve and maintain a rigid erection. During major pelvic trauma, the hypogastric artery, internal pudendal artery, or the distal branches may be injured. The internal pudendal and common penile arteries are most commonly injured with blunt pelvic trauma, particularly those resulting in pelvic fractures.[17] Blunt perineal trauma may lead to intimal injury, shearing injury, disruption of vessels, injury by bony spicules, or a combination of any of these. Young men with traumatic disruption of the proximal penile blood supply usually have normal distal penile vasculature, as the occlusion is usually focal, and are ideal candidates for revascularization procedures.

ANATOMY AND PHYSIOLOGY OF THE PENIS IN THE FLACCID AND ERECT STATE

The descending aorta bifurcates into the two common iliac arteries, which further divide into the external iliac and internal iliac (hypogastric) arteries. The arterial blood supply to the penis is delivered through the paired internal pudendal arteries, the terminal branches of the internal iliac (hypogastric) arteries. The internal pudendal artery runs in a curve in the dorsolateral pelvic wall remotely from the viscera. It enters the lesser pelvis, accompanied by the nerve, through the lesser sciatic notch. It enters the ischiorectal fossa where it courses along in Alcock's canal along the inferior insertion of the obturator internus muscle. In men the internal pudendal gives rise to scrotal and bulbar branches (via a perineal branch) before continuing as the common penile artery. The latter pierce the urogenital diaphragm and continue along the medial margin of the inferior ramus of the pubis. In the anterior perineum near the bulbospongiosus, the penile artery divides into its terminal branches (trifurcation), the bulbourethral, cavernous artery (central or deep penile), and the dorsal artery (superficial penile) of the penis. The cavernosal artery is responsible for flow to the corporal bodies. The cavernosal artery enters the hilum of the penis adjacent to the junction of both cavernous bodies on either side. It gives off a short branch to the crus and then passes throughout the cavernous body almost to the tip. Along its course it gives off two types of branches. One supplies the smooth muscle and nerve fibers and the other divides into a series of helicine arteries. Blood flow in the helicine arteries passes directly into the cavernous sinusoidal spaces, allowing the penis to elongate and dilate without compromising the blood supply to the corpora cavernosa.[18] In many instances accessory arteries exist, arising from the external iliac, obturator, and other arteries occasionally becoming the dominant or the only arterial supply to the corpus cavernosum.[19] The bulbourethral artery is short and of large caliber and passes medially to enter the urethral bulb. It supplies the bulb, then continues distally within the corpus spongiosum alongside the urethra. The dorsal artery passes anteriorly to the crus and courses distally along

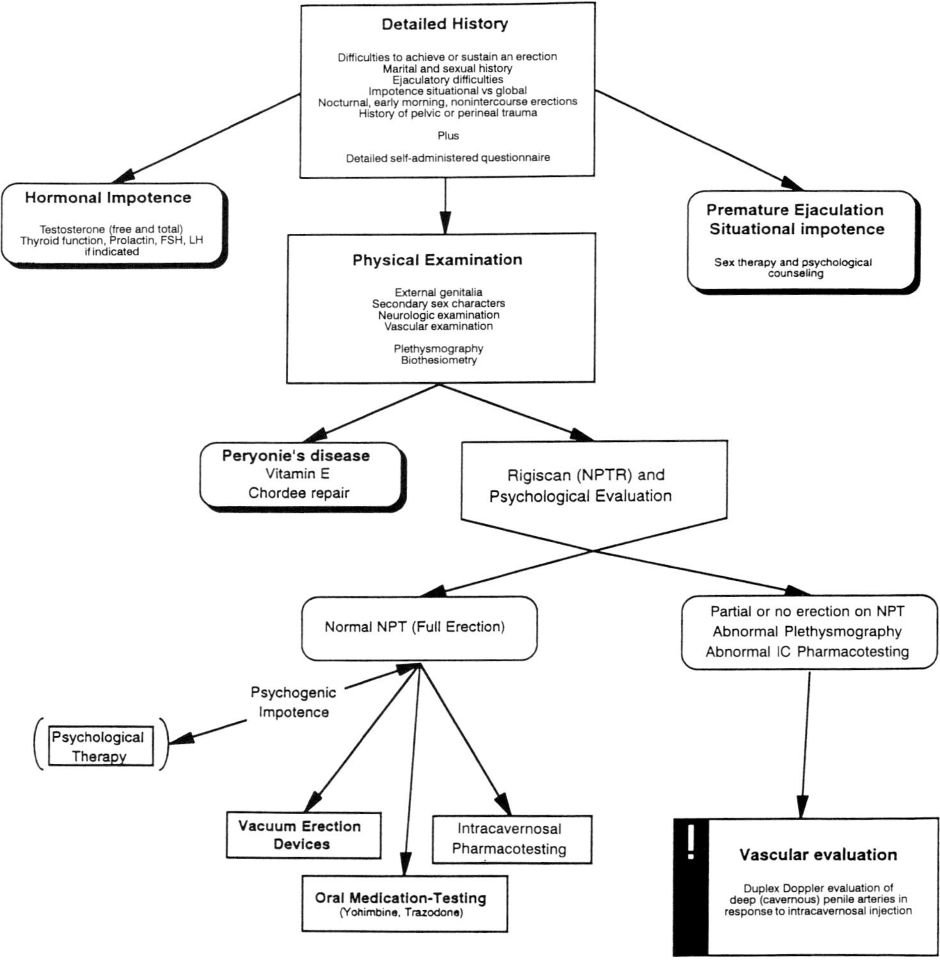

Fig. 7.1. Workup algorithm.

the dorsum of the penis under Buck's fascia between the deep dorsal vein medially and the dorsal nerve laterally toward the glans penis. It gives off several circumflex branches (from 3 to 10) to the mid-dorsal corpora cavernosa and, for this reason, bypass into a proximally occluded dorsal penile artery can improve flow into the corpora cavernosa. Anatomic variants are the rule and include both cavernous arteries originating from the same side, hypoplasia or absence of one dorsal penile artery, and accessory penile arteries. The latter may occur in 6–9%. Connective branches exist between the different penile arteries, and collateral vessels may open up in the presence of obstruction.

The penis is drained by three venous systems: the superficial, intermediate, and deep drainage systems. The superficial drainage system is formed from multiple superficial veins located between Colles' and Buck's fascia, merging near the root of the penis to form a single superficial dorsal vein, which usually drains into the saphenous veins. The intermediate drainage system is formed by the retrocoronal venous plexus forming the deep dorsal vein. The deep dorsal vein receives several circumflex and emissary veins that provide the main venous drainage of the glans penis, corpus spongiosum, and the distal two-thirds of the corpora cavernosa. The deep dorsal vein becomes the periprostatic venous plexus. The deep drainage system is draining the proximal corpora cavernosa and drains into the internal pudendal veins. Numerous communications exist among the three systems. For an erection to occur there are four crucial physiologic requirements: intact neurohormonal system, sufficient arterial supply, appropriate smooth muscle relaxation, and functional veno-occlusive system.[20] Assuming that the neurohormonal system and the corporal smooth muscle are intact, blood flow must increase 5- to 10-fold to attain an erection. Except for the increase in arterial inflow, the veno-occlusive mechanism is mandatory for the creation of a fully rigid erection. The veno-occlusive mechanism is dependent upon the normal function of the corporal smooth muscle. As the sinusoids dilate, and arterial flow increases, the relaxed trabecular walls are forced against the tunica albuginea compressing the subalbugineal venous plexus and subsequent reduction in venous outflow.

THE WORKUP ALGORITHM

The most important step in the diagnosis of erectile dysfunction is the history and physical exam. The history may be enhanced by the use of a sexual function questionnaire and by interviewing the sex partner.[21] The history should include the different disorders of sexual dysfunction, including desire, ejaculatory, orgasmic, and erectile dysfunction. In addition medical as well as social risk factors should be investigated (see questionnaire). The physical exam is a regular urologic physical exam including digital rectal examination, concentrating on the evaluation of the external genitalia and the peripheral pulses. During the physical exam two noninvasive tests may be performed, biothesiometry and plethysmography, which will give a hint as to the nervous sensory integrity and screening for arterial pathology.[22] After this initial exam, the patient will be evaluated by means of nocturnal penile tumescence for two nights,[23] and will have a thorough psychological evaluation which will include his sex partner[21] (Fig. 7.1).

PENILE VASCULAR EVALUATION

Several tests have been developed to evaluate the penile vascular function including intracavernous pharmacotesting with or without stimulation, radionuclear imaging,[24] dynamic infusion cavernosometry and cavernosography, penile Doppler ultrasound, and selective pudendal angiography. Candidates for penile bypass surgery should be evaluated initially by penile Doppler ultrasound, followed by pudendal angiogram. The other tests evaluate erectile capability and not specifically arterial incompetence.

PENILE DOPPLER ULTRASOUND

The modern pulsed Doppler ultrasound for the evaluation of penile blood flow was introduced by Lue et al.[25] The test is performed using a 10 to 13 MHz imaging frequencies and 5 to 7 Doppler frequencies. The major advantage of duplex/color ultrasound is the ability to visualize penile anatomy and measure arterial flow velocity and assess arterial compliance simultaneously (*Anatomy*, *Blood* flow, *Compliance*, *Drainage* of venous efflux of *ABCD* of penile ultrasound). Over the past decade, several Doppler parameters have been added to improve its accuracy and assess functions. These parameters include: end diastolic flow velocity, acceleration, acceleration time, and resistance index (RI). The examination is performed with the patient in the supine position, and the penis placed on the abdomen. A comfortable, warm secure setting is essential to reduce anxiety and thus sympathetic cavernous smooth muscle tone. Scanning should be performed several times to assess arterial diameter and compliance, peak flow velocity as well as waveform changes before and after intracavernosal pharmacotherapy. The initial exam is performed in the flaccid state. Both longitudinal and transverse planes are evaluated to detect structural and blood flow anomalies. The examination in the flaccid state is used to determine the echo texture of both corpora cavernosa, and the diameter and blood flow in the cavernosal arteries. Blood-filled sinusoids are relatively hypoechoic and form the background. Hyperechoic lesions of the tunica albuginea represent fibrosis and plaques. These parameters serve as baseline values for the values obtained after intracavernous pharmacotherapy. The location of the arteries is close to the septum near the hilium, and assumes a central position distally. They appear tortuous in the flaccid state and straight when the penis is stretched or in full erection. Communications between the paired cavernous arteries and between the cavernous and the dorsal arteries are common. When multiple arteries are present, they should be assessed individually (Fig. 7.2).

After the intracavernous injection, the examination is continued in the same fashion to observe the progression of the normal phases of the spectral waveform. The time of the injection is noted. Real-time sonographic imaging is repeated continuously, switching from side to side during erection until the maximum cavernosal artery diameter and cavernosal artery peak systolic velocity and end diastolic velocity measurements are recorded. Flow velocities should be measured immediately after injection. During the exam specific notation is made of erectile quality, penile curvature, and fibrotic bands that become apparent during the erection. In the flaccid state, cavernosal artery velocities range from 5 to 12 cm/sec; following intra-

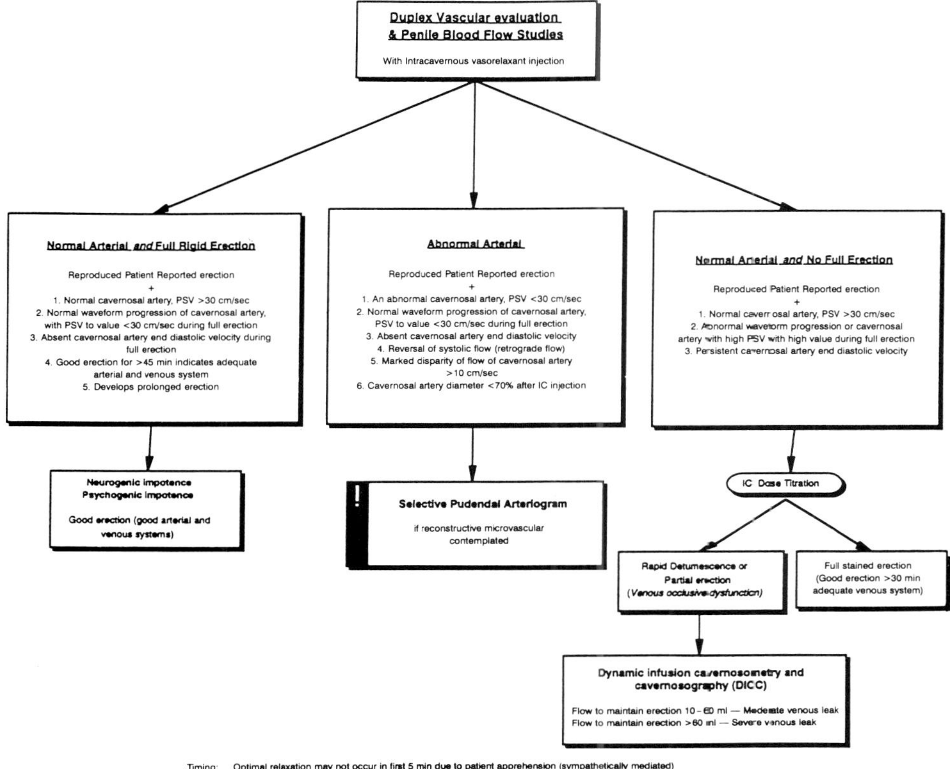

Fig. 7.2. Vascular evaluation.

cavernosal pharmacotherapy arterial velocities normally increase in the range of 30 to 120 cm/sec. Men with vasculogenic impotence do not exhibit this increase in flow after penile injection. Atherosclerotic or traumatic lesions to the arterial tree that keep the perfusion of the cavernosal bodies below this rate will cause erectile dysfunction. The high flows are usually reached during the tumescence phase prior to achievement of the rigid erection. In a normal erection, as the intracavernosal pressure approaches the mean systolic blood pressure, arterial inflow decreases from its maximal inflow value to virtually the arterial inflow during the flaccid state. This temporal relationship of arterial inflow to the corpora cavernosa is also observed during penile Doppler ultrasonography as a progression of velocity waveforms from minimal to maximal to minimal peak-systolic cavernosal artery velocities during the pharmacologic erection. The duplex ultrasound is also used to gain insight into the integrity of corporal veno-occlusive function. Physiologically, veno-occlusion and venous outflow resistance are the result of subtunical venule luminal narrowing from elongation and compression during erection. In normal veno-occlusion, following trabecular smooth muscle relaxation, the outflow from the corporal bodies is zero or even negative. Under such conditions, the corpora are virtually closed spaces which allow for only arterial inflow during cardiac systole. Thus, the study in normal corporal veno-occlusion should reveal absent end diastolic velocity. If the

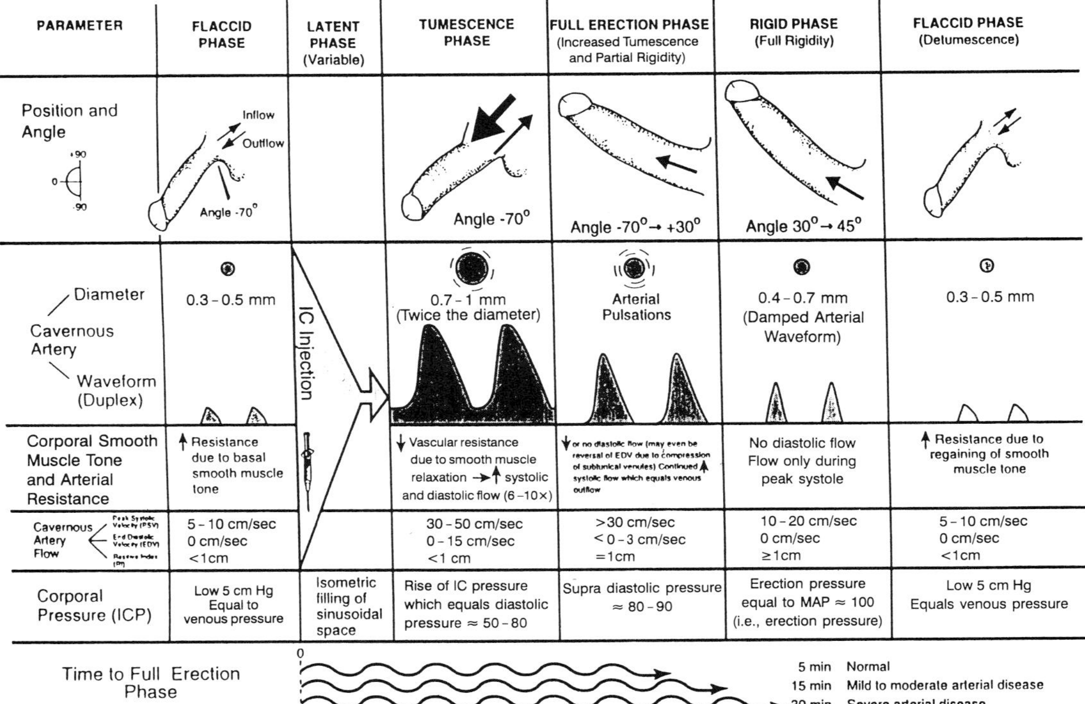

PARAMETER	FLACCID PHASE	LATENT PHASE (Variable)	TUMESCENCE PHASE	FULL ERECTION PHASE (Increased Tumescence and Partial Rigidity)	RIGID PHASE (Full Rigidity)	FLACCID PHASE (Detumescence)
Position and Angle	Inflow / Outflow; Angle -70°		Angle -70°	Angle -70° → +30°	Angle 30° → 45°	
Diameter / Cavernous Artery / Waveform (Duplex)	0.3 – 0.5 mm	IC Injection	0.7 – 1 mm (Twice the diameter)	Arterial Pulsations	0.4 – 0.7 mm (Damped Arterial Waveform)	0.3 – 0.5 mm
Corporal Smooth Muscle Tone and Arterial Resistance	↑ Resistance due to basal smooth muscle tone		↓ Vascular resistance due to smooth muscle relaxation → ↑ systolic and diastolic flow (6–10×)	↓ or no diastolic flow (may even be reversal of EDV due to compression of subtunical venules) Continued ↑ systolic flow which equals venous outflow	No diastolic flow Flow only during peak systole	↑ Resistance due to regaining of smooth muscle tone
Cavernous Artery Flow — Peak Systolic Velocity (PSV) / End Diastolic Velocity (EDV) / Resistive Index (RI)	5 – 10 cm/sec / 0 cm/sec / <1cm		30 – 50 cm/sec / 0 – 15 cm/sec / <1 cm	>30 cm/sec / <0 – 3 cm/sec / =1cm	10 – 20 cm/sec / 0 cm/sec / ≥1cm	5 – 10 cm/sec / 0 cm/sec / <1cm
Corporal Pressure (ICP)	Low 5 cm Hg Equal to venous pressure	Isometric filling of sinusoidal space	Rise of IC pressure which equals diastolic pressure ≈ 50 – 80	Supra diastolic pressure ≈ 80 – 90	Erection pressure equal to MAP ≈ 100 (i.e., erection pressure)	Low 5 cm Hg Equals venous pressure

Time to Full Erection Phase: 5 min — Normal; 15 min — Mild to moderate arterial disease; 30 min — Severe arterial disease.

Fig. 7.3. Penile duplex ultrasound and blood flow studies.

arterial response is adequate but the erection is poor or short-lived, penile veno-occlusive dysfunction is suspected and dynamic infusion cavernosometry cavernosography would then be recommended. On the other hand, if duplex ultrasound reveals poor arterial function in a young patient who is interested in arterial bypass, selective pharmacologic pudendal arteriography may be indicated (Fig. 7.3).

From the parameters available, cavernous arterial dilatation seems to be an unreliable parameter and in addition to peak systolic and end diastolic velocities, acceleration and acceleration time are used in the diagnosis of arteriogenic erectile dysfunction. During the test the flows in the dorsal arteries are determined as well as the patency and flow in the deep dorsal vein. The results of this test will determine if the patient has functional arterial pathology and should undergo selective pudendal angiogram prior to bypass surgery.

FUNCTIONAL SELECTIVE PHARMACOPUDENDAL ANGIOGRAPHY

Hemodynamic Versus Morphologic Lesion

Pharmacopudendal angiogram is usually performed after penile Doppler ultrasound in patients who are candidates for penile bypass surgery. The introduction of intracavernous injection of vasoactive medications (ICI) has improved the quality of the study so much that only local anesthesia with sedation and one percutaneous femoral puncture is now needed. The test should include a nonselective pelvic angiogram with a catheter above the aortic bifurcation — the pelvic flush, and selective pudendal angiogram on each side. The nonselective pelvic angiogram is used for the diagnosis of pathologic findings in the common iliac arteries or the origin of the hypogastric arteries and for the visualization of the inferior epigastric arteries — the future donor vessels for penile bypass surgery (Fig. 7.4). Those pathologies may be amenable to balloon dilatation,[26] or surgery on larger blood vessels.[16] An angiographic sheath is introduced into the right femoral artery. A pigtail catheter is placed in the low abdominal aorta, and bilateral oblique flush pelvic angiograms are obtained using a mixture of Hexabrix and ioxaglate sodium 30 ml at 12 ml/sec, filming at one per second. After the pelvic flush is completed, an intracavernous injection of 0.2 Trimix is injected. A smaller pigtail catheter is then advanced into the origin of the internal pudendal artery using 24 ml Hexabrix at 4 ml/sec and the ipsilateral anterior oblique projection at a slant of 45° of axis filming at one per second. Timing of the arteriogram is very important as it should be done after the drug has relaxed the corporal smooth muscles by simultaneous intracavernous pharmacotherapy. Poor visualization of the cavernous artery may result in false interpretation of arterial disease.

- Simultaneous intracavernosal pharmacologic injection is necessary and in certain cases intra-arterial vasodilators may be required
- The test includes pelvic flush study, bilateral hypogastric arteries, and selective internal pudendal arteriography

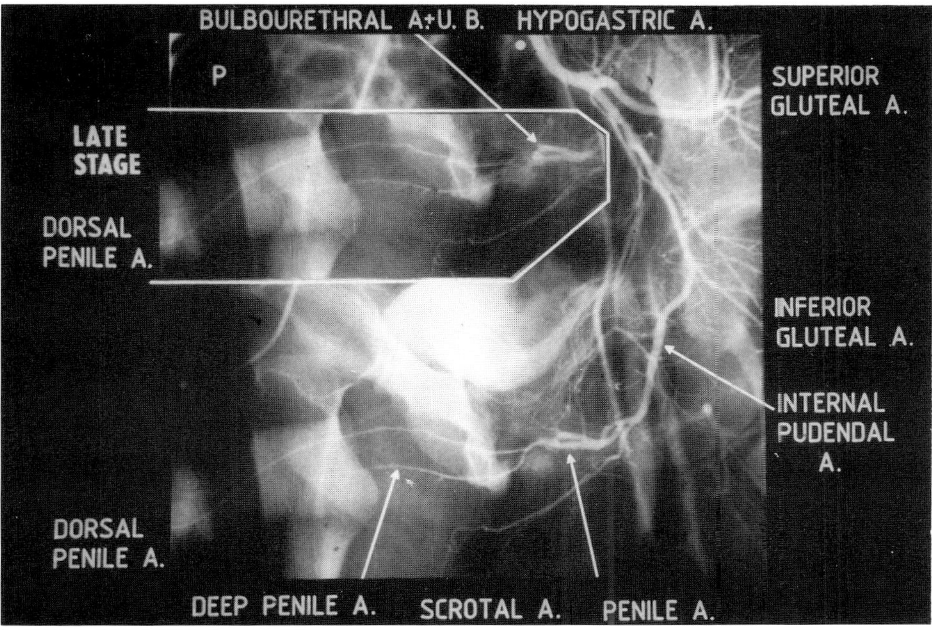

Fig. 7.4. Selective pudendal angiogram. Courtesy of Dr. Vaclav Michal. From *Clin Endocrinol Metab*. With permission.

- During the study, donor (inferior epigastric) and recipient arteries (dorsal arteries) are visualized

- Magnification views or subtraction studies may aid in visualization of these small arteries.

- The positioning used is left anterior oblique for left artery study and right anterior oblique for right artery study

Arteriographic Signs of Significant Vascular Disease

- Bilateral occlusion of the common penile artery in Alcock's canal
- Delay in filling of cavernosal arteries compared to other penile vessels
- Abrupt termination of arteries, particularly in the perineal segment of the penile artery
- Late collateral filling
- Retrograde filling of the cavernous artery from the dorsal artery
- Nicking, beading, or narrowing of the deep penile or cavernous artery and tributaries

Arterial disease may involve any part of the vessel, but the distal pudendal artery or proximal penile branches are more frequently involved. It needs to be emphasized that significant bilateral arterial obstruction needs to be present for arteriogenic impotence and thus unilateral revascularization may restore potency. The selective arteriogram may be limited to the one side if a normal ipsilateral cavernosal and dorsal artery is demonstrated and no collateral flow is shown to indicate contralateral disease,[27] otherwise both sides have to be visualized. Erectile dysfunction associated with pudendal arteriovenous malformation will demonstrate early passage of contrast medium from the bulbar artery to a large tortuous vein or veins in the pelvis. In cases of noniatrogenic trauma, arterial obstruction may be at variable and multiple levels. These may be from the internal iliac artery to the penile artery and its terminal branches. If collateral arteries fill the cavernosal and dorsal arteries but both fail to opacify distally, the presence of isolated stenosis in the common or internal iliac arteries makes percutaneous transluminal angioplasty (PTA) a feasible option. However, before attempting PTA the distal arterial tree must be shown to be intact as the success of the procedure depends to a large degree on a normal distal internal pudendal artery and its branches.

TREATMENT

Disease Proximal to Origin of Internal Pudendal Artery

Aortoiliac Reconstruction

Aortoiliac reconstruction is generally performed for conditions other than isolated erectile dysfunction. Although aortoiliac surgery may provide an opportunity to improve blood flow to the penis and thus improve erectile function, the surgical procedure may make sexual function worse.[28] Simple aortic replacement or bypass of the diseased aorta into the common iliac arteries in the absence of outflow disease should allow hypogastric perfusion to take place normally. However, if the distal limbs of an aortic bypass graft are placed into the external iliac arteries to bypass proximal disease or if the distal anastomoses are performed in an end-to-end fashion, thus preventing retrograde flow to the hypogastric arteries, the hypogastric arteries will not be perfused by the neoarterial inflow. In this case the need for reimplantation of the hypogastric arteries into the graft is essential. Attention should be paid to prevent damage to the superior hypogastric plexus, and revascularization of the hypogastric arteries has led to a higher success rate in restoring erectile function.

Angioplasty

Percutaneous transluminal angioplasty is widely used in focal vascular occlusive disease. Improvement of sexual potency following angioplasty was reported by several authors.[26,29,30] Angioplasty of the internal pudendal arteries, or internal iliac arteries, or both improves the blood inflow and often restores or improves erectile function. Angioplasty should be performed during the pudendal angiogram in vessels that are amenable to balloon dilatation.

Disease Distal to Origin of Internal Pudendal Artery

The procedure is selected depending upon the arteriographic pattern. The inferior epigastric artery is usually used as the donor artery (Table 7.2).

Methods of Penile Arterial Surgery

All the procedures listed are based on two parts of the surgical procedure; the first part is the harvesting of the inferior epigastric artery and the second part is the anastomosis between the inferior epigastric artery and the penile dorsal arteries or the deep dorsal vein. Historically attempts have been made to create anastomoses between the inferior epigastric artery and the corpus cavernosum[10] or to anastomose the inferior epigastric artery to the cavernosal arteries.[31] These methods have been abandoned because of their low success rate. Nowadays the anastomoses are performed mainly between the inferior epigastric artery and the dorsal arteries or the dorsal vein or both in different combinations.

Harvesting of the Inferior Epigastric Artery

With the patient under general anesthesia in the supine position, a midline incision extending from the umbilicus to the superior rim of the pubic bone is made. This approach enables the surgeon to use the best artery or both arteries in certain cases. The linea alba is incised and one rectus muscle is retracted to expose the inferior epigastric artery and its two accompanying veins. During the dissection of the inferior epigastric artery, thermal or other physical injury should be avoided. The dissection is done with the aid of magnifying loupes. The length of the arterial stump should exceed the distance measured since the artery tends to shrink after it is dissected, and a tension-free anastomosis should be used. The uppermost part of the

TABLE 7.2. Surgical Approach

Arteriographic Level of Obstruction	*Microvascular Bypass Procedure of Choice*
1. Proximal disease Bilateral focal disease proximal to cavernosal artery in the internal pudendal or common penile artery prior to bifurcation to dorsal or cavernosal artery	Inferior epigastric artery to dorsal penile artery to increase perfusion pressure and inflow to cavernosal arteries either retrograde through the proximal dorsal arteries or through the distal dorsal artery branches to cavernosal artery.
2. Distal disease Arterial occlusive disease in both cavernosal arteries and dorsal arteries	Inferior epigastric artery to an isolated dorsal vein to increase perfusion pressure and inflow to the corpora in a retrograde fashion from the deep dorsal vein graft through the emissary vein and subtunical vein.
Unilateral cavernosal artery occlusion with an ipsilateral occluded dorsal artery in conjunction with the contralateral dorsal proximal arterial occlusive disease and a communication between the contralateral dorsal, penile artery and the contralateral cavernosal artery	Inferior epigastric artery to isolated deep dorsal vein segment in a side to side fashion and dorsal penile artery (jump anastomosis) in end to end or end to side fashion. Location of anastomosis depends on the location of the dorsal artery to cavernosal artery communication. This increases perfusion pressure and inflow to corpora using both available pathways, through the dorsal artery to cavernosal artery and retrograde through the emissary vein off the deep dorsal vein graft.
Bilateral cavernosal artery occlusion with an ipsilateral normal dorsal artery	Direct or jump artery-venous shunt created of normal dorsal artery to an isolated deep dorsal vein segment. This increases perfusion pressure and inflow to corpora retrograde from the deep dorsal graft through the emissary and subtunical veins.
Absence of suitable dorsal penile arteries.	Virag V procedure is recommended.

artery is dissected up to the point where the artery perforates the rectus muscle. This part usually is at the level of the umbilicus. The artery is then ligated with a 2-0 silk tie that will be used to pull the artery to the anastomotic site. A second incision on the dorsal base of the penis is performed. A passage is created between the lower part of the midline incision and the penile incision. The artery is then pulled through the passage to the anastomotic site and either papaverine or 2% xylocaine is applied topically to the inferior epigastric artery to promote relaxation of the blood vessel.

Revascularization of the Dorsal Penile Artery

The most common technique employed is the neoarterial inflow into the dorsal penile artery (modified Michal II) to eventually access the deep penile artery via a patent common penile artery bifurcation. The eventual success of this artery-to-artery approach is dependent not only upon an adequate flow of perfusion pressure in the neoarterial inflow source but also upon the presence of a patent bifurcation and adequate distal arterial runoff. As a result, the ideal candidate for such a revascularization has to date been the young patient suffering from focal cavernosal artery occlusive disease following blunt perineal or pelvic trauma. An attempt should be made to anastomose the inferior epigastric artery to both dorsal arteries, one end to side and the other side to side. The adventitia should be preserved in all vessels by minimizing the surgical dissection to the vessel except at the site of vascular anastomosis. This helps preserve vasa nervosum, preventing denervation supersensitivity and vasa vasorum supplying arterial wall nutrition. With the aid of the operating microscope a 10-0 nylon suture is used for the anastomosis between the inferior epigastric and the dorsal arteries.

Dorsal Vein Arterialization

Various venous arterialization procedures have been developed to increase the caliber of the anastomotic site as well as the flow, perfusion pressure, and thus distal runoff at the anastomosis. The development and utilization of a venous access for corpus cavernosum revascularization obviates the prerequisite for focal arterial occlusive disease and as a result has enabled the application of penile revascularization procedures to a much larger patient population, i.e., the more commonly seen, relatively younger patient with a history of atherosclerotic vascular risk factors and diffuse arteriosclerotic occlusive disease of the hypogastric–cavernous arterial bed. With deep dorsal vein arterialization, neoarterial blood supply is brought into the corporal space in a retrograde fashion through the deep dorsal vein. The modified Virag I procedure consisted of anastomosis of the inferior epigastric artery to the deep dorsal vein in an end-to-side fashion. Subsequent modifications were made to the operative technique. The Virag I–III[32,33] procedures differ in what serves as the arterial source and whether or not the proximal dorsal vein is ligated. The Virag IV–VI[34,35] procedures differ from the earlier variations in that a direct shunt from the dorsal vein of the penis into the cavernous body is also created. The choice to perform the dorsal vein–cavernous anastomosis is made if the patient has inflow disease. Furlow and Fisher[36] modified the Virag procedures in which they arterialized a segment of the deep dorsal vein between distal and proximal ties with the route to the cavernous bodies being only the perforating emissary vein. The advantage of deep dorsal vein arterialization is that the anastomosis is technically easier because the dorsal vein is larger than the dorsal or central penile arteries. Another advantage is that penile arterial blood flow that is present is allowed to continue unimpeded, since no surgery is being performed on the arteries. Furthermore, when deep dorsal vein arterialization is used, the hemodynamics of the venous system are altered in a potentially advantageous way. Ligation of the proximal vein may prevent some degree of venous leak. During the dissection of the deep dorsal vein care is taken not to damage the vessels, emissary vein branches, or the adjacent dorsal nerve. Topical papaverine is used to prevent vascular spasm. Distal branches are ligated to prevent postoperative glans hyperemia. Exposure of the proximal deep dorsal vein is ultimately gained within the suspensory ligament. The vessel is ligated proximally under the pubic symphysis between the onset of the suspensory ligament and the urogenital diaphragm. At this proximal location, there are usually no emissary branches draining into the deep dorsal vein as the separate crural venous system drains the penile crura. In certain cases the crural and cavernosal veins are ligated, especially in patients who could not achieve a fully rigid erection. This deep dorsal vein segment may have several valves within the lumen. The most common pattern of valves includes one proximal valve at the junction of the suspensory and fundiform ligaments and one distal valve near the glans penis. Valve ablation is now carried out very gently with 2-F valvulotome.

Longitudinal venotomy is done with a microscalpel to create a window. The anastomotic site of the inferior epigastric artery is spatulated. The sutures are placed initially at each apex of the anastomosis and then subsequently 3 to 4 interrupted sutures are placed in between. A second anastomosis may be subsequently completed between the distal aspect of the inferior epigastric artery and the dorsal artery in an end-to-side or end-to-end fashion. Modifications of the above described procedure are used depending upon the location of the blockage (Fig. 7.5).

Surgical Candidates

The ideal candidate is a young patient with a history of blunt trauma and a minimum of modifiable vascular risk factors. The patient should demonstrate a hemodynamic abnormality of arterial inflow in the presence of normal corporal veno-occlusive function. The following questions need to be answered before deciding on therapy: (1) Will the patient benefit from arterial revascularization? (2) What surgical technique to use? (see Table 7.2)

Patient selection criteria:

1. Age less than 60 yr.
2. Absence of diabetes.
3. Delayed or absent response to intracavernous injection of vasoactive agents.
4. Penile duplex documenting cavernosal flows below 30 cm/sec during the first 5 min.
5. Pudendal angiogram documenting dysfunctional or absent cavernosal arteries.
6. Minimal or no veno-occlusive dysfunction

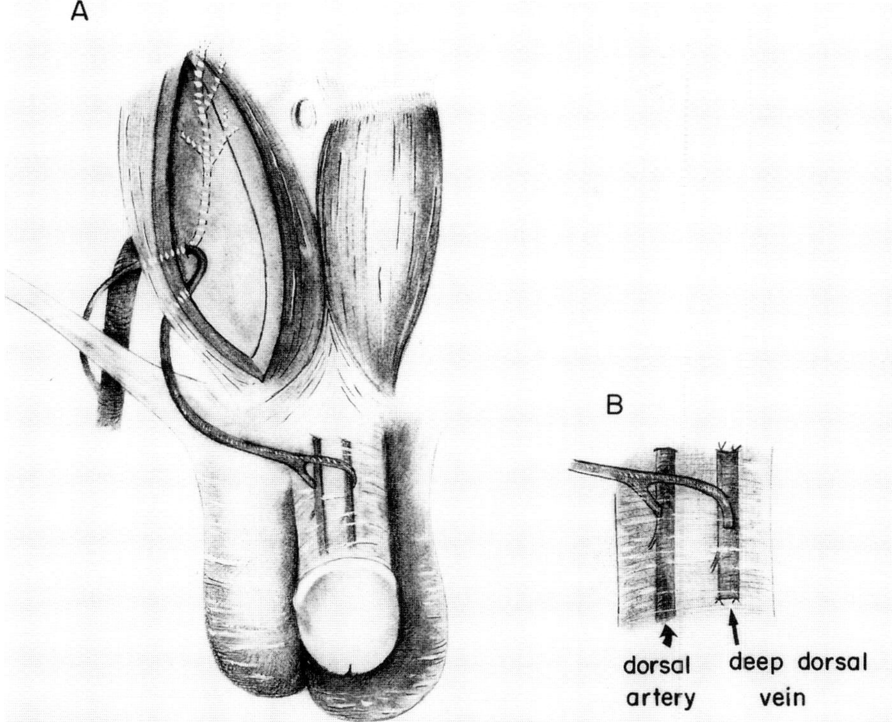

Fig. 7.5. Inferior epigastric to dorsal artery and deep dorsal vein anastomosis. From Melman A. Surgery of Impotence. In Droller M (eds) Surgical Management of Urologic Disease—An Anatomic Approach, Mosby—Year Book, St. Louis, MO, 1992, p. 887. Reproduced with permission.

Factors Affecting Long-term Patency

1. Prevention of ischemic, mechanical, or thermal injury to the vascular endothelium of the donor or recipient vascular structures.

2. Adventitia should be preserved in all vessels by minimizing the surgical dissection to the vessel because vasa vasorum supply blood to the layers of the vessel and vasa nervosum preservation prevents denervation supersensitivity.

3. Perfect transmission of systolic arterial inflow pressures and flow (i.e., no anastomotic strictures) with good arterial runoff into the penile vessels.

4. Patients are maintained on baby aspirin, a tablet daily beginning in the recovery room.

Complications

1. Mechanical disruption of the microvascular anastomosis and subsequent uncontrolled arterial hemorrhage may occur from blunt trauma in the first few postoperative weeks following coitus, masturbation, or from accidents. We recommend abstinence from sexual activities involving the erect penis until 6 wk postoperatively.

2. Glans hyperemia is a complication that occurs in 2% of patients who undergo deep dorsal vein arterialization. This occurs when unrecognized collateral veins communicate from the dorsal vein to the glans penis or from a direct cavernosal/spongiosal communication. The distal penile skin and glans become abnormally engorged with blood. After several days of elevated pressure, local edema develops, and skin breakdown can occur. Embolization of the inferior epigastric artery is an available option. Surgical exploration and subsequent ligation of all distal branches in the deep dorsal vein segment may solve the problem. Ligating the distal end of the deep dorsal vein usually prevents the occurrence of this complication.

3. Anastomotic occlusion. Early occlusion due to technical errors and late occlusion due to myointimal proliferation. Vein grafts have been proposed as optimal conduits for small vessel arterial occlusive disease since they possess native endothelium with intrinsic biologic properties which modulate the blood–graft interface and thus maintenance of vascular patency. Postoperatively, baby aspirin is administered daily for 6 months.

4. Diminished penile sensation or penile pain from injury to the nearby dorsal nerve.

5. Penile length loss due to fibrosis of the suspensory and fundiform ligaments postoperatively may lead to diminished penile length. Preserving the two ligaments has markedly minimized these complications.

Results

Our first follow-up results[37] were published in 1993. Since then we follow our operated patients and update our follow-up results.[38–40] From 1987 to 1995, 36 patients were diagnosed as having decreased vascular inflow as the main cause for their erectile dysfunction. The mean age was 46 yr with age range from 21 to 62 yr. The average follow-up time was 38 months.

All patients underwent an extensive workup to determine the cause of their problem.[22] Seven patients had medical history significant for hypertension, 2 patients for diabetes mellitus, 6 patients for pelvic trauma, 15 patients a significant history for smoking, 4 patients for alcohol, and 4 patients for peripheral vascular disease. Of the 36 patients who underwent a revascularization procedure for their erectile dysfunction, 8 patients were lost to follow-up. The selective pudendal angiography was used to help to decide which revascularization procedure was to be attempted. The final decision was made, however, after direct visualization of the status of the dorsal arteries with the operating microscope. The two operative procedures done were inferior epigastric artery to the deep dorsal vein in an end-to-side fashion (18 patients) or inferior epigastric artery to the dorsal artery (side-to-side) and deep dorsal vein (end-to-side) (18 patients). Because of the reported success in improving the patency of the microanastomotic sites with the use of plasma expanders, we have added the use of hetastarch during our surgery. For this report, patients were then asked to return for follow-up and to answer a questionnaire regarding their satisfaction with the procedure. Early in the series, patients with adult onset diabetes were included. Soon thereafter, however, it was decided that men with diabetes mellitus were to be excluded because surgical failures might have been a result of pathology from the diabetes and not as technical failures of the

TABLE 7.3. Results

Surgical Procedure	Cure	Improvement	Failure	Lost to Follow-up	Total
Procedure I Inferior epigastric artery to deep dorsal vein	7	4	3	4	18
Procedure II Inferior epigastric artery to dorsal artery and to deep dorsal vein	6*	4	4	4	18

*One patient had inferior epigastric artery to bilateral dorsal arteries and deep dorsal vein.

surgery. Therefore, only two patients with diabetes mellitus had a revascularization procedure performed at our center. Of the 28 patients observed, 13 patients experienced total return of their erections. Eight patients had improvement of their erections but required adjuvant intracorporal injection therapy to obtain a rigid erection. Seven of the eight patients who had improvement had the onset of a spontaneous erection for a short period postoperatively; however, they lost the ability for spontaneous rigid erection. The remainder of the patients, 7 of the 28, had no improvement of erectile function after surgery and were thus classified as failures. Of the 13 patients cured, 3 patients had a medical history significant for hypertension and one of these also had an additional history of peripheral vascular disease and alcohol abuse. Two patients had a medical history for pelvic trauma in addition to a smoking history. Of the remaining 8 patients, 1 patient had medical history significant for peripheral vascular disease and smoking, whereas 3 other patients had medical history only for smoking. Four patients had no medical history. Of the 13 patients cured, 7 patients had an inferior epigastric artery to deep dorsal vein whereas 6 patients had inferior epigastric artery to deep dorsal vein and dorsal artery. Of the 8 patients who had shown improvement after surgery, 2 patients had medical history significant for hypertension and smoking whereas one had history of alcohol abuse and the other had a history of pelvic trauma. One of the remaining 6 had a history of alcohol abuse in addition to a smoking history. One patient had a history that only included smoking. Four others had no medical history. Of those who had improved erections after surgery, 4 had an inferior epigastric artery to deep dorsal vein anastomosis, whereas the other 4 had an inferior epigastric artery to dorsal artery and deep dorsal vein anastomosis. Of those 7 patients who had no improvement, 2 patients had a medical history significant of hypertension and peripheral vascular disease and 1 of them had, in addition, a medical history of diabetes mellitus and smoking. Of the remaining 5 patients, one had a significant history of diabetes mellitus and smoking, one only of smoking and the remaining 3 with no significant medical history. Two patients after having their revascularization surgery eventually had a penile prosthesis placed. One patient now uses a vacuum device. Of the 8 patients who were lost to follow-up, 3 patients had a medical history of pelvic trauma, 2 patients had a history of smoking; 1 of these also had a history of alcohol abuse. Three patients had no significant medical history. Of the total 36 patients who underwent revascularization procedures, only three complications were observed. One patient experienced glans hypervascularization requiring distal deep dorsal vein ligation, 1 patient had a wound hematoma that needed to be drained, and 1 patient complained of severe postoperative pain (Table 7.3).

CONCLUSION

The outcome of a surgical procedure in general is dependent on correct diagnosis, surgical technique, and the processes that occur during healing. Arterial insufficiency as a cause of erectile failure is one of the few disease processes that allow specific correction of the problem. The option of resumption of erection without the need for interventional aides is an attractive one to many suffering from erectile dysfunction. Further improvement in the surgical success rate will be achieved with improved understanding of erectile physiology, diagnostic methodology, and both microsurgical and radiologic techniques. It is our conclusion that penile revascularization is an effective treatment alternative in a select group of patients with pure arteriogenic erectile dysfunction, particularly in young men.

REFERENCES

1. Lerner S, Melman A, Christ G: A review of erectile dysfunction: new insights and more questions. *J Urol* 149:1246–1255, 1993.

2. Feldman H, Goldstein I, Hatzichristou D, et al: Impotence and its medical and psychological correlates: results of the Massachusetts male aging study. *J Urol* 151:54–61, 1994.

3. Benet AE, Melman A: The epidemiology of erectile dysfunction. *Urol Clin North Am* 22:699–709, 1995.

4. Dennis M, Benet AE, Melman A: Patient's preference in the treatment of erectile dysfunction. *J Urol* (*in press*).

5. Carrel A: La technique des anastomoses vasculaires et la transplantation de visceres. *Lyon Med* 98:859–864, 1902.

6. Howell W, Holt E: Two new factors in blood coagulation—heparin and prothrombin. *Am J Physiol* 47:328–341, 1918.

7. Nylen C: The microscope in aural surgery, its first use and later development. *Acta Otolaryngol Supple* 116:226–240, 1954.

8. Chenvechai C, Irarrazaval M, Loop F, et al: Aorta-coronary bypass grafting with the internal mammary artery: clinical experience in 70 patients. *J Thorac Cardiovasc Surg* 70:278–281, 1975.

9. Isom O, Spencer F: The current status of bypass grafting for coronary artery disease [Review]. *South Med J* 68:897–907, 1975.

10. Michal V, Kramer R, Pospichal J, et al: Direct arterial anastomosis on corporal cavernosa penis in therapy of erectile impotence. *Rozhledy V Chirugii* 52:587–593, 1973.

11. Michal V, Kramar R, Pospichal J: Femoro-pudendal bypass, internal iliac thromboendarterectomy and direct arterial anastomosis to the vacernous body in the treatment of erectile impotence. *Bull Soc Int Chirurgie* 33:343–350, 1974.

12. Michal V, Kramar R, Pospichal J, et al: Vascular surgery in the treatment of impotence; its present possibilities and prospects. *Czechoslovak Med* 3(3):213–217, 1980.

13. Rosen M, Greenfield AJ, Walker TG, et al: Arteriogenic impotence: findings in 195 impotent men examined with selective internal pudendal angiography. Young Investigator's Award. *Radiology* 174:1043–1048, 1990.

14. Virag R, Brouilly P, Frydman D: Is impotence an arterial disorder? A study of arterial risk factors in 440 impotent men. *Lancet* 1:181–184, 1985.

15. Leriche R: Des obliterations arterielles hautes comme cause d'une insuffisance circulatoire des membres inferieurs. *Bull Soc Chirurgie* 49:1404, 1923.

16. DePalma RG, Olding M, Yu GW, et al: Vascular interventions for impotence: lessons learned. *J Vasc Surg* 21:576–584; discussion 584–585, 1995.

17. Levine F, Greenfield A, Goldstein I: Arteriographically determined occlusive disease within the hypogastric–cavernous bed in impotent patients following blunt perineal and pelvic trauma. *J Urol* 144:1147–1153, 1990.

18. Newman HF, Northup JD: Mechanism of human penile erection: an overview. *Urology* 17(5):399–408, 1981.

19. Breza J, Aboseif S, Orvis B, et al: Detailed anatomy of penile neurovascular structures: surgical significance. *J Urol* 141:437–443, 1989.

20. Melman A, Christ G, Hirsch M: Anatomy and physiology of the penis. In: Bennett A (ed). *Impotence*: Philadelphia, WB Saunders, 1994, pp 18–30.

21. Tiefer L, Melman A: Interview of wives: a necessary adjunct in the evaluation of impotence. *Sex Disabil* 6:167–175, 1983.

22. Benet AE, Sharaby J, Melman A: Male erectile dysfunction assessment and treatment options. [Review]. *Compr Ther* 20:669–673, 1994.

23. Benet AE, Rehman J, Melman A: The correlation between the new RigiScan plus software summary of the RigiScan recording and the final diagnosis. *J Urol* (*in press*).

24. Zuckier LS, Kikut J, Benet A et al: Quantitative analysis of tTc-99m red cell (RBC) washin time-activity curves (TACs) for determination of cavernosal blood volume (BV) and blood flow (BF) in the flaccid penis. 42nd Annual Meeting of the Society of Nuclear Medicine Society, Minneapolis, MN, June 12–15, 1995, Vol 36.

25. Lue TF, Hricak H, Marich KW, et al: Vasculogenic impotence evaluated by high-resolution ultrasonography and pulsed Doppler spectrum analysis. *Radiology* 155:777–781, 1985.

26. Castaneda-Zuniga WR, Smith A, Kaye K, et al: Transluminal angioplasty for treatment of vasculogenic impotence: *AJR Am J Roentgenol* 139:371–373, 1982.

27. Bookstein JJ, Valji K, Parsons L, et al: Pharmacoarteriography in the evaluation of impotence. *J Urol* 137:333–337, 1987.

28. Machleder HI, Weinstein M: Sexual dysfunction following surgical therapy for aorto-iliac disease. *Vasc Surg* 9:283–287, 1975.

29. Angelini P, Fighali S: Early experience with balloon angioplasty of internal iliac arteries for vasculogenic impotence. *Cathet Cardiovasc Diagn* 13:107–110, 1987.

30. Becker GJ, Rowe DM, Holden RW, et al: Percutaneous transluminal angioplasty for vasculogenic impotence. *Indiana Med* 79:256–262, 1986.

31. Crespo E, Soltanik E, Bove D, et al: Treatment of vasculogenic sexual impotence by revascularizing cavernous and/or dorsal arteries using microvascular techniques. *Urology* 20:271–275, 1982.

32. Virag R, Zwang G, Dermange H, et al: [Investigation and surgical treatment of vasculogenic impotency (author's transl)]. *J Mal Vasc* 5:205–209, 1980.

33. Virag R, Zwang G, Dermange H, et al: Vasculogenic impotence: a review of 92 cases with 54 surgical operations. *J Vasc Surg* 15:9–17, 1981.

34. Virag R, Saltiel H, Floresco J, et al: Surgical treatment of vascular impotence by arterialization of the dorsal vein of the penis. Experience of 292 cases. *Chirurgie* 114(9):703–714, 1988.

35. Virag R, Bennett AH, Shoukry K: Arterial and venous surgery for vasculogenic impotence: a combined French and American experience. *J Urol* 141:289A, 1989.

36. Furlow W, Fisher J: Deep dorsal vein arterialization: clinical experience with a new technique for penile revascularization. *J Urol* 139:298A, 1988.

37. Melman A, Riccardi RJ: The success of microvascular penile revascularization in treating arteriogenic impotence. *Int J Impot Res* 5:47–52, 1993.

38. Sharaby JS, Benet AE, Lazar S, et al: Revascularization: a five year follow-up study. *J Urol* 153:369A, 1995.

39. Sharaby JS, Benet AE, Melman A: Penile revascularization. *Urol Clin North Am* 22:821–832, 1995.

40. Rehman J, Benet AE, Melman A: Penile revascularization. In Culley C, Carson I (eds): *Mediguide in Urology.* New York, Lawrence DellaCorte Publications, 1996.

8

Venous Impotence

James J. Chang
Tom F. Lue

Since the discovery of the mechanism of venous occlusion, much effort has been spent on perfecting the technique of penile vein ligation for the identified cases of venous leakage. These efforts are thwarted by higher than expected rates of failure with many initial responders becoming impotent by 1-yr follow-up. While almost all patients show immediate improvement after surgery, only about half enjoy spontaneous erections long-term. Recent works document the disappointing long-term results after surgical vein ligation and attempt to identify the subset who will most likely benefit. With better understanding comes the finding that veno-occlusive dysfunction is probably the terminal pathway of multiple separate pathologic mechanisms of which primary venous pathology is a small subset. Current diagnostic techniques probably are not rigorous enough to reliably identify this last group of patients. Only through better elucidation of these differing etiologies can treatment be better tailored for the specific causes with resultant improvement in outcome.

PENILE VENOUS ANATOMY

Penile venous drainage consists of four primary pathways divided into three systems: superficial, intermediate, and deep drainage systems[1] (Fig. 8.1A, B). The skin and superficial fascia layers are drained by multiple small veins which coalesce at the base of the penis to form the superficial dorsal vein. This vein is often single but can be paired and it joins the external pudendal vein which drains into the saphenous vein in the thigh. The intermediate drainage system consists of the deep dorsal vein and its tributary circumflex veins. Multiple small veins draining the glans join to form the retrocoronal plexus. These veins coalesce to form the deep dorsal vein which is usually single but can be multiple. As this vein courses proximally beneath Buck's fascia in the groove between the two corporal bodies, it is joined by several penile circumflex veins draining the distal two-thirds of the corpora cavernosa. The deep dorsal vein then continues below the pubic bone to form the periprostatic plexus of Santorini. Several valves are present in the deep dorsal vein usually located at the level of the glans as well as before formation of the

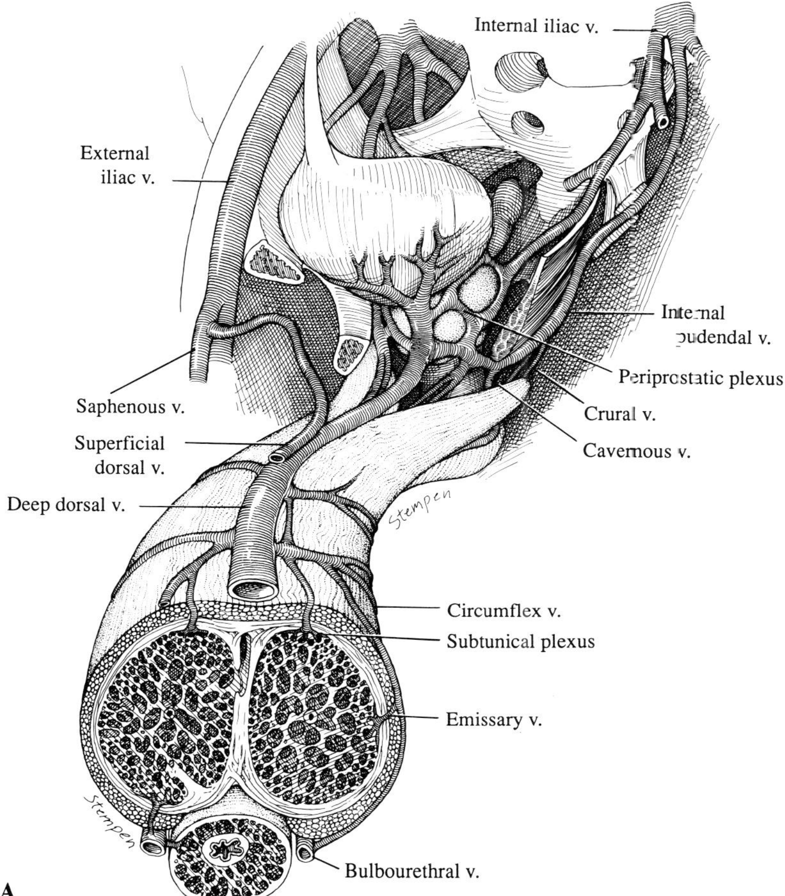

Fig. 8.1. A: Cross-section of the penis showing penile venous drainage and the inner circular and outer longitudinal layers of the tunica albuginea. The longitudinal layer is absent between the corpus cavernosum and the spongiosum. **B:** Longitudinal view of penile venous return. (Reprinted with permission from Lue TF: Physiology of penile erection and pathophysiology of impotence and priapism. In Walsh PC, Retik AB, Stamey TA, et al (eds): *Campbell's Urology*, ed 7. Philadelphia, WB Saunders [*in press*].)

periprostatic plexus, and these function to prevent retrograde flow. The proximal third of the corpora cavernosa is drained by the cavernosal vein which exits the dorsomedial penis at the hilum and continues to form the internal pudendal vein. Several small crural perforators directly drain the penis dorsolaterally and join the internal pudendal vein. The cavernosal vein and the crural veins make up the deep drainage system.

The corpus spongiosum should be considered separately since it lacks veno-occlusive function. It is drained by the bulbourethral vein which also joins the internal pudendal vein.

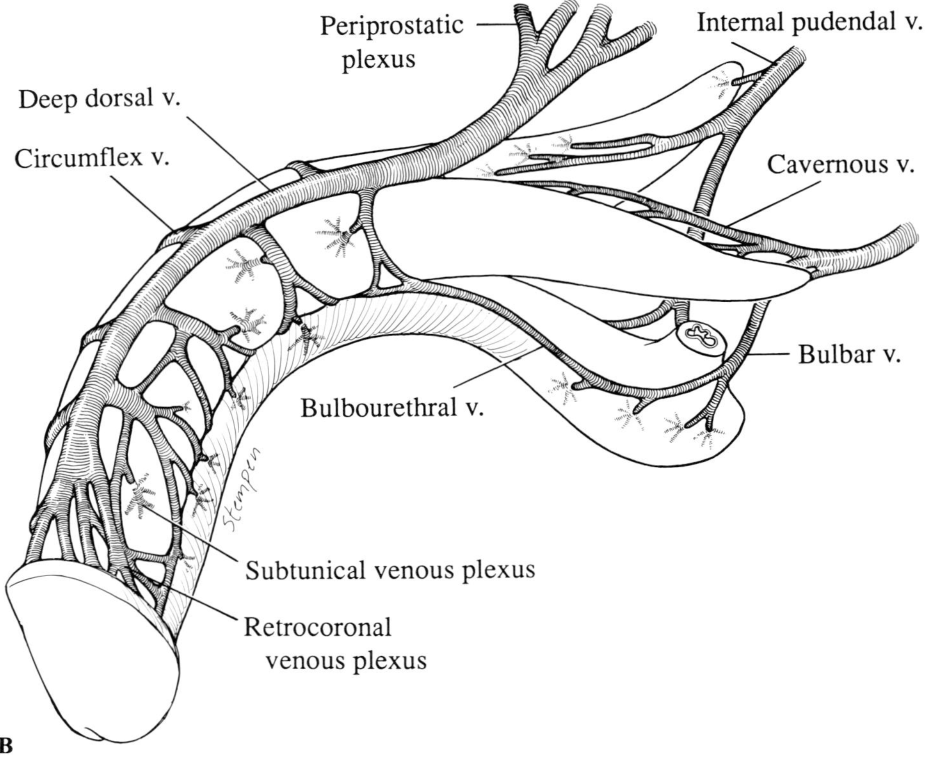

Fig. 8.1. Continued.

Both physiologic and pathologic collaterals between the drainage systems have been identified. The superficial and deep dorsal veins may communicate. The circumflex veins also drain into the bulbourethral vein, thereby connecting the deep dorsal vein to the spongiosal drainage system. The periprostatic plexus can have communication with the internal pudendal vein as well.[2] All of these drainage pathways and their collaterals must be controlled to optimize the outcome.

The intrinsic drainage system of the corpora cavernosa is unique. The venules that drain the sinusoidal spaces and the smooth muscles of the penis coalesce as they approach the periphery of the corpora cavernosa and form the subtunical venular plexus.[3] These then exit as the emissary veins and drain into the circumflex veins or directly into the deep dorsal vein for the distal two-thirds of the penis. In the proximal one-third, they directly form the cavernosal vein and the smaller crural veins. The position of the subtunical venular plexus between the sinusoids and tunica albuginea allows for their compression and occlusion as the smooth muscle and sinusoids relax and expand against tunica albuginea during tumescence. This occlusion traps the blood within the penis. The loss of this function results in leakage of blood from the penis and subsequent impotence.

PHYSIOLOGY OF VENO-OCCLUSIVE DYSFUNCTION

While the mechanism has only recently been demonstrated, the concept of venous outflow occlusion is not new. Early observation in mammals led to theories of "sluice channels" and "sluice valve".[4] Obstruction of the smaller sluice channels by these muscular, artery-like veins would block drainage and create erection. Venous valves were also thought to contribute to outflow obstruction.[5] Probably the most widely held belief was that of arterial inflow overwhelming the drainage capacity of penile veins with subsequent trapping of blood in the penis.[6]

Evidence of venous occlusion was first demonstrated in the canine. Blood flow and intracorporeal pressures were performed after producing erections by cavernosal nerve stimulation. Once an erection was achieved, only minimal inflow was required to maintain an erection. Constant flow infusion studies with and without cavernous nerve stimulation showed marked increase in corporeal pressure after stimulation.[7] A venous occlusion mechanism is necessary to account for these findings.

The anatomy of this occlusion mechanism was demonstrated using corrosion casts of canine and human penises.[3] During erection the arterioles dilate and blood inflow increases. The smooth muscles of the penis relax and expand, and the sinusoids engorge with blood. This expansion of smooth muscle and sinusoids compresses the subtunical venular plexus against the relatively noncompliant tunica albuginea and occludes venous outflow. Distention may cause the inner circular and outer longitudinal fibrous coats of tunica albuginea to slide upon each other and serve to obliterate the perforating emissary veins, further contributing to the occlusion of venous outflow.

Impotence results when the occlusion mechanism fails to properly function. This failure may result from any multitude of causes, and most of these are probably not of primary venous origin. While true anomalous venous drainage channels probably do exist, they are likely to make up only a small subset of the patients with veno-occlusive dysfunction. Venous occlusion relies on functioning cavernosal tissue to expand and compress against tunica albuginea. Any abnormality in corporeal sinusoid or smooth muscle function or in tunical integrity will prevent this from occurring.

Studies of penile ultrastructure of potent and impotent men have demonstrated significant differences in the quantity of smooth muscle fibers and in the integrity of the cellular structure. Impotent men show decreased smooth muscle content with the largest losses seen in those with severe arterial insufficiency.[8] The cell losses were replaced by connective tissue, and the remaining smooth muscles were abnormal with decreased contractile elements.[9] Mild atherosclerosis with subclinical arterial insufficiency may create enough atrophic changes to prevent proper occlusive function especially when combined with other concomitant disorders.

Neuropathic disorders can also cause atrophy and improper function. The cavernosal smooth muscles from diabetic patients show diminished capacity to relax. Multiple different neurotransmitters are present within the penis, including acetylcholine, calcitonin gene-related peptide, and vasoactive intestinal peptide. Of interest is the finding of nitric oxide synthase activity in penile neurons. Nitric oxide is a potent vascular smooth muscle relaxant that may be the mediator in nonadrenergic, noncholinergic neurotransmission. Cavernosal smooth muscle cell relaxation in vitro to electrical stimulation was blocked by nitric oxide synthase inhibitors implicating nitric oxide in a modulatory role. Defects in endothelial cell function could result in depressed nitric oxide synthesis with subsequent reduction in smooth muscle relaxation and failure of the veno-occlusive mechanism. The difficulty in treating veno-occlusive disease stems from its wide number of possible causes. Current surgical treatment is still limited to controlling the symptom rather than the cause of the dysfunction.

DIAGNOSTIC EVALUATION

While a wide variety of diagnostic evaluations are available, proving the diagnosis of veno-occlusive dysfunction should be straightforward. The desires and motivations of the patient should dictate the aggressiveness of the individual workup. A thorough medical and sexual history and physical exam are performed, and selective laboratory tests are done looking primarily for endocrinologic abnormalities. If the history raises the possibility of psychogenic pathology, nocturnal tumescence testing should be performed to confirm or rule out organic impotence.

Once organic impotence is diagnosed, a vascular evaluation is then performed. The best test looking for vasculogenic impotence is the intracavernous injection and self-stimulation test. If a sustained and rigid erection is achieved within 10 min after the injection of 10 μg of alprostadil, venous and arterial insufficiency is unlikely. Those with moderate to severe venous insufficiency will have difficulty achieving a pharmacologic erection. If a full erection is not seen or if the erection lasts only a short period, the patient is then asked to stimulate himself in an attempt at improving the response. Again if a good sustained erection is achieved, then a severe arterial or venous insufficiency is unlikely. If the response is poor, duplex ultrasound with intracavernous injection is then performed to evaluate for vasculogenic impotence.

Duplex ultrasound with gray scale or color-coded Doppler evaluation can readily diagnose arterial insufficiency and may suggest venous insufficiency. Full evaluation of the penis is performed to look for any anatomic abnormalities. Cavernosal artery diameter and thickness is noted at the base of the penis. After injection of 10 μg of alprostadil, the cavernosal arteries are reexamined. Normal arterial response to pharmacotherapy is a cavernous artery peak flow velocity greater than 30 cm per second. This finding correlates well with normal pudendal artery angiography results. Veno-occlusive dysfunction is suggested if diastolic flow persists, and the erection is not rigid or poorly sustained. If an inadequate erection is confirmed on Rigiscan testing, the patient should then be evaluated with dynamic pharmacocavernosometry and cavernosography to confirm the diagnosis and to document the anatomic sites of leakage. In a subset of patients in whom arterial insufficiency is found but who are under consideration for arterial revascularization, evaluation for venous leakage should be performed. If a combined arterial and venous insufficiency exists, these patients may be candidates for combined dorsal vein arterialization and vein ligation.

PHARMACOCAVERNOSOMETRY/ CAVERNOSOGRAPHY

Ebbehoj described the use of infusion cavernosography with audiovisual stimulation to detect three cases of corporoglandular leak and one case of corporovenous leak.[10] Dynamic infusion cavernosometry creates passive veno-occlusion by dilating the cavernosal sinusoids with saline infusion. An induction rate is required to initiate the occlusion process, then a lower rate can be infused to maintain the erection. The parameters of interest are the maintenance flow rate, the rapidity of pressure decline when the infusion is stopped, and the cavernosographic localization of the sites of leakage. Penile arterial flow occlusion pressures can be used to evaluate cavernosal artery function although this is redundant once the duplex Doppler ultrasound exam has confirmed adequate arterial function. Patients with venous occlusion defects will require higher induction and maintenance flow rates, and those with severe defects may be unable to obtain an erection even with infusion rates greater than 200 ml per minute. Normal erection pressures and infusion flow rates required to produce passive erection in men with and without venous leak have been described.[11,12] These evaluations were further modified with the use of papaverine.[13–15] Vasodilator injection activates the erectile tissues so that lower rates of infusion result in an erection. Pharmacocavernosometry and cavernosography have the advantage of being more physiologic compared with simple saline infusion alone.[16,17] The venous occlusion mechanism is more complex than just mechanical compression of subtunical venules, and the use of injectable vasodilators intuitively makes good sense.

A 21-gauge butterfly needle is inserted into one corpus cavernosum, and 0.5 ml of a mixture of papaverine, phentolamine, and alprostadil is injected after placing a rubber band tourniquet at the base of the penis. The tourniquet, used to prevent rapid washout of the drug from the penis, is removed after 2 min. A 21-gauge butterfly needle is inserted into the opposite side after 10 min, and the baseline pressure is measured. If the intracorporeal pressure does not exceed 90 mm Hg, saline is infused at 60 to 120 ml per minute until the pressure of 90 mm Hg is achieved or the pressure is stable for several minutes. Once 90 mm Hg pressure is achieved, the flow is recorded as the maintenance flow. The rate of pressure decline can then be measured by increasing the infusion rate until corporeal pressure equals 150 mm Hg. The infusion is then stopped and the rate of pressure decline over 30 sec is measured. Cavernosography can then be performed with the injection of 60 ml of 50 : 50 dilute radiographic contrast. Intracorporeal pressure should be monitored during and after injection. Radiographic clarity is enhanced when intracorporeal pressure is maintained at less than 60 mm Hg. Sufficient films are taken in anterior-posterior as well as oblique views to document the presence or absence and locations of the venous leakage. Patients are observed for 1 hr or until the erection declines. If the erection persists, this is treated by aspiration followed by injection of neosynephrine in 250–500 µg aliquots until the erection abates. Ecchymosis and occasional transient hypertension with palpitation are the only complications.

Cavernosography has demonstrated potential leakage into all the penile venous drainage systems. In one study the breakdown of the incidence of leakage by sites after papaverine injection was 50% superficial dorsal vein, 70% deep dorsal vein, and 70% cavernosal and crural veins. Multiple sites of leakage are noted in over two-thirds of the patients and this is the rule rater than the exception.[2]

Two principal numbers are obtained during pharmacocavernosometry. Induction flow is highly dependent upon the size of the penis and therefore offers very little information regarding venous competence. Maintenance flow rates, on the other hand, show high correlation. Each series has produced normal potent men showing rates between 20 and 50 ml per minute. The maintenance flow rate after injection of the Trimix solution is significantly reduced with normal rates of 4–5 ml per minute. The abnormal cutoff varies from study to study. Pharmacocavernosometry maintenance flow rate greater than 12 ml per minute is considered abnormal,[2] although a cutoff of 40–50 ml per minute has been recommended by others to improve specificity.[12,18,19] The rate of pressure fall in 30 sec greater than 45 mm Hg is considered abnormal as well.

While pharmacocavernosometry and cavernosography remain the optimal tests for detecting venous incompetence, the influence of the α-adrenergic tone must always be considered. Patients should try injections at home in comfortable surroundings to truly test the effects of the medications because there may be a subset with normal occlusion mechanism who respond poorly due to adrenergic tone.[20] Few cases have been documented where venous leak was diagnosed in patients with normal Rigiscan results, and therefore we recommended nocturnal testing for all patients contemplating venous surgery.[21] The other complication of vasodilator injection in patients with massive venous incompetence is transient systemic vasodilatation due to rapid efflux of injected drug from the penis. This can be circumvented by placing a tourniquet at the base of the penis prior to the injection, and the tourniquet is taken off after a few minutes once the medication has had a chance to be absorbed.

Multiple options are available to treat venous impotence, but due to the underlying pathology, the outcome is often less successful than expected. By definition this subset of patients respond poorly to single agent intracavernous drug injections. Combination drug injections should produce better results while minimizing side effects. Different combination have been tried but the most commonly used is the Trimix solution of alprostadil, papaverine, and phentolamine. A synergistic effect results with papaverine blocking phosphodiesterase function, PGE_1 promoting adenylate cyclase activity, and phentolamine inhibiting adrenergic stimulus to the corporal arteries and smooth muscle.[22] Atropine in higher doses releases the nitric oxide. There may be a role for the inclusion of this agent into the combination protocols.[23] If the erection obtained remains inadequate, intracavernous injection can be combined with the use of a vacuum device to further assist in tumescence, and obviously the vacuum device can be tried alone. Many patients may achieve success through the use of combination drug regimens with only those having the most severe insufficiency failing. Vacuum devices can be used successfully by up to 69% of the patients although therapeutic rates as low as 27% have been reported.[24,25]

The other principal options are surgical. After careful selection, penile vein ligation can be a reasonable choice, and the technique and results of this procedure are described below. If successful, this is the most natural and physiologic result that can be achieved. Long-term results have been somewhat disappointing, however, with frequent transient improvements that show deterioration over 1 yr. Interventional radiologists show success rates similar to open surgery, and these improvements also tend to deteriorate over time. For patients with focal arterial insufficiency who have a coincident venous insufficiency, a dorsal vein arterialization with vein ligation can be an option as well. If all else fails, the placement of a penile prosthesis is the final option.

VENOUS SURGERY

The approach to penile venous ligation should have sound basis in anatomy. All veins draining from the penis need to be ligated to prevent future collateralization and optimize outcome. This dictates that the deep dorsal vein, cavernosal veins, and crural veins must all be occluded. While several incisional approaches have been used, the most flexible appears to the inguinoscrotal incision.[26] With the patient in a low lithotomy position, the incision is made lateral to the base of the penis along the tract of the spermatic cord and carried obliquely onto the anterior surface of the scrotum. This incision preserves the lymphatic drainage and minimizes postoperative edema. Cord damage can be avoided by staying within the dartos layer. The distal aspect of the incision can be lengthened if further exposure is needed. The penis can be bluntly dissected free below the level of superficial fascia and delivered through the incision by invagination. The fundiform and suspensory ligaments of the penis are taken down to expose the most proximal portions of the penis. Careful dissection is necessary at this level to avoid injury to the neurovascular bundles. Both crura are freed off of the ischial bone.

Having fully mobilized the penis, the next step is to dissect free the dorsal vein. Loop magnification is used to avoid injury to the paired dorsal neurovasculature lying lateral to the dorsal vein. The most proximal aspect of the dorsal vein below the pubic bone is double ligated with 2-0 silk ties and transected. The dorsal vein is then dissected free distally for 4 to 5 cm and resected so the underlying penile hilum can be exposed. Rather than resect out the whole dorsal vein, the distal portion is left in place and injected with sclerosing agent to decrease the risk of subsequent collateral formation. The most distal portion of the dorsal vein just proximal to the glans is dissected free and ligated. This reduces the risk of retrograde reflux of sclerosing agent into the glans. A rubber band is also placed tightly at the level of the corona to prevent flux. The remaining dorsal vein is then cannulated and injected with 2 ml of 3% sodium tetradecyl sulfate mixed with methylene blue. The dorsal vein and circumflex veins filling with the sclerosing agent can then be monitored by tracking the methylene dye. The rubber band is taken off about 10 min later. If blue dye appears in the glans, a butterfly needle is placed into the glans and saline irrigation is performed to prevent glans necrosis. There should be less risk of subsequent cavernospongiosal collateralization after the sclerosis of the circumflex veins.

With the deep dorsal vein drainage controlled, the next step is to disrupt the deep venous drainage system. Prior technique was directed at identification of the individual cavernous and crural veins under operating microscope magnification and individually ligating the many small veins. In addition to being tedious, veins can be missed by this technique. Total ligation can be achieved more easily by removing the ischiocavernosus muscle. The paired cavernous arteries branch from the penile artery and enter the corpora cavernosa at the penile hilum. Careful dissection of the dorsal neurovasculature under loop magnification can identify where the cavernosal artery enters the penis. En bloc occlusion of the cavernous bodies proximal to the insertion of the arteries will disrupt venous drainage through the cavernous and crural veins while leaving the arterial inflow intact.

The cavernous artery is identified where it separates from the penile artery and inserts into the penis. The neurovasculature is dissected clear off the cavernous bodies proximal to where the penile artery divides. Clear understanding of the neurovascular anatomy at this level is critical to avoid injury to the cavernous artery and the dorsal nerve and artery. A plane is developed between the corpus spongiosum and the corpora cavernosa and between the two corpora. A doubled segment of umbilical tape is then passed circumscribing the corpus cavernosum, and the tape is then passed under the dorsal neurovasculature to exclude it from the ligation. Careful inspection notes that only the corpus cavernosa proximal to the insertion of the cavernosal artery is contained within the umbilical tape (Fig. 8.2). This maneuver is repeated for the opposite corpus cavernosum. Each corporeal body is double ligated with the umbilical tape. The ties should be snug to restrict outflow through the deep venous system. Doppler ultrasound can be used to confirm the patency of the deep dorsal and cavernosal arteries. A Foley catheter must be placed before development of the plane between the corpora cavernosa and the corpus spongiosum to lessen the risk of injury and to better delineate the path of the corpus spongiosum.

Throughout the course of the case, any superficial vein encountered should be ligated. Spongiolysis can be readily performed through this approach if leak to the

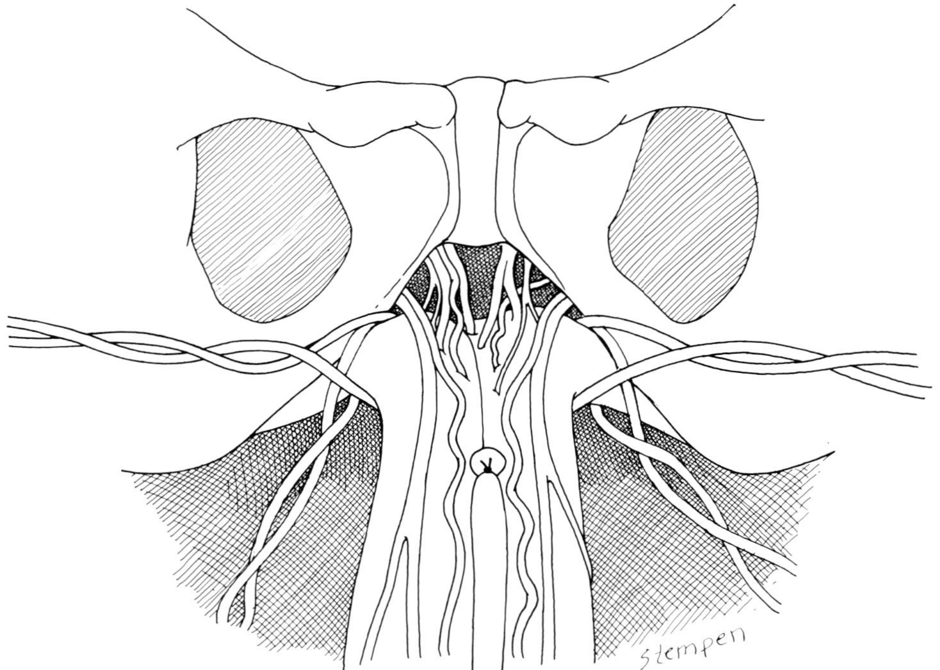

Fig. 8.2. Dissection of neurovascular bundles off the tunica albuginea and ligation of both crura with double umbilical tapes.

corpus spongiosum is noted on preoperative workup. The whole pendulous penis is exposed and readily accessible through this approach.

Prior to closure the suspensory ligament is reapproximated to the periosteum of the pubic bone using 2-0 silk ligature. This may help to reduce the penile contracture that has been described in other studies. Since the dissection can be quite extensive, a 7-French Jackson–Pratt closed suction drain is placed into the subcutaneous layer. This is removed the next day prior to discharge. The closure is completed with 3-0 Dexon for the subcutaneous tissue and interrupted 4-0 chromic for the skin. A nonadhesive dressing is applied over the incision and Coban dressing (elastic tape) is applied loosely over the penile shaft to prevent edema, and an athletic supporter is placed.

The patient is admitted overnight for pain control and discharged home the next day after removal of the Foley catheter and the drain. The Coban dressing on the penis is reapplied each day by the patient for 1 wk. Tylenol with codeine usually suffices for pain control. An ice pack applied is good for the control of both swelling and pain.

RESULTS

The outcome from vein ligation surgery has fallen short of revolutionary. In general, nearly all patients experience immediate improvements in their potency. However, this effect is lost over the course of time from the multiplicity of the causes of veno-occlusive dysfunction since not all can be expected to respond favorably to a single type of procedure. While the immediate improvement may be encouraging, the underlying pathology may then progress which facilitates the development of new collateral veins and negates the initial effect.

The results at the University of California, San Francisco roughly parallel those reported in the literature (Table 8.1). Approximately 56% of the patients are capable of spontaneous erections of sufficient tumescence and rigidity for intercourse. Another 27% of the patients now respond to intracavernous injections with good erections. These results are comparable to those achieved by extensive vein resection and ligation. The overall spontaneous erection rate is about 44%.

The goal of venous ligation is to achieve spontaneous erection. With this as the objective, the outcome from the current form of treatment is suboptimal. The critical question that must be asked is whether this is failure of treatment or failure of diagnosis. Up to 83% of the patients benefit from the surgery if improvement in response to intracavernous injection is included. Only 17% appear to completely fail remaining refractory to intracavernous injections of vasodilators. Postoperative cavernosography usually documents newly incompetent sites although occasional persistent leakage is also seen. Most of these patients are probably not treatment failures but rather diagnosis failures. Also not uncommon are the patients who remain persistently impotent despite the absence of further leakage. In addition, many patients who previously could not respond to intracavernosal injection enjoy a good response after venous ligation.

Intraluminal attempts at venous obliteration have been reported.[27,28] Multiple routes of vascular access have been tried including cut down exposure of the dorsal vein and percutaneous deep dorsal and femoral vein punctures. Placement of coils

TABLE 8.1. Surgical Results of Venous Surgery

Reference	Investigator	Technique	Case	Spontaneous	Inject	Fail	F/U
34	Wespes and Schulman (1985)	DV Ligation	20	16 (80%)		4 (20%)	3–24 months
35	Bennett et al (1986)	DV Ligation	8	6 (75%)		2 (25%)	6–18 months
36	Austoni et al (1987)	DV Ligation	234	129 (55%)		108 (45%)	9 months
37	Puech-Leao et al (1987)	Crural ligation	8	7 (88%)		1 (12%)	"short term"
38	Bar-Moshe and Vandendris (1988)	Crural vein ligation; Prn DV ligation	13	9 (69%)	3 (23%)	1 (8%)	2–12 months
39	Lewis (1988)	DV Resection	50	12 (24%)	12 (24%)	25 (50%)	15 months
40	Lunglmayr et al (1988)	DV Resection	29	9 (31%)	1 (3%)	19 (66%)	4–24 months
41	Williams et al (1988)	DV Resection	13	9 (69%)		4 (21%)	2–10 months
26	Lue (1989)	DV Resection; crural/cavernosal vein ligation	64	36 (56%)	17 (27%)	11 (17%)	12–26 months
42	Treiber and Gilbert (1989)	DV Ligation	115	28 (24%)	39 (34%)	48 (52%)	13 months
42	Treiber and Gilbert (1989)	Spongiolysis	11	4 (36%)	5 (45%)	2 (19%)	14 months
43	Rossman et al (1990)	DV Ligation; Prn crural vein ligation and spongiolysis	16	2 (16%)	2 (16%)	12 (68%)	>9 months
44	Wespes (1990)	DV Resection	67	31 (46%)		36 (54%)	24–72 months

45	Knispel (1991)	DV Ligation	12	1 (8%)	4 (33%)	7 (58%)	12.8 months
46	Hauri et al (1992)	DV Arterialization; cavernosal band	40	21 (53%)	10 (25%)	9 (22%)	>12 months
29	Yu et al (1992)	DV Ligation; Prn crural/ cavernosal vein ligation	11	2 (18%)		9 (82%)	>3 months
47	Freedman et al (1993)	DV Resection; Prn crural/ cavernosal vein ligation	46	11 (24%)	8 (17%)	27 (59%)	>12 months
48	Hirsch et al (1993)	DV Resection; cavernosal vein ligation; Prn crural vein ligation and spongiolysis	24	10 (41%)	2 (9%)	12 (50%)	6 months
49	Montague et al (1993)	DV Resection; crural/cavernosal vein ligation	18	11 (61%)		7 (39%)	12–37 months
50	Kerfoot et al (1994)	DV Resection; crural vein ligation	36	15 (42%)	10 (28%)	11 (30%)	1–31 months
51	Stief et al (1994)	DV Resection	77	31 (40%)	8 (10%)	38 (49%)	6–47 months
52	Wespes et al (1994)	DV Resection; Prn cavernosal vein ligation	23	12 (52%)		11 (48%)	12–26 months
Overall			935	412 (44%)	121 (13%)	404 (43%)	

DV = Dorsal Vein; Prn = as needed

and balloons and injections of sclerosing agents have been tried with greater than 90% radiographic success. Up to 85% show initial improvement, but many of these do not endure over time. The Schwartz group report 70% improvement with 25% of patients having spontaneous erections. Considering the small numbers, this correlates well with operative rates of improvement. One group followed up surgical failures with intraluminal venous obliteration and achieved some successful salvage.[29] With the difficulty encountered due to scarring and loss of fascial planes during reexplorations, the intraluminal approach may yield equal results with less complication for patients with history of prior penile surgery. Pulmonary migration of coils has been reported with this procedure as is the risk with all intraluminal interventional procedures, and this should be considered.[30]

More recent works attempt to further differentiate the subset who will best benefit from surgical intervention. Patients with isolated venous anomalies should have normal penile parenchyma with intact smooth muscle and sinusoid function. Penile biopsy has been suggested and normal results do appear to show correlation to better surgical results. A less invasive evaluation under consideration is cavernosal electrical activity.[31–33] Smooth muscle function requires electrical activity, and those patients with normal penile parenchyma would be expected to have normal electrical activity. Improved success with vein ligation surgery can probably be obtained through better patient selection rather than through further improvements in technique.

CONCLUSION

Despite growing knowledge and evolving techniques, venous ligation procedures restore spontaneous erections in only 50% of the patients. This probably reflects the fact that causes of veno-occlusive dysfunction are still poorly understood. Penile venous ligation merely treats the symptom without addressing the causes. The failures probably represent diagnostic errors far more often than surgical failures. The areas that appear to hold promise look at the tunica albuginea and corporeal smooth muscle of the penis and its electrical and mechanical function. Better understanding of the underlying pathology may help to improve focusing of the treatment to the principal cause.

REFERENCES

1. Breza J, Aboseif SR, Orbis BR, et al: Detailed anatomy of penile neurovascular structures: surgical significance. *J Urol* 141:437–443, 1989.

2. Aboseif SR, Breza J, Lue TF, et al: Penile venous drainage in erectile dysfunction. Anatomical, radiological, and functional considerations. *Br J Urol* 64:183–190, 1989.

3. Fournier GR, Juenemann K, Lue TF, et al: Mechanisms of venous occlusion during canine penile erection: an anatomic demonstration. *J Urol* 137:163–167, 1987.

4. Deysach LJ: The comparative morphology of the erectile tissue of the penis with especial emphasis on the probable mechanism of erection. *Am J Anat* 64: 111–131, 1939.

5. Fitzpatrick TJ: The Penile intercommunicating venous valvular system. *J Urol* 127:1099–1100, 1982.

6. Newman HF, Northup JD, Devlin J: Mechanism of human penile erection. *Invest Urol* 1:350–353, 1964.

7. Juenemann KP, Luo JA, Lue TF, et al: Further evidence of venous outflow restriction during erection. *Br J Urol* 58:320–324, 1986.

8. Wespes E, Goes PM, Schiffman S, et al: Computerized analysis of smooth muscle fibers in potent and impotent patients. *J Urol* 146:1015–1017, 1991.

9. Persson C, Diederichs W, Lue TF, et al: Correlation of altered penile ultrastructure with clinical arterial evaluation. *J Urol* 142:1462–1468, 1989.

10. Ebbehoj J, Wagner G: Insufficient penile erection due to abnormal drainage of cavernous bodies. *Urology* 13:507–510, 1979.

11. Wespes E, Schulman CC: Parameters of erection. *Br J Urol* 56:416–417, 1984.

12. Wespes E, Delcour C, Struyven J, et al: Cavernometry-cavernography: its role in organic impotence. *Eur Urol* 10:229–232, 1984.

13. Virag R, Frydman D, Legman M, et al: Intracavernous injection of papaverine as a diagnostic and therapeutic method in erectile failure. *Angiology* 35:79–87, 1984.

14. Brookstein JJ, Valji K, Parsons L, et al: Penile pharmacocavernosography and cavernosometry in the evaluation of impotence. *J Urol* 137:772–776, 1986.

15. Puyau FA, Lewis RW, Balkin P, et al: Dynamic corpus cavernosography: effect of papaverine injection. *Radiology* 164:179–182, 1987.

16. Stief CG, Diederichs W, Benard F, et al: The diagnosis of venogenic impotence: dynamic or pharmacologic cavernosometry? *J Urol* 140: 1561–1563, 1988.

17. Stief CG, Benard F, Diederichs W, et al: The rationale for pharmacologic cavernosography. *J Urol* 140:1564–1566, 1988.

18. Wespes E, Delcour C, Struyven J, et al: Pharmacocavernometry-cavernography in impotence. *Br J Urol* 58:429–433, 1986.

19. Lewis RW: This month in investigative urology: venous impotence. *J Urol* 140:1560, 1988.

20. Freidenberg DH, Berger RE, Chew DE, et al: Quantitation of corporeal venous outflow resistance in many by corporeal pressure flow evaluation. *J Urol* 138:533–538, 1987.

21. Montague DK, Lakin MM: False diagnosis of venous leak impotence. *J Urol* 148:148–149, 1992.

22. Von Heyden B, Donatucci CF, Kaula N, et al: Intracavernous pharmacotherapy for impotence selection of appropriate agent and dose. *J Urol* 149:1288–1290, 1993.

23. Montorsi F, Guazzoni G, Bergamaschi F, et al: Four-drug intracavernous therapy for impotence due to corporeal veno-occlusive dysfunction. *J Urol* 149:1291–1295, 1993.

24. Blackard CE, Borkon WD, Lima JS, et al: Use of vacuum tumescence device for impotence secondary to venous leakage. *Urology* 41:225–230, 1993.

25. Meinhardt W, Nijeholt AABLA, Kropman RF, et al: The negative pressure device for erectile disorders: when does it fail? *J Urol* 149:1285–1287, 1993.

26. Lue TF: Penile venous surgery. *Urol Clin North Am* 16:607–611, 1989.

27. Courtheoux P, Maiza D, Henriet JP, et al: Erectile dysfunction caused by venous leakage: treatment with detachable balloons and coils. *Radiology* 161:807–809, 1986.

28. Schwartz AN, Lowe M, Harley JD, et al: Preliminary report: Penile vein occlusion therapy: selection criteria and methods used for the transcatheter treatment of impotence caused by venous-sinusoidal incompetence. *J Urol* 148:815–820, 1992.

29. Yu GW, Schwab FJ, Melograna FS, et al: Preoperative and postoperative dynamic

cavernosography and cavernosometry: objective assessment of venous ligation for impotence. *J Urol* 147:618–622, 1992.

30. Moriel EZ, Mehringer CM, Schwarts M, et al: Pulmonary migration of coils inserted for treatment of erectile dysfunction caused by venous leakage. *J Urol* 149:1316–1318, 1993.

31. Wagner G, Gerstenberg T, Levin RY: Electrical activity of corpus cavernosum during flaccidity and erection of the human penis: a new diagnostic method? *J Urol* 142:723–725, 1989.

32. Stief CG, Djamilian M, Schaebsdau F, et al: Single potential analysis of cavernous electric activity—a possible diagnosis of autonomic impotence. *World J Urol* 8:75–79, 1990.

33. Yarnitsky D, Sprecher E, Barilan Y, et al: Corpus cavernosum: electromyogram: spontaneous and evoked electrical activities. *J Urol* 153:653–654, 1995.

34. Wespes E, Schulman CC: Venous leakage: surgical treatment of a curable cause of impotence. *J Urol* 133:796–798, 1985.

35. Bennett AH, Rivard DJ, Blanc RP, et al: Reconstructive surgery for vasculogenic impotence. *J Urol* 136:599–601, 1986.

36. Austoni E, Bellorofonte C, Mantovani F: Improved results with intracavernous vasoactive drug infusion following new surgical techniques for vasculogenic impotence. *World J Urol* 5:182–189, 1987.

37. Puech-Leao P, Reis JMSM, Glina S, et al: Leakage through the crural edge of corpus cavernosum. *Eur Urol* 13:163–165, 1987.

38. Bar-Moshe, O. and Vandendris, M. Treatment of Impotence due to perineal venous leakage by ligation of crura penis. *J. Urol* 139:1217, 1988.

39. Lewis RW: Venous surgery for impotence. *Urol Clin North Am* 15:115–121, 1988.

40. Lunglmayr G, Nachtigall M, Gindl K: Long-term results of deep dorsal penile vein transection in venous impotence. *Eur Urol* 15:209–212, 1988.

41. Williams G, Mulcahy MJ, Hartnell G, et al: Diagnosis and treatment of venous leakage: a curable cause of impotence. *Br J Urol* 61:151–155, 1988.

42. Treiber U, Gilbert P: Venous surgery in erectile dysfunction: a critical report on 116 patients. *Urology* 34:22–27, 1989.

43. Rossman B, Mieza M, Melman A: Penile vein ligation for corporeal incompetence: an evaluation of short-term and long-term results. *J Urol* 144:679–682, 1990.

44. Wespes E: Penile venous surgery for cavernovenous impotence. *World J Urol* 8:97–100, 1990.

45. Knispel HH: Penile venous surgery in impotence: results in highly selected cases. *Urol Int* 47:144–148, 1991.

46. Hauri D, Alund G, Spycher M, et al: Venous leakage—a new therapeutical concept. *Urol Int* 49:56–62, 1992.

47. Freedman AL, Costa Neto F, Mehringer CM, et al: Long-term results of penile vein ligation for impotence from venous leakage. *J Urol* 149:1301–1303, 1993.

48. Hirsch M, Lubetsky R, Goldman H, et al: Dorsal vein sclerosis as a predictor of outcome in penile venous ligation surgery. *J Urol* 150:1810–1813, 1993.

49. Montague DK, Angermeier KW, Lakin MM, et al: Penile venous ligation in 18 patients with 1 to 3 years of follow-up. *J Urol* 149:306–307, 1993.

50. Kerfoot WW, Carson CC, Donaldson JT, et al: Investigation of vascular changes following penile vein ligation. *J Urol* 152:884–887, 1994.

51. Stief CG, Djamilian M, Truss MC, et al: Prognostic factors for the postoperative

outcome of penile venous surgery for venogenic erectile dysfunction. *J Urol* 151:880–883, 1994.

52. Wespes E, Moreira de Goes P, Sattar AA, et al: Objective criteria in the long-term evaluation of penile venous surgery. *J Urol* 152:888–890, 1994.

9

Peyronie's Disease: Etiology, Diagnosis, and Treatment

Culley C. Carson

Peyronie's disease is a localized disorder of the connective tissue of the penis producing changes in collagen composition of the tunica albuginea of the corpus cavernosum and the adjacent areolar space. These tissue changes result in deformity of penile shape, especially during erection (Fig. 9.1). This penile deformity was described as early as 1561 by Fallopius, but Francois, Gigot de la Peyronie, the founder of the French College of Surgeons and Surgeon to King, Louis XV of France first published a series of patients with this condition in 1743 giving us the currently used eponym.[1] Since early reports of this condition, theories of its etiology have continued to evolve and medical and surgical alternatives for the treatment of the symptoms associated with this condition have varied. Each of these medical and surgical alternatives has attempted to improve penile curvature, penile pain, plaque size and composition, and ultimately erectile function. Currently, no single approach appears to be appropriate for all patients, but medical and surgical alternatives can be chosen systematically in an effort to treat these signs and symptoms.

Studies of the pathophysiology of Peyronie's disease have long focused on an inflammatory reaction characterized histologically by lymphocytic and plasmacytic infiltration of the perivascular spaces of the tissue of the tunica albuginea. Smith demonstrated that the mature scarred portion of the Peyronie's plaque is rich in hyaluronic acid, characteristic of a postinflammatory process of progressive fibrosis which usually includes perivascular fibrosis and abnormal elastic fibers.[3] The rigid fibrotic scarring shortens one side of the corpus cavernosum producing curvature toward the area of plaque because of the loss of ipsilateral corpus cavernosum elasticity. As a result of this progressive fibrosis, early medical treatment should be focused toward the inflammatory reaction while subsequent intervention should be concerned with mature fibrosis and possible calcification.

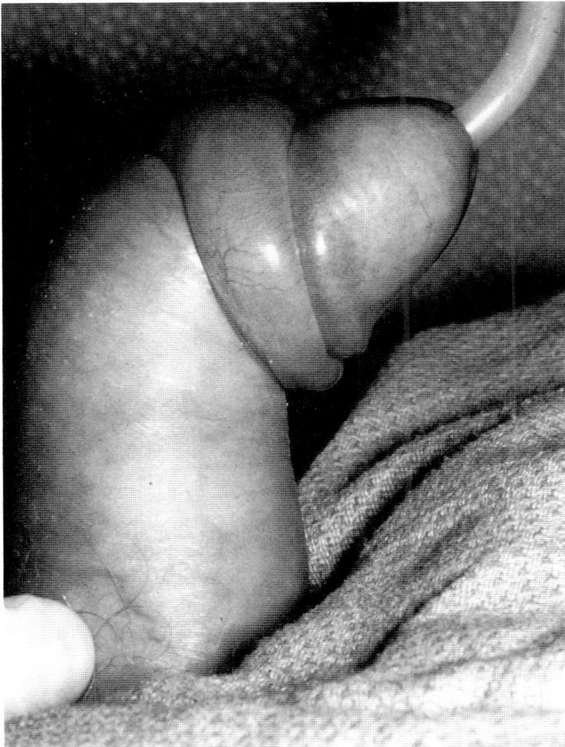

Fig. 9.1. Peyronie's disease with artificial erection prior to surgical intervention. Significant dorsal penile curvature on erection.

ETIOLOGY

The cause of the initial inflammatory process which produces the subsequent fibrosis and collagen changes of the tunica albuginea resulting in Peyronie's plaques continues to be an enigma. Devine et al, have proposed the most plausible theory by describing the initiation of abnormal fibrosis as a result of minimal penile trauma caused by bending or stretching. This injury causes delamination of the layers of the tunica albuginea at the septum with subsequent microvascular damage between the layers of the tunica albuginea.[4] This microvascular trauma results in a small hematoma and subsequent inflammation, fibrosis, and possible calcification. In men susceptible to these traumatic events, an initial episode predisposes the future trauma with retained fibrin between the layers of the tunica albuginea activating the proliferation of fibroblast and leukocyte infiltration. The inflammatory reaction may involve the corpus cavernosum tissue in its entirety and produce inflammation and fibrosis of Buck's fascia and around the structures between Buck's fascia and the tunica albuginea, including the dorsal neurovascular bundle of the penis, the intracorporal septum and the corpora spongiosa surrounding the urethra. In many patients, this inflammatory reaction may resolve completely with minimal fibrosis and deformity.[5,6] Chiang et al, have described the changes in collagen content and type in the tunica albuginea of patients with Peyronie's disease.[7] Type 3 collagen, which is found in abundance in Peyronie's plaques, is also identified in the tunica albuginea of patients with venogenic impotence.[8] In normal control patients without Peyronie's or venogenic impotence, however, type 3 collagen in infrequently identified in the tunica albuginea. These authors also identified a decrease in glycine and alanine contents of collagen in patients with Peyronie's plaque reinforcing the concept of an abnormal collagen composition.[9] Luangkhot et al have also reported alterations in the collagen of Peyronie's plaque in the tunica albuginea of patients with Peyronie's disease and priapism in comparison with normal controls.[10] These studies which have been demonstrated alterations in areas of the corpora cavernosa away from the Peyronie's plaques may account for the penile shortening identified in many patients with chronic Peyronie's disease.[8] This generalization of abnormal collagen formation has been supported by Anafarta et al in a histopathologic study comparing normal tunica albuginea in patients with Peyronie's disease with control patients.[11] These findings have also been supported by Iacono et al who evaluated the tunica albuginea of patients with Peyronie's disease away from the definitive plaque.[12] While these areas of tunica had no evidence for fibrocalcific formations, there was a statistically significant decrease in the elastic fiber concentration compared with normal control patients. Furthermore, patients with Peyronie's disease and impotence had a statistically significant decrease in elastic fiber concentration when compared with potent Peyronie's patients. The fibrotic and calcific plaques and dystrophic calcification within the tunica albuginea may be associated with similar fibrotic conditions occurring elsewhere in the body. As many as 10% of patients with Peyronie's disease also have Duypuytren's contracture while 3% of males with Duypuytren's contracture also have Peyronie's plaques. Furthermore, as many as 15% of patients with Peyronie's disease have excessive scarring or keloid formation elsewhere in the body. Patients with scleroderma have an increased incidence of Peyronie's disease. Thus, abnormal fibrosis characterizing the healing process in certain patients may be associated with the congenital familial trait that produces Peyronie's disease in suitable circumstances.

A variety of conditions have also been associated with Peyronie's disease, including early reports of vitamin E deficiency interfering with normal connective tissue repair as well as medications such as barbiturates and β-blocking agents.[13–15] Bivins et al reported 2 of 6 patients with carcinoid syndrome and Peyronie's disease, and proposed that an increased level of serotonin has a contributory factor to the fibrosis encountered in the retroperitoneum, endocardium, and tunica albuginea of these patients.[2]

VandeBerg et al suggested that Peyronie's disease is an autoimmune response to vascular trauma. Using scanning and transmission electromicroscopy, they demonstrated calcification originating from the vascular lumen producing osteoblastic cells associated with calcific plaque.[16] Willscher et al suggested a familial relationship to Peyronie's disease and histocompatibility antigens of the B7 cross reacting group, suggesting that Peyronie's disease may represent a pathologic response to an unidentified infective agent similar to the B7 antigen.[17] Subsequent studies have questioned this association and failed to identify these B7 antigens.[18,19] Nyberg et al studied three families with a possible inherited form of Peyronie's disease transmitted by an autosomal dominant trait also associated with Duypuytren's contracture.[20] These patients all exhibited the HLA-B27 cross-reacting antigens.

Subsequent studies by Rompel et al have suggested that HLA class 2 antigens in association with HLA-DR3 and HLA-DQW2 are more frequently identified with Peyronie's disease than with control patients.[18] These antigens are frequently identified with organospecific autoimmune disorders.[21] HLA-related changes, however, have been disputed by Leffell et al who carefully investigated 28 patients with Peyronie's disease and demonstrated no association with any of the previously described HLA antigens.[22]

While the etiology of Peyronie's disease remains controversial, there is little question that retained fibrin between the layers of tunica albuginea with excessive fibroblast activation and proliferation with increased leukocyte deposition forms the early lesion leading to the fibrotic Peyronie's plaque. Trauma from coitus, constriction rings, self-injection therapy, or other injuries may initiate this cascade of abnormal healing in susceptible patients.[23,24] Conditions associated with systemic fibrosis are also associated with Peyronie's disease.[2,25,26]

EVALUATION

The patient who presents with Peyronie's disease generally complains of pain, angulation, palpable plaque, or decreased erectile function. Diagnostic evaluation for these patients should be focused at potential treatment alternatives with an understanding of the etiology and natural history of Peyronie's disease. While the natural history of Peyronie's disease continues to be elucidated, Gelbard et al suggested the ultimate outcome in following a group of 97 patients for as long as 8 yr using questionnaires.[27] In their study, 3% of patients reported that pain, curvature, and erectile ability changed little during the course of disease. An additional 40% reported worsening of both curvature and erectile dysfunction while 6% of patients reported increasing pain. Seventy-seven percent of these patients had significant psychologic effects from their disease with only 28% improving spontaneously. There was no statistically significant difference in ultimate outcome of those patients treated conservatively versus those who underwent no treatment. Lindsay et al investigated 101 Peyronie's patients who are residents of Rochester, Minnesota during a 34-yr period.[28] The median age of these patients was 53 yr with an age-adjusted annual incidence of 25.7 yr and a prevalence rate of 388.6/100,000 male population. Their study suggested an increase in incidence during recent years without apparent explanation.

Most patients present to their urologist with complaints of penile pain, erectile curvature, palpable plaque, or erectile dysfunction. Erectile dysfunction which may occur in as many as 20% of patients may be caused by the Peyronie's disease itself, vascular disease associated with Peyronie's disease, or by a variety of other causes including psychogenic impotence.[29] Vascular abnormalities have been frequently reported as associated with Peyronie's disease. Identification of these abnormalities using color Doppler ultrasonography and dynamic infusion cavernosography and cavernosometry (DICC) procedures will not only assist in the diagnosis of Peyronie's disease but also select those patients most likely to benefit from reconstructive procedures and those in whom penile prosthesis implantation would be more effective[30] (Fig. 9.2). Lopez and Jarow studied 95 patients with Peyronie's disease using duplex ultrasonography.[31] Of the potent patients with Peyronie's

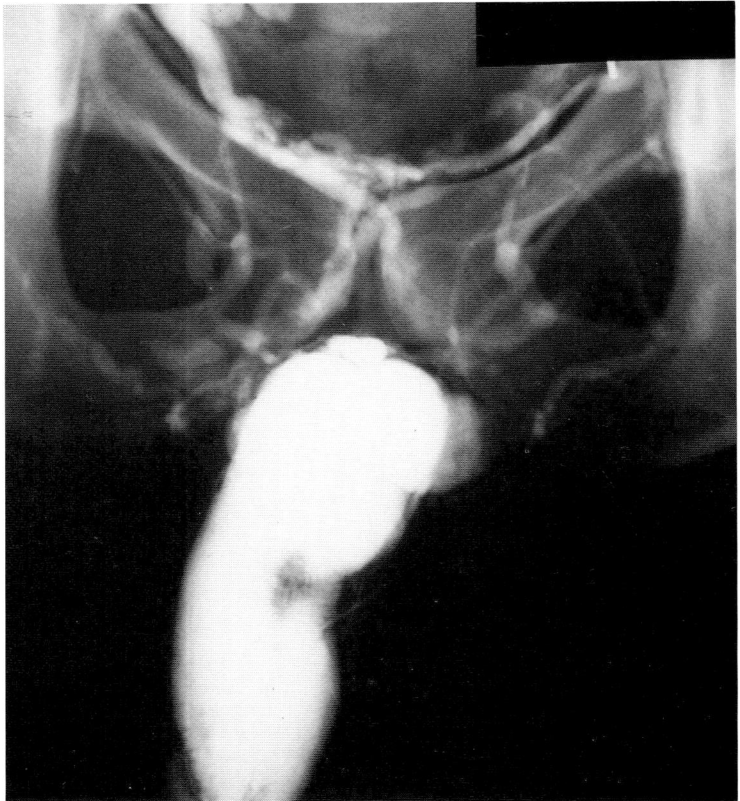

Fig. 9.2. Cavernosogram of Peyronie' disease. Inadequate filling of left corpus cavernosum caused by Peyronie's plaque. Significant venous leakage is identified.

disease, only one had abnormal arterial blood flow while 36% of impotent patients with Peyronie's disease had grossly abnormal arterial blood flow and 59% had evidence of high-grade veno-occlusive dysfunction. The incidence of veno-occlusive dysfunction in these impotent Peyronie's patients was statistically significantly different from control patients. Ralph et al confirmed this increased incidence of venogenic impotence associated with Peyronie's disease using color Doppler ultrasonography.[30] Amin et al also identified 18% of Peyronie's patients with impotence having associated venogenic abnormalities.[32] This increased incidence of venogenic abnormalities may well account for erectile dysfunction following penile reconstructive procedures. Dalkin and Carter as well as Jordan and Angermeier identified veno-occlusive dysfunction in patients with Peyronie's disease following plaque excision and grafting suggesting that simple repair of penile curvature and plaque alone may not produce a satisfactory result in all patients.[33,34] Many patients with erectile dysfunction and associated Peyronie's disease may require preoperative DICC to identify veno-occlusive dysfunction. If these patients are treated with plaque excision and grafting, consideration should be given to simultaneous deep dorsal penile vein ligation or penile prosthesis implantation with curvature straightening.

Peyronie's inflammation and fibrosis may produce pre- and postoperative decreases in distal penile sensation as documented by Amarenco and Casanova.[35] These investigators studied a group of patients with Peyronie's disease with neurophysiologic investigation of the dorsal nerve of the penis and demonstrated a significant reduction in nerve conduction, velocity, and amplitude in those patients with dorsal penile plaques. Many of these patients were identified as having sensory reabnormalities probably as a result of Peyronie's plaque surrounding the dorsal nerve of the penis. Preoperative biothesiometry studies at the University of North Carolina Hospitals has confirmed this increased incidence of abnormal distal penile sensation in both treated and untreated patients with dorsal Peyronie's plaques.

TREATMENT

A conservative initial approach to the treatment of Peyronie's disease will result in a satisfactory outcome in many patients. Patients with minimal or moderate curvature, no penile pain, and continued normal sexual activity require no invasive diagnostic procedures or treatment. Surgical alternatives must be considered only for those patients with erectile dysfunction precluding satisfactory sexual activity. Patients with mild curvature and erectile dysfunction from other causes may be considered for intercavernosal self-injection or a vacuum constriction device. Since both of these methods of treatment have resulted in increasing penile curvature in reported patients, patients must be advised that further curvature or aggravation of Peyronie's disease and its penile curvature may occur from these nonsurgical treatment modalities.

While nonsurgical treatment alternatives are widely used and discussed, no significant advances have been made with these techniques.[36,37] Because of the rarity of Peyronie's disease and the poor understanding of its ultimate natural history, the value of these treatment options continues to be controversial. Oral agents have been used widely for the treatment of Peyronie's disease. While these agents may simply allow patients to experience spontaneous resolution, reports of salutary effects from vitamin E, potassium para-aminobenzoate, and colchicine have led to their wide use of oral therapy of Peyronie's patients. Scardino and Scott in 1949 first reported the beneficial effects of vitamin E on Peyronie's plaques.[38] Subsequent noncontrol studies have reported success rates as high as 91% but most studies suggest little effectiveness of this vitamin supplement.[39,40] Potassium para-aminobenzoate acid (Potaba) has also been used but without control studies to confirm its success rates. Reported success rates as high as 88% have not been confirmed with controlled studies.[41] In vitro studies using cultured fibroblasts have demonstrated anti-inflammatory activity through stimulated polymorphonucleocytes and a limitation in the production of glycosaminoglycan (GAG).[42] The observation that Potaba limits collagen synthesis in fibroblast cell culture may explain its therapeutic effect.[18,43] Because of gastrointestinal side effects and medication costs, however, many patients find long-time use of potassium para-aminobenzoate difficult and the absence of controlled studies for confirmation of its effect discouraged urologists from the widespread use of this medication. More recently, colchicine has been suggested as an alternative for treatment of Peyronie's disease. Akkus et al in a recent pilot study administered colchicine to 24 Peyronie's patients for 3–5 months.[39] Improvement in Peyronie's plaque was identified in 12 of 24 patients with resolution of penile discomfort in 7 of 9 patients with penile pain. Penile curvature was reported to improve in 7 of 19 cases. While this study suffers from the limitations of no control group, colchicine theoretically induces collagenase activity and may decrease collagen synthesis in early Peyronie's plaques. Ralph and associates have also used tamoxifen, an agent which decreases the inflammatory response in fibroblast collagen production, with some early reported success.[44]

Intralesional injection with a variety of medications has also undergone investigation.[45–47] Injections with dimethyl sulfoxide and parathyroid hormone were tried without significant success.[48,49] Corticosteroids locally injected into the plaque also produce little improvement in pain, curvature, or plaque size. Collagenase which softens collagen-related fibrosis has been used for Peyronie's plaque intralesional treatment.[50,51] In a carefully performed prospective randomized study, Gelbard et al compared placebo with collagenase injection in patients with Peyronie's disease.[45] Although the response to collagenase injection for the whole group significantly outperformed placebo, when patients were stratified according to disease severity, it was apparent that patients with slight deformity were more likely to respond than those with severe deformity. Unfortunately, however, angular change in penile curvature was not statistically significant. Levine et al utilized the calcium channel block of verapamil as an intralesional injection agent.[47] Calcium channel blockers have been shown to alter fibroblast metabolism with decreased collagen secretion and increased collagenase activity. They studied 14 men who received biweekly injections of verapamil into the Peyronie's plaques for 6 months. There was improvement in penile narrowing in 100% of patients with curvature improvement in 42%. Plaque softening was likewise noted in all patients. Before intralesional therapy can be recommended, however, further study and long-term follow-up in controlled conditions should be evaluated.

Radiation therapy has also been frequently used for the treatment of Peyronie's disease.[6,52] Significant improvement in penile pain has been reported with little change in curvature or plaque size and no change in erectile function.[52] Rodrigues et al recently combined radiation therapy with vitamin E in a noncontrolled study and demonstrated reasonable effectiveness in diminishing penile pain with less effect on curvature, plaque, size, and erectile dysfunction.[53] No patient in their study, however, demonstrated deterioration of erectile function or other significant radiation-induced morbidity. Recent reports of corpora cavernosum fibrosis following low-dose radiation therapy for Peyronie's disease, however, raise significant concerns about using this modality for patients with penile pain from Peyronie's diseases since the pain from Peyronie's disease generally resolves spontaneously.

SURGICAL TREATMENT

The surgical treatment of Peyronie's disease must be reserved for those patients with severe disabling deformities precluding sexual activity. It is most appropriate to choose candidates for surgery with stable disease, waiting approximately 12 months after onset until plaque and curvature progression have ceased and pain has diminished. If patients continue to complain of significant curvature precluding sexual intercourse or inadequate penile rigidity, surgical intervention may be the only alternative. Patients with inadequate penile rigidity who prefer to avoid penile prosthesis implantation should undergo DICC, duplex Doppler ultrasound, and perhaps, nocturnal penile tumescence monitoring to fully evaluate erectile function. In patients with compromised vascular function in whom erection is poor or in whom pharmacoactive intercavernosal injection or vacuum constriction device is unsuccessful, reconstructive surgery without penile implantation is unlikely to be successful. If such patients demonstrate significant veno-occlusive abnormalities, reconstruction with venous ligation may result in restoration of erectile function. Because these reconstructive surgical procedures are frequently significant, penile incisions and plaque exposure may be difficult. Miller et al have reported a modification of the surgical incision of the penis to allow an adequate approach to the entire penile shaft and corpora cavernosa.[54] This extensive penile shaft exposure involves a circumcoronal incision and lateral scrotal incision to expose the penis adequately for more extensive reconstructive procedures. The penile shaft can be delivered through the lateral scrotal incision to reconstruct the penis in its entire length.

An appropriate procedure for reconstruction of the penis is best chosen by attention to the deformity associated with an individual's Peyronie's disease. In patients with excellent erections, minimal penile shortening, and mild to moderate curvature, simple penile straightening procedures with plication or Nesbit procedures are lowest in morbidity and preserve erectile function most adequately.[55-58] Plication procedures are the simplest to perform and involve creation of an artificial erection using the Gittes technique or the injection of papaverine or prostaglandin E prior to surgery. For a dorsal curvature, a ventral longitudinal incision can be carried out to expose the area opposite the curvature (Fig. 9.3A). Using nonabsorbable sutures only, multiple deep through-and-through sutures are placed into the tunica albuginea approximately 2–3 mm from the corpora spongiosum. These sutures are then tied and the erection again recreated to assess further curvature (Fig. 9.3B). For ventral curvature, a similar procedure is performed, however, a dorsal skin incision is uncomfortable and unsightly postoperatively and a circumcoronal incision with penile skin retraction is the most satisfactory method for exposure of the area for plication. Plicating sutures are placed lateral to the dorsal artery and vein but medial to the dorsal nerves which lie 1–2 cm lateral to the dorsal midline. Skin closure is carried out on both incisions using 4.0 chromic catgut sutures or other absorbable suture. Patients are provided with Valium for decreasing sleep rapid eye movement (REM), amylnitrite for decreasing erections, and, perhaps, diethylstilbestrol to eliminate nighttime erections during the healing period. In the recovery room, an ice pack is applied along with a light noncompressive dressing. Poulsen and Kirkeby retrospectively evaluated a series of patients undergoing tunica albuginea plication compared with the Nesbit procedure.[59] Of 32 patients undergoing plication procedures, 38% reported good results after first operation, with an additional 22% following a second plication procedure. Of 103 patients undergoing the Nesbit procedure, 88% obtained good or acceptable results after a first operation with an additional 5% success after a second operation. Failures from the plication group were primarily caused by recurrences of angulation, whereas those from the Nesbit group were accounted for primarily by erectile dysfunction. Other studies have strongly suggested that plication procedure provides excellent penile straightening with preserved erectile function.[60-62]

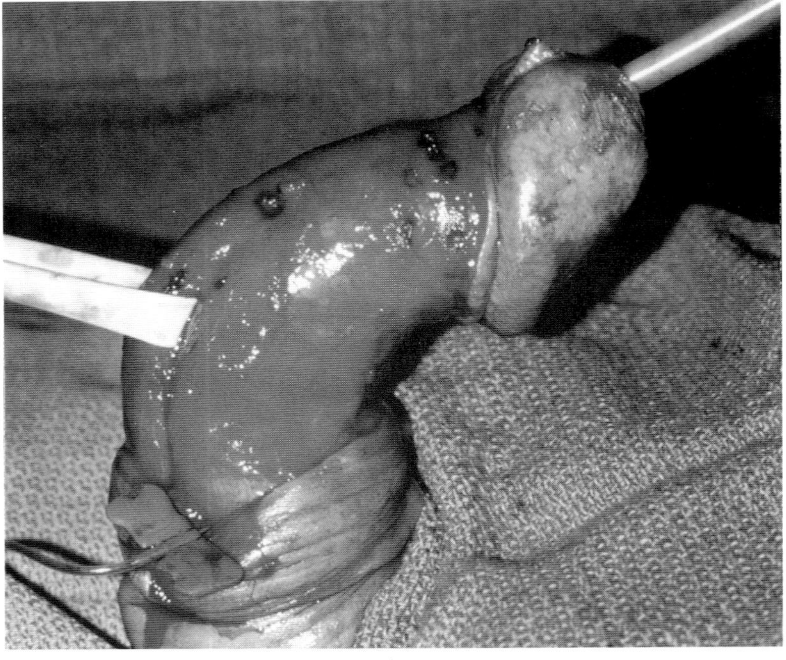

A

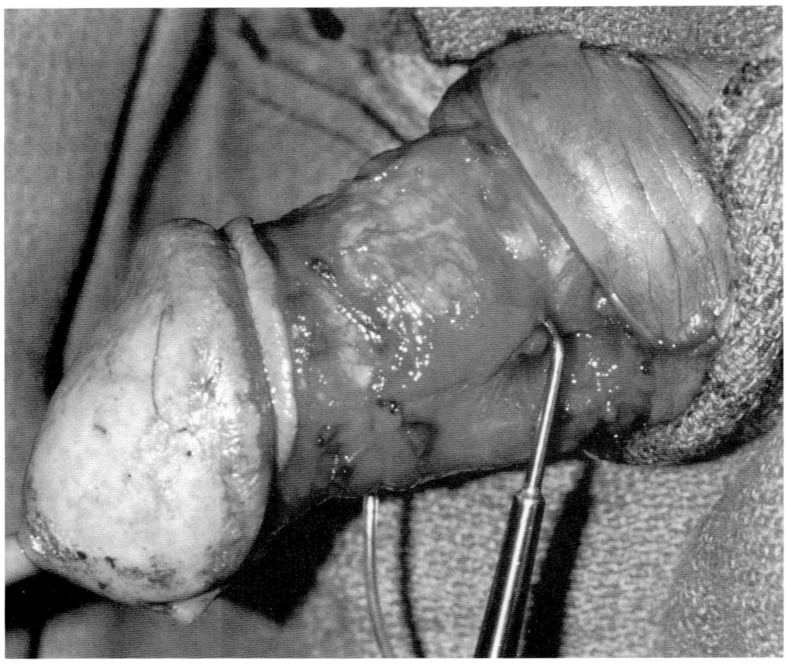

B

Fig. 9.3. A: Dorsal penile curvature at artificial erection prior to Nesbit procedure. **B:** After Nesbit ellipse has been removed and defect closed with running suture, artificial erection demonstrates straight penis. Surgical equipment marks the area of ellipse closure.

The Nesbit procedure has long been for correction of penile curvature and angulation. This conservative surgical procedure is performed in a fashion similar to that of corporal plication, however, an ellipse of tunica albuginea is removed to facilitate straightening.[63,64] The incisions previously described are appropriate for the Nesbit procedure as is the artificial erection created by the Gittes technique or papaverine injection. An ellipse of tunica albuginea is excised from the area opposite the point of greatest curvature with the amount of excision decided by approximating Alice clamps proximal and distal to the area to be excised. Once the ellipse is removed, the resultant defect is closed using continuous sutures of 4.0 polypropylene. Absorbable suture are not appropriate for either of these procedures since disolution during healing may result in curvature recurrence. Surgical knots are inverted to decrease postoperative palpation of suture material. Additional artificial erections are carried out following correction to ensure adequate straightening. If a sizable ellipse has been removed, a small suction drain may be left beneath the flap of penile skin to eliminate fluid collection. Usually 24 hr of suction drainage accompanied by an ice pack is adequate for healing and decreases subsequent pain, edema, and ecchymosis. A light nonconstriction dressing is applied and a Foley catheter is left in place if the patient had preoperative voiding difficulty. If venous excision and ligation are necessary or suggested by preoperative studies, incision should be carried out superior or lateral to the base of the penis such that the dorsal surface of the corporal bodies can be easily exposed to the level of the suspensory ligament of the penis. Ligation and an excision of abnormal venous structures are carried out in the standard fashion.[65]

Frequently, patients complain of "hinging" or the hourglass deformity which occurs in association with curvature or inadequate penile rigidity. Treatment of these areas of constriction may be surgically carried out using a corporoplasty as described by Sassine et al.[66] This corporoplasty is carried out by creating a longitudinal corpus cavernosum incision and closing it horizontally on a more complex flap using nonabsorbable suture. Yachia et al report 91% functional success in 41 patients undergoing incisional corporoplasty for penile curvature. Seven patients reported penile shortening without interference with coitus, whereas 11 patients complained of glans hypoesthesia which resolved within 6 months.[67]

For patients with significant penile curvature or short penises, plication or Nesbit procedures may result in unsatisfactory functional results. With these patients, plaque incision or excision and grafting may be necessary. These procedures, first popularized by Horton and Devine, initially were described using complete excision of the Peyronie's plaque and grafting using a graft of dermis.[68] This continues to be the gold standard treatment of many patients with Peyronie's disease. Patients with significant penile curvature, calcified plaque, and/or short penis in whom plication would result in unacceptable result are best suited to plaque excision and grafting. These patients should have adequate erectile function to be considered for these procedures. Recent modifications of this procedure have led to facilitation of surgery and some increased success.[69-71] Sapaio et al describe a newer method for plaque incision without plaque excision using an H-shaped incision to allow distention of the area of curvature followed by graft placement.[72] They report seven cases of Peyronie's disease treated with incision of Peyronie's plaque without excision of the tunica albuginea tissue. Once the incision was carried out, the penis was straightened and a patch of human lyophilized dura mater was placed. Surgical and functional results were reported as excellent.

Plaque incision without excision has been confirmed as effective using the carbon dioxide laser and grafting techniques in series of both Fournier et al and McVary and Kim.[71,73] Fournier et al described complete ablation of the entire palpable plaque using the carbon dioxide laser with excellent preservation of underlying corpus cavernosal tissue with vein grafting.[71] Plaque excision may be carried out using standard surgical dissection carbon dioxide laser. It is important, however, to begin dissection of Buck's fascia well lateral to the dorsal neurovascular bundle remembering that dorsal nerves to the penis may be 1–3 cm lateral to the deep dorsal artery and vein. Elevation of Buck's fascia from the plaque is carried out using sharp and blunt dissection and may be quite difficult because of reaction of the Peyronie's plaque to these structures. The dorsal neurovascular bundle or corpus spongiosum is mobilized thoroughly to an area approximately 1–2 cm proximal and distal to the plaque to be excised. The tunica albuginea once exposed is dissected free and all palpable plaque removed. Once the plaque has been excised and removed, relaxing incisions are carried out in each of the four corners of the defect to permit further penile straightening.[74] It may be necessary to further incise the Peyronie's plaque in the intracorporal septum in order to relax the penile curvature fully.

Once the dissection has been completed and straightening confirmed, graft material is chosen to close the defect. Reports by Wild et al described use of a dermal graft with excellent results for many patients.[75] A dermal graft can be obtained from groin or ventral forearm skin using either a dermatome or free hand excision of the epidermis.[68] I prefer a free hand harvest of groin skin because it is easily accessible, usually hairless, and closes well after skin removal. Other authors have described the use of tunica albuginea from the scrotum, dura mater, temporalis fascia, or saphenous vein with excellent results.[48,76–79] UNC Urology currently prefer the use of saphenous vein which is easily harvested through an incision superior to the medial malleolos of the patient's ankle. This venous patch provides an elastic, well-tolerated graft material. I suggest that the vein graft is better tolerated and that, perhaps through nitrite oxide production, healing and erectile function are stimulated. My experience is similar and finds that induration, inflammation, and graft contraction are less frequent with the saphenous vein patch in comparison with dermis, temporalis fascia, or artificial materials. Alternatives for graft materials include artificial graft material such as Gor-Tex (W.L. Gore & Associates, Baltimore MD) or Dacron (Dail Chemical, Goleta, CA).[49,56] Faerber and Konnak report that all nine men treated with incision and a Dacron patch had resolution of penile curvature and maintenance erectile function.[56] Treiber and Gilbert also report excellent results in 6 of 11 patients with an additional 3 patients requiring pharmacoactive injection therapy to maintain erectile function, but with preservation of normal erectile function and excellent penile straightening using plaque incision and Dacron grafting.[26] Ganabathi et al used polytetrafluoroethylene (Got-Tex) graft material in 16 men followed for an average of 47 months.[80] All 16 reported excellent erections with satisfactory intercourse although seven men had continued but mild penile curvature. Because impotence rates following plaque excision or incision and graft procedures may be as high as 70%, patients must be instructed thoroughly in the possible outcomes of these procedures, including the possibility of additional therapy being necessary following these plastic procedures. Preoperative evaluation to rule out veno-occlusive dysfunction and venous ligation at the time of reconstruction may decrease these postoperative failures. Patients must understand, however, that subsequent intracavernosal injection therapy, vacuum constriction device, or penile prosthesis implantation may be required for adequate erection.

Krishnamurti has recently reported an interesting method for reconstruction of the defect produced by excision of Peyronie's plaque.[81] He reports 17 patients in whom vascularized dermal flaps are created from penile skin. In the uncircumcised patient, an area of skin with the dorsal prepuce is infiltrated with saline and the epidermis removed by dermabrasion. An incision is carried out in the inner prepuce and a portion of preputial skin isolated on its vascular pedicle. This vascularized graft is than positioned over the area of plaque excision with its pedical distally. The graft is placed beneath the dorsal neurovascular bundle and the circumcoronal incision closed in the standard fashion. In patients who have been previously circumcised, a portion of dorsal penile skin is isolated with a lateral and distal vascular pedicle and again positioned over the area of plaque excision following dermabrasion removal of the epidermis. While this technique has not been confirmed by larger studies, the use of vascularized graft material may help reduce the incidence of graft contracture after surgical intervention.

If patients with Peyronie's disease have significant erectile dysfunction and lack of rigid erection or if other surgical procedures have failed to produce adequate results, penile prosthesis implantation, with or without penile straightening may be required to return patients to normal sexual activity.[29] Excellent results have been reported by a number of investigators using penile prosthesis implantation with or without plaque incision for correction of the corpus cavernosum.[82,83] Corpus cavernosum reconstruction after penile prosthesis implantation can be successfully carried out with simple plaque incision or with plaque incision and placement of natural or artificial graft material for filling the incisional defect (Fig. 9.4A, B). Complete plaque excision is rarely necessary. Several series have reported excellent results combining penile prosthesis implantation with plastic surgical correction of penile curvature.[84–87] Of 35 patients reported by Eigner et al, 88% were satisfied with the result of their treatment and were able to engage actively in sexual intercourse after mean follow-up of 6.9 yr.[85] Montorsi et al report poor patient satisfaction with semirigid prostheses and frequent requests to substitute three piece penile prostheses.[88] Further alternatives for penile prosthesis using Peyronie's disease were described by Wilson and Delk. They report 138 patients with severe Peyronie's disease implanted with penile prostheses who underwent modeling of the erect penis after prosthesis placement.[89] Modelling requires manual manipulation of the erect penis following prosthesis implantation until a straight penis results. This modelling which produces Peyronie's plaque relaxation was successful in 86% of patients with straight rigid erections with only 8% of patients requiring subsequent plaque incisions. In patients with significant and difficult penile shortening from Peyronie's disease, Rigaud and Berga have suggested procedures to produce penile lengthening after penile prosthesis implantation has been carried out.[90] These procedures require incision of the Peyronie's plaque, and in some cases, circumferential incision of the tunica albuginea and its septum with patching and placement of a penile implant. They report an average length gain of 1.5 inches with a circumferential incision in five patients undergoing this procedure. These more radical plastic reconstructive procedures require significant experience with Peyronie's surgery, penile

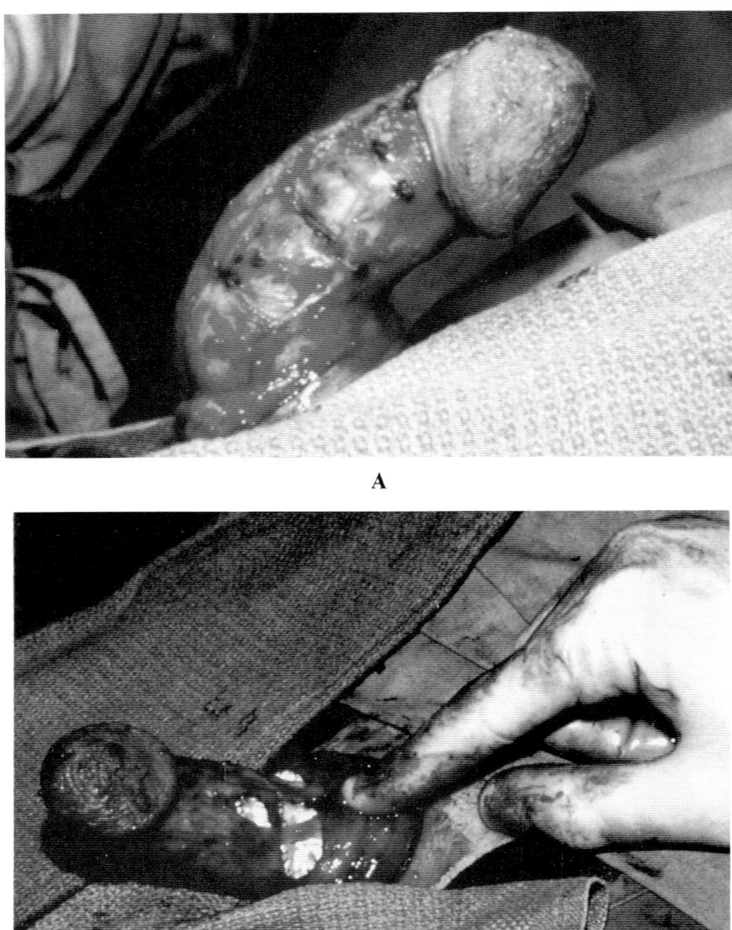

Fig. 9.4. A: Penile curvature following implantation of penile prosthesis in patient with severe Peyronie's disease. Continued dorsal penile curvature requires additional penile straightening. **B:** After isolation of dorsal neurovascular bundles, Peyronie's plaque is incised and Gor-Tex graft placed in the defect. Two Gor-Tex grafts have been sutured to the corpus cavernosum using Gor-Tex suture.

reconstructive surgery, and prosthesis implantation. Although results are generally good, morbidity and adverse outcomes restrict these procedures from patients with sever Peyronie's curvature and penile shortening.

CONCLUSION

The treatment of Peyronie's disease must be individually tailored to the patient and his complaints. Early Peyronie's disease before stabilization should be treated conservatively with watchful waiting, medical or injection techniques, or radiation therapy. Once the curvature, plaque, and pain have stabilized, the patient should be stratified for surgical intervention based on the severity of his complaints. Patients with minimal curvature and normal erection are best served by conservative procedures such as corpus cavernosum plication or the Nesbit procedure. With normal erectile function and short penis, or significant penile curvature, patients should be selected for plaque incision or excision, and grafting. Grafting material must be chosen based on the surgeon's experience. A complaint material is best selected and includes saphenous vein, dermis, dura mater, tunica vaginalis, temporalis fascia, and other similarly dualistic grafting tissues. Plaque excision and grafting can be combined with venous ligation surgery if veno-occlusive incompetence is diagnosed preoperatively. In those patients with significant erectile dysfunction and penile curvature, penile prosthesis implantation, with or without penile straightening, appears to be the procedure of choice.

REFERENCES

1. Carson CC: Francoix, Gigot de La Peyronie. *Invest Urol* 19:62–63, 1981.

2. Bivins CH, Marecek RL, Feldman JM: Peyronie's disease-presenting complaint of carcinoid syndrome. *N Engl J Med* 289:844–845, 1973.

3. Smith BH: Peyronie's disease. *Am J Clin Pathol* 45:670–677, 1966.

4. Devine CJ, Somers KD, Ladaga LE: Peyronie's disease: pathophysiology. *Prog Clin Biol Clin Biol Res* 370:355–358, 1991.

5. Gelbard MK: Dystrophic penile calcification in Peyronie's disease. *J Urol* 139:738–739, 1988.

6. Viljoen IM, Goedhals L, Domann J: Peyronie's disease: a perspective on the disease and the long term results of radiotherapy. *S Afr Med J* 83:19–20 10, 1993.

7. Chiang PH, Chiang CP, Shen MR, et al: Study of the changes in collagen of the tunica albuginea in the venogenic impotence in Peyronie's disease. *Eur Urol* 21:48–51, 1992.

8. Mersdorf A, Goldsmith PC, Diedrichs W: Ultrastructural changes in impotent penile tissue: comparison of 65 patients. *J Urol* 145:749–754, 1991.

9. Somers KD, Sismour EN, Wright GL: Isolation and characterization of collagen in Peyronie's disease *J Urol* 141:629–635, 1989.

10. Luangkhot R, Rutchik S, Agarwal V, et al: Collagen alterations in the corpus cavernosum of men with sexual dysfunction. *J Urol* 146:467–471, 1992.

11. Anafarta K, Beduk Y, Uluoglu O, et al: The significance of histopathological changes of the normal tunica albuginea in Peyronie's disease. *Int Urol Nephrol* 26:71–77, 1994.

12. Iacono F, Barra S, DeRosa G, et al: Microstructural disorders of the tunical albuginea in patients affected by Peyronie's disease with or without erection dysfunction. *J Urol* 150:1806–1809, 1993.

13. Mattson RH, Cramer JA, McCutchen CB: Barbiturate related connective tissue disorder. *Arch Int Med* 149:911–912, 1989.

14. Osborne DR: Propranolol and Peyronie's disease. *Lancet* 1:1111–1112, 1977.

15. Yudkin JS: Peyronie's disease in association with metoprolol. *Lancet* 2:1355, 1977.

16. VandeBerg JS, Devine CJ, Horton CE: Mechanisms of calcification in Peyronie's disease. *J Urol* 127:52–56, 1982.

17. Willscher MK, Cwazka WF, Novicki DE: The association of histocompatibility antigens of the B7 cross reacting group with Peyronie's disease. *J Urol* 122:34–36, 1979.

18. Rompel R, Meller-Eckhardt G, Schroeder-Printzen I, et al: HLA Antigens in Peyronie's disease. *Urol Internat* 52:34–37, 1994.

19. Somers KD, Winters PA, Dawson DM: Chromosomal abnormalities in Peyronie's disease. *J Urol* 137:672–676, 1987.

20. Nyberg LM, Bias WB,Hochberg MC, et al: Identification of an inherited form of Peyronie's disease with autosomal dominant inheretance in association with Duypuytren's contracture in histocompatibility B7 cross reacting antigens. *J Urol* 128:48–57, 1982.

21. Stewart S, Malto M, Sandberg L, et al: Increased serum levels of antielastin antibodies in patients with Peyronie's disease. *J Urol* 152:105–106, 1994.

22. Leffell MS, Devine CJ, Horton CE: Non-association of Peyronie's disease with HLA B7 cross reactive antigens. *J Urol* 127:1223–1226, 1983.

23. Desai KM, Gingell JC: Penile corporal fibrosis complicating papaverine self-injection therapy for erectile impotence. *Br J Urol* 15:132–136, 1988.

24. Kim JH, Carson CC: Development of Peyronie's disease with the use of vacuum constriction device. *J Urol* 149:1314–1315, 1993.

25. Gauldieri L, Valentini G, Lupolli S, et al: Peyronie's disease in systemic sclerosis: report of two cases. *J Rheumatol* 15:380–384, 1988.

26. Treiber LL, Gilbert P: Surgical treatment of Peyronie's disease. *Urol Int* 47:240–244, 1991.

27. Gelbard MK, Dorey F, James K: The natural history of Peyronie's disease. *J Urol* 144:1376–1380, 1990.

28. Lindsay MB, Shain DM, Granbach P, et al: The incidence of Peyronie's disease in Rochester, Minnesota, 1950 through 1984. *J Urol* 146:1007–1009, 1991.

29. Pryor JP: Peyronie's disease and impotence. *Acta Urol Belg* 56:317–325, 1988.

30. Ralph DJ, Hughes T, Lees WR, et al: Preoperative assessment of Peyronie's disease using color Doppler sonography. *Br J Urol* 69:629–632, 1992.

31. Lopez JA, Jarrow JP: Penile vascular evaluation of men with Peyronie's disease. *J Urol* 149:53–55, 1993.

32. Amin A, Patel U, Friedman EP, et al: Color Doppler and duplex ultrasound assessment of Peyronie's disease in impotent men. *Br J Radiol* 66:398–402, 1993.

33. Dalkin BL, Carter MF: Venogenic impotence following dermal graft repair of Peyronie's disease. *J Urol* 146:849–851, 1991.

34. Jordan GH, Angermeier KW: Preoperative evaluation of erectile function with dynamic infusion cavernosemetry/cavernosography in patients undergoing surgery for Peyronie's disease: correlation with postoperative results. *J Urol* 150:1138–1142, 1993.

35. Amarenco G, Casanova JM: Lesion of the dorsal nerve of the penis in Peyronie's disease. *Prog Urol* 1:906–910, 1991.

36. Morales A, Bruce AW: The treatment of Peyronie's disease with parathyroid hormone. *J Urol* 114:901–902, 1975.

37. Scheinman LJ, Miller EV: The use of dimethylsulfoxide (DMSO) and Peyronie's disease: a preliminary report. *Bac Med Surg* 75:61–62, 1967.

38. Scardino PL, Scott WW: The use of tocopherols in the treatment of Peyronie's disease. *Ann N Y Acad Sci* 52:390–392, 1949.

39. Akkus E, Carrier S, Rehman J, et al: Is colchicine effective in Peyronie's disease? A pilot study. *Urology* 44:291–295, 1994.

40. Pryor JP, Fitzpatrick JM: A new approach to the correction of the penile deformity of Peyronie's disease. *J Urol* 122:622–625, 1979.

41. Hasche-Klunder R: Treatment of Peyronie's disease using para-aminobenzoate potassium (Potaba), para-aminobenzoic acid potassium. *Urologe (A)* 17:224–227, 1978.

42. Sagone AL, Husney RM, Davis WB: Biotransformation of para-aminobenzoic acid and salicylic acid by PMN. *Free Rad Biol Med* 14:27–35, 1993.

43. Griffiths MR, Priestley GC: A comparison of morphea and lichen sclerosis et atrophicus in vitro: the effects of para-aminobenzoate on skin fibroblast. *Acta Derm Venereol* 72:115–118, 1992.

44. Ralph DJ, Brooks MD, Botazzo GF, Pryor JP: The treatment of Peyronie's disease with tamoxifen. *Br J Urol* 70:648–651 561, 1992.

45. Gelbard MK, James K, Reich P, et al: Collagenase versus placebo in the treatment of Peyronie's disease: a double-blind study. *J Urol* 146:56–58, 1993.

46. Jadot G, Vaille A, Maldonado J, et al: Clinical pharmacokinetics and delivery of bovine superoxide dismutase. *Clin Pharmacokinet* 28:17–25, 1995.

47. Levine LA, Merrick PF, Lee RC: Intralesional verapamil injection for the treatment of Peyronie's disease. *J Urol* 151:1522–1524, 1994.

48. Moriel VZ, Grinwald A, Rajfer J: Vein grafting of tunical incisions combined with contralateral plication in the treatment of penile curvature. *Urology* 43:697–701, 1994.

49. Schiffman ZJ, Gursel EO, Laor E: Use of Dacron patch graft in Peyronie's disease. *Urology* 25:38–41, 1995.

50. Gelbard MK, Lindner A, Kaufman JJ: The use of collagenase in the treatment of Peyronie's disease. *J Urol* 134:280–284, 1983.

51. Hamilton RG, Mintx GR, Gelbard MK: Humoral immune responses in Peyronie's disease patients receiving clostridial collagenase therapy. *J Urol* 135:641–644, 1986.

52. Carson CC, Coughlin PWF: Radiation therapy for Peyronie's disease: is there a place? *J Urol* 134:684–687, 1985.

53. Rodrigues CI, Njo KH, Karim AB: Results of radiotherapy and vitamin E in the treatment of Peyronie's disease. *Int J Rad Onc Biol Physics* 31:571–576, 1995.

54. Miller EB, Schlossberg SM, Devine CJ: New incision for penile surgery. *J Urol* 150:179–180, 1993.

55. Erpenbach K, Rothe H, Derschum W: The penile plication procedure: an alternative method for straightening penile deviation. *J Urol* 146:1276–1278, 1991.

56. Faerber GJ, Konnak JW: Results of combined Nesbitt plication with plaque incision and Placement of Dacron patch in patients with severe Peyronie's disease. *J Urol* 149:1319–1320, 1993.

57. Ludwig G: Evaluation of conservative therapeutic approaches to Peyronie's disease. *Urol Int* 47:236–239, 1991.

58. Mufti GR, Atchison M, Bramwell SP, et al: Corporal plication for surgical correction of Peyronie's disease. *J Urol* 144:281–282, 1991.

59. Poulsen J, Kirkeby HJ: Treatment of penile curvature—a retrospective study of 175 patients operated with plication of the tunica albuginea or the Nesbitt procedure. *Br J Urol* 75:370–374, 1995.

60. Austoni E, Colombo F, Mantovani F: Evaluation of corpora alterations and erectile dysfunction following radical surgery for Peyronie's disease and long term follow-up on 152 operated patients. *J Androl* 15(ASN):57–62, 1994.

61. Claes H, VanPoppel H, Baert L: Nocturnal penile tumescence evaluation before and after corporal plication for Peyronie's disease. *Acta Urol Belg* 62:57–60, 1984.

62. Nooter RI, Baosch JL, Schroeder FH: Peyronie's disease and congenital penile curvature: long term results of operative treatment with a plication procedure. *Br J Urol* 74:497–500, 1994.

63. Coughlin PWF, Carson CC, Paulson DF: Surgical correction of Peyronie's disease: the Nesbit procedure. *J Urol* 131:282–286, 1984.

64. Ralph DJ, Al-akraa M, Pryor JP: The Nesbitt operation for Peyronie's disease: 16 year experience. *J Urol* 154:11362–11363, 1995.

65. Kerfoot WW, Carsosn CC, Donaldson JT, et al: Investigation of vascular changes following penile vein ligation. *J Urol* 152:884–887, 1994.

66. Sassine AM, Wespes E, Schulman CC: Modified corporoplasty for penile curvature: ten years experience. *Urology* 44:419–421, 1994.

67. Yachia D, Aridogan IA, Erlich N, et al: Patient satisfaction after incisional corporoplasty and Peyronie's disease curvature. *J Urol* 153:272a, 1995.

68. Devine CJ, Horton CE: Surgical treatment of Peyronie's disease with dermal graft. *J Urol* 111:44–55, 1974.

69. Abe S, Takami Y, Yamaguchi Y, et al: Penile reconstruction with de-epithelized superficial external pudendal arterial flap. *J Urol* 147:155–157, 1992.

70. Costello RT: Laser vaporization of Peyronie's plaques. *Lasers Surg Med* 13:246–247, 1993.

71. Fournier GR, Lue TF, Tanagho BA: Peyronie's plaque: Surgical treatment with a carbon dioxide laser and deep dorsal vein patch graft. *J Urol* 149:1321–1325, 1993.

72. Sapaio JS, Passarino A, Oliveira AG, et al: Surgical correction of severe Peyronie's disease without plaque excision. *Eur Urol* 22:130–133, 1992.

73. Kim ED, McVary KT: Long term follow-up of treatment of Peyronie's disease with plaque incision, carbon dioxide laser plaque ablation and placement of a deep dorsal vein patch graft. *J Urol* 153:1843–1846, 1995.

74. Gelbard MK: Relaxing incisions in the correction of penile deformity due to Peyronie's disease. *J Urol* 145:1457–1460, 1995.

75. Wild RM, Devine CJ, Horton CE: Dermal repair of Peyronie's disease: survey of 50 patients. *J Urol* 121:47–51, 1979.

76. Brock G, Kadioglu A, Lue TF: Peyronie's disease: a modified treatment. *Urology* 42:300–304, 1993.

77. Fallon B: Cadaveric dura mater graft for correction of penile curvature in Peyronie's disease. *Urology* 35:127–129, 1990.

78. Helal MA, Lockhart JL, Sanford E, Persky L: Tunica vaginalis flap for the management of disabling Peyronie's disease: surgical technique, results, and complications. *Urology* 46:390–392, 1995.

79. Gelbard MK, Hayden B: Expanding contractures of the tunica albuginea due to Peyronie's disease with temporalis fascia free grafts. *J Urol* 145:772–776, 1991.

80. Ganabathi K, Demochowski R, Zimmern PE, et al: Peyronie's disease: surgical treatment based on penile rigidity. *J Urol* 153:662–666, 1995.

81. Krishnamurti S: Penile dermal flap for defect reconstruction in Peyronie's disease: operative technique in four years experience in 17 patients. *Int J Impot Res* 7:195–208, 1995.

82. Bertram RA, Carson CC, Altaffer LF: Severe penile curvature after implantation of an inflatable penile prosthesis. *J Urol* 139:743–748, 1988.

83. Kulaksizoglu H, Hakim LS, Hamill BK, et al: The first guide to safe electrocautery use with Bioflex inflatable cylinders: results of in vitro tests and in vivo studies in patients undergoing tunical incisions for Peyronie's disease following implantation of mentor alpha-1 inflatable penile prosthesis. *J Urol* 153:360a, 1995.

84. Carson CC, Hodge GB, Anderson EE: Penile prosthesis in Peyronie's disease. *Br J Urol* 55:417–420, 1983.

85. Eigner EB, Kabalin JN, Kessler R: Penile implants in the treatment of Peyronie's disease. *J Urol* 145:69–71, 1991.

86. Knoll LD, Furlow WL, Benson RC: Management of Peyronie's disease by implantation of inflatable penile prosthesis. *Urology* 36:406–409, 1990.

87. O'Donnell PD: Results of surgical management of Peyronie's disease. *J Urol* 148:1184–1187, 1992.

88. Montorsi F, Guazoni G, Bergamaschi F, et al: Patient partner satisfaction with semi-rigid rod penile prosthesis for Peyronie's disease: a five year follow-up study. *J Urol* 150:1819–1821, 1993.

89. Wilson SK, Delk JR: A new treatment for Peyronie's disease: modelling the penis over an inflatable penile prosthesis. *J Urol* 152:1121–1123, 1994

90. Rigaud G, Berga RE: Corrective procedures for penile shortening due to Peyronie's disease. *J Urol* 153:368–370, 1995.

<h1 style="text-align:center">10</h1>

Minimally Invasive Therapy for Erectile Dysfunction: Intracavernosal, Oral, Transdermal/Transglanular, and Intraurethral Approaches

Harin Padma-Nathan

Erectile dysfunction is a significant public health issue affecting nearly 10–20 million American men.[1] It is perhaps best defined functionally as the inability to obtain and maintain an erection sufficient for satisfactory intercourse or other sexual expression.[2] It is a para-aging phenomenon that affects nearly 52% of men between the age of 40 and 70 yr.[1] It is exacerbated in the presence of such patient profile factors as diabetes, heart disease, hypertension, cigarette smoking, hyperlipidemia, and cardiovascular medication. There exists a direct correlation between potency and quality of life.[3] The social and behavioral costs of erectile dysfunction are staggering. It has been demonstrated to adversely impact self-esteem, anxiety, depression, work capacity, alcohol and illicit drug use as well as the ability to maintain social, family, and intimate interpersonal relationship roles.[4] Recent quality-of-life assessments of the impact of successful erectile dysfunction therapy by intracavernosal alprostadil have demonstrated not only improved erection, orgasm, and sexual satisfaction but also improved long-term (18 months follow-up) mental health and interpersonal sensitivity and decreased anxiety.[5]

Historically, the advent of the penile prostheses enabled for the first time the effective treatment of organic impotence by facilitating a "hard penis" (not a physiologic erection). However, the modern era of intracavernosal pharmacotherapy enabled not only the re-creation of a physiologic erection but also the ability to understand and manipulate the corporal trabecular smooth muscle. Intracavernosal pharmacotherapy is now the cornerstone of therapy for erectile dysfunction and it is the gold standard by which all alternative pharmacologic therapies are measured. This era began somewhat serendipitously with the observation by Brindley, a neuropsychiatrist, that the self-injection of an irreversible-adrenergic antagonist, phenoxybenzamine, into the corpora produced a rigid erection on demand.[6] Virag independently at about the same time demonstrated that papaverine hydrochloride was able to do the same when injected into the corpora of a patient with erectile dysfunction.[7] Zorgniotti and Lefleur suggested that the combination of vasoactive substances with differing mechanisms of action, including papaverine hydrochloride (a direct smooth muscle relaxant) and phentolamine mesylate (an α-adrenergic antagonist), may have synergistic effects.[8] This combination of papaverine and phentolamine remained the most commonly utilized intracavernosal pharmacotherapy approach in the United States until the late 1980s.[9] Ishii and Shirai,[10] Virag and Adaikin,[11] and Stackl[12] each contributed to the clinical experience that ultimately demonstrated that alprostadil, the synthetic formulation of prostaglandin E1 was indeed the pharmacologic agent that most closely approximated the ideal pharmacologic agent for intracavernosal pharmacotherapy. Alprostadil produces corporal smooth muscle relaxation by increasing the concentration of adenosine $3':5'$-cyclic phosphate (cAMP) via modulation of adenyl cyclase. This in turn stimulates proteininase A and ultimately, via the voltage dependent L-type calcium ion channels, decreases the intracellular free calcium concentration and produces smooth muscle relaxation. It is rapidly metabolized primarily by a dehydrogenase system in the corporal tissue. Any systematically transferred drug is metabolized nearly completely within two passes through the lungs. It is associated with an overall response rate of 75% and this is increased to 85% and 92% when combined with phentolamine[13] (bi-mix) and papaverine/phentolamine[14] (tri-mix). The FDA approval on July 6, 1995 of a proprietary formulation of alprostadil sterile powder (Alprostadil S.Po.) or Caverject (Pharmacia and Upjohn Inc., Kalamazoo, MI), heralded a new era of intracavernosal pharmacotherapy. Alprostadil sterile powder or Caverject contains in addition to alprostadil, lactose, sodium citrate, and benzyl alcohol. It has a pH ranging between 4.4 and 7.05 when reconstituted with sterile water. It appears to be room temperature stable for at least 3 months until reconstitution. The stability of the reconstituted solution is at least 24 hr but is probably similar to the previous diluted solutions of Prostin VR pediatric (Pharmacia and Upjohn Inc.) i.e., 3 months. In comparative studies it appears to be identical in effect to Prostin. It is currently available in 10- and 20-µg vials with a plan to introduce a 5-µg vial in the near future. In Australia a frozen sterile solution is employed that appears to be more user-friendly. This solution will probably be the next generation of Caverject introduced in the United States. Additionally, a proprietary formulation of alprostadil with a unique α-cyclodextrin ring (a cyclic glucose oligomer), alprostadil alphadex, is being investigated by Schwarz Pharma AG (Mannheim, Germany). It may be more heat stable as a result of the modification of its chemical structure. Initial clinical trials results appear to be similar to those from the Alprostadil S. Po. trials. Alprostadil S. Po. has undergone rigorous clinical investigation in 12 different studies encompassing over 1,800 patients.[15] A summary of the salient points of these studies is as follows:

1. A single dose of Alprostadil S. Po. is effective over the range of 2.5 to 20 µg. Even at 2.5 µg Alprostadil S. Po. was more effective than placebo. In open label, long-term studies the effective dose ranged between 0.2 and 140 µg.

2. There is a dose response to Alprostadil S. Po. with respect to both the erectile rigidity, evaluated clinically or by RigiScan (Dacomed Corp.), and the duration of erectile response.

3. Regardless of the etiology, 75–79% of patients will achieve an optimal dose sufficient for intercourse.

4. In patients who were titrated in-office, achieved an optimal response and subsequently injected at home, 89–99% reported an adequate at-home response. The mean optimal dose in-office in one long-term study was 17.7 µg. The majority (75%) did not alter this does at home—17% increased the dose and 8% decreased the dose. The final mean dose was 20.7 µg.

5. Patient and partner acceptance (satisfaction) was high. Patients reported 73–87% of injections resulted in satisfactory intercourse. Partners reported 72–86% of injections resulted in satisfactory intercourse.

6. When median "minimum effective" doses were examined, patients with psychogenic effective dose (ED; 4 µg) tended to respond at lower doses than those with neurogenic ED (7.5 µg), vasculogenic ED (7.5 µg), or mixed etiology ED (10 µg). Patients with arteriogenic ED (median "minimum effective" dose: 2.5 µg) responded to lower doses than those patients with venogenic ED (median "minimum effective dose: 7.5 µg). The most pure neurogenic patients, the spinal cord injured patients, responded in 50% of cases to a 1.0-µg dose and no spinal cord injured patient required more than 7.5 µg. However, regardless of the etiology, patients may respond to Alprostadil S. Po. in doses as low as 0.5 µg and therefore all patients should be carefully titrated in the office. The recommended initial titration dose of Alprostadil S. Po. for pure neurogenic patients or for patients of unknown etiology is 1.25 µg and 2.5 µg for all others.

The introduction of an FDA-approved pharmacologic agent for intracavernosal therapy has scientifically (via placebo-controlled, randomized and blinded as well as open label clinical trials) established efficacy and safety parameters. At a practical level I continue to offer either Alprostadil S. Po./Caverject alone or more commonly a combination of Alprostadil S. Po./Caverject (20 µg/ml) and phentolamine mesylate (0.5 µg/ml). This solution is produced by reconstituting ten 20-µg vials of Caverject and one 5-mg vial of phentolamine mesylate in 10 ml of sterile water. This bi-mix has an overall response rate of 85% and significantly reduces the alprostadil requirement by 50% in a patient, thereby decreasing the incidence of dose-related side effects as pain and possibly corporal scarring. It is also associated with a lower incidence of pain than is prostaglandin alone because the two pharmacologic agents act synergistically and as a result, lower doses of alprostadil are required to achieve a rigid erection. If a patient fails, the bi-mix 50–65% can be salvaged by tri-mix combinations of alprostadil, phentolamine, and papaverine. I do not attempt to salvage patients further with the addition of atropine (quad-mix) because of the potential for severe cardiac collapse.[16] It should be noted that if any combinations other than Caverject alone are employed the package insert will no longer serve as adequate informed consent and the patient must be formally consented.

Priapism is readily avoided by careful titration. We routinely employ a 29-gauge needle for injection. There have been reports of finer needles (30-gauge) which have broken in the corpora. The patients should inject along the proximal two-thirds of the penis and alternate sides if able. I usually initiate titration, utilizing my bi-mix, at 0.1 to 0.3 ml depending on the age of the patient and the estimated adequacy of their corporal veno-occlusive mechanism. In young patients with a history of penile perineal or pelvic trauma as well as in psychogenic or neurogenic patients, test dosing is initiated at 0.05 to 0.1 ml. In older patients with atherosclerotic vascular risk factors or metabolic diseases such as diabetes, the corporal smooth muscle is abnormal in number and function. This smooth muscle degeneration will be clinically manifest as corporal veno-occlusive dysfunction. These patients will require much higher doses of intracavernosal vasoactive agents and may even fail to respond to medication. I usually initiate test dosing in these patients at 0.3 ml or higher if invasive testing has been performed and has demonstrated the presence of severe corporal veno-occlusive dysfunction. Regardless, the maximum dose I employ is 1.0 ml (i.e., 20 µg alprostadil and 0.5 mg phentolamine). In select patients who fail to respond or those who experience significant pain; nearly 50% can be salvaged with the employment of a three-drug combination of alprostadil (10–20 µg/ml), papaverine (15 mg/ml), and phentolamine (0.5 mg/ml). The other agents currently available include moxisylate, vasoactive intestinal polypeptide, calcitonin gene-related peptide, and nitric oxide donors such as linsidomine hydrochloride.[17–21] However, none of these to date have demonstrated adequate clinical efficacy as a single agent.

These patients should be followed at regular intervals. It is now known that corporal fibrosis in patients on long-term alprostadil injection therapy will increase progressively over time. I instruct patients on regular self-examination (in the erect state) and perform a formal color duplex ultrasound evaluation annually. The latter is done in conjunction with a physical examination in the erect state and provides early detection of echo-dense microscopic scar tissue and an assessment of the hemodynamic improvement or deterioration from the baseline.

In my practice, intracavernosal pharmocotherapy plays a critical role in managing patients who have undergone a nerve-sparing radical prostatectomy.[22] In a recent study at our institution, nearly 90% of patients following a nerve-sparing radical prostatectomy responded to intracavernosal alprostadil in contrast to only 66% of patients following a non-nerve-sparing radical prostatectomy. In addition, nearly 25% of the nerve-sparing prostatectomy patients who responded did so at 2 µg of alprostadil or less (when combined with phentolamine). In contrast, patients having undergone a non-nerve-sparing procedure required significantly higher doses of the same drug. These results, in combination with the relatively low overall potency restoration rate of the nerve-sparing approach to radical prostatectomy, have prompted us to present this surgical procedure to most patients as one that will more likely facilitate subsequent pharmacotherapy even in the absence of restored potency.

Recently we have had the opportunity to examine the ultrastructure (by electron microscopy) of corporal tissue biopsies at the time of radical pelvic surgery and again 3 months later when the patient returned for the placement of penile prosthetic cylinders (see below). In this interim the corporal ultrastructure demonstrated severe smooth muscle loss and degeneration. Therefore we hypothesize that, in part, the failure of potency restoration following a nerve-sparing radical prostatectomy is the result of end organ degeneration during the period of repair of a neuropraxia. This degeneration of corporal smooth muscle may be initiated by the loss of neurotropic factors or by the loss of oxygenation of the corpora during spontaneous and nocturnal erections. Regardless, this may be prevented by early institution of intracavernosal pharmacotherapy. As a result of this preservation, the ultimate potency restoration rate of a nerve-sparing radical prostatectomy may increase dramatically. Such studies are currently underway at our institution.

INDICATIONS AND CONTRAINDICATIONS FOR INTRACAVERNOSAL PHARMACOTHERAPY

Patients with the following demonstrate true and absolute contraindications to intracavernosal pharmacotherapy with alprostadil or any other vasoactive substances: patients on monoamine oxidase (MAO) inhibitors, patients with a known hypersensitivity to alprostadil, patients with a propensity toward secondary forms of priapism such as those with sickle cell disease or trait, multiple myeloma, or leukemia. The patient with Peyronie's disease indeed presents a therapeutic dilemma. We urologists have long employed intracavernosal pharmacotherapy as a means of treating the erectile dysfunction associated with Peyronie's disease that demonstrates minimal to moderate curvature. Currently, the Caverject insert considers this an exclusion to its use. Therefore, if it is employed in such patients, it must be considered an off label indication that requires specific consent. Informed consent, either written or verbal, should include the following: a discussion of safe and relatively sterile injection techniques, injection site compression (including more prolonged compression in patients on acetylsalicylic acid (ASA) and anticoagulants—which are otherwise not a contraindication to intracavernosal injection therapy), the practice of safe sex, injection frequency of 3 to 5 times per week and no more than once in a 24-hr period of time, the safe single use and disposal of needles, and the adverse medical events discussed below.

ADVERSE MEDICAL EVENTS RELATED TO INTRACAVERNOSAL PHARMACOTHERAPY

As a result of both intracorporal metabolism and rapid systemic metabolism (lungs), systemic adverse events are virtually nonexistent with intracavernosal alprostadil therapy. The most significant adverse medical effects issues are local and include principally penile pain, prolonged erections, and corporal fibrosis.

Penile Pain

Penile pain occurred in 34% of patients but only in 11% of injections, i.e., not all injections resulted in pain. Penile pain is more frequently a diffuse ache within the penis (63%) than needle site pain related to injection (37%). The intensity but not the duration of the former is dose-dependent and occurs in about 5–20% of patients receiving less than 10 μg of straight alprostadil S. Po. and in 30–40% of patients receiving 20–40 μg of the same. This pain is most frequently described as minimal to moderate. Only 3% of patients discontinued therapy as a result of pain. It has been suggested that, in those patients in whom this pain prevents comfortable intercourse, one consider the addition of a local anesthetic (procaine)[23] or buffering agent (sodium bicarbonate).[24] I, however, am concerned about the possible increase in corporal fibrosis as a result of the addition of these agents. I therefore attempt to address this innocuous local adverse event by the employment of polypharmacotherapy to minimize the total dose of alprostadil delivered. The exact mechanism of pain induced by prostaglandins is incompletely understood. It may be related to the carrier or preservative, the alcohol (Prostin), or most likely to the nocioceptive nerve fiber interaction with the drug. Prostaglandins can cause hyperalgia—they appear to lower the threshold of the pain fiber to mechanical, thermal, or chemical stimulation.[25] Some specific patient groups appear to be more sensitive to this event, particularly diabetic patients. I have found systemic oral prostaglandin inhibitor therapy (e.g., ASA, ibuprofen etc.) to be of no benefit in treating or preventing this pain.

Prolonged Erections and Priapism

Prolonged erections (>4 hr and <6 hr) and priapisms (>6 hr) represent urgent medical events that potentially may result in irreversible corporal smooth muscle loss. Significant smooth muscle and eventually endothelial ultrastructural changes are observed at 24 and 48 hr respectively. However, the progressive loss of smooth muscle from ischemic injury may occur even earlier and therefore prolonged erections must be avoided if at all possible by careful dose titration, particularly in high-risk patients, and if they occur they must be treated early (5–8 hr) and aggressively.

Priapism related to intracavernosal pharmacotherapy may either be, more commonly, low-flow (veno-occlusive) or high-flow (arterial). The latter may occur if a branch of the cavernosal artery is lacerated by the needle. This is exceedingly uncommon. It may be suspected if the erection is painless, partial and associated with arterial red blood on aspiration. It is best screened for by color flow duplex ultrasonography and definitively diagnosed and treated by interventional selective internal pudendal arteriography.

Veno-occlusive low-flow priapisms resulting from intracavernosal alprostadil or alprostadil bi-mix are significantly less resistant to intracavernosal α-adrenergic therapy than those associated with papaverine bi-mix, timix, or idiopathic priapisms if treated within 6–8 hr of onset. If treated within 3–4 hr, simple α-adrenergic injection without large needle aspiration and irrigation are often completely effective. The drug of choice is a pure α-adrenergic agonist, phenylephrine (Neosynephrine). Mixed α- and β-agonists, such as adrenaline, are less effective and ganglionic agents such as metaraminol may cause refractory hypertension that may be severe enough to rupture cerebral and abdominal aneurysms. Phenylephrine is available as a 1% solution (i.e., 10 mg in a milliliter vial). This is diluted 1 : 10 to produce a 1,000 µg/ml solution. This is done as follows: in a 10- or 12-ml syringe withdrew 9 ml of normal saline and then withdraw the 1-ml solution of phenylephrine. The resultant solution is then of the desired concentration following mixing. Now have your assistant remove the needle from the syringe, hold it upside down and withdraw 0.4–0.5 ml into a U100 insulin syringe with an ultrafine needle (29G). Inject this following measurement and monitoring of the patient's blood pressure and heart rate. Repeat at intervals of 10 to 15 min if the blood pressure has not elevated. If 3–6 administrations have not achieved detumescence, particularly in prolonged cases, consider aspirating a corpora with the aid of a 19–21G butterfly needle. Once arterialized red blood has reentered the corpora, the smooth muscle may become rapidly responsive again to α-agonists. Therefore be cautious not to be overly aggressive with phenylephrine therapy following aspiration—utilize the same small repetitive doses described above while continuing to monitor the patient's cardiovascular status. Be persistent, virtually all pharmacologically induced priapisms of less than 12–24 hr duration will respond and will not require surgical shunting. Do not overcorrect! This may result in a rapid systemic flush of phenylephrine and subsequent hypertension, headache, chest pain, etc. Following the treatment of the priapism, determination of the cause is necessary if the patient was not titrating but rather on home maintenance—was this related to inadvertent or intentional overdosing or double dosing, etc.

Corporal Fibrosis

Corporal fibrosis is the most significant chronic complication of intracavernosal pharmacotherapy. The clinical and histopathologic incidence of corporal fibrosis with the intracavernosal administration of alprostadil is significantly different than that observed with previous generations of pharmacologic agents. Papaverine was associated with a clinical and histopathologic incidence of fibrosis of 30(50)% and nearly 100% respectively in animal models[26] and in men following at least 2 yr of therapy. Alprostadil, however, in animal models appears to demonstrate necropsy findings indistinguishable from saline administration.[27] These findings were primarily related to needle trauma and resolved rapidly. In fact, in recent cell culture studies at our institution, we demonstrated that transforming growth factor-β_1 (TGF-β_1)-mediated collagen synthesis is repressed by alprostadil. Therefore, prostaglandins may protect the corporal tissue from fibrosis. The long-term phase 3 Caverject clinical trials in both the United States (683 patients) and Europe (863 patients) have demonstrated that the incidence of corporal fibrosis at 6 months is 2.2–4.0% and at 18 months is 6.0–7.8%.[28] In contrast to the previous generation of pharmacologic agents, the clinical manifestation of the fibrosis (130 patients) was most frequently as a curvature without any detectable plaque or nodule (39.2%) or as a Peyronie's-like plaque in the tunica albuginea (35.4%) as opposed to disfiguring intracavernosal nodules (25.4%). The incidence of corporal fibrosis was slightly greater in diabetic patients and may theoretically be greater in patients at risk for Peyronie's disease. It is otherwise unrelated to the primary diagnosis. Although the overall incidence of fibrosis in the above two clinical trials increased with time, corporal fibrosis does not appear to be related to the frequency of injection. It may, however, be related to false (intratunical, intratrabecular, intraseptal) injections and hematoma formation. It may also be related to the trauma of intercourse in a similar fashion to the delamination injury theory associated with Peyronie's disease. The site of the fibrosis is rarely at the injection site. Ultimately, the pathogenesis of alprostadil-associated corporal fibrosis may demonstrate itself to be related to a complex combination of drug effect, mechanical trauma, genetic predisposition, and altered wound healing. Additionally, the ischemic injury of a priapism (particularly if over 12 hr duration) may result in smooth muscle degeneration and fibrosis. Corporal fibrosis in its various manifestations is best diagnosed by physical examination in the erect state. This is best done following an injection by both the patient at-home and by the physician in-office at least annually. Ultrasound may assist in early detection of echo-dense areas that may ultimately become areas of fibrosis.

The management principles applied to corporal fibrosis related to intracavernosal pharmacotherapy have been significantly influenced by the clinical experience with Peyronie's disease. In a manner similar to Peyronie's disease, there is frequently a spontaneous resolution of the fibrosis. In fact, 15.2% of Peyronie's-like plaques,

36.4% of intracorporal nodules, and 49% of curvatures resolved spontaneously with (31.8%) or without (68.2%) temporary termination of injection therapy. The overall spontaneous resolution rate was 33.8% (44 of 130). It is not unreasonable to reinstitute intracorporal pharmacotherapy following resolution of the fibrosis. If the fibrosis does not resolve, however, a clinical decision must be made as to whether the fibrosis is functionally significant. If the curvature, deformity, or shortening does not preclude comfortable intercourse for both the patient and partner, then continued intracavernosal pharmacotherapy with informed consent is not unreasonable. If, however, this is not the case, the patient's options are limited and involve penile prosthesis insertion with corporal reconstruction and plastic procedures for penile straightening.

Corporal fibrosis related to intracavernosal alprostadil therapy is uncommon and associated with a relatively high spontaneous resolution rate. It may rarely, however, be unremitting, functionally disfiguring and ultimately require reconstructive surgery. Therefore, each patient selecting this treatment option must be cognizant of corporal fibrosis (by informed consent) and must exercise the appropriate preventative measures and aid in the early diagnosis by continuous self-examination and routine follow-up with his treating physician.

Long-term Patient Acceptance and Return of Spontaneous Erections

Although the patient and partner satisfaction rate is about 80–85%, the drop-out during test-dosing is generally 10% to 30%, in even those patients that respond with a rigid erection. In these patients, the primary reason for drop-out in this phase is related to fear or disinterest in needle-injection. The drop-out rate following institution of home self-injection is about 50% (30–80% in various series).[29] In a well-motivated group of patients in the Caverject trials the drop-out rate was still 25–30%. This later drop-out may be related to a waning interest on the part of the patient or his partner, loss of response to medication, cost, intercurrent illness or most interestingly the return of spontaneous erections. The latter is believed to occur in 8–15% of patients and in one small Upjohn Caverject study it represented the most frequent cause for drop-out. The progressive return of spontaneous erections is best and most consistently seen in psychogenic patients as opposed to arteriogenic or venogenic patients over a 6-month follow-up as demonstrated by McMahon.[30] The return of spontaneous erections therefore most likely reflects a decrease in the psychogenic component of the patient's erectile dysfunction. However, it is theoretically possible that the increased oxygenation of the corporal[31] resulting from the pharmacologic stimulation may aid in the preservation of the corporal smooth muscle and, in some early cases of smooth muscle myopathy, it may reverse the pathology. This remains to be proven, however.

The high drop-out related to intracavernosal pharmacotherapy in part reflects normal human sexual behavior. Many patients, following a "honeymoon period" of frequent use, will ultimately inject only once a month or less. However, many patients drop-out as a result of factors related to the need to inject. An impetus therefore exists for the development of less invasive drugs and delivery systems. As previously mentioned, alprostadil appears to be an ideal drug for corporal pharmacotherapy. However, less invasive routes of delivery are now being explored and are in varying states of clinical development. The following is a discussion of these novel delivery routes and novel drugs that demonstrate the promise of expanding our therapeutic armamentarium by the turn of the century.

ORAL CORPORAL PHARMACOTHERAPY

Adrenergic Antagonists

α_2-Adrenoceptor Antagonists

Yohimbine hydrochloride is an α_2-adrenoceptor antagonist that demonstrates both central and peripheral action. The α_2 presynaptic receptor appears to be located on nonadrenergic (nitrergic) nerves particularly localized to the cavernosal artery, and its blockade may augment the release of nitrergic neurotransmitters and thus increase intracorporal blood flow. To date, yohimbine appears to be no more effective than placebo in the treatment of organic erectile dysfunction.[32] It may, however, benefit that specific subgroup with early arteriogenic impotence and patients with psychogenic erectile dysfunction.[33] It is utilized in a 10-mg three times daily dosage. It is associated with tremulousness, insomnolence, headache, palpitations, minor elevations in blood pressure, and gastric intolerance. Larger on-demand doses (20–30 mg) have been reported anecdotally to be more effective. Delequamine hydrochloride (Syntex Pharmaceuticals, recently acquired by Hoffman-LaRoch) is a similar α_2-adrenoceptor antagonist that is associated with a 1000-fold greater affinity for this receptor than yohimbine. It was recently dropped from clinical trials as a result of inadequate efficacy.

α_2-Adrenoceptor Antagonists

Transbuccal phentolamine mesylate was recently reexamined in a small multicenter controlled pilot study by Wagner et al.[34] A dose of 20–40 mg thus delivered produced a 30–40% erectile response compared to a 15–20% response for placebo. The only side effect was a sensation of burning at the application site. These trials are currently being expanded.

Dopamine Agonists

Transbuccal apomorphine delivery by a novel buccal tablet is being investigated by Heaton and associates.[35] It has been examined primarily in men with nonorganic erectile dysfunction. They have demonstrated a dose-dependent (10, 20, 100 mg/ml) erectogenic efficacy greater than that of placebo when examined by real-time rigidity monitoring. It is taken "on demand." Overall a 70% response rate has been observed. The response appears to be dependent upon sexual stimulation as evidenced by a significant augmentation of the effect when exposed to visual sexual stimulation. Side effects of apomorphine therapy include persistent yawning, nausea, vomiting, and hypotension. Its role in the management of organic erectile dysfunction is yet to be defined, however, large-scale phase 3 clinical trials evaluating the role of this proprietary formulation, currently called Med-Po, in the management of psychogenic and mild organic erectile dysfunction are underway. I personally believe this novel therapeutic approach is very promising. It may well enter the market by 1998.

Serotonin Agonist

Trazadone (Desyrel) is both a central acting seratonin agonist and a peripheral sympatholytic. It has been reported to be "effective" in 60% of patients.[36] It has been demonstrated to decrease peripheral sympathetic tone[37] and it has been associated anecdotally with erectogenic activity in impotent men in doses of 100–200 mg/day or on demand. There may exist a synergistic effect when combined with yohimbine.[38] Adverse side effects include drowsiness, hypertension, orthostatic hypotension, nausea, and vomiting. It is rarely able to produce adequate erections in the absence of severe sedation and therefore has not played a significant role in my therapeutic armamentarium.

Nitric Oxide Precursors

The amino acid L-arginine is a NO precursor that was examined by Zorgniotti and Lizza in a small group of 20 impotent men.[39] A daily dose of 2,800 mg was administered for 2 wk. Six of the 15 men who completed the study reported improved erections. This is a non toxic drug that requires further exploration.

Type V Phosphodiesterase Inhibitor

Phosphodiesterase enzymes (PDE) break down cyclic neucleotides cAMP and cyclic guanosine monophosphate (cGMP). The corporal smooth muscle has predominantly the type III and V isozymes as well as type II. Type V PDE is also found in the retina. Inhibition of this PDE would result in a greater erectile response to NO-mediated cGMP. Papaverine is a nonspecific PDE inhibitor effecting primarily cAMP. UK 92,480 is an oral cGMP specific type V PDE inhibitor that in pilot trials in England appears to be more effective than placebo in small numbers of nonorganic and diabetic patients. Clinical phase 3 trials are currently ongoing in the United States and initial data indicates that it may be significantly effective in organic disease. This is obviously very promising.

TRANSDERMAL/TRANSGLANULAR CORPORAL DRUG DELIVERY

Preliminary trials examining the efficacy of transdermal or transglanular (minoxidil) delivery of nitroglycerin paste (Heaton),[40] minoxidil with or without a percutaneous absorption enhance (2-nonyl-1,3-dioxalane) or capsaicin (Cavallini),[41] papaverine (McVary),[42] and prostaglandin E1 (McVary)[43] have demonstrated some degree of drug delivery to the corporal smooth muscle sufficient to elicit Doppler-detected increased arterial inflow and penile tumescence. However, rigid erections have only been produced in the rare spinal cord injured neurogenic patient. New drug formulations, drug carriers, and iontophoresis may ultimately make this route of drug delivery clinically efficacious.

TRANSURETHRAL CORPORAL DRUG DELIVERY

The distal urethral mucosa has demonstrated itself to be an excellent route for absorption and transfer of vasoactive substances to the corpora cavernosa. This transfer occurs by direct venous communications between the corpus spongiosum and the corpora cavernosa.[43] The transurethral route of vasoactive drug delivery is able to produce hemodynamic alterations in the corpora cavernosa similar to that of direct intracavernosal injection.[44] The novel delivery system, MUSE (Vivus, Menlo Park, CA), consists of a polypropylene applicator with a hollow stem measuring 3.2 cm in length and 3.5 mm in diameter, the tip of which contains a semisolid pellet of medication—either alprostadil alone or in combination with an α-adrenergic antagonist (Fig. 10.1). Initial results indicate that this therapeutic option promises to be an early or first-line therapy because of its relatively noninvasive delivery.[45]

CONCLUSION

The future of erectile management lies in the arena of pharmacotherapy. Intracavernosal pharmacotherapy is the cornerstone of the current management of erectile dysfunction. There exists, however, an inherent impetus for the development of less invasive delivery systems and routes. The therapeutic armamentatrium for erectile dysfunction by the turn of the century will include effective oral and transurethral approaches.

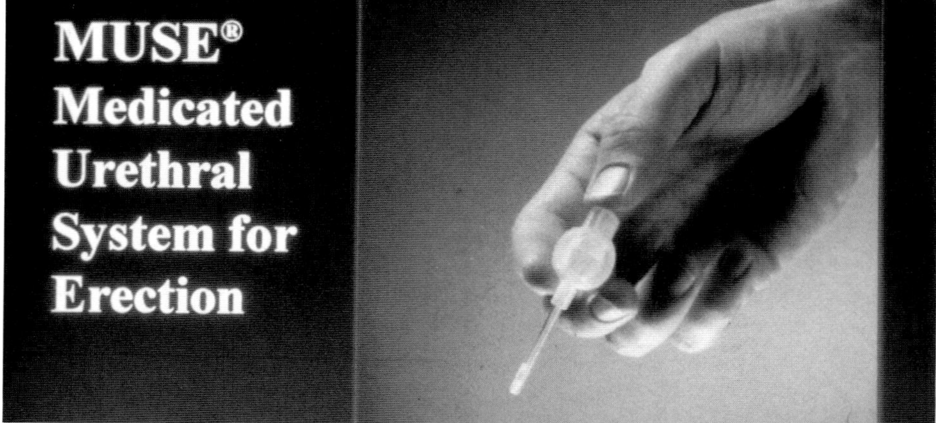

Fig. 10.1. The MUSE delivery system utilized for intraurethral drug adminsitration and transurethral drug delivery to the corpora cavernosa.

REFERENCES

1. Feldman HA, Goldstein I, Hatzichristou D, et al: Impotence and its medical and psychosocial correlates: results of the Massachusetts male aging study. *J Urol* 151:54–61, 1994.

2. Impotence. NIH concensus conference statement. Dec 7–9; 10(4):1–31, 1992.

3. Jonler M, Moon T, Brannan W, et al: The effect of age, ethnicity, and geographical location on impotence and quality of life. *Br J Urol* 75:651–655, 1995.

4. Zurowski K, Kayne H, Goldstein I: The social and behavioural costs of organic impotence, *J Urol* 151(5):319A, 1994.

5. Glick HA, McCarron TJ, Wilkie RJ, et al: Quality of life effects of alprostadil therapy for erectile dysfunction. *Int J Impot Res* 7(1):4, 1995.

6. Brindley GS: Cavernosal alpha-blockade: a new technique for investigating and testing erectile impotence. *Br J Psychiatry* 143:322, 1983.

7. Virag R: Intracavernous injection of papaverine for erectile failure. Letter to the editor. *Lancet* 2:938, 1982.

8. Zorgniotti AW, Lefleur RS: Auto-injection of the corpus cavernosum with vasoactive drug combination for vasculogenic impotence. *J Urol* 133:39, 1985.

9. Padma-Nathan H, Goldstein I, Payton T, et al: Intracavernosal pharmacotherapy: the pharmacologic erection program. *World J Urol* 5:160, 1987.

10. Ishii N, Watanabe H, Irisawa C, et al: Studies on male sexual impotence. Report 18. Therapeutic trial with prostaglandin E1 for organic impotence. *Jap J Urol* 77:954, 1986.

11. Virag R, Adaikin PG: Effects of prostaglandin E1 on penile erection and erectile failure. Letter to the editor. *J Urol* 137:1010, 1987.

12. Stackl W, Hasun R, Marberger M: Intracavernous injection of prostaglandin E1 in impotent men. *J Urol* 140:66, 1988.

13. Padma-Nathan H. The efficacy and synergy of polypharmacotherapy in primary and salvage therapy of vasculogenic erectile dysfunction. *Int J Impot Res* 2(2):257–258, 1990.

14. Bennett AH, Carpenter AJ, Barada JH: An improved vasoactive drug combination for a pharmacological erection program. *J Urol* 146:1564–1565, 1991.

15. Linet O: Upjohn NDA for Caverject, PDR formulary information, and teaching material, 1995.

16. Montorsi F, Guazzoni G, Bergamaschi F, et al: Four-drug intracavernous therapy for impotence due to corporeal veno-occlusive dysfunction. *J Urol* 149:1291–1295, 1993.

17. Gerstenberg TC, Metz P, Ottesen B, et al: Intracavernous self-injection with vasoactive intestinal polypeptide and phentolamine in the management of erectile failure. *J Urol* 147(5):1277, 1992.

18. Schwarzer JU, Hofmann R, Pickl U, et al: Calcitonin-gene-related-peptide for therapy of erectile impotence. *Int J Impot Res* 4:219, 1992.

19. Costa P, Sarrazin B, Bressolle F, et al: Efficiency and side effects of intracavernous injections of moxisylyte in impotent patients: a dose-finding study versus placebo. *J Urol* 149:301, 1993.

20. Stief CG, Holmquist F, Djamilian M, et al: Preliminary results with the nitric oxide donor linsidomine chlorhydrate in the treatment of human erectile dysfunction. *J Urol* 148:1437, 1992.

21. Porst H: Prostaglandin E1 and the nitric oxide donor linsidomine for erectile failure: a diagnostic comparative study of 40 patients. *J Urol* 149:1280, 1993.

22. Chung WS, Lieskovsky G, Skinner DG, et al: The value of a nerve-sparing approach in post-operative response to intracavernosal pharmacotherapy following radical prostatectomy. *J Urol* 149(4):231A, 1993.

23. Schramek P, Plas EG, Hubner WA, et al: Intracavernous injection of prostaglandin E1 plus procaine in the treatment of erectile dysfunction. *J Urol* 152:1108, 1994.

24. Moriel EZ, Rajfer J: Sodium bicarbonate alleviates penile pain induced by intracavernous injections for erectile dysfunction. *J Urol* 149:1299, 1993.

25. Ferreira SH: Prostaglandins: peripheral and central analgesia. In Borrea JJ (ed): *Advances in Pain Research and Therapy* 5:627–633, 1983.

26. Aboseif SR, Breza J, Bosch RJLH, et al: Local and systemic effects of chronic intracavernous injection of papaverine, prostaglandin E1, and saline in primates. *J Urol* 142:403–407, 1989.

27. Kolaja GJ, Kirton KT: Toxicology studies with alprostadil. In Goldstein I, Lue T (eds): The role of alprostadil in the diagnosis and treatment of erectile dysfunction. Princeton, NJ, Excerpta Medica, 1993, pp 40–50.

28. Linet O: Personal communication regarding Caverject phase 3 clinical trial results.

29. Witjes WPJ, Meuleman EJH, Nijeholt GABL, et al: The efficacy and acceptance of intracavernous autoinjection therapy with the combination of papaverine/phentolamine. *Int J Impot Res* 4:65–72, 1992.

30. McMahon CG: The return of spontaneous erections after self-injection of prostaglandin E1. *Int J Impot Res* 4:179–186, 1992.

31. Kim N, Vardi Y, Padma-Nathan H, et al: Oxygen tension regulates the nitric oxide pathway. *J Clin Invest* 91:437–442, 1993.

32. Morales A, Surridge DH, Marshal PG, et al: Non-hormonal pharmacologic treatment of organic impotence. *J Urol* 128:45–47, 1982.

33. Reid K, Surridge DH, Morales A, et al: Double blind trial of yohimbine in the treatment of psychogenic impotence. *Lancet* 151:1225–1226, 1987.

34. Wagner G, Lacy, Lewis R, et al: Buccal phentolamine: a pilot trial for male erectile dysfunction at three separate clinics. *Int J Impot Res* 6(1):D78, 1994.

35. Heaton JPW, Morales A, Adams MA, et al: Recovery of erectile function by the oral administration of apomorphine. *Urology* 45:200, 1995.

36. Saenz de Tajada I, Ware JC, Blanco R, et al: Pathophysiology of prolonged erection associated with trazadone use. *J Urol* 165:60–63, 1991.

37. Chiang PH, Tsai EM, Chiang CP: The role of trazadone in the treatment of erectile dysfunction. *Kao Hsiung I Hsueh Tsa Chih* 10:287–294, 1994.

38. Montorsi F, Strambi LF, Guazzoni G, et al: Effect of yohimbine-trazadone in psychogenic impotence: a randomized double-blind, placebo-controlled study. *Urology* 44:732–736, 1994.

39. Zorgniotti AW, Lizza AF: Effect of large doses of nitric oxide precursor L-arginine on erectile failure. *Int J Impot Res* 6:33, 1994.

40. Heaton JPW, Morales A, Owen J, et al: Topical glyceryltrinitrate causes measurable penile arterial dilation in impotent men. *J Urol* 143:729–731, 1990.

41. Cavallini G: Minoxidil and capsaicine: an association of transcutaneous active drugs for erection facilitation. *Int J Impot Res* 6(1):D71, 1994.

42. Kim ED, El-Rashidy R, McVary K: Papaverine Topical gel for treatment of erectile dysfunction. *J Urol* 153:361–365, 1995.

43. Kim ED, McVary K: Topical prostaglandin E1 for the treatment of erectile dysfunction. *J Urol* 153:1828–1830, 1995.

44. Padma-Nathan H, Keller T, Poppiti R, et al: Hemodynamic effects of intraurethral alprostadil: the medicated urethral system for erection (MUSE). *J Urol* 151(5):469, 1994.

45. Padma-Nathan H, Bennett A, Gesundheit N, et al: Treatment of erectile dysfunction by the Medicated System for Erectile Dysfunction. *J Urol* 153(4):975, 1995

11

Premature Ejaculation

Allen D. Seftel

Stanley E. Althof

INTRODUCTION

Oral pharmacotherapy for premature ejaculation has just begun. In the past, various behavioral and psychotherapeutic regimens were promulgated as the treatment of what was thought to be a psychological or environmental problem. This chapter will review the data available on pharmacotherapy for rapid ejaculation and offer suggestions for combining the psychological and pharmacologic approaches to treatment.

HISTORICAL PERSPECTIVE

There is no agreement on the definition of quick ejaculation. A number of studies have defined the dysfunction in terms of time from intromission to climax, number of coital thrusts, partner satisfaction, and degree of voluntary control. The most recent criterion set appearing in the fourth edition of the American Psychiatric Associations *Diagnostic and Statistical Manual*[1] outlines three criteria for premature ejaculation (302.75):

A. Persistent or repeated ejaculation with slight stimulation before, on, or shortly after penetration and before the person wishes it. The clinician must take into account factors that affect duration of the excitement phase, such as age, new sexual partner or situation, and recent frequency of sexual activity.

B. The disturbance causes considerable anguish or interpersonal difficulty.

C. The premature ejaculation is not due exclusively to the direct effects of a chemical (e.g., withdrawal from opioids).[1]

The physician must make three additional observations. First, whether the problem is lifelong or acquired; second, whether it is of a generalized or specific type; and third, whether it is due to psychological or combined factors. While this criterion set uses a multidimensional definition employing time and voluntary control, it provides few measurable points of reference. For instance, what is meant by minimal sexual stimulation and how much time after penetration should one consider ejaculation to be dysfunctional?

Individual, conjoint, and group psychotherapy approaches combined with behavioral strategies such as stop-start or squeeze techniques have all been utilized to treat premature ejaculation.[2-9] It is now known that the initial post-treatment success rates ranging from 60% to 95%[7,10] were not sustainable; 3 years after treatment, success rates diminished to 25%.[11,12] This data suggests that clinicians have failed to develop long-term plans that allow patients to maintain their initial therapeutic successes. It would be interesting to see information on the efficacy of treatment where therapists use periodic booster or maintenance sessions after the termination of the original treatment.

This psychological/behavioral approach to rapid ejaculation, which has been on the rise for over 20 years became challenged by data that suggested that ejaculatory latency could be prolonged by clomipramine or the selective serotonin reuptake inhibitor drugs (SSRIs)—fluoxetine, sertraline, and paroxetine—without bothersome side effects.[13-17] These early reports led to our conducting the trial described below.

CLOMIPRAMINE

Our group[18] conducted a double-blind, randomized, placebo-controlled study using strict dosages in a carefully chosen population to find out if clomipramine was biologically and psychologically effective in delaying ejaculation The results with 15 couples were that 25 mg of clomipramine prolonged ejaculatory latency 249% while 50 mg of the drug increased time to climax by 517%. However, when the men stopped the medication the success disappeared and their ejaculatory latencies returned to baseline. Placebo administration (nonsignificantly) increased ejaculatory latency 30% over baseline. These results were consistent with prior studies conducted by Segraves et al[15] and Assalian.[13]

Psychosocially, there were significant improvements in male and female sexual gratification, male relationship satisfaction, and male emotional well-being. Three women partners who never achieved coital orgasm became orgasmic while the man was taking medication. Six of ten women who commonly reached orgasm reported this occurred with greater frequency when their partners were taking the medication.

Side effects were generally mild, dose-dependent, and tended to decrease with time. Dry mouth, constipation, and feeling "unusual" were the longest lasting effects on 50 mg, but were not generally clinically significant at 25 mg. Nausea, sleep disturbance, fatigue, and hot flashes were infrequently observed at 50 mg.

A second open label study was undertaken to determine: (1) whether lengthy treatment with clomipramine could lead to continued ejaculatory control discontinuation of medication; (2) whether men can take the drug on less than a daily basis; and (3) characteristics of those subjects who remain on pharmacologic treatment and those that dropout.[19]

Of 37 men contacting our Center, 27 men with a mean age of 45 agreed to treatment. They were begun on a daily regimen of 25 mg of clomipramine and asked to fill out sexual and side effect logs on five coital episodes. Based on their self-report, medication was increased to 50 mg daily, 50 mg every other day (qod), 50 mg as needed (prn), decreased to 25 mg qod, 25 mg prn, or left unchanged. Each time the medication schedule was changed, subjects were asked to complete sexual and side effect logs on five more coital experiences. Each subject's dose continued to be adjusted upward or downward until some reasonable effectiveness was achieved. Those subjects who could not tolerate the side effects of clomipramine or who did not adequately, respond were offered trials on fluoxetine or paroxetine. Patients continued on medication for 7 months at which point they were asked to take a 1-month drug holiday while reporting on ejaculatory latency and sexual satisfaction.

After 7 months, 14 men continued to take medication while 13 dropped out. The baseline ejaculatory latencies of those remaining on the drug were shorter than those of the dropouts (64 sec versus 81 sec). The stayers' mean estimated ejaculatory latencies on 25 mg was 403 sec; the latencies of the dropouts averaged 206 sec. Five of 13 dropouts noted no efficacy on 25 mg. All 14 stayers reported an improvement of at least 55 secs. Equal numbers of dropouts and stayers noted side effects.

Sexual satisfaction scores at baseline were lower for stayers than dropouts. However, on a daily dose of 25 mg the stayers' satisfaction levels had improved more than twofold while the dropouts' levels had decreased (3.2 versus 2.07). At 50 mg daily and 50 mg prn satisfaction levels for the stayers increased to 3.8 and 4.2 respectively.

By 7 months the 14 subjects were distributed among seven medication schedules (in mg): 1–25 (qd); 2–25 qod; 1–25 prn; 7–50 qd; 2–50 qod; 1–50 prn. Only 2 of 14 subjects achieved success with taking the medication the day of intercourse; the other 12 required more intensive programs.

Eleven of 14 men went on drug holiday, three by protocol plan at 7 months and eight by themselves at varied intervals ranging from 2 to 7 months. None of the four men who went on holiday by design at 7 months were able to sustain the increases in ejaculatory latency. Two of the four men returned to baseline; the other two noted losing 25% to 50% of the ejaculatory improvements. All the men who placed themselves on holiday returned to baseline ejaculatory latencies. This open label trial reaffirmed our group's previous findings regarding the efficacy of clomipramine in the treatment of rapid ejaculation. Seven months of treatment was not successful in allowing men to maintain their gains off medication. Only a small number of subjects were able to delay ejaculation on less than a daily dose of medication. This would indicate a lifelong dependency on oral therapy for premature ejaculation.

The results of the second study should be viewed as preliminary and interpreted with caution because of the small sample size, the lack of control groups, objective timing, or blinding of the investigators or subjects. We believe the 48% dropout rate was in part due to our failure to closely observe the patients' progress. We suggested that initially patients be followed at least monthly. Dropouts should be expected because some patients unrealistically expect the medication to remedy relationship problems as well as cure rapid ejaculation.

A note of caution regarding the use of clomipramine. One study[20] reports that a daily dosage of 75 mg of clomipramine taken for 3 months in a series of 11 depressed patients resulted in pathologic spermiograms in all patients in terms of volume, sperm motility, and sperm morphology. This important finding warrants further documentation and research into the possible effects on male fertility of pharmacotherapy with clomipramine and/or other antidepressant drugs.

SERTRALINE

In a double-blind, randomized, placebo-controlled study, Mendels et al[21] reported that sertraline produced clinically and statistically significant improvements relative to placebo in time to ejaculation and number of successful attempt at coitus. The average daily dose was 121 mg/day. Similarly, in an open label trial, Swartz[22] reported on ten patients who were prescribed either 25 mg or 50 mg of sertraline. The average ejaculatory delay was 20 mins. Side effects were infrequent and consisted of transient anorexia and headaches.

FLUOXETINE AND PAROXETINE

Waldinger et al[17] studied the effect of paroxetine on ejaculation in a double-blind, placebo-controlled trial in men with rapid ejaculation. The dose of paroxetine was increased from 20 mg and 40 mg after the first week. Successful results were noted in most patients and side effects were minimal. Presently, there are no double-blind, placebo-controlled studies regarding the efficacy of fluoxetine in treating rapid ejaculation; however, several anecdotal reports and the authors' clinical experience suggest that it may also be useful at doses ranging from 20 to 40 mg daily.[23]

PRELIMINARY GUIDELINE FOR PATIENT SELECTION

The key to patient satisfaction lies in selecting the right candidates who have realistic expectations of treatment outcome. Based on the authors' limited clinical experience, the following guidelines were developed. Further investigation is needed to validate these as useful and over time the guidelines will continue to evolve.

The lifelong versus acquired classification of rapid ejaculation may prove to be a useful marker for developing treatment recommendations. The ideal candidate for drug therapy might be a man with several years of sexual experience with a lifelong pattern of rapid ejaculation who is free of substance abuse, depression, and psychosis and capable of developing stable, satisfying, nonsexual relationships. Drug treatment can also be considered for those patients who have not benefited from a competently conducted psychological treatment. In contrast, acquired rapid ejaculation begs the clinician to be interested in the forces that brought about the new symptom. Given a relatively recent onset and some degree of psychological mindedness these men/couples might, in the long run, do better with a behavioral or psychological treatment.

Sexual Experience Level

Pharmacologic intervention should not be a first-line consideration for the young or inexperienced man who in the first sexual encounters rapid ejaculation. Reassurance and counseling are likely to be worthwhile; hopefully in time these men will develop increased confidence and learn to control ejaculation.

Quality of the Nonsexual Relationship

Whether lifelong or acquired caution is warranted in offering drug therapy alone to men where the symptom clearly reflects intrapsychic or interpersonal conflict, therapists must not lose sight of the time-honored dynamic maxim that symptoms exist for reasons. Rapid symptom removal may interrupt the individual's or couple's equilibrium. This advice is not simply a restatement of the psychoanalytic theory of symptom substitution, but a concern based on our experience where treatment in a small minority of cases resulted in destructive acting out.

CASE WESTERN RESERVE UNIVERSITY (CWRU) EXPERIENCE WITH CLOMIPRAMINE FOR PREMATURE EJACULATION

The Urologists' Perspective

As the treatment of erectile dysfunction has become less surgical, urologists are faced with new challenges in the treatment of male sexual dysfunctions. Pharmacotherapy of rapid ejaculation is one such new horizon. The urologist must now become facile and knowledgable with diagnosis and management of this dysfunction. A sample questionnaire is included as an addendum. To this end, an ongoing trial of clomipramine was initiated for those patients with primary, lifelong premature ejaculation, based upon the above work, and remains in effect. The selection process was a careful one. Excluded were those patients who were suspected of secondary or acquired premature ejaculation or those patients with accompanying erectile dysfunction. Superficial psychosocial screening excluded patients with overt psychopathology. To date, we have accrued ten patients with an average follow-up of 1.5 years. Five of the patients were happily married, and the remaining five patients had a stable relationship with only one partner. The subjects did not perceive that the dysfunction had negatively impacted the nonsexual relationship although they were dissatisfied with the quality of their sexual life. Other patients not accepted in the study had unrealistic expectations that rapid ejaculation would lead to marital harmony. To date, seven of ten patients continue on pharmacotherapy and find it helpful and satisfying. The one treatment "failure" was due to the deterioration of the relationship rather than the lack of efficacy of the drug. This treatment is not a substitute for marital counseling; should not be used for treatment of erectile dysfunction; and should not be offered to men anticipating new relationships concerned about their possible sexual performance (performance anxiety). The two other failures with clomipramine were middle-aged men, both married. One man found the clomipramine of no help and has been changed to paroxetine. A second man tried oral clomipramine for 2 wk, 25 mg qd for the first week, and 25 mg qod, the second week. He developed headaches, nausea, and chest flushing and was switched to paroxetine. Thus, we have seven patients on long-term therapy with good results. Two of seven men were able to be maintained on an as needed schedule as opposed to a more intensive regimen.

In addition, those patients with erectile dysfunction, who have developed premature ejaculation secondarily are generally not helped by SSRI therapy. In our anecdotal experience, these patients' premature ejaculation improves with treatment of the erectile dysfunction.

Treatment Experience

Initially, we treated these patients with clomipramine, 25 mg qd. Early on, this regimen produced significant side effects for many of these patients, which contrasts with some of the data presented above. Side effects included headache, hot flashes, nausea, vomiting, and fatigue. Subsequently, we have altered the oral therapy to every other day or twice a week or even to the day of anticipated intercourse. This has significantly reduced the incidence of side effects and appears to have reasonable efficacy. The urologist currently uses this regimen for all new patients.

Side Effects

The side effects of clomipramine treatment are generally mild, dose related, and tended to diminish over time. There were 5 of 27 patients in the aforementioned study who could not tolerate even low doses of clomipramine and would not consider switching to another drug.

Patient Acceptance Rates

In carefully selected research populations, the patient acceptance rate was over 79%. However, it appears that in less carefully selected samples the patient acceptance rate markedly drops to 52%. This treatment is likely to negatively impact on non-physician therapists who would lose potential therapy patients and slightly less negatively impact physician therapists who would see patients for a medication-only treatment. The economics might benefit both the patient and third-party payers.

In sum, oral therapy for premature ejaculation is just beginning. It is exciting to be able to provide oral therapy for these men. Analogous to all other oral therapies, clinical use will ultimately indicate the optimal drug dose as well as point out the appropriate patient for treatment. An understanding of the psychobiology of the effects of the oral therapy is needed to better understand the ejaculation relax arc and the central pathways that effect it, allowing us to alter therapy and produce drugs with greater specificity. The final chapter for oral therapy in the management of premature ejaculation is far from complete.

APPENDIX
UROLOGIC HISTORY FOR
PREMATURE EJACULATION

I. Complaint and Duration of Complaint

Have patient describe "premature ejaculation" in his own terms.

a. When did it start—acquired or lifelong? If acquired, was there a precipitating event or life circumstance that was temporally related to the onset?

b. Assess mean ejaculatory latency with intercourse, manual and oral stimulation, and masturbation.

c. Does the man sense that he has voluntary control over the ejaculatory reflex even if it is rapid?

d. Patient's attribution for the rapid ejaculation.

e. What solutions has the patient undertaken to remedy the dysfunction?

f. Are there other sexual dysfunctions present in the patient or partner?

g. What is the quality of the nonsexual relationship?

II. Partner's Assessment of Ejaculation

a. Is this a problem for her/him? How so?

b. Do they view it as a lifelong or acquired dysfunction?

c. Have patient and partner ever had successful intercourse?

d. What is the quality of the nonsexual relationship?

e. What do they believe is causing the problem?

From Seftel AD, Althof SE: For premature ejaculation, clomipramine shows promise, Contemporary Urology 1996; (8):25–35, Copyright Medical Economics.

REFERENCES

1. American Psychiatric Association: *Diagnostic and Statistical Manual of Mental Disorders*, ed 4. American Psychiatric Association, Washington, DC 1994, p 511.

2. Halvorsen J, Metz M: Sexual dysfunction, part I: classification, etiology and pathogenesis. *J Am Board Family Pract* 5:51–61, 1992.

3. Kaplan H: *Overcoming Premature Ejaculation.* New York, Brunner-Mazel, 1989.

4. Levine S: *Sexual Life: A Clinician's Guide.* New York, Plenum, 1992.

5. LoPiccolo J, LoPiccolo I: *Handbook of Sex Therapy.* New York, Plenum, 1978.

6. McCarthy B: Cognitive-behavioral strategies and techniques in the treatment of early ejaculation. In Leiblum SR, Rosen R (eds): *Principles and Practice of Sex Therapy: Update for the 90's.* New York, Guilford Press, 1990, pp 143–167.

7. Masters W, Johnson V: *Human Sexual Inadequacy.* Boston, Little, Brown, 1970.

8. St. Lawrence J, Madakasira S: Evaluation and treatment of premature ejaculation: a critical review. *Int J Psychiatry* 22:77–97, 1992.

9. Semans J: Premature ejaculation: a new approach. *South Med J* 49:353–358, 1956.

10. Hawton K, Catalan J: Prognostic factors in sex therapy. *Behav Res Ther* 24:377–385, 1986.

11. Bancroft J, Coles L: Three years experience in a sexual problems clinic. *Br Med J* 1:1575–1577, 1976.

12. DeAmicus L, Goldberg D, Lopiccolo J, et al: Clinical follow-up of couples treated for sexual dysfunction. *Arch Sex Behav* 14:467–489, 1985.

13. Assalian P: Clomipramine in the treatment of premature ejaculation. *J Sex Res* 24:231–251, 1988.

14. Goodman RE: Premature ejaculation. *Br Med J* 282:1796–1797, 1981.

15. Segraves RT, Saran A, Segraves K, et al: Clomipramine versus placebo in the treatment of premature ejaculation: a pilot study. *J Sex Marital Ther*, 19:198–200, 1993.

16. Kaplan P: The use of serotonergic uptake inhibitors in the treatment of premature ejaculation. *J Sex Marital Ther* 20:321–324, 1995.

17. Waldinger M, Hengeveld M, Zwinderman A: Paroxetine treatment of premature ejaculation: a double-blind randomized placebo-controlled study. *Am J Psychiatry* 151:1377–1379, 1994.

18. Althof S, Levine S, Corty E, et al: Clomipramine as a treatment for rapid ejaculation: a double-blind crossover trial of fifteen couples. *J Clin Psychiatry* (*in press*).

19. Althof S, Resnick K, Levine S, et al: Early experience with clomipramine for rapid ejaculation. Paper presented to the Annual Meeting of the American Urological Association, Las Vegas, Nevada, 1995.

20. Maier U, Koinig G: Andrological findings in young patients under long-term anti-depressive therapy with clomipramine. *Psychopharmacology* 116:357–359, 1994.

21. Mendels J, Camera A, Sikes C: Sertraline treatment for premature ejaculation. *J Clin Psychopharmacol* 15:341–346, 1995.

22. Swartz D: Sertraline hydrochloride for premature ejaculation (Abstract 471). In: Programs and Abstracts of the 89th Annual Meeting of the American Urological Association, San Francisco, 1994, p 345A.

23. Levine S. Personal communication, 1996.

12

Vacuum Devices

Ronald W. Lewis

In medicine, it is always surprising to discover that a treatment has been described long ago. Such is the case of using a vacuum pump to enhance penile function described by John King, M.D. in 1874. He used a "small exhausting pump" (vacuum) to excite new activity in the blood vessels of the penis.[1] A United States patent was issued to Dr. Otto Lederer in 1917 for a device to produce erection by vacuum but this was not accepted by his medical peers.[2] The modern treatment of erectile difficulties with a vacuum pump and a tension band was developed in 1982. An Augusta, Georgia businessman, Geddings D. Osbon, Sr., received the first permission by the Food and Drug Administration to distribute and market a noninvasive treatment for impotence. He developed this device in 1960 for his own personal need which was unmet by other medical treatment options. By 1974, he had formed a company to market the device. Two urologists instrumental in scientific presentations for the use of this type of therapy (met with early skepticism) were Drs. Perry Nadig and Roy Witherington. Both physicians published the first two articles evaluating this type of treatment for erectile dysfunction in 1986 and 1989 respectively.[3,4]

PATIENT SELECTION

Almost all patients suffering from erectile dysfunction are eligible candidates to use vacuum therapy for treatment. In the scheme of goal-directed therapy, a term first proposed by Tom Lue,[5] this type of treatment option is chosen by the patient, and preferably his sexual partner, after the evaluating history and physical is accomplished with little need for any further testing to uncover the etiology of the erectile dysfunction. Some patients desire more evaluation to determine what other options are available for treatment of their particular condition, but external vacuum therapy is always an option. Even patients who have failed other therapeutic choices, including those who have had penile prostheses fail or removed because of infection, have this type of therapy as a choice for continued treatment of their erectile dysfunction. Patients who have had previous implants removed have been satisfied with subsequent use of the vacuum device.[6,7] Moul and McLeod reported that 71% (10 of 14) explant patients engaged in regular successful intercourse using a vacuum device, including 5 of 6 who had the penile prosthesis removed for infection.[6] Interestingly, 6 of 11 (55%) patients who tried home use stated that the vacuum device was much better or better than the previous penile implant. Korenmann and Viosca similarly reported good success with the vacuum device in 4 of 5 patients who had a penile prosthesis explanted and enhancement of sexual activity in four patients with an indwelling semirigid implant.[7] In this same report, eight patients who were impotent secondary to pelvic cancer surgery were also successfully sexually rehabilitated with the vacuum device. There was one report of low satisfaction in patients with psychogenic impotence and patients who had previously used or were using injection therapy but the authors admitted that this particular group of patients were poorly selected and had failed other types of therapy.[8] The vacuum device has been recommended for patients with a veno-occlusive disorder with a 69% success rate reported (20 of 29).[9]

Patients who have severe penile scarring of the corpora cavernosa (such as priapism secondary to sickle cell disease or trait or a severe intracavernosal infection associated with removal of a penile prosthesis) may not get an acceptable penile engorgement with the vacuum device.[8] Some patients with severe Peyronie's curvature with penile erection are unable to use the vacuum device because of lack of freedom of movement of the penis within the cylinder. If the patient has severe phimosis, a circumcision may be necessary before the patient can successfully use the vacuum device. Relative contraindications to the use of the vacuum therapy for erectile dysfunction are few. Those patients with a history of unexplained intermittent priapism or diseases prone to priapism and patients with bleeding disorders or on anticoagulation therapy, particularly those with enhanced capillary fragility, are not candidates for vacuum therapy.

CHOICES AVAILABLE FOR VACUUM THERAPY

Table 12.1 lists the different types of vacuum therapy offered in the United States market. One published paper compared the responses of 10 novice and 20 regular users to different devices.[10] There are differences among the individual devices which will not be specifically elaborated but these differences will be presented as each of the components of the vacuum device is described in the following discussion. Costs of the different devices vary and the physician may determine this for

TABLE 12.1. External Vacuum Devices

- Catalyst vacuum system (Dacomed Corporation, Minneapolis, MN)
- E/P System (NuMedTec, Inc., Vernon Hills, IL)
- ErecAid system (Osbon Medical Systems, Ltd., Augusta, GA)
- Post-T-Vac vacuum therapy (Post-T-Vac, Dodge City, KS)
- Response/Touch vacuum constriction (Mentor, Goleta, CA)
- VED vacuum erection device (Mission Pharm, San Antonio, TX)
- VET vacuum erection technologies (Vetco, Birmingham, AL)
- VTU system (Encore, Louisville, KY)

his particular geographic area. Some of the larger companies cite the availability of a 24-hr telephone line for consultation by a trained professional staff for patient questions and support as justification for the higher cost of their units. They may also provide pre-purchase, in-office training demonstrations for the individual

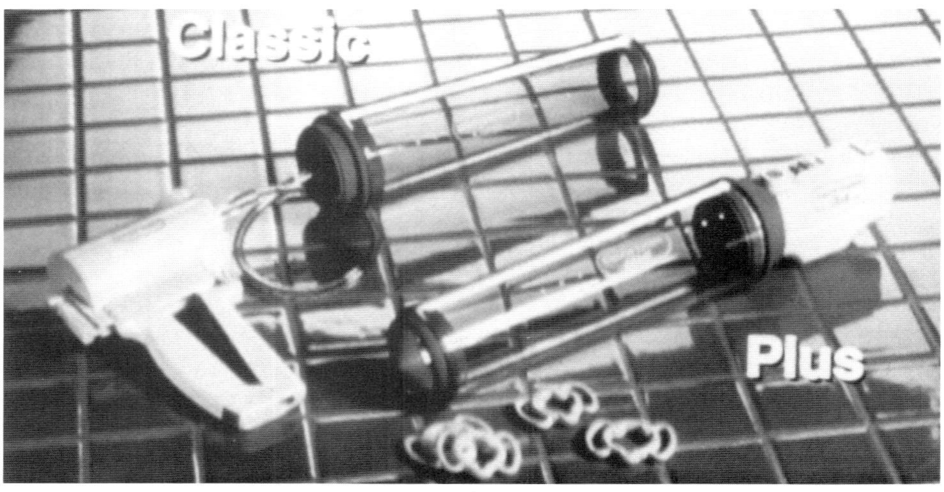

A

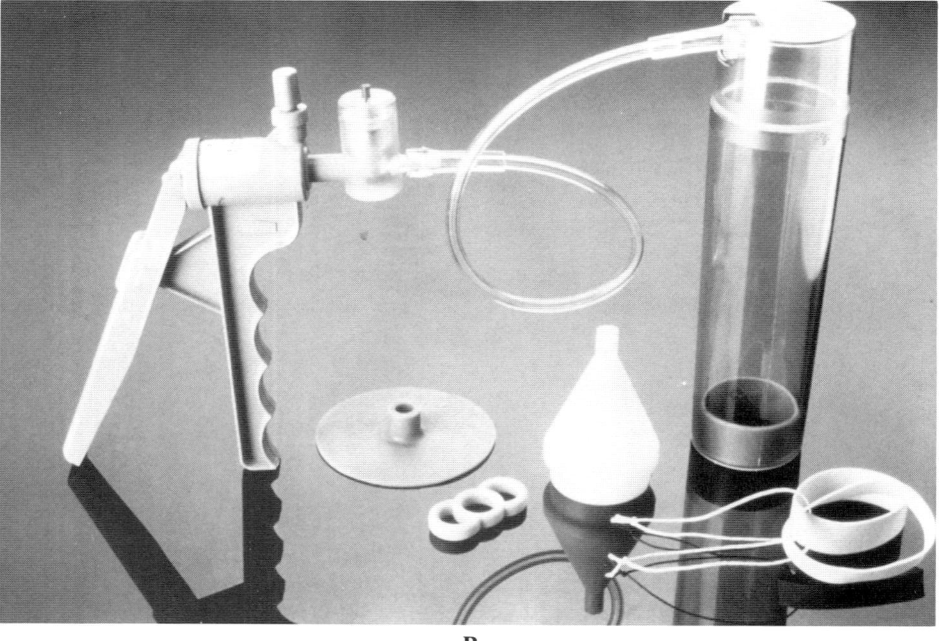

B

Fig. 12.1. Four examples of vacuum therapy devices. **A:** Osbon Medical Systems manual (Classic) and battery-powered pump (Plus) ErecAid models. **B:** Mission Pharmaceuticals VED system shown with three types of tension devices. **C:** Vetco VET system. **D:** Mentor Response and Touch systems showing two types of manual pump systems and their battery-powered pump (central unit).

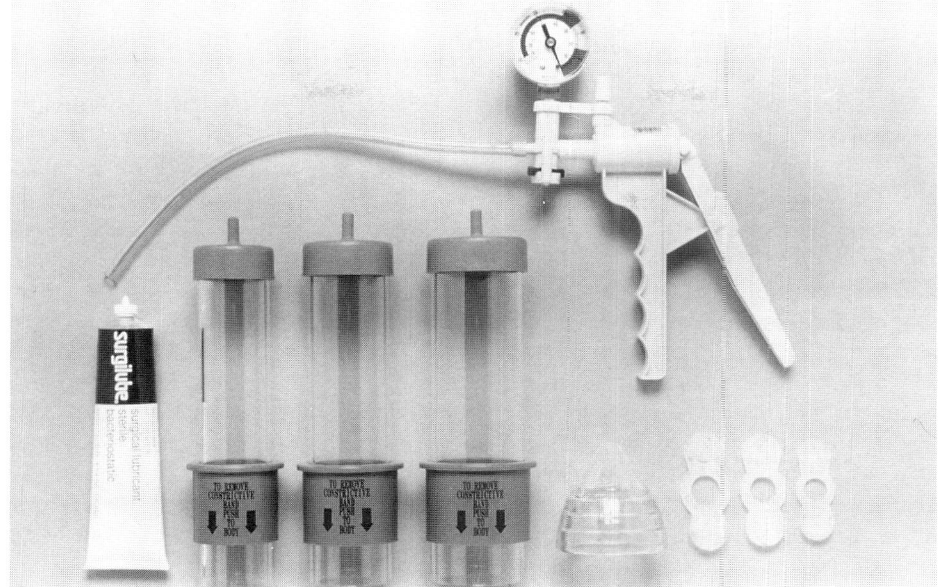

C

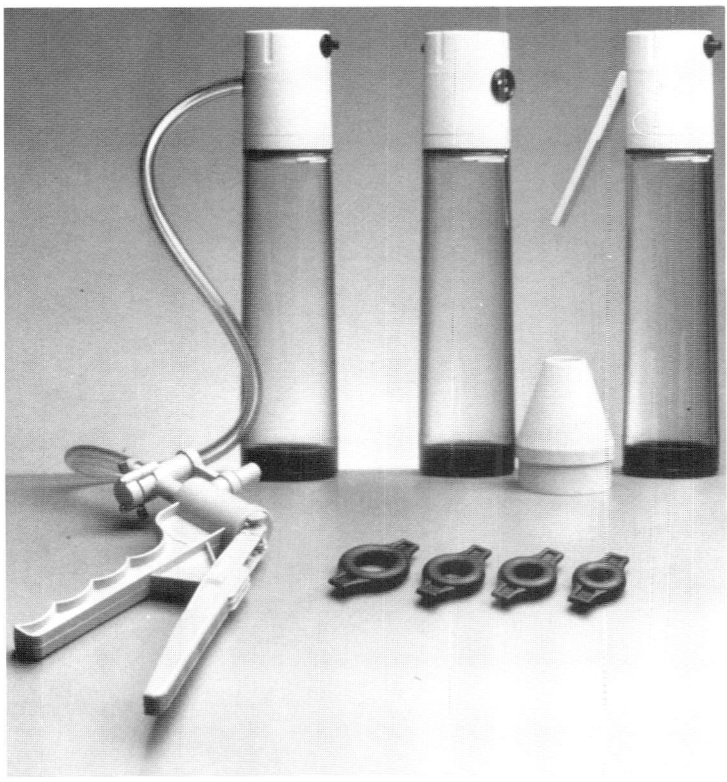

D

Fig. 12.1. Continued

patient. They feel that this availability for counseling greatly aids in patient satisfaction with this type of therapy. Most of the devices come with a video tape to demonstrate proper preparation, care, and use of the device.

The components of the vacuum system are essentially three: the cylinder, the pump, and the tension or occlusion bands or rings (Fig. 12.1). Basically, the cylinders are constructed of clear plastic, some tapering out distally, with an extension connection to attach tubing which connects to a hand held vacuum pump. Some cylinders are open-ended at the distal end for direct attachment of the pump. Some companies provide different cylinder choices with each unit to allow for the variance in penile size. Some companies have larger cylinders available for the rare patient who obtains significantly greater penile circumference with application of the vacuum device. These may also be necessary for patients with severe penile angulation from Peyronie's who have difficulty removing the cylinder once engorgement is obtained. The vacuum pump is hand held and connected to the cylinder either by a plastic tubing or attached to the distal end of the cylinder with a pump handle or has an outer pumping cylinder over an inner cylinder. Most devices have a release valve which activates after a certain negative pressure is reached (200 to 300 mm Hg), as a safety feature built into the pump. To produce adequate rigidity of the penis, the vacuum pressure must exceed 90 mm Hg. Several companies produce a battery-driven pump particularly designed for the patient who does not have the mechanical facility or strength to produce hand motion vacuum pumping. All devices have a release mechanism built into the pump for release of the negative pressure when adequate penile engorgement has occurred and tension rings or bands have been placed around the base of the penis (Fig. 12.2). After use, all parts

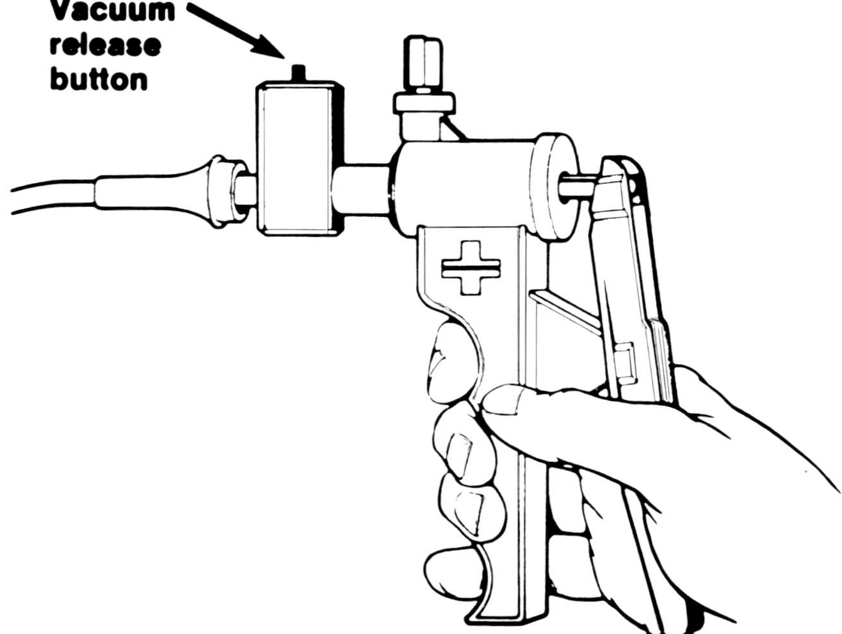

Fig. 12.2. An example of a vacuum release button (Mission Pharmaceuticals).

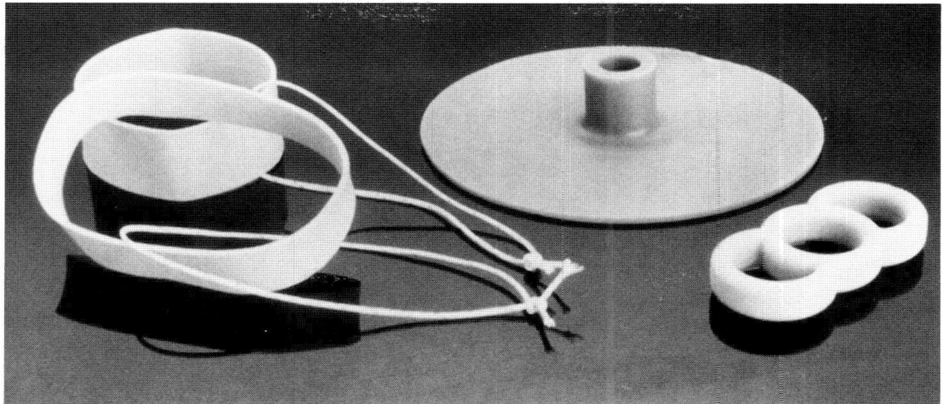

Fig. 12.3. Examples of three different types of tension components: rubber bands, a plastic cylinder disc, and molded plastic ring (Mission Pharmaceuticals).

of the vacuum devices except for the pump itself are able to be submerged for cleaning. Constriction or tension devices can be wide width rubber bands, rings of varying size and tension, or plastic discs with a central opening (Fig. 12.3). Some companies produce round tension bands of varying width and others produce rings molded to have a urethral sparing area on the inside curve of the ventral position of the ring (Fig. 12.4). The constriction devices have tabs or strings to ease removal after use.

Fig. 12.4. A specially notched tension ring with a ventral tension notch for the urethra which produces less tension at this site (Osbon Medical Systems).

Several companies market tension rings alone for patients to use who can not maintain rigidity despite being able to achieve an initial good erection. Examples are the Osbon Sta-Erec system (Osbon Medical Systems, Ltd., Augusta, GA) which comes with an applicator cone and plastic ring in order to facilitate placement of the tension device around the base of the penis or Pro-Long rings (NuMedTec Inc., Vernon Hills, IL).

USE OF THE VACUUM DEVICE

The patient assembles the device, connecting the pump to the cylinder, loads the cylinder with the constriction apparatus (sometimes using more than one tension band), and lubricates the proximal open end of the cylinder with a water-soluble lubricant in order to obtain a better seal to the skin surrounding the base of the penis. Sometimes patients have a difficult time obtaining a tight seal because of excessive pubic hair. They may have to shave or cut some of this hair away. With one hand around the cylinder the patient presses the device against the skin surrounding the base of the penis. When the design of the particular cylinder allows it, the user may press the distal end of the cylinder against a table or counter allowing a free hand to pump the vacuum or activate the pump switch with the battery-powered devices (Fig. 12.5). The number of pumps necessary with manual pumping

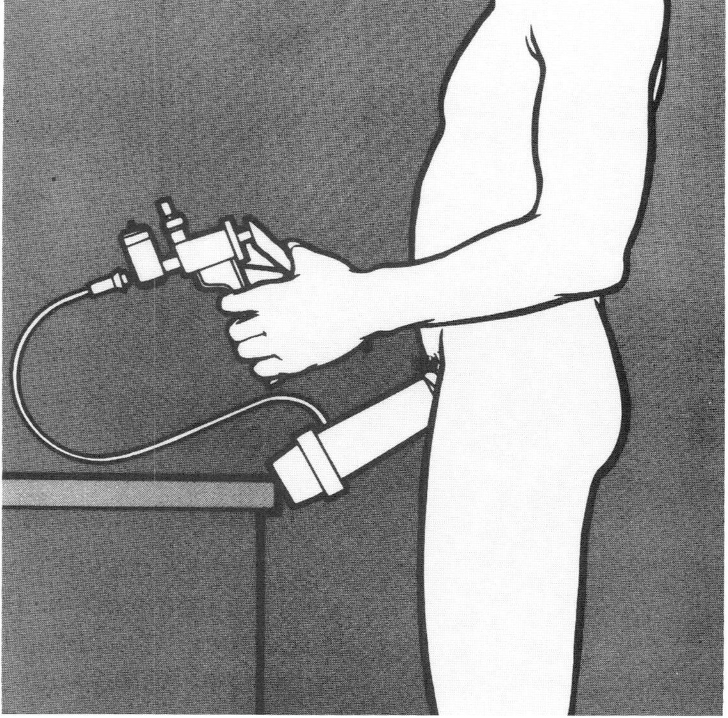

Fig. 12.5. Example of single handed use of a vacuum system (from the manual of VED system of Mission Pharmaceuticals).

devices and time to produce an adequate erection varies. Roy Witherington report-
ed that the average time to obtain a usable penile engorgement was 2.5 min (range
30 sec to 7 min).[4] Sidi and associates reported that 88% of 100 patients obtained
optimum tumescence and rigidity by 30 sec to 2 min.[11] Many manufacturers advise
pumping for 1–2 min, releasing pressure, and then resuming pumping for 3–4 min.
Intermittent pumping may result in a more engorged penis producing a more satis-
factory rigidity for vaginal penetration. Once adequate penile rigidity is obtained,
the preloaded constriction bands or loops are slid off the proximal end of the cylin-
der and onto the base of the penis. The vacuum is released by a valve or button on
the pump, the cylinder removed and the patient is ready for intercourse. It is not
recommended that the tension bands or rings be left in place for longer than 30 min
(Fig. 12.6).

The "erection" obtained with a vacuum device is different from an erection
obtained normally. There is no initial relaxation of the sinus smooth muscle so the
circumference of the corpora cavernosa does not enlarge as much as with a natural
erection. Instead, there is engorgement of all tissue of the penis with trapped blood.
Because the buried portion of the corpora cavernosa does not become tumescent

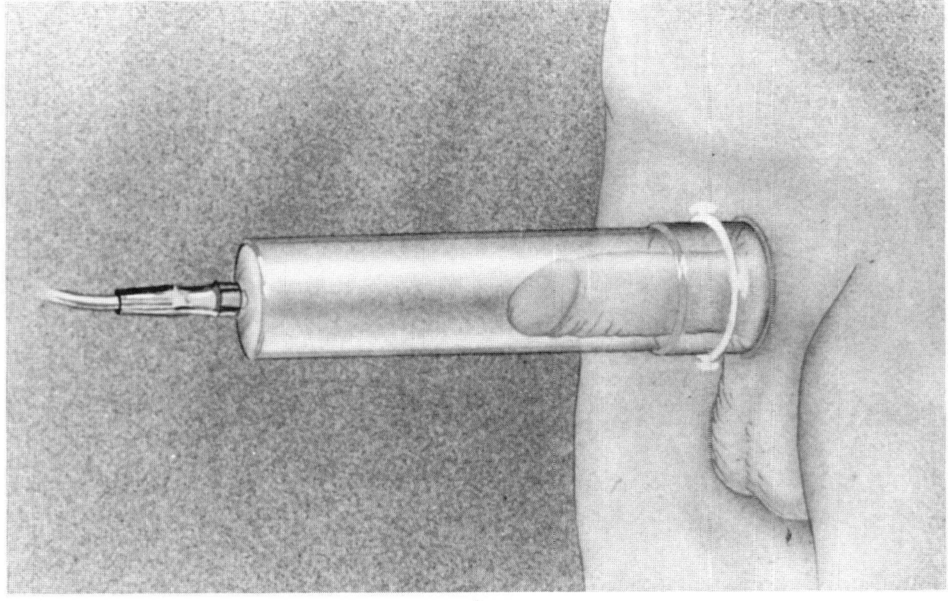

A

Fig. 12.6. Steps in the use of the vacuum system. **A:** Initial placement over the flaccid penis of
the cylinder which has one tension band loaded around the cylinder against the lower pubic
region. (This drawing shows no pubic hair.) The tubing from the distal cylinders goes to the
hand held manual vacuum pump. **B:** Similar step with a battery-powered pump attached to
the distal end of the cylinder. (This drawing shows pubic hair which sometimes has to be
trimmed or shaved to obtain a good seal.) **C** and **D:** Once a vacuum is obtained by the pump,
the penis becomes engorged with blood. **E:** The tension ring has been slipped off the cylinder
onto the base of the penis once adequate erection is obtained. The tension band should not
be left in place for longer than 30 min. Sometimes more than one tension band is needed.

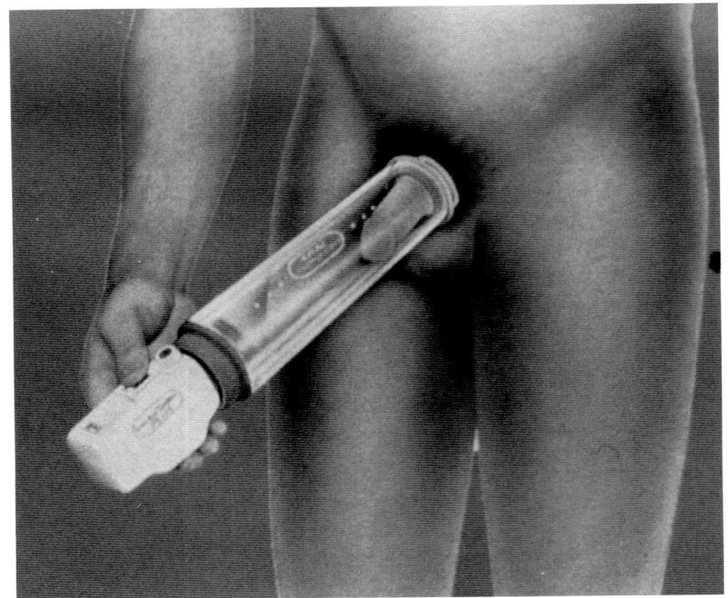

B

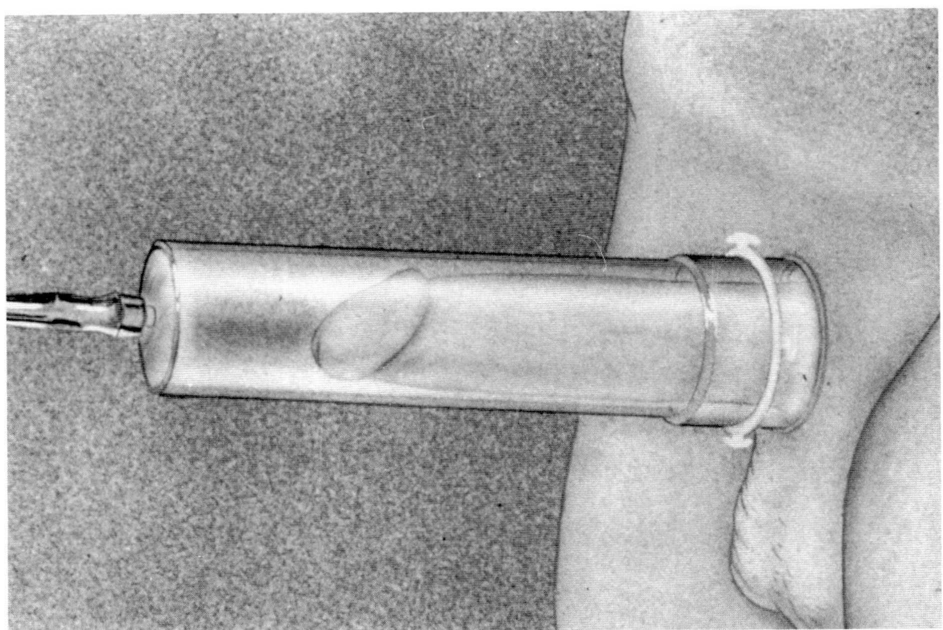

C

Fig. 12.6. Continued.

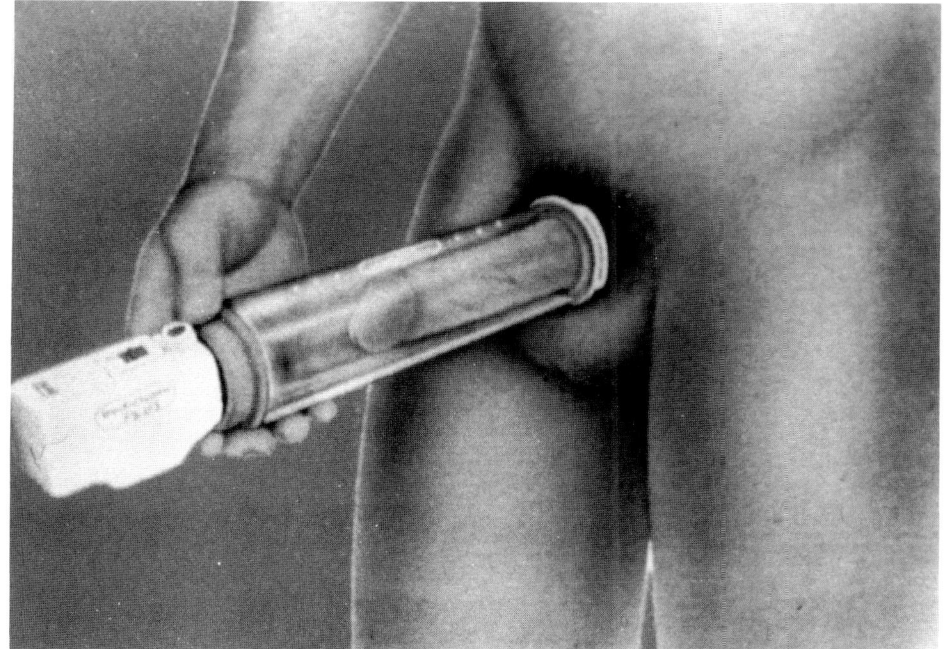

D

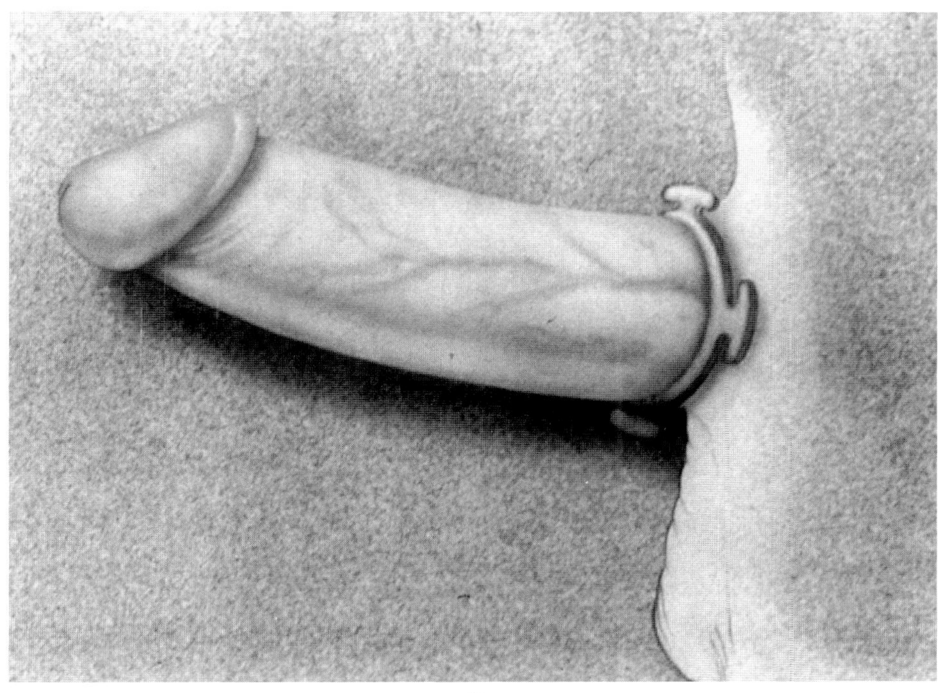

E

Fig. 12.6. Continued.

below the constriction band, there usually is lack of fixation of the penis compared to normal erection. The penis may become slightly cool, obtain a slightly bluish color due to cyanosis, and be slightly numb. Pain with penile engorgement and application of the constriction device is rare and mostly of a mild nature which is not a concern for the patient. With orgasm and ejaculation, there may not be expulsion of fluid from the penis because of the constriction device around the shaft of the penis. This is not always the case but is commonplace and not a problem, especially if the patient has been forewarned. When the bands are removed after intercourse and ejaculation, the seminal fluid will usually run or drip from the penile meatus. Pain with ejaculation related to trapping of the ejaculatory fluid is extremely rare. It is recommended to the patient and his partner that the device be used in practice sessions before trying to have intercourse since some practice is needed for facility of use. The videos supplied with the devices are quite helpful in answering problem areas and, as mentioned earlier, some companies maintain health care professionals available by telephone for help when using the device. It should be recommended by the treating physician that the patient use these services when available.

Nadig has stated that the most frequent complaint by men using vacuum therapy is the unnatural interruption of the act of lovemaking.[2] Some partners are unhappy with the coldness of the penis and the need to use lubricating jelly.

RESULTS OF USE OF VACUUM DEVICES FOR TREATMENT OF ERECTILE DYSFUNCTION

Dr. Perry Nadig, as earlier mentioned, published one of the first scientific reports regarding vacuum therapy for impotence and has continued to update his patients' results.[3,12] His most recent review compared results in two groups: those responding to a short-term evaluation (161 of 216 patients (75%) with 2 to 6 month follow-up, average 3 months) and those responding for long-term evaluation (115 of 202 (57%) with an 11 to 63 month follow-up, average 29 months).[13] Regular use was reported in 69% of group 1 and 70% of group 2. Patient and partner satisfaction for groups 1 and 2 were 82% and 87% and 84% and 89% respectively. Overall quality of erection was greater than 90% in both groups for the following three parameters: hardness of erection, length of penis, and circumference of penis. As for side effects, the following were reported respectively in groups 1 and 2: (1) occasional numbness, 48% and 49%, as a major problem, 6% and 5%; (2) increased climax or orgasm, 38% and 50%; (3) decreased climax or orgasm, 23% in both; (4) pivoting of base of penis, 35% and 29%; (5) bruising of the penis, 32% in both; (6) penile petechiae, 32% and 38%; (7) pain or swelling after device use, 16% and 28%; and (8) pain with orgasm related to the constriction device, 19% in both. The last five were often-occurring or major in less than 6% for each side effect in both groups. Median times per month of successful intercourse were 1, 4, and 4 for the year before, during, and after obtaining the vacuum constriction device in group 2. It was felt by the authors that this study substantiated data, shown by previous reports, that regular use of the vacuum device is continued by the majority of patients who use the device successfully for 3 months.

In 1990, Sidi et al[11] reported a 68% success rate in 100 patients, followed for 2–14 months (average 7.9 months), who used the Osbon ErecAid device. Eleven patients continued to use the device but were neutral regarding satisfaction; 21% discontinued use of the device. Reasons for discontinuance included the following: inability to achieve and maintain a full erection (12), pain and discomfort (4), inconvenience and awkwardness of the device (4), and reasons not related to the device such as poor health or marital problems (5). Eight patients used vacuum devices in conjunction with intracavernous pharmacotherapy (4) or semirigid penile prostheses (4).

In 1991 Turner and associates reported the results of a year long prospective study in which patients used the external vacuum device for treatment of erectile dysfunction. Results showed that 87% of 36 men achieved erections sufficient for intercourse. There was a 20% dropout rate.[14]

Others have not reported such good results. One study from the Netherlands reported only 22 of 72 patients considered vacuum device therapy successful, however these patients had all failed previous therapy. None of the nine psychogenic impotent patients in this series liked the device as a treatment although all acknowledged function. Of four patients in this series who felt their Jonas prosthesis was too short, three were satisfied with the enhancement afforded by the vacuum.[8] In an earlier published study, Gilbert and Gingell noted only a 26.7% rate of satisfactory intercourse in 12 of 45 patients.[15]

Recently, the Impotence Resource Center of the Geddings Osbon Foundation conducted a questionnaire survey of 34,777 registered owners of the Osbon vacuum products. The survey was a stratified disproportionate sample of owners (100% of owners acquiring the device between 1974 and 1988; 50%, 1989; 35%, 1990; 30%, 1991; 25%, 1992). A total of 7,075 (20.3%) returned the questionnaire, and of these 5,847 were considered valid and results were compiled from them. When training and support were utilized, it was supplied by the prescribing physician in 24.9% of respondents, by certified technicians in 19.8%, and by telephone hotline in 26.6%. Over 75% (76.8%) of the responders remain continuous users, 83.5% have sex as often as desired, 65.4% reported improved self-image, and 69.6% reported an improved relationship with their partner. Of 1,357 responders who had ceased using the device, 42.9% reported a reason for cessation not related to the device (no partner, 17%; natural erections returned, 10.8%; health problems, 9.3%; no desire for sex, 5.8%). See Table 12.2 for numbers and percentages of the 1,377 responders who ceased using the device due to dissatisfaction with it. In summary, if early use of the device is good, it is sustained with training and support contributing significantly to patient satisfaction.

TABLE 12.2. Ceased Use of Erection Vacuum Device—1,377

Reason	Number	%
Inability to achieve adequate erection	580	42.7
Pain or discomfort	555	40.9
Too much trouble	487	35.9
Partner nonacceptance	280	20.6
Switched to other therapies	214	15.8

Roy Witherington published the first results of a retrospective survey of Osbon vacuum devices in 1989.[4] Ninety-two percent of the 1,517 patients who used the device from 1974 to 1987 and mailed in a questionnaire reported satisfactory erection and 77% stated that they used it at least every 2 wk. Patients reported that for successful use, an average time of 1 wk with an average of 4 practice sessions was required to gain facility for device use.

Complications from use of the vacuum devices are minor and rare. Some patients develop minimal bruising or petechiae of the superficial shaft of the penis. Some patients complain that their scrotum is drawn into the cylinder when the vacuum is applied. If the bands are left on for prolonged periods of time there can be potential severe ischemic damage to the penis, which is why the time limit of 30 min of constriction band use is made by the manufacturers of the devices. Skin necrosis was reported in a paraplegic man who used a vacuum device three times daily on three successive days.[16] Kim and Carson reported development of Peyronie's disease in a patient who had used a vacuum device for 4 yr on a weekly basis as a treatment for his impotence.[17]

COMPARISON REPORTS OF VACUUM THERAPY VERSUS OTHER TREATMENT

Gould et al presented a study comparing external vacuum device use with pharmacologic erection therapy. There were three groups studied: 21 men who failed pharmacologic stimulation, 12 men who successfully used pharmacologic treatment for at least 6 months at home, and 13 men who never used pharmacologic treatment. Seventy-one percent of the first group chose continued vacuum device treatment after 3 months of a successful trial at home. Fifty-eight percent of the 12 who successfully used injection therapy previously elected to continue therapy with the vacuum device alone. Sixty-two percent of the 13 patients in the last group chose continued vacuum therapy.[18] Marmar and colleagues suggested that a vacuum device may augment a partial erection following an intracavernous injection.[19] Recently Chen and colleagues reported similar findings.[20] Turner and associates compared a group of 42 patients using self-injection with papaverine and phentolamine to 36 patients using the Osbon ErecAid, both followed for 12 months. Both treatments were used with equal frequency and rates of success. In this particular report, there was a 20% dropout rate with the vacuum device compared to 60% with the injection therapy.[21] In another publication by the same group, sexual, marital, and psychological responses of women to their partner's use of two different treatments, pharmacologic injection and vacuum tumescence therapy, were reported. Statistical analysis indicated that the women responded equally well to both treatments.[22]

REFERENCES

1. King J: *American Family Physician/Domestic Guide to Health.* Indianapolis, Streight/ Douglass, 1874, p 384.

2. Nadig PW: External devices for erectile dysfunction. In Whitehead ED, Nagler HM (eds): *Management of Impotence and Infertility*. Philadelphia, JB Lippincott, 1994, p 99.

3. Nadig PW, Ware JC, Blumoff R: Noninvasive device to produce and maintain an erection-like state. *Urology* 27:126–131, 1986.

4. Witherington R: Vacuum constriction device of management of erectile dysfunction. *J Urol* 141:320–322, 1989.

5. Lue TF: Impotence: a patient's goal directed approach to treatment. *World J Urol* 8:67–74, 1990.

6. Moul MW, McLeod DG: Negative pressure devices in the explanted penile prosthesis population. *J Urol* 142:729–731, 1989.

7. Korenmann SG, Viosca SSP: Use of a vacuum tumescence device in the management of impotence in men with a history of penile implant or severe pelvic disease. *JAGS* 40:61–64, 1992.

8. Meinhardt W, Lycklama a Nijeholt AAB, Kropman RF, et al: The negative pressure device for erectile disorders: when does it fail? *J Urology* 149:1285–1287, 1993.

9. Blackard CE, Borkon WD, Lima JJ, et al: Use of vacuum tumescence device for impotence secondary to venous leakage. *Urology* 41:225–230, 1993.

10. Salvatore FT, Sharman GM, Hellstrom WJ: Vacuum constriction devices and the clinical urologist: an informed selection. *Urology* 38:323–327, 1991.

11. Sidi AA, Becher EF, Zhang G, et al: Patient acceptance of and satisfaction with an external negative pressure device for impotence. *J Urol* 144:1154–1156, 1990.

12. Nadig PW: Six years experience with the vacuum constriction device. *Int J Impot Res* 1:55–58, 1989.

13. Cookson MS, Nadig PW: Long-term results with vacuum constriction device. *J Urol* 149:290–294, 1993.

14. Turner LA, Althof SE, Levine SB, et al: External vacuum devices in the treatment of erectile dysfunction: a one-year study of sexual and psychosocial impact. *J Sex Marital Ther* 17:81–93, 1991.

15. Gilbert HW, Gingell JC: Vacuum constriction devices: second-line conservative treatment for impotence. *Br J Urol* 70:81–83, 1992.

16. Meinhardt W, Kropman RF, Lycklama a Nijeholt AA, et al: Skin necrosis caused by use of negative pressure device for erectile impotence. *J Urol* 144:983, 1990.

17. Kim JH, Carson CC: Development of Peyronie's disease with the use of a vacuum constriction device. *J Urol* 149:1314–1315, 1993.

18. Gould JE, Switterd DM, Broderick GA, et al: External vacuum devices: a clinical comparison with pharmacologic erections. *World J Urol* 10:68–70, 1992.

19. Marmar JL, DeBenedictis TJ, Praiss DE: The use of a vacuum constrictor device to augment a partial erection following an intracavernous injection. *J Urol* 140:975–979, 1988.

20. Chen J, Godschalk MF, Katz PG, et al: Combining intracavernous injection and external vacuum as treatment for erectile dysfunction. *J Urol* 153:1482, 1995.

21. Turner LA, Althof SE, Levine SB, et al: Twelve-month comparison of two treatments for erectile dysfunction: self-injection versus external vacuum devices. *Urology* 39:138–144, 1992.

22. Althof SE, Turner LA, Levine SB, et al: Through the eyes of women: the sexual and psychological responses of women to their partner's treatment with self-injection or external vacuum therapy. *J Urol* 147:1024–1027, 1992.

13

Overview of Penile Implants

John J. Mulcahy

The treatment of erectile dysfunction has mushroomed with the widespread acceptance of medications and vacuum devices as effective, less aggressive, and less invasive options than surgical alternatives. Clinics touting a nonsurgical approach to this problem have proliferated in major cities in the United States and reports indicate that they are doing a brisk business. Despite the shift to medications and vacuum erection devices to restore erectile ability, penile implants are still a widely chosen option for managing this problem. Vendors claim that sales of these devices are steady in most areas and increased usage as a treatment option is occurring in some locations. The widespread marketing of impotence as a treatable problem has brought many more patients to physicians' offices for help in resolving this condition.

Since attitudes changed about 25 yr ago with a more open discussion of sexuality, there has been a shift in the type of patient who has chosen a penile implant as the treatment of his erectile dysfunction. Often we are now seeing patients with scar tissue forming in the penis as a result of Peyronie's disease where the implant tends to both straighten and strengthen the erection. Patients with venous leak impotence who do not respond well to intracorporal injections have selected a penile prosthesis when a vacuum erection device has proven unsatisfactory. Often a patient with physical impotence is influenced by a neighbor, coworker, or relative who has had a pleasing result in restoring his erections with a penile implant. The overall satisfaction rate has been very good with at least 4 out of 5 patients and partners happy with the results of their implant.[1-3] Disappointment in the remaining 20% may be decreased by thorough discussion beforehand which will allay apprehension and lessen the chance of unrealistic expectations regarding the result. A natural erection occurs as blood fills the corpora cavernosa, stretching the elastic tunica albuginea to the point where it will stretch no more, giving an increase in the diameter and length of the penis. When implant cylinders are placed in these erectile bodies, a nonstretchable sheath of scar tissue forms around these cylinders. This limits their expansion as scar tissue stretches very little or not at all. If scar tissue is already present in the penis from a previous injury such as priapism, intracorporal injections, or Peyronie's disease, this adds to the restriction in length and girth so that the resulting erection after penile implantation is usually shorter than the patient's former natural erection. The degree of loss in size is unpredictable, and this is the most frequent source of dissatisfaction with the outcome of prosthesis surgery. If one were to try and place a larger cylinder in an effort to overcome this, it would only result in pain, curvature, and possibly erosion of the prosthesis through the tunica.

Some patients relate that sensitivity is decreased following implantation but testing will almost always show that the nerves to the distal skin area are intact. Ability to appreciate pain, touch, and vibration persists. The reason for this reduced sensitivity is unclear. It may be related to changes in the nerve endings resulting from surgery and with time it may improve. Ejaculation is not directly influenced by the implant procedure and any change that the patient experiences in this physiologic function is due to stimulation or environmental influences. Couples should be counseled that the implant erection will be somewhat different from the patient's natural erection, especially in size and firmness. Positions for intercourse may need to be modified and if vaginal lubrication is scant, it may need to be supplemented, especially in older women. A modest degree of pain is to be expected after the surgery and the degree of pain varies from patient to patient. Diabetics who are experiencing peripheral neuropathy may have a higher incidence of prolonged pain than other groups of patients who are receiving a penile implant.

Patients should be made aware that there are two types of prosthesis, semirigid rods and inflatable cylinders, with the features of each of these discussed. As time progresses there is a possibility that the device may need to be repaired or replaced and the chance of this occurring within the first 5 yr is in the range of 5–10%. Beyond this time period no good studies are available and most of the manufacturers have changed their implant by this time to eliminate or reinforce areas that have tended to wear. Competition in the penile implant market has been keen and a number of the prototype models such as the Small-Carrion and Jonas prostheses are no longer available on the American market. Surgitech, which marketed the Flexirod, Flexiflate, and Uniflate 1000 prostheses, ceased manufacturing these devices in 1992. Bard Urological, which markets a number of products for use in the urinary tract, made a modest attempt to introduce an inflatable device in the late

TABLE 13.1. Hydraulic Penile Prostheses

	Prosthesis	Vendor	Wholesale Cost in USA (Dollars)—1996
Unitary	Dynaflex	AMS	$3,695.00
Two-piece	Mark II	Mentor	$4,357.00
	Ambicor	AMS	$4,195.00
Three-piece	700 Ultrex		
	(Three connectors)	AMS	$4,145.00
	700 Ultrex Plus		
	(One connector)	AMS	$4,265.00
	700 CX	AMS	$4,145.00
	700 CXM	AMS	$4,145.00
	Inflatable		
	(Three connectors)	Mentor	$4,000.00
	Alpha-1		
	(One connector)	Mentor	$4,383.00

TABLE 13.2 Semirigid Penile Prostheses

	Prosthesis	*Vendor*	*Wholesale Cost in USA (Dollars)—1996*
Mechanical	Dura II	UroHealth	$2,695.00
Malleable	Mentor Malleable	Mentor	$1,450.00
	Accuform	Mentor	$1,695.00
	650	AMS	$1,795.00
	600M	AMS	$1,595.00

1980s but the complexity of the product and competition made this impractical. Currently there are two categories of penile implants, the hydraulic or inflatable (Table 13.1), and the semirigid rod (Table 13.2), with three vendors in the United States: America Medical Systems, a subsidiary of Pfizer; Mentor Corporation; and UroHealth. The last company, UroHealth, recently acquired Dacomed Corporation and Osbon and is transferring sales of the Dura II, its penile implant, from the Dacomed division to Osbon.

SEMIRIGID RODS

Semirigid rod prostheses encompass two types, the mechanical and the malleable. American Medical Systems sells two malleable devices, the 650 and the 600M, while Mentor Corporation offers a malleable and an Accuform. The only mechanical device is the Dura II of UroHealth (Fig. 13.1). The Dura II replaced its precursor, the Duraphase, in 1993.[4] It consists of a body of articulating segments composed of

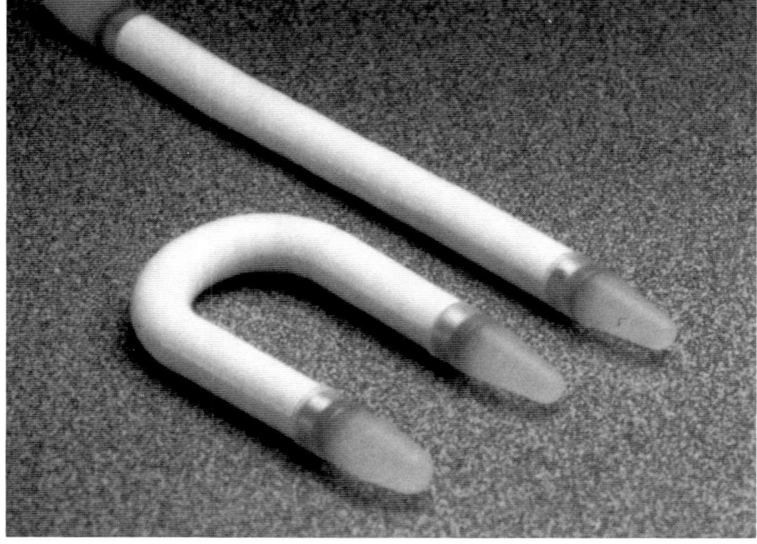

Fig. 13.1. Dura II penile implant. (Courtesy of UroHealth).

high-molecular-weight polyethylene. Through the center of these segments courses a cable which is attached to fixed posts on each end by a spring. The high-molecular-weight polyethylene is more durable than the polysulfone of the original Duraphase. With time the articulation of the segments composed of polysulfone would cause this material to wear with resulting shortening of the segments and reduced tension on the spring. Substituting the more durable polyethylene should reduce the incidence of this problem. The cable is composed of a stainless steel alloy with seven wires and 19 strands each. Bench testing of this cable has shown it to be extremely durable. In addition the reconfiguration of the design of the segments to minimize friction against the cable will hopefully prolong the life of this device. A polytetrafluoroethylene sleeve covers the body and a thin film of silicone is placed over this sleeve to prevent ingrowth of body tissues into the device.

The Dura II is easy to manipulate, with no springback following bending which does occur to some degree with the malleable rods. Insertion can be performed by a subcoronal or ventral penile incision. The latter is the favored approach and consists of a proximal shaft skin incision and more distally placed corporotomies (Fig. 13.2). One then lifts the distal end of the corporotomy over the cylinder with mild bending of the distal trips.[5] The Dura II cylinder does not bend easily and excessive angulation of this device may cause possible damage to the mechanism. For this reason it is difficult to place through penoscrotal or infrapubic incisions.

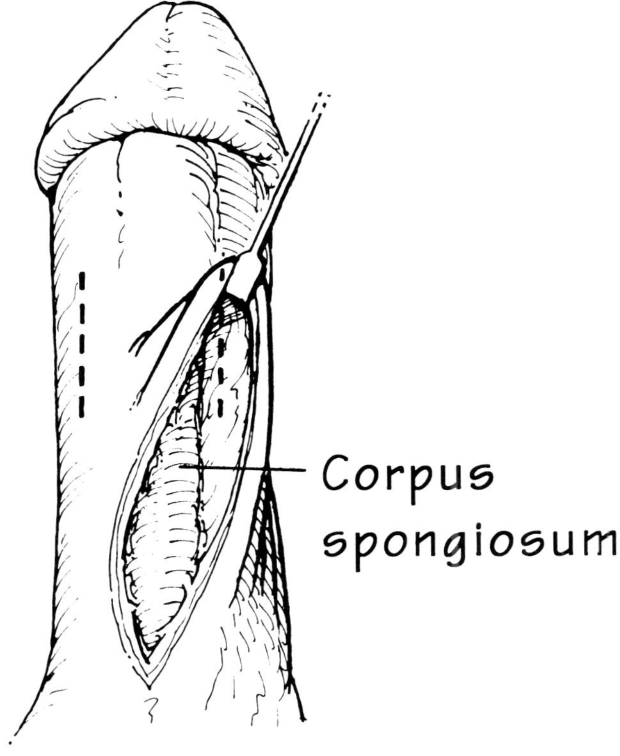

Fig. 13.2. Ventral penile incision. Proximal shaft midline skin incision. Distal shaft lateral corporotomies.

Local anesthesia is readily used for placing the Dura II as it is with any of the unitary prosthetic devices. One simply infiltrates the base of the penis circumferentially with the anesthetic as in performing a penile block for circumcision. A tourniquet is then placed around the base of the penis and 25 cc of 0.5% lidocaine solution without epinephrine is placed intracorporally as if one were performing an artificial erection. In a minute or two the tourniquet is released and the anesthetic is allowed to flow proximally to anesthetize the entire extent of both corpora cavernosa. One should not use bupivacaine which is a longer lasting local anesthetic but may be cardiotoxic when given systematically in high doses.

MALLEABLE RODS

There are four varieties of malleables to choose from. American Medical Systems markets the 650 and the 600M. The 650 comes in two sizes, 13 and 11 mm (Fig. 13.3). By stripping an outer jacket of silicone from the 13-mm device one now has the 11-mm version. The 600M is a narrower version of the 650 supplied in 11.5 mm width which is trimmable to 9.5 mm by removing the outer jacket. The AMS 650 introduced to the American market in early 1996 is an improvement in design over its precursor, the AMS 600. There are more numerous and thinner strands per core wire, making bending easier and with less springback. It is provided in the same sizes as the AMS 600 model.

The Mentor malleable rods consist of a single silver coil surrounded by a silicone jacket. The Accuform rods are comprised of paired silver coils which make the device more easily bendable and with less springback after bending. Each of these

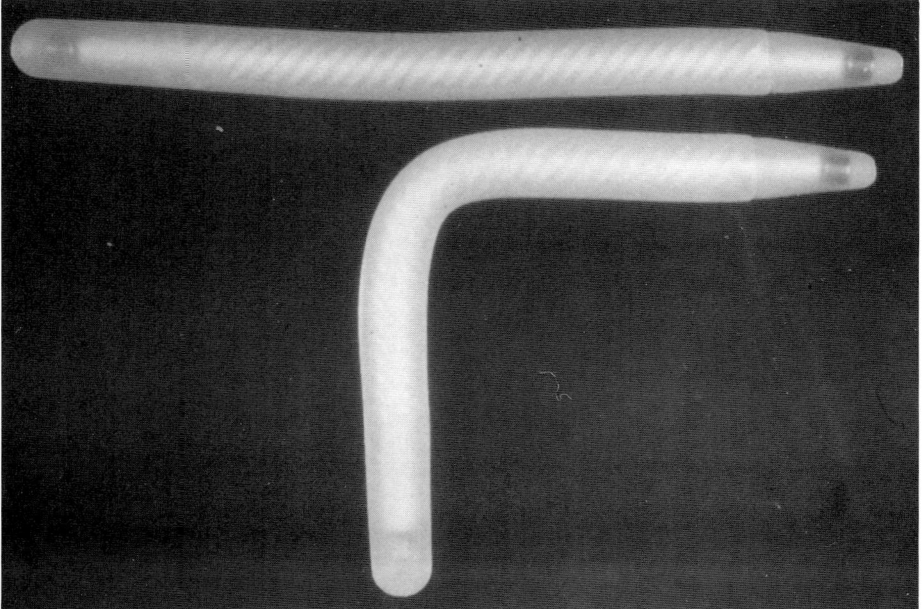

Fig. 13.3. AMS 650 malleable penile implant. (Courtesy of American Medical Systems)

two models comes in 9.5 mm, 11 mm, and 13 mm widths with the silver segment located at the bend angle of the penis. The Mentor rods come in one length but the proximal portion of each rod can be trimmed and a tapered cap added to produce the desired length that would fit the patient's corporal bodies appropriately. When sizing semirigid rods or hydraulic cylinders which are supplied in more than one fixed girth size, it is necessary to determine before opening the sterile package which width size is appropriate for implantation. An easy method for deciding the best fit would be to place two dilators of the same size as the cylinders into each corporal body side by side. One then apposes the thumb to the index finger between the dilators. If one is able to touch the thumb to the index finger, a loose fit will be achieved with that size cylinder and a larger one should be selected. Slight separation of the dilators while apposing the fingers between them would indicate an ideal fit of that size cylinders, whereas no movement of the dilators would suggest a snug fit.

Malleable rods require some manual dexterity to bend and some degree of springback after bending is seen. With these devices in place, the penis should be worn in the upward position or in the crease of the leg, especially in the long penis, to prevent friction against the patient's undergarments during day-to-day activities. They intrinsically provide good support to the erection but better support and bendability are achieved by appropriate sizing. The malleables have been very durable with reports of wire breakage being extremely rare. With any of the semirigid rods the length size should be about 1/2 cm less than the measured corporal length. This tends to give better bendability, less pain, and less chance of erosion. During ventral bending if a consistent springback or tendency to become S-shaped or snaking is noted, a smaller length cylinder may be a more appropriate fit.

UNITARY INFLATABLE DEVICES

The Dynaflex from American Medical Systems is the only unitary hydraulic device. It consists of a distal pump which is somewhat difficult to operate, a central

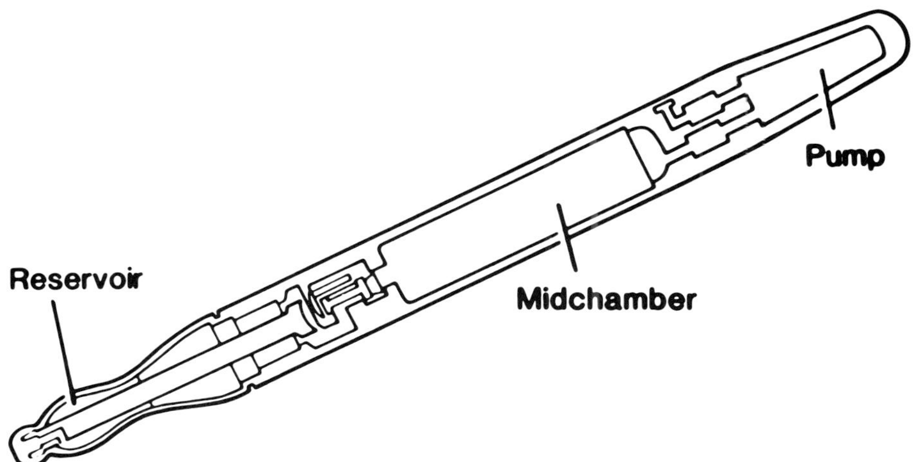

Fig. 13.4. Diagram of Dynaflex penile implant. (Courtesy of American Medical Systems)

chamber which always remains partially filled with fluid, and a proximal reservoir cavity from which fluid is transferred through side channels to the central chamber when rigidity is desired (Fig. 13.4). A small volume shift, in the range of 2–3 cc changes the status of the cylinder from flaccid to rigid. Deflation is easily accomplished. One simply bends the cylinder and holds it in the bent position for a short period of time. Fluid then flows back to the reservoir area by simply manually compressing the central portion of the device. Simplicity of insertion using a local anesthetic through any type of penile incision and the absence of extra penile parts are positive features. The Dynaflex comes in two widths, 11 and 13 mm diameter. From experience we have found that the support given to the erection by a hydraulic prosthesis is determined by the degree of filling of the corporal body, the more complete the filling the better the support given. A good analogy when discussing with patients how a hydraulic device works would be to compare it with the inner tube on a bicycle tire. The more completely the inner tube fills the tire, the better the firmness of the tire. In the penis if there is room for the cylinder to shift, less optimal support is achieved. In the very broad penis, the Dynaflex with maximum girth of 13 mm would not give as complete filling and hence less optimal rigidity.

TWO-PIECE INFLATABLE IMPLANTS

Two models are available in this category, the Mark II of Mentor (Fig. 13.5) and the Ambicor of AMS (Fig. 13.6). Each consists of two inflatable cylinders connected to a pump-reservoir located in the scrotum. The Mark II cylinders are made of Bioflex

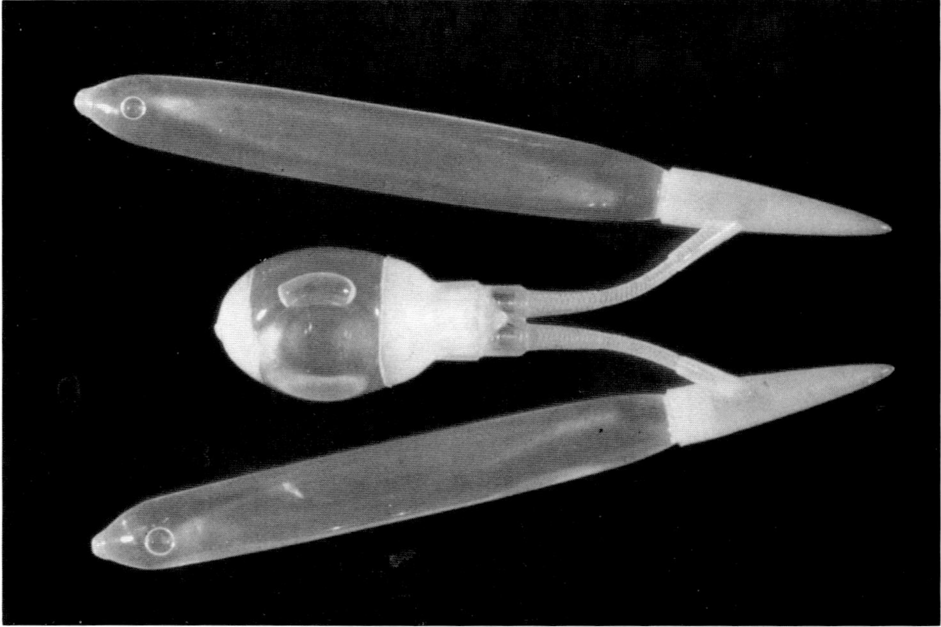

Fig. 13.5. Mark II penile implant. (Courtesy of Mentor Corporation)

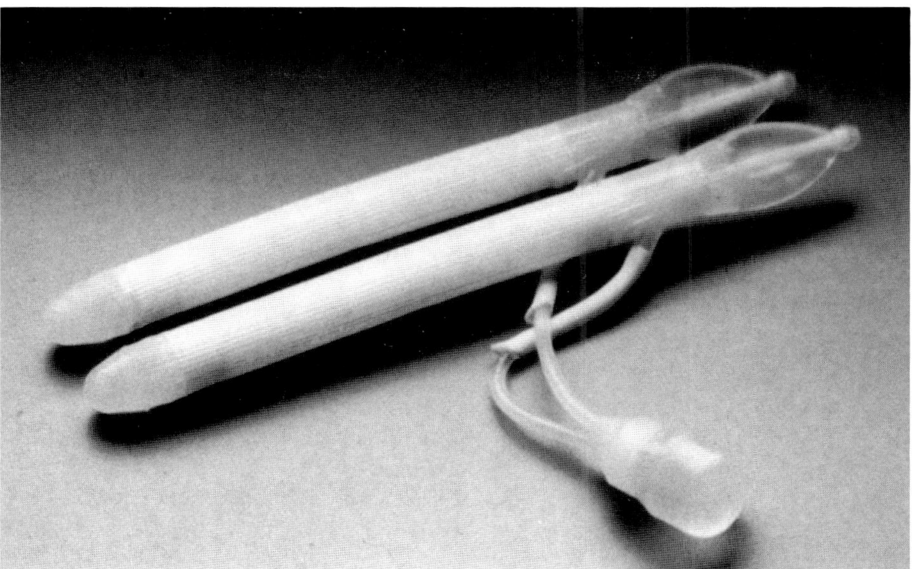

Fig. 13.6. Ambicor penile implant. (Courtesy of American Medical Systems)

(polyurethane) and the resipump volume is 20 cc.[6] In the very broad or long penis, rigidity or flaccidity may be compromised as only 15 cc is available for transfer. This resipump is relatively large and is best positioned between the testicles. The penoscrotal approach is easiest and placement of an intra-abdominal reservoir is avoided which is advantageous in patients who have had previous pelvic surgery. The Ambicor has storage capacity in the proximal part of the device, and a small pump is located in the scrotum. A small volume of fluid, about 3 cc, is transferred when alternating between rigidity and flaccidity. Three width sizes, 11 mm, 13 mm, and 15 mm, give flexibility between insertion in the narrow and the broad penis. When flaccid the penis appears full but bendable. Both the Mark II and Ambicor have relatively easy inflate and deflate mechanisms and neither requires tubing adjustment or connectors interposed in the tubing. The Ambicor comes prefilled and pre-packaged in a saline medium with tubing lengths appropriate for the penoscrotal approach only. The Mark II is filled through a self-sealing penetrable port located on the inferior side of the pump. Transcutaneous fluid adjustment through this port in the postoperative period is possible. Two lengths of tubing are provided for the Mark II, the longer length for infrapubic insertion and the shorter length for the penoscrotal approach.

THREE-PIECE INFLATABLES

The original inflatable penile prosthesis was introduced in 1972 by American Medical Systems and was the three-piece model consisting of a scrotal pump, prevesicle reservoir, and a cylinder in each erectile body.[7] With time the occurrence of cylinder aneurysms and the wearing of silicone parts led to malfunction in a high percentage of patients. The manufacturer attended to design problems and the current three-piece inflatable devices have proven to be very reliable. Both American Medical Systems and Mentor Corporation market three-piece devices. The American Medical Systems' cylinders come in three types, Ultrex, CX, and CXM. Each of these consists of an inner silicone cylinder, a middle layer of woven Dacron Lycra, and an outer silicone sheath to prevent ingrowth of tissues into the Dacron Lycra weave. In the Ultrex device the Dacron Lycra layer is woven in two directions which allows expansion in both length and width. In the CX and CXM cylinders the Dacron Lycra weave is in one direction allowing expansion in girth only. The Ultrex and CX expand from 12 to 18 mm diameter, the CXM stretches from 9.5 to 14 mm at maximum inflation. This narrow cylinder is more suitable for placement when there is less width to the corporal bodies and is very helpful in situations of previous surgery where the erectile cavities have been scarred. As mentioned earlier, the degree of rigidity depends on the completeness of filling of the erectile body. If a finger-in-glove like fit occurs, good support is achieved; a looser fit would result in suboptimal support. Since the reservoir is inside the body cavity, it can have a very large capacity and complete removal of fluid from the penis is possible in the flaccid state. In addition, the very large penis can be completely filled with this device. It has been said that length expansion of the Ultrex cylinders permit elongation of penis in a few patients but the degree has been small.[8]

In 1982 the Mentor Corporation introduced a three-piece device similar in design to the American Medical Systems product. The Bioflex cylinders have proven to be more durable in resisting wear and intrinsically are less prone to aneurysm formation. This material, however, is more prone to thermal injury and care should be taken when using electrocautery near these polyurethane type cylinders.[9] Currently there are two types of Mentor three-piece prostheses, the Alpha I (Fig. 13.7) which has one connection between the pump and reservoir, and the Mentor inflatable which has three connections. In 1993 a clinical trial on a distally expanding cylinder called Excel was successfully completed by Mentor and the device is now pending FDA approval.[10] The mechanism of distal expansion is an accordion or bellows configuration of the cylinder located just distal to the input tube. This will permit length as well as girth increase as with the AMS Ultrex. The advantage of the distal expanding cylinders is that they will make up for short sizing and permit one to use a slightly shorter cylinder. These cylinders will completely fill the corporal bodies and if scar tissue is present they will tether the penis to the side of the curve. With the girth only expanding cylinders (CX or Alpha I), good intrinsic rigidity is achieved and the end of the corporal body is allowed to shift over the end of the cylinder which tends to straighten the erection. Hence, in situations where scar tissue is present or there is a tendency of the penis to curve, the CX or Alpha I would be a more appropriate choice for implantation than the Ultrex or the Excel cylinders.[11] The pump of either three-piece inflatable prosthesis is somewhat difficult to operate and is not recommended for the patient with impaired manual dexterity. Mild autoinflation is seen with each device. The manufacturers have attempted to reduce this phenomenon by introducing a lock-out mechanism on the pump or increasing tension on the spring in the pump but these modifications have proven difficult for the patients to operate and were abandoned. This autoinflation remains state-of-the-art and may be minimized by creating an adequately large

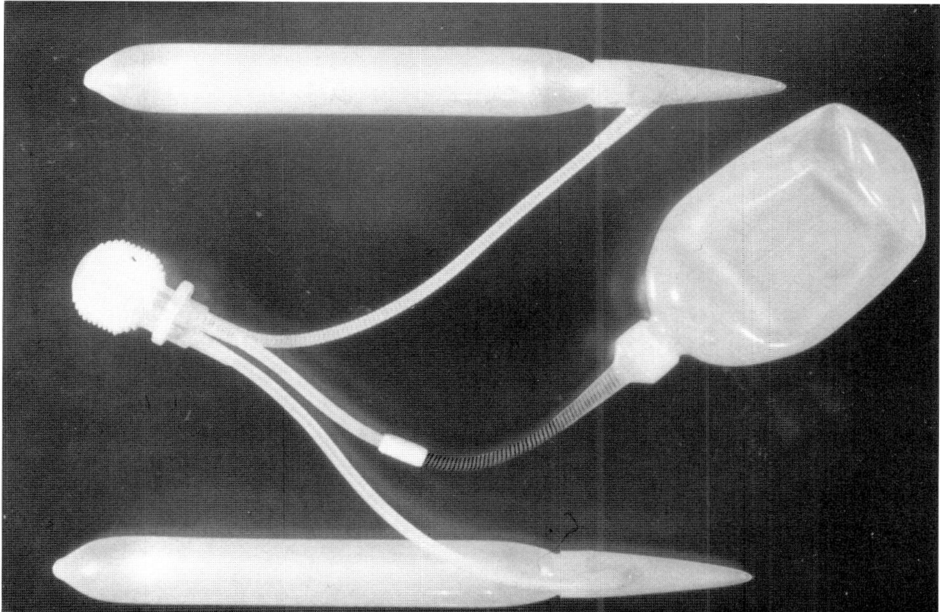

Fig. 13.7. Mentor Alpha-1 penile implant. (Courtesy of Mentor Corporation)

cavity for the balloon reservoir within the abdomen, by decreasing the fluid volume
of the reservoir to 5–10 cc less than the capacity, and by frequent complete deflation
of the cylinders to prevent the capsule of scar tissue which forms around the
reservoir as the body's reaction to healing to encase this structure in the partially
filled condition. The reservoirs may be placed intraperitoneally or in an epigastric
location if the pelvis is excessively scarred.[12]

PREOPERATIVE PREPARATION

After thoroughly discussing the expectations, features, and results of implant surgery
with the patient and his partner, the operation should be scheduled. Time should be
permitted for precertification or prior approval from insurance if this is pertinent.
The urine should be sterile if possible. This is difficult in patients with neurogenic
bladder or indwelling suprapubic tubes. In such cases, oral antibiotics are started 1
wk preoperatively to maintain a sterile urine. The skin of the perineum and pelvis
should be washed thoroughly with a strong antiseptic soap for 3 days and shaving
of pubic hair carried out in the operating room. At a previous office visit the skin
should be inspected for lesions such as comedomes or sebaceous cysts which harbor
pathogenic organisms. These should be eliminated prior to surgery. Most urologists
favor the use of prophylactic antibiotics in association with implant surgery. If one
wishes to use these, they should be started 1 hr preoperatively and continued for 48
hr in the postoperative period. The rationale for using prophylactic antibiotics is to

provide good tissue levels during the time the wound is open to neutralize any bacteria that may stray into the wound during this time. By 48 hr the wound is sealed and there is no further need for these compounds. Some infectious disease experts have a different view of this approach. The operating field is sterile to begin with, the surgeon is unusually cautious during insertion of the device with copious wound irrigations which may contain antibiotics, and he sees no need for using extensive antibiotics which may increase the chance of resistant organisms developing. No control study has been performed which shows the effectiveness of use versus nonuse of prophylactic antibiotics during prosthesis insertion. A thorough skin preparation with a strong antiseptic solution such as povidone–iodine is performed. In cases where a urethral catheter has been indwelling, or in which patients are at greater risk for urethral perforation during the procedure such as where the corporal bodies are scarred from previous surgery, a urethral preparation by instilling antiseptic solution should be considered. During the procedure, frequent wound irrigations with a sterile solution with or without antibiotics will reduce the concentration of environmental pathogens which may stray into the operating field. The best antibiotic regimen is currently vancomycin and gentamicin. Vancomycin is effective against 99% of *Staphylococcus epidermidis*, the most common organism found to be associated with prosthetic infections. Gentamicin is effective against most Gram-negative organisms which may also be associated with prosthetic infections. Other antibiotics that are useful in treating such infections are the third-generation cephalosporins and the quinolones. The overall infection rate with primary implant procedures is in the range of 1–3%.[13] With secondary procedures for repair or reinsertion of these devices, the incidence of infection becomes greater. If infection associated with an implant does occur, one has two options. The prosthesis can be removed, the wound cleansed, drains placed, and the situation allowed to heal for 6 months at which time consideration for another implant may be made. The other alternative is termed a *salvage* or *rescue procedure* which entails removing the prosthesis and all foreign materials, washing the wound thoroughly with antiseptic solutions, and inserting a new prosthesis during the same procedure. The purpose of salvage is to maintain penile length and make cylinder insertion easier. Success in the range of 80–90% of cases has been achieved by using this alternative approach.[14–16]

POSTOPERATIVE CARE

A urethral catheter may be placed during the procedure and may be helpful in identifying the corpus spongiosum if this is a problem. It is not necessary, though many urologists favor draining the bladder by this method for the first 24 hr after surgery. Cycling of hydraulic devices begins at 5–6 wk. During the healing phase until cycling begins patients are encouraged to keep the prosthesis pointing upward to preserve the natural upward tilt of the erection. A scrotal supporter or other device which gently restricts the penis against the body has been helpful for this purpose. Patients may begin using the implant for intercourse at about 5–6 wk if they wish. Frequent cycling of hydraulic devices, at least two times a week, is encouraged thereafter to prevent additional contracture of scar around the cylinders.

SILICONE ISSUE

Recent furor over silicone prostheses as a possible detriment to body health has occurred. Breast implants have been accused in courtrooms and in the media of causing pain, disfiguration, and autoimmune diseases. Most of the problems have occurred with gel-filled prostheses that extruded a foreign substance into the breast tissue when the capsule ruptured. This created an inflammatory response with pain, nodules, and disfiguration. In a large series no increased incidence in the occurrence of collagen diseases or even the symptoms of these illnesses was seen in women with silicone breast implants when compared with an age-matched control group without implants.[17] Barrett and coworkers examined the tissues of 26 patients with genitourinary silicone prosthetic devices and found silicone particles in the peri-prosthetic sheath and regional lymph nodes of some of these patients.[18] None of these patients showed symptoms or signs of autoimmune disease and no other study has documented an association of silicone implants with autoimmune disease. The Food and Drug Administration still considers this issue controversial and has insisted that the two vendors of inflatable implants, American Medical Systems and Mentor Corporation, conduct prospective clinical trials documenting the safety, efficacy, patient satisfaction, and incidence of concomitant disease documented by laboratory studies and questionnaires in a group of patients with these devices.

LONG-TERM SURVIVAL

As the time interval from the placement of a penile prosthesis increases, the more difficult it is to collect reliable data on the function of these devices. A number of features account for this. Patients may move from the area or die. The partner or spouse may be lost and sexual activity discontinued. Design changes in a particular model have occurred at a frequency of every 5–8 yr making the old model obsolete. These changes usually include improvements which replace or reinforce areas that tended to wear or break down. The polyurethane material of the Mentor cylinders has been very durable with few instances of wear occurring. Tubing connectors have been problematic with these devices, and these have now been eliminated in many cases or improved in the design to prevent disruption or tubing fracture. The silicone coating of the AMS inflatable cylinders tended to wear with time, and replacing the prototype model with the triple layered CX and Ultrex cylinders has improved longevity. The Hydroflex unitary inflatable, the precursor of the Dynaflex, had a high replacement rate at 5–7 yr. The Dynaflex has not shown this propensity as yet although long-term evaluation is still pending. The Duraphase segments wore with frequent bending and this device was replaced with the Dura II. Stainless steel malleable devices have proven to be very wear resistant. The original malleable Jonas prosthesis showed fractures in the silver core developing with time. Individually wrapping the silver strands has improved the longevity of silver core malleable rods. In general when discussing repair rates with patients the figure of 5–15% in the first 5 yr is reasonable.[19] By 15–20 yr the majority of the devices, especially the inflatables, will need to be replaced. With repeat surgery for repair, replacement, or reinsertion of penile prostheses, patient satisfaction rates decline due mainly to the smaller size of the penis which occurs with each procedure.

REFERENCES

1. Fallon B, Ghanem H: Sexual performance and satisfaction with penile prostheses in impotence of various etiologies. *Int J Impot Res* 2:35–42, 1990.

2. Garber BB: Mentor Alpha-1 penile prosthesis: patient satisfaction and device reliability. *Urology* 43:214–217, 1994.

3. McLaren RH, Barrett DM: Patient and partner satisfaction with the AMS 700 penile prosthesis. *J Urol* 147:62–67, 1992.

4. Mulcahy JJ: Mechanical penile prostheses. *Prob Urol* 7:311–316, 1993.

5. Wahle GR, Mulcahy JJ: Ventral penile approach in unitary component penile prosthesis placement. *J. Urol* 149:537–538, 1993.

6. Fein RL: GFS Mark II inflatable penile prosthesis: four-year clinical study. *Urology* 43:209–213, 1994.

7. Scott FB, Bradley WE, Timm GW: Management of erectile impotence: use of implantable inflatable prosthesis. *Urology* 2:80–82, 1973.

8. Montague DK, Lakin MM: Early experience with the controlled girth and length expanding cylinders of the American Medical Systems Ultrex penile prosthesis. *J Urol* 148:1444–1446, 1992.

9. Halsim LS, Kulaksizoglu H, Hamill BK, et al: A guide to safe corporotomy incisions in the presence of underlying inflatable penile cylinders: results of in vitro and in vivo studies. *J Urol* 155:918–923, 1996.

10. Nejad SH, Nehra A, Williams C, et al: Three year multi-institutional prospective study of the Mentor Alpha Excel: an investigative inflatable penile prosthesis with a wave-shaped expandable retractable cylinder section. *J Urol* 153:4(Abstract 360A), 1995.

11. Wilson SK, Cleves MA, Delk JR: Ultrex cylinders: problems with uncontrolled lengthening (the S-shaped deformity). *J Urol* 155:135–137, 1996.

12. Riemenschneider HW: Epigastric placement of reservoir for inflatable penile prosthesis. *Urology* 17:79–81, 1981.

13. Carson CC: Infections in genitourinary prostheses. *Urol Clin North Am* 16:139–147, 1989.

14. Fishman, IJ, Scott FB, Selim AM: Rescue procedure: an alternative to complete removal for treatment of infected penile prostheses. *J Urol* 137:4(Abstract 202A), 1987.

15. Furlow WL, Goldwasser B: Salvage of the eroded inflatable penile prosthesis: a new concept. *J Urol* 138:312–314, 1987.

16. Brant MD, Ludlow JK, Mulcahy JJ: The prosthesis salvage operation: immediate replacement of the infected penile prosthesis. *J Urol* 155:155–157, 1996.

17. Sherine GE, O'Fallon WM, Kurland LT, et al: Risk of connective tissue diseases and other disorders after breast implantation. *N Engl J Med* 330:1697–1702, 1994.

18. Barrett DM, O'Sullivan DC, Malizia AA, et al: Particle shedding and migration from silicone genitourinary prosthetic devices. *J Urol* 146:319–322, 1991.

19. Lewis RW, McLaren R: Reoperation for penile prosthesis implantation. *Prob Urol* 7:381–401, 1993.

14

Management of Penile Implant Complications

Steven Karl Wilson

Penile prosthesis implantation, an operation formerly done only in large American centers, is now performed in most countries of the world. Penile implant surgery has evolved from an experimental, time-consuming procedure to a routine surgical operation often accomplished in less than an hour. Despite widespread acceptance of the efficacy of prosthesis implantation as a correction for erectile dysfunction, less than 10% of urologists worldwide do 90% of the world's penile implants. Why do so few urologists implant?

It is not due to fear of unreliability of the product. Since 1986 the implants manufactured by American Medical Systems, Mentor Corporation, and UroHealth are remarkably dependable. Much like military aviation, where pilot error exceeds mechanical failure as a cause of crash, the human factor is more often the cause of implant reoperation than mechanical problems.[1] Physician error, patient dissatisfaction, and infection are more usual causes of reoperation than mechanical breakage. Recently, in the United States, litigation arising from prosthesis implantation has supplanted vasectomy as the number one cause of malpractice suits involving urologists.

This chapter is a practical "how to do it" guide to the correction of common penile implant complications. Many of the complications can be corrected at the time of surgery if only recognized! Tips for minimizing complications are included in each of the sections. It is our hope that this chapter will stimulate implant abstainers and occasional implanters to participate more often in this satisfying field of surgical correction of erectile dysfunction.

INTRAOPERATIVE COMPLICATIONS

Most intraoperative complications occur during dilatation of the corpora cavernosa. The corpora can be ruptured proximally or distally resulting in either urethral laceration or crural perforation. Additionally, the intracorporal septum may be violated resulting in a crossover of the implanted cylinder. With the exception of urethral laceration in the distal penis, all complications can be corrected at the time of implantation. The problem is failure to recognize them.

Corporal Dilation Problems: Urethral Laceration, Perforation, and Crossover

Urethral Laceration

Should urethral laceration occur during the course of prosthesis implantation, treatment depends on the location of the laceration. Proximal lacerations can be repaired upon discovery and the implantation completed. Unfortunately, the most common location of urethral laceration is at the meatus. For these cases it is necessary to abort the procedure and allow the laceration to heal over a Foley catheter for 3–5 days. Suprapubic drainage is not necessary and reoperation can occur in 4–6 wk. It is not necessary (or even possible) to repair the meatal laceration. One should not leave the implant in place and divert the urine. The chronic pressure of the implant prevents urethral healing, even with urinary diversion. Experienced implanters are wary of distal urethral laceration and attempt to detect it by always irrigating the corpora via asepto syringe following corporal dilatation. Irrigation fluid visible around the Foley catheter at the meatus indicates distal urethral laceration (Fig. 14.1A).

If the cylinder is visible at the meatus within 3 months after implantation, it usually indicates delayed presentation of urethral trauma that was sustained at operation.[2] In the absence of purulence, these cases can be handled by removing only the offending cylinder and capping off the tubing leading to it. The cylinder can be replaced in 4–6 wk. Some patients with inflatable mentor Alpha I cylinders (which have tunical-dependent expansion) will be satisfied with the erection afforded by only a single cylinder and will defer replacement. If cylinder erosion into the urethra presents beyond 6 months, an infectious etiology can be suspected and the entire prosthesis must be removed. Infected implants with urethral or penile erosion are specific contraindications to salvage (rescue) procedures.[3]

Crural Perforation

Crural perforation occurs during vigorous proximal dilatation, particularly in fibrotic corpora. If proximal dilatation is difficult, one should extend the corporotomy proximally rather than attempting to force small dilators into the unyielding corporal tissue. Should a proximal corporal body perforation occur, it can be identified by a discrepancy of greater than 1 cm in the proximal intracorporal measurements. It may also be recognized by placing dilators in each corporal body proximally and noticing that the angles of presentation are different and that one dilator is deeper than the other (Fig. 14.1B, 1C). Proximal corporal rupture can be confirmed the morning after surgery by the detection of perineal bruising—the "blue butterfly sign" (Fig. 14.1C).

There are several techniques to correct proximal corporal perforation. The easiest technique is nothing more than the selection of the proper type of prosthesis. If a

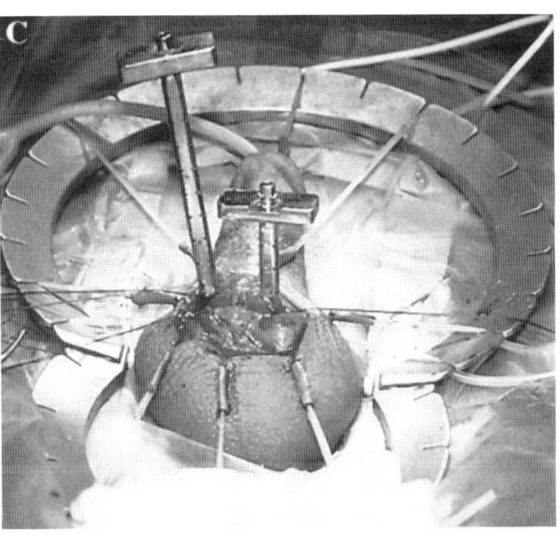
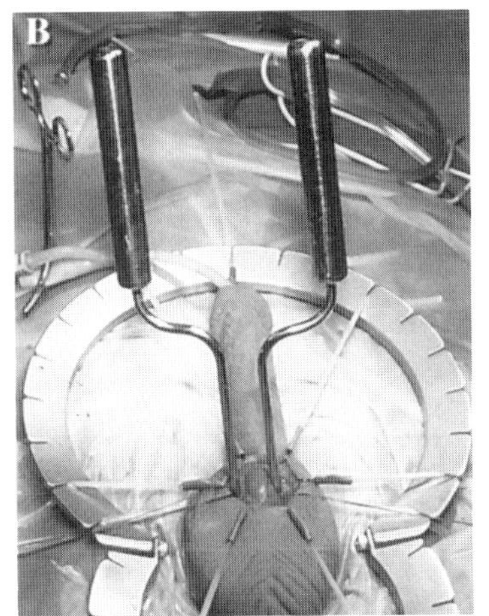
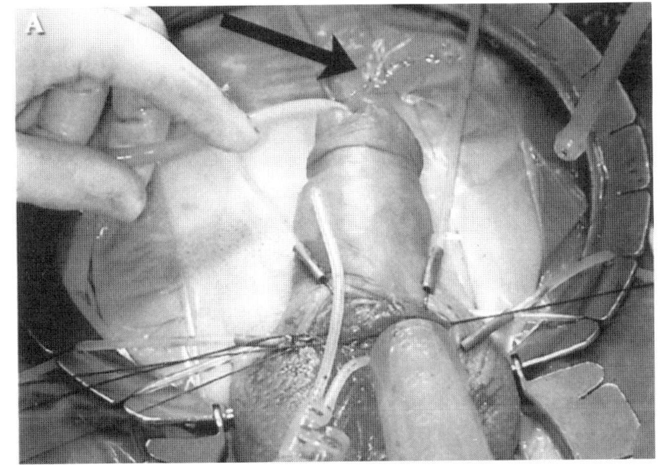

Fig. 14.1. A: Irrigation of corpora demonstrating fluid around catheter–urethral laceration. **B:** Dilators in both corpora demonstrating correct dilatation. **C:** Furlow insertion tools in both corpora demonstrating unilateral corporal rupture.

multiple component prosthesis is used, no special correction is necessary. The cylinder input tubing will anchor the prosthesis in place if care is taken to tether the input tubing with tight corporal sutures. If using an AMS 700 cylinder, additional security can be obtained by suturing the polytetrafluoroethylene tubing sleeve to the tunica. With time, scar tissue will form around the base of the prosthesis closing the defect. It is also effective to suture the rear tip extender of the prosthesis to tunica albuginea or pelvic bone. Many times both tight corporal closure and suture fixation of the rear tip extender may be used.

If a self-contained or semirigid rod prosthesis is used, it is necessary to construct a cup or "wind sock" of synthetic material (Gor-Tex or Dacron), resting the prosthesis base in the sock, and anchoring the sleeve to the corpora with nonabsorbable sutures. It is a better idea to substitute a multiple component prosthesis since most authorities believe that the introduction of additional synthetic material may increase the risk of infection.[4]

It is a mistake to attempt primary repair of ruptured crus. Exposure is arduous and very little suitable tissue is available to construct the closure. If the cylinder is secured by any of the above methods, a combination of capsule formation and scar tissue will prevent subsequent proximal migration of the newly implanted cylinder.

Unrecognized corporal body perforation will result in proximal migration of the cylinder in the postoperative period. This will often appear as a supersonic transport (SST) deformity. The glans of the penis droops over the prosthesis rather than being supported by the tip. The development of an SST deformity from proximal corporal perforation is more commonly seen when self-contained prostheses or semirigid rods are used. The correction of the SST deformity is addressed later in the chapter.

Septal Crossover

Septal crossover can occur proximally or distally. The septum is inconstant in the distal penis and may have areas of thinning or even outright gaps. It is surprisingly easy to be deflected to the opposite corporal compartment during dilatation or cylinder insertion. The operator must be alert to the problem of distal crossover since it may only be evident upon inflation of the prosthesis (Fig. 14.2A, 2B). If distal crossover occurs, the correction is simple. The corpora are redilated and a large dilator is placed in the opposite corpus during repeat cylinder insertion. It is not necessary to repair the corporal septum and, in fact, is virtually impossible.

Proximal crossover can be suspected when difficulty is encountered during insertion of the second cylinder. It can be diagnosed by placing dilators in both corpora proximally at the same time. In fact, many experienced implanters do this both proximally and distally to routinely check for both septal crossover and crural perforation (Fig. 14.1B, 1C). As with distal crossover, proximal crossover requires only recognition and rerouting of the cylinders into their proper locations. Failure to recognize either of these conditions results in an unhappy patient who certainly will have no difficulty recognizing that something is amiss.

Prevention of Corporal Problems

Most episodes of urethral trauma or corporal rupture are associated with passage of small dilators. We make it a practice to always begin dilatation with size 11 dilator

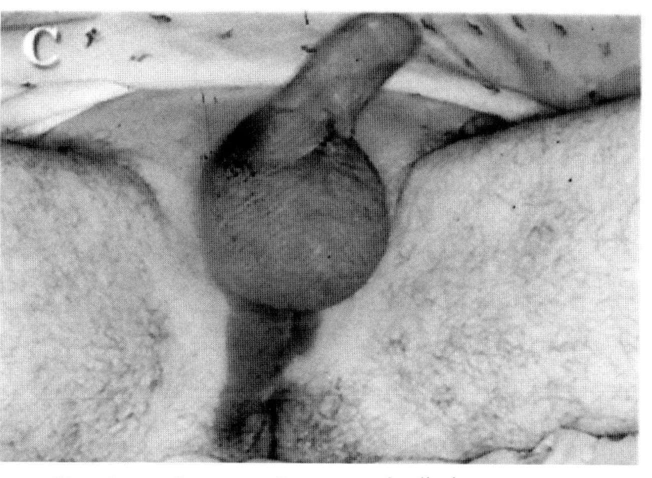

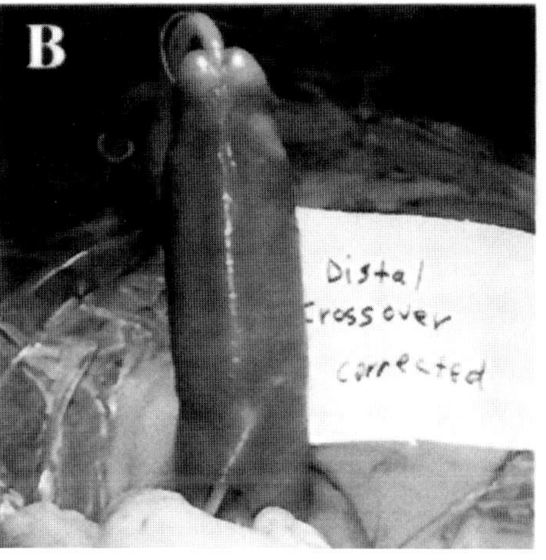

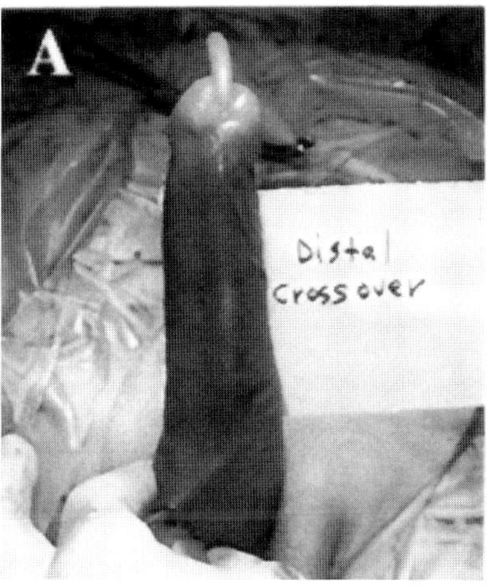

Fig. 14.2. A: Distal cylinder crossover. **B:** Same patient after correction by redilatation and correct placement of cylinders.

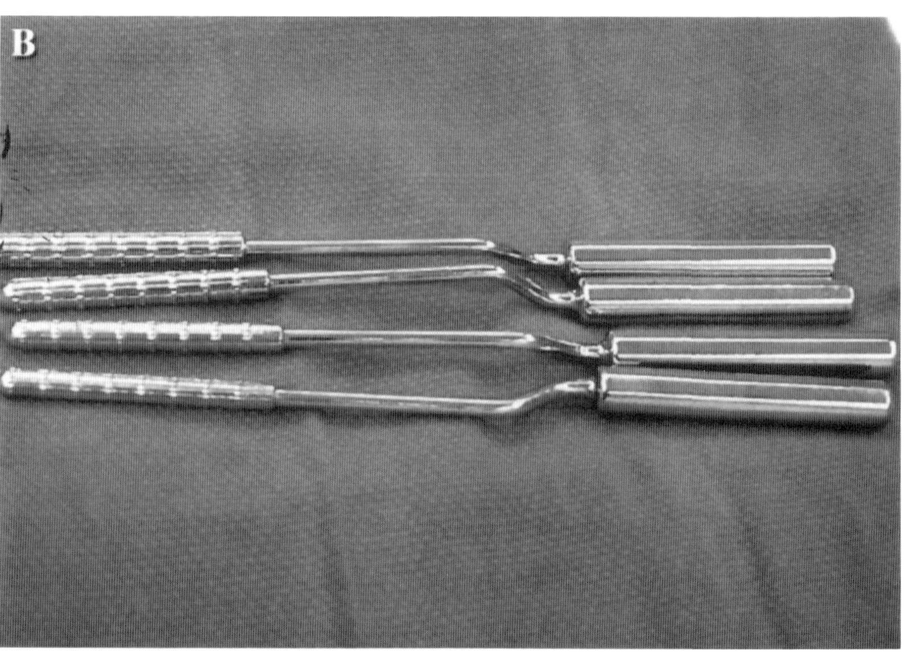

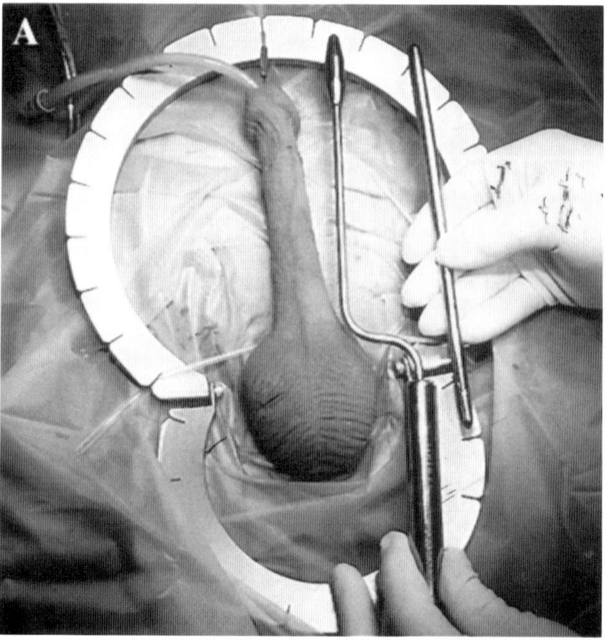

Fig. 14.3. **A:** Comparison of Brooks and Hegar dilators. Note also correct configuration of Scott retractor. **B:** Carrion-Rossello Cavernotomes size 9–12 mm.

instead of sizes 8–10. Even in the thin penis seen in some Asian and Caucasian men, it is usually possible to easily pass size 11 as the initial dilator. If resistance is met to size 11, it is better to pass the Metzenbaum scissors first, rather than a smaller dilator. The surgeon will have more control of the scissors and can keep them pointed in a lateral direction away from all the trouble. We have found the Brooks dilators (Mentor Corporation) to be safer than the commonly available Hegar. The dilating end of the Brooks dilator is shaped like a blunt-nosed bullet and the handle has a bayonet configuration. Both of these characteristics coupled with size 11 initial corporal dilatation make overzealous dilatation less likely (Fig. 14.3A).

Detection of corporal problems such as urethral perforation, crossover, and crural rupture can be facilitated by following a ritual in each case (similar to the pilot's preflight checklist). Valuable maneuvers are:

1. Irrigation of both corpora after dilatation to check for urethral damage.

2. Placement of two dilators distally and proximally to diagnose rupture or crossover.

3. Inflation of the implant to the maximum to check for lopsidedness after placement.

MECHANICAL COMPLICATIONS

Inflatable penile prostheses manufactured in the 1970s were notoriously unreliable. Virtually all of those implants have been removed or revised.[5] Most of the problems were related to silicone wear or aneurysm of the cylinders. The year 1986 is considered a watershed year for improved longevity of penile implants. This was the year American Medical Systems introduced a 3-ply cylinder designed to eliminate aneurysm formation and improve longevity. Three years earlier Mentor Corporation had introduced a multicomponent implant similar in design to the AMS 700 but with cylinders constructed of a polyurethane material called Biodex. Since 1986 these two companies have continued to improve their inflatable models. In our series utilizing the Mentor Alpha I and AMS 700 CX, five-year survival (freedom from mechanical revision) is now better than 90%.[6,7]

It is beyond the scope of this chapter to analyze specific causes of mechanical failure with the various models of prostheses. Some generalizations based on two decades of literature can be made. Malleable and semirigid rods have very few mechanical problems but are associated with higher rates of patient dissatisfaction and erosion. Self-contained prostheses have more mechanical problems than three-piece devices. They also have a higher rate of patient dissatisfaction. Similarly, two-piece devices have less patient satisfaction than three-piece prostheses. The classic three-piece prosthesis as designed by Dr. Brantley Scott and marketed by AMS and Mentor has better mechanical reliability, greater patient satisfaction, and no statistical difference in infection rates when compared with malleable, semirigid, self-contained inflatable and two-piece devices.[8]

Revisions for Mechanical Breakage

If a prosthesis fails, repair or replacement will be necessary. If the device is either a self-contained or two-piece prosthesis, the entire prosthesis must be removed since there are no connectors. If revision is required for an AMS 700 or Mentor Alpha I, it is possible to remove and replace only the defective component. Often it is difficult to diagnose the actual point of leakage. If there is any doubt, the entire prosthesis should be replaced. Nothing is as disappointing to the patient as for one to "guess" it is fixed and then to have the prosthesis go down again. Revision of the AMS 700 and the Mentor Alpha is approached differently.

AMS 700 Revisions

The three most common problems with the AMS 700 prosthesis revolve around silicone wear. The old suture tie connectors caused silicone tubing shear at the connection site. The new Quick Connect connectors have eliminated this common problem. The majority of mechanical problems with newer AMS 700's is now related to silicone wear of cylinders or reservoir. Since the entire prosthesis is constructed of silicone, our present policy is to replace all components during an AMS 700 revision. Silicone surfaces of the cylinders and reservoir continue to wear and single component replacement risks the possibility of another revision all too soon. During revisions involving cylinders, it is necessary to remove the fabric "boots" which cover the input tubing where it inserts into the corpora. This can be difficult due to tissue ingrowth into the polytetrafluoroethylene material. Additionally, it is necessary to remove all rear tip extenders. These can be extracted by distending the proximal corpora with irrigating fluid and then probing a Yankoff suction tip (with suction on) deep into the corpora.

Revisions of the AMS 700 prosthesis which are necessary after 2–3 yr should involve total replacement of the components.[9] If single component replacement is to be done for early failure, the use of "Quick Connect" connectors is favored since the Quick Connect connectors are remarkably free from revision. American Medical Systems product literature counsels using the suture tie connectors for any revision involving component replacement. This recommendation should be ignored since the experience with suture tie connectors has been discouraging.

Mentor Alpha I Revisions

Mentor Corporation began manufacturing a three-piece inflatable prosthesis in 1983. The design was similar to the original Scott concept featuring paired cylinders, a scrotal pump, and an abdominal reservoir. The pump and tubing were silicone but, unlike the AMS 700, the cylinders and reservoir were constructed of Bioflex, a polyurethane polymer. Initially the Mentor IPP was plagued by mechanical failure due to silicone tubing shear at the connector junction. In 1990 the current model, Mentor Alpha I, was introduced featuring only one connector of a new design. These Tru-lock connectors were a vast improvement and problems of tubing wear at the connector have been virtually eliminated. The Bioflex material has also proven to have remarkable longevity. In large series reported in the literature, cylinder and reservoir fatigue occurred very rarely.[6]

In our series of over 1,000 Mentor Alpha I implants we note an infrequent, but recurrent, cause for revision. A fracture of the silicone tubing may occur where the tubing exists the pump. It occurs more often on the outside cylinder tubing but may also be evident on the inside cylinder tubing and very rarely the reservoir tubing.

Because the Mentor Alpha I cylinders are preconnected, separate models meant for penoscrotal and infrapubic implantation are marketed. The only difference in the models is tubing length. Tubing fracture at the pump happens more often with the penoscrotal model with its shorter tubing than with the infrapubic model.[10] The present policy on revision of the Mentor Alpha I recognizes the remarkable durability of the Bioflex cylinders and reservoir. The problem necessitating revision is invariably silicone tubing fracture. Unlike the AMS 700, we feel no obligation to replace all components.

To revise the Mentor prosthesis, a small scrotal incision is made and then the pump is cut down upon with the electrosurgical unit set on pure #1 cutting current. All three tubings are traced out and the pump is removed distal to the tubing fracture. The cylinders and reservoir are aspirated free of residual fluid. The system is purged with antibiotic irrigant. The reservoir is filled with the proper amount of saline and a new pump is installed with three new connectors. It is a good idea to drain this revision for 12–24 hr with a closed drainage system since the capsule that formed around the implant is frequently quite vascular. This revision is quick and easy on both patient and surgeon. It does not risk the chance of a repeat revision due to the demonstrated durability of Bioflex and the Tru-lock connectors.

Revision Operation Caveats

The patient should be made aware that revision operation increases the risk of implant infection to 8% and multiple revisions carry a risk of 12%. Revision in a diabetic patient has a rate of infection of 18%.[2] Revision operations should be done through the original incision since it is difficult to access the reservoir through a different exposure. The electrosurgical unit with the current on the pure #1 cutting setting is used to expose the components. Silicone (all components of the AMS 700 and the pump and tubing of the Mentor Alpha) is unaffected by the electosurgical unit and exposure with the cautery is very quick. It is possible to injure Bioflex with the cautery but it requires a forceful application of a high current. Taking a small amount of care when exposing Mentor cylinders allows the use of this time-saving tool during the revision of Mentor prostheses. A word of warning: it is surprisingly easy to get disoriented during revision surgery since the anatomy is no longer pristine. If a penoscrotal incision is used, a Foley catheter is placed to identify the urethra. If the exposure is infrapubic, one must be aware of the dorsal nerves' location. Fear of inadvertent dorsal nerve injury during revisions is the reason many experienced implanters prefer the penoscrotal approach. It is virtually impossible to injure the dorsal nerves through this exposure.

PATIENT DISSATISFACTION

There are few things in medicine more disturbing to the physician than a patient who is unhappy despite a good surgical result. This distressing occurrence is usually the result of a combination of unrealistic patient expectations and failure to communicate on the surgeon's part. It is extremely important to spend time with the patient (and possibly his partner) discussing what may be expected postoperatively. It is also imperative that other, more conservative, therapeutic options for treatment of impotence be thoroughly reviewed and documented before proceeding with implantation. It is a good idea for most prospective implant patients to receive an injection of PGE_1 in the office prior to making the informed consent to receive the implant. Since there are only three therapies for impotence commonly available (vacuum device, injection erection, and implant), an increasing number of authorities feel more time should be spent on instruction and promotion of realistic expectations than elaborate diagnostic algorithms.[11]

Full Disclosure

The patient should be warned that the erection achieved with an implanted penile prosthesis will not be quite as long as his natural erection. The prosthetic erection does not cause lengthening of the penis, as occurs with physiologic penile tumescence. In addition, there is no engorgement of the glans penis as occurs naturally. Should the patient have concerns with regard to penile size during consultation, the use of semirigid rods, self-contained or two-piece devices should be discouraged. Superior erection and flaccidity is achieved with three-piece devices and the discerning patient will question the wisdom of the implantation of a compromised model.

It seems elementary to stress that erection has nothing to do with libido or orgasm, but the implanting physician will save himself heartache if this point is emphasized preoperatively. Many patients will initially have difficulty achieving orgasms when using their prosthesis. They should be counseled that it may take up to 1 yr before they will be able to relax enough to reach a climax with the prosthesis in place. Prolonging foreplay to achieve greater intimacy will help hasten the return.

A fully informed patient is a satisfied customer. We make it a point to cover the following checklist preoperatively:

1. Impotence can also be treated by vacuum device or "injection erection."
2. The penis is not going to be as long as a natural erection.
3. The cylinders will autoinflate for the first 3 months (see below).
4. The implant may break or infection may occur requiring revision or removal.
5. It may take up to a year to achieve orgasm.

Autoinflation

The preoperative consultation with the patient should include a discussion of the fact that *all* three-piece inflatable devices will automatically inflate in the immediate postoperative period. This peculiar phenomenon is caused by abdominal pressure on the reservoir forcing fluid past the pump into the cylinders. This results in a spontaneous partial erection. The manufacturers have attempted to use lock-out devices to prevent the problem, but the resultant device was too difficult to use.[12] For the first 3 months, autoinflation will necessitate the patient's letting some fluid out of the cylinders several times a day in order to encourage maximum capacity of the capsule which will form around the reservoir. The patient will accept autoinflation in the first 3 months if he is warned in advance that it will occur. If this warning is omitted, he may be distressed and forever believe something is wrong. If the patient maximizes deflation for 3 months, the reservoir capsule capacity will usually be adequate and autoinflation is subsequently unusual.

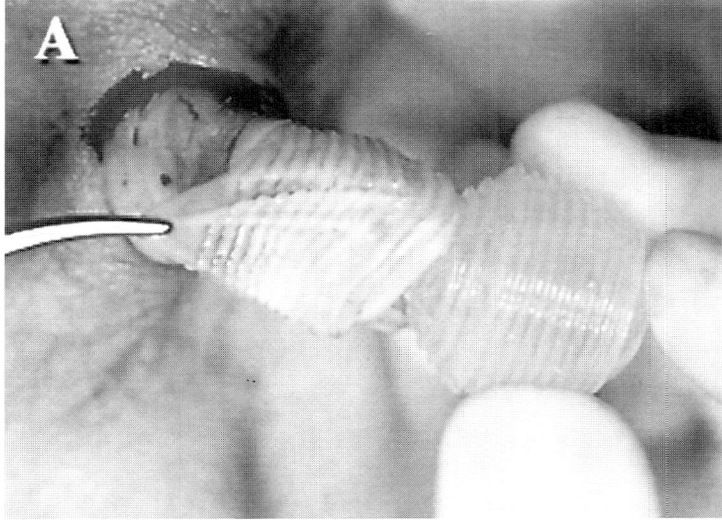

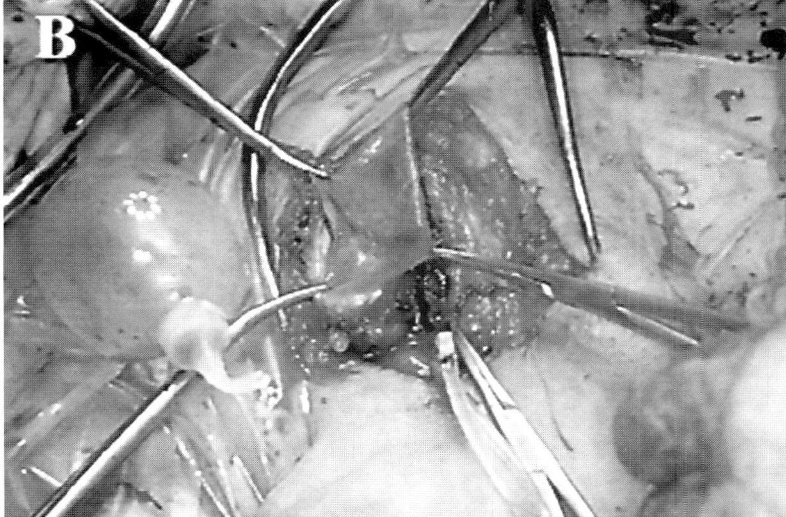

Fig. 14.4. A: Capsule around Mentor pump. B: Capsule from AMS reservoir.

Cases of autoinflation that persist after 6 months may require surgical attention. All implanted materials stimulate fibrous capsule formation in the human body (Fig. 14.4). Excessive periprosthetic capsule formation may form around the reservoir and simply prohibit full deflation. The plastic surgery literature calls this *capsular contraction*. The spherical, smooth silicone reservoir used in AMS prostheses seems more likely to cause the excessive periprosthetic capsule than the cylindrical, textured Bioflex reservoir of Mentor devices.[13] Formal resection of the tight capsule can be a formidable surgical exercise. Fortunately, it is rarely necessary as there is a very simple surgical correction.

Surgical Correction of Autoinflation

The repair is simple; it is not necessary to resect the excessive capsule. A small scrotal incision is made and dissection continued with the cautery. The reservoir tubing (notable because of its black striping) is isolated and severed. With a hand placed suprapubically, the reservoir is overdistended with up to twice its rated capacity. A palpable bursting of the capsule is felt with both Mentor and AMS reservoir. Frequently the surgeon will hear a "pop" with AMS devices. After palpably rupturing the capsule, normal reservoir capacity is reestablished and the system is reconnected. It is tempting to decrease the amount of fluid in the system but this may contribute to crease fold failure in the silicone of the AMS reservoir. There is no reason the fluid capacity of the Mentor device cannot be decreased. The patient must religiously maximize deflation for 3 months after revision in order to encourage maximum capsule capacity. This repair has been successful in over 50 cases with only one complication (bladder laceration in a post radical prostatectomy patient). Recurrence of the autoinflation after the revision has not been detected.

POSTOPERATIVE COMPLICATIONS

Glans Bowing–SST Deformity

Hypermobility of the glans over the end of the prosthesis is a rare complication. It may be seen when the implant is improperly sized (too short) due to inadequate distal dilatation. Other cases result from unrecognized proximal corporal perforation allowing migration of the cylinder. This is more common with rods and self-contained prostheses. Finally SST deformity may result in cases of correct implantation for unknown reasons (Fig. 14.5A). Sometimes, after a routine implantation, the glans appears to be too mobile. Despite encouragement in the literature to perform immediate glans fixation, the subsequent capsule formation around the cylinder often corrects the problem.[14] If the glans still appears floppy after healing, it can be corrected easily.

Undersized cylinders should be corrected by redilatation and the addition of rear tip extenders. If the problem is proximal migration of a rod or self-contained prosthesis, the prosthesis should be replaced with an inflatable one and the cylinder tethered to the corpora with nonabsorbable suture. If dilatation and sizing were correct, glans fixation may be accomplished.[15] A hemi-circumcising incision is made proximal to the glans and dissection is carried down to tunica albuginea. The tunica is not opened but used as a guide for dissection deep beneath the glans on each side. The dissection is kept lateral to the dorsal neurovascular bundle. Two nonabsorbable sutures are placed deep into glans tissue on each side. The deflated prosthesis cylinder tip is displaced proximally with a milking motion in order to secure these sutures to distal tunica without injuring the prosthesis. Tying the sutures should correct the floppy glans. Figure 14.5 illustrates the surgical technique.

Penile Prosthesis Infections

Development of infection following implantation of penile prosthesis is a feared complication. The removal of an infected prosthesis is followed by significant penile

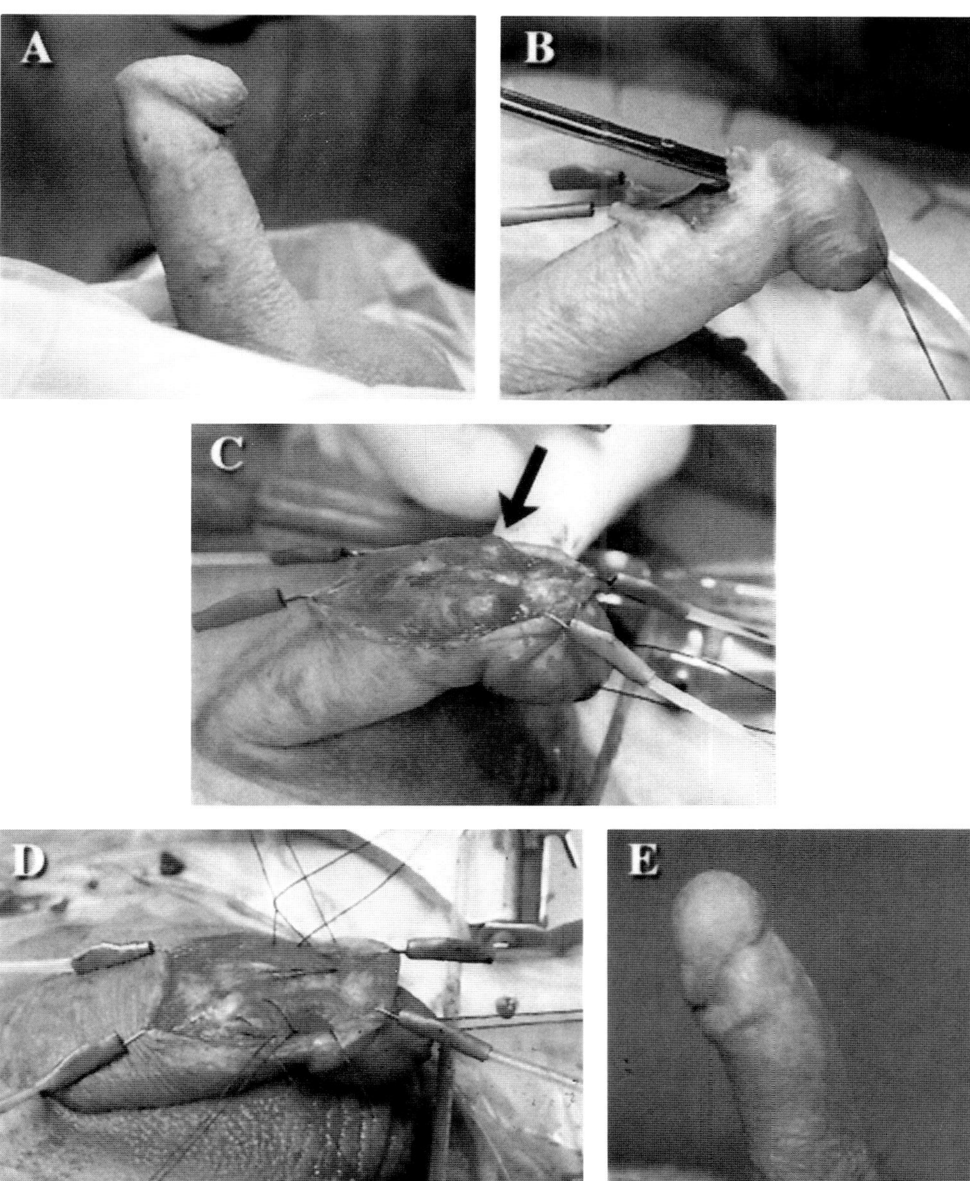

Fig. 14.5. A: SST preoperatively. **B:** Dissection underneath glans. **C:** Dissection complete; note tips of cylinders (*arrow*). **D:** Nonabsorbable sutures in place. **E:** SST corrected.

shortening secondary to corporal fibrosis. Reimplantation is extremely difficult. Since the development of corporal fibrosis always follows removal of an infected prosthesis, experienced implanters have long experimented with salvage/rescue procedures to avoid this dreaded complication.

Fortunately, infection occurs infrequently. Predisposing factors for infection were significant for spinal cord injury (9% of the cases) and steroid use (50%). Diabetes had a statistically insignificant 3% risk of infection. Revision operations carry a 10% risk ranging from 8% in nondiabetics to 18% in diabetics. Patients with no identifiable risk factors had a 1% incidence of infection. Staphylococcal species are the most commonly cultured organisms (65%) followed by Group B *Streptococcus* and *Escherichia coli*. The predominant staphylococci were low-toxicity skin organisms such as *Staphylococcus epidermidis* and *Staphylococcus saprophytica*. Most infections are indolent, presenting with mild symptoms, frequently 3–6 months after implantation. Occasionally, these infections present years after the implantation. The hallmark of these opportunistic staphylococcal infections was persistent pain without visible signs of infection or significant toxicity. Other frequent symptoms were skin attachment to an underlying component, tiny sinus tracts, and mild swelling of the penis (Fig. 14.6A–C). These symptoms persisted for weeks until finally drainage or component erosion prompted the diagnosis of infection. Fever, leukocytosis, positive blood cultures, or toxicity occurred late, if at all.[2]

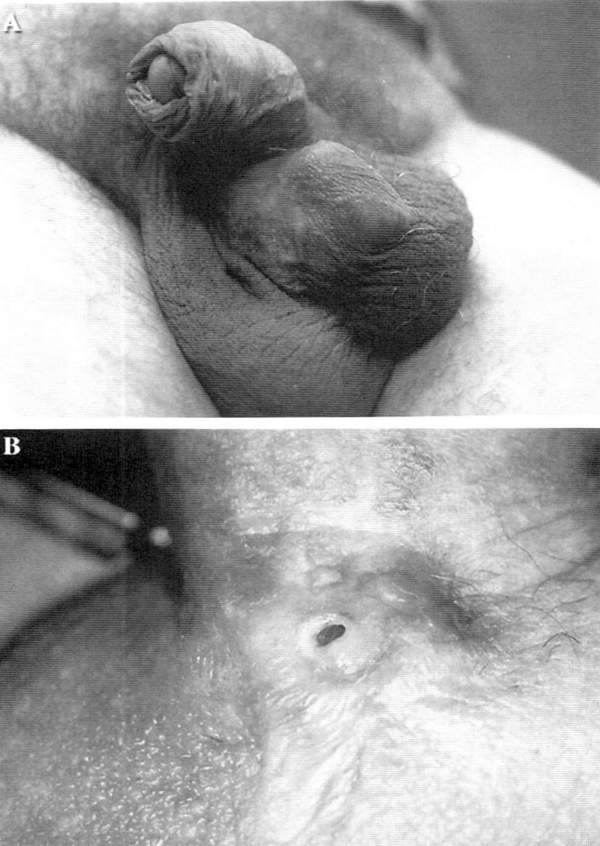

Fig. 14.6. A: Component stuck to skin. **B:** Tiny sinus tract; note lack of scrotal swelling. **C:** Tubing erosion. **D:** Mucopolysaccharide glycomatrix—"slime". **E:** Cylinder erosion at meatus.

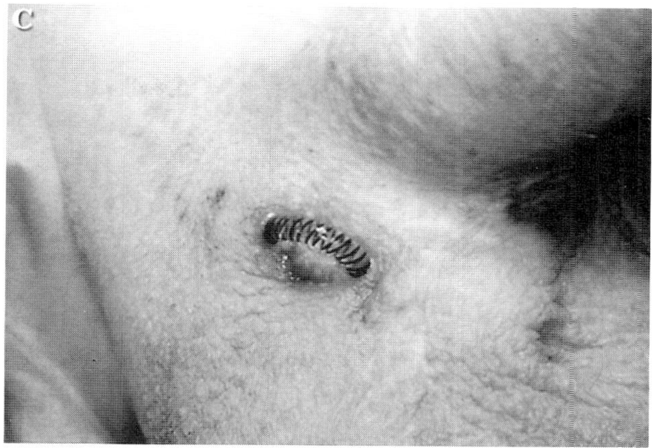

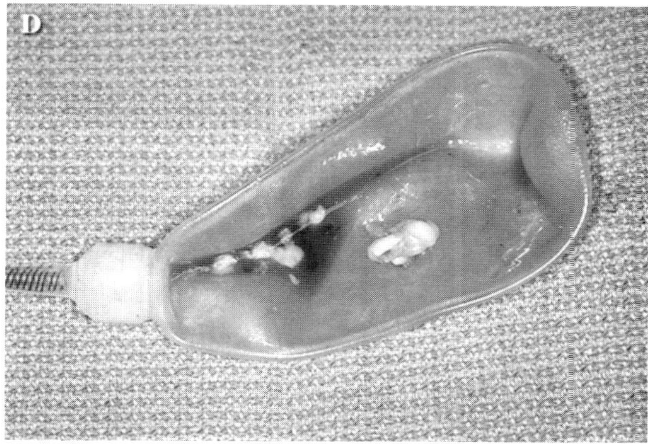

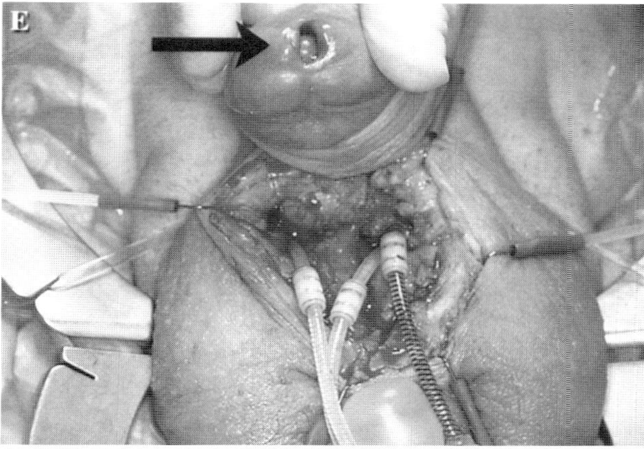

Fig. 14.6. Continued.

Pain that persists greater than 45 days after surgery is presumed to be a subclinical staphylococcus infection. These patients may be treated with intravenous vancomycin for 3 days followed by 1 month of oral trimethoprim-sulfamethoxazole or rifampin. There is no formal study to substantiate the success rate of this empirical therapy but anecdotal evidence is abundant. The theory is that the bacteria have not had sufficient time to secrete the mucopolysaccaride matrix which protects fully mature infections from antibiotic eradication.

Prosthesis Removal for Infection

When prosthesis infection is evident, the wound should be explored and the prosthesis completely removed. The surgeon should not be tempted to remove or to replace only the infected component. Lack of success with piecemeal removal/ substitution is well documented.[2] Infections caused by low-toxicity, opportunistic organisms can be treated by removal, irrigation, drain insertion, and primary wound closure. It is not necessary to pack the wound open or leave drains longer than 24 hr. The patient can usually be discharged the next day and the morbidity of open wound granulation can be avoided.[11] For infections with significant purulence, the wound is still closed primarily, but drainage may be necessary for longer periods.

Salvage Operations

Removal of the prosthesis for infection is followed by corporal fibrosis and penile shortening. Delayed reimplantation is difficult because of the fibrotic and stenotic corpora. Salvage procedures have been proposed to avoid corporal fibrosis by preserving the intracorporal space in the face of infection. The underlying principle of these rescue procedures is complete exchange of the prosthesis and copious irrigation of all tissues surrounding the infected components. The theory is that the bacteria secrete an extracellular mucopolysaccharride matrix which coats the prosthesis and protects the bacteria from antibiotic therapy (Fig. 14.6D). By removing the prosthesis and irrigating out this slime, a new prosthesis can be placed and the infection is eradicated. Several variations of salvage operations have been published.[16] The literature reports 32–90% success.[17]

Salvage operation is not recommended in cases of gross purulence, component erosion through corpora, and in insulin-dependent diabetics[18] (Fig. 14.6E). All salvage operations should be approached with caution. One should thoroughly discuss the expectation and possible lack of success with the patient before embarking on such a course.

We have published our poor results (38%) with older salvage techniques.[2] We have recently been encouraged by much better success using a multiple solution method.[3] This variation irrigates with large quantities of four different solutions in seven applications. The implant is exchanged for a new one and primary closure is used without drainage. While we still remove the majority of our infected implants, this method has been effective in 12 of 14 patients. Both of our failures with this method occurred in early (<15 days postimplant) infections due to Group B streptococcus.

There is a certain ambivalence with regard to salvage. The avoidance of corporal fibrosis and penile shortening is a strong incentive to attempt a salvage operation.

While the prosthesis literature supports these rescue procedures, the practice is not standard surgical textbook doctrine. In addition, the patient will accept the fact that he has had the misfortune of having an infection if the prosthesis is removed immediately. However, he may question the doctor's judgment and wisdom if a salvage attempt is made and is ultimately unsuccessful. Caution is advised. Our caveat remains: When in doubt, take it out!

Scrotal Hematoma

Hematoma of the scrotum seems to occur more often following penoscrotal implantation than via the infrapubic incision. Blood collects around the pump and often dissects up the reservoir tubing into the inguinal canal. Hematomas almost always result from corporal bleeding rather than from scrotal dissection. The exception to this rule is following revision operations. These hematomas occur as a consequence of bleeding from the cut surface of the capsule surrounding the components. This fibrotic tissue growth is accompanied by neovascularity and precise hemostasis is difficult.

Scrotal hematomas can be managed conservatively. Most will be absorbed with little consequence except a delay in teaching the patient how to use his prosthesis. Rarely the hematoma will stimulate a thickened capsule making pump manipulation difficult or adhering the pump to adjacent structures. If drainage is noted, the scrotum must be explored and the hematoma evacuated. In these reoperations, the pump is moved to a new location and walled off from the space of the previous collection of bloodclot using absorbable sutures. The old hematoma site is drained for 24 hr.

The complication of hematoma following prosthesis implantation can be significantly diminished by partially inflating the cylinders for 24 hr and using a small closed drain for the same time period. It is notable that some cases will drain over 100 cc in the first 24 hr despite careful hemostasis and partial inflation. In our series of over 1,000 implants we decreased our hematoma occurrence rate from 3% to 0.7% (P < 0.005) with these maneuvers. There was no significant increase in infection rate using this short drainage period.[19] Both drainage and partial inflation are necessary since each maneuver separately did not result in a significant decrease in the rate of hematoma formation.

Simultaneous Operations with Penile Prosthesis

At the time of penile prosthesis implantation, it is permissible to simultaneously perform circumcision, hernia repair, hydrocele, orchiectomy, epididymectomy, vasectomy, penile straightening, artificial urinary sphincter placement, penile lengthening, penile widening, or transurethral resection of bladder neck. When possible, the use of different incisions is encouraged to isolate the second operation from the implant. The additional operation is usually performed *after* complete closure of the implant incision. An exception to this rule is transurethral incision of bladder neck. Simultaneous transurethral resection of prostate and visual internal urethrotomy have increased complication rates and these procedures are best avoided.[11] If a prosthesis patient needs subsequent scrotal or inguinal surgery, one should attempt to keep the dissection away from the components to avoid possible contamination of the implant by ubiquitous skin organisms.

COMPLICATED PENILE IMPLANTS

Peyronie's Disease

This benign condition is characterized by the formation of fibrotic plaques in the tunica albuginea of the corpora cavernosa. These patients have erectile deformity with the penis bending to the side of the lesion. The lesions may be so extensive that erectile insufficiency may result. The usual complaint is distal flaccidity. Peyronie's disease when associated with impotence has several operative solutions.[20] If the penis is still bent after prosthesis placement, corporoplasty both with and without grafting has been advocated.[21] This additional dissection risks dorsal nerve injury and the addition of graft material may increase the risk of infection. A new and remarkably simple method of treating Peyronie's disease in the impotent patient has been described.[22] It is believed that the original idea for this modeling procedure was conceived by F. Brantley Scott, M.D., the father of the inflatable prosthesis.

The Modeling Procedure

Often simple placement of a pair of semirigid rods or an inflatable prosthesis is enough to straighten the penis. If not, the modeling procedure can be done following three-piece prosthesis implantation. After placement of all components and closure of the corporotomies, the prosthesis is inflated to the maximum. The pump is protected with rubbershod clamps and the penis is forcibly bent in a direction opposite the curvature. The maneuver is similar to breaking a twig over one's knee and the pressure on the penis is held for 90 sec. An audible snapping may be heard and movement of the cylinders is felt. After the pump protection is removed, more fluid can be added to the prosthesis and the modeling procedure can be repeated several times until the desired straightening is achieved. Persistence is the key and several modeling attempts of 90 sec each may be necessary. Satisfactory straightening ($<30°$) with modeling alone can be achieved in 89% of patients. The most difficult curvature to correct is in the patient with a short penis and distal upward curvature. The surgeon should always check corporotomies after vigorous modeling. Sometimes the increased pressure will open these incisions. If the modeling procedure does not result in sufficient straightening, a circumcising incision can be made and corporoplasty performed with the electrosurgical unit (Fig. 14.7).

For optimum results, the AMS 700 CX or Mentor Alpha I cylinders should be used. Both have advantages and disadvantages. The Mentor cylinders have the advantage of their expansion being tunical-dependent and may generate more power to overcome the curvature. A disadvantage of the Mentor cylinders is that the defect following corporoplasty (if necessary) must be covered with graft material. The CX cylinders do not generate as much straightening power and the outer layer of silicone can be damaged (rarely) by the forcible bending. The CX cylinders have the advantage of withstanding direct exposure to the electrocautery with impunity and grafting is not necessary to cover corporal defects. The Ultrex cylinders should not be implanted in Peyronie's disease patients because their lengthening characteristic may exaggerate the Peyronie's curvature.[23]

The real advantage of the modeling procedure is that it is simple and usually effective. The only significant complications have been urethral erosion of the cylinder (4%) and partial splitting of tunica albuginea (2%). Dorsal nerve injury or glan-

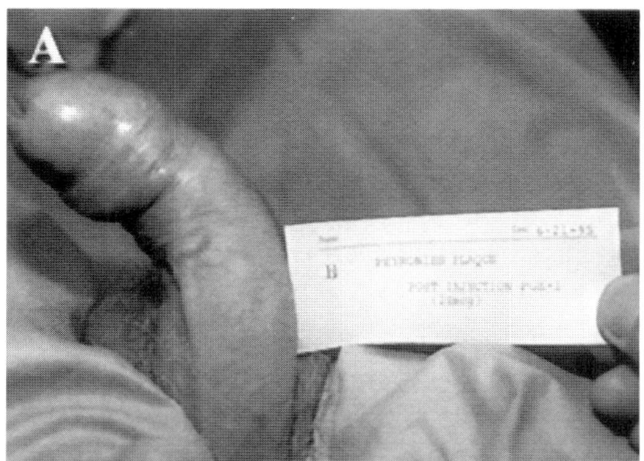
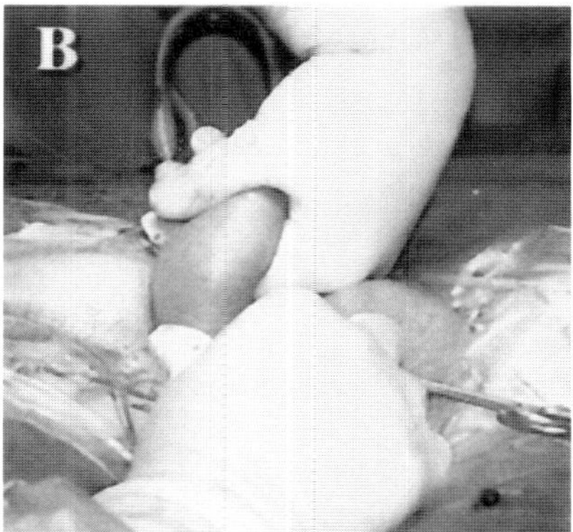
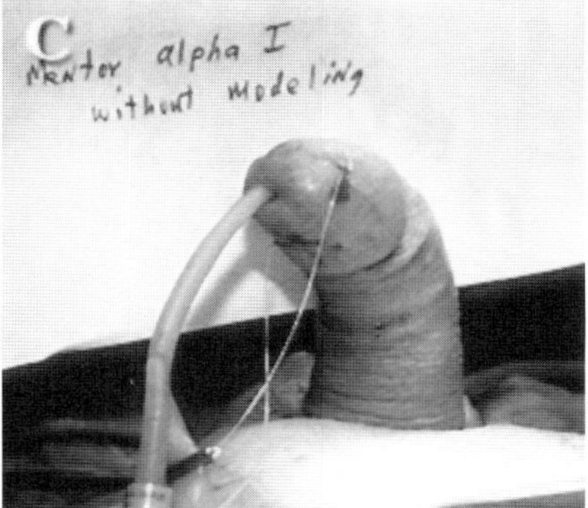

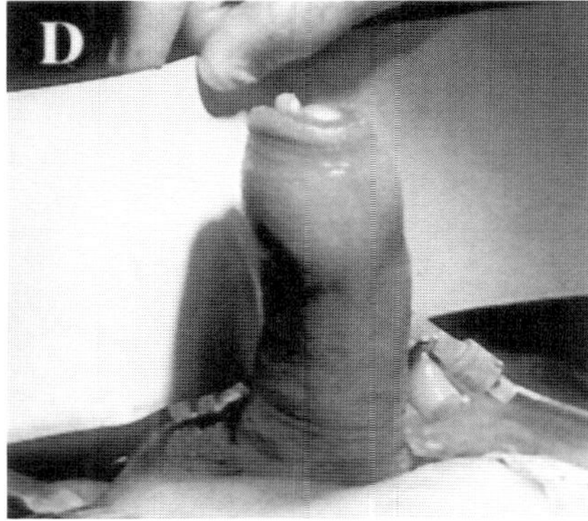

Fig. 14.7. A: Peyronie's disease before correction. **B:** The modeling procedure: hold pressure opposite curvature for 90 sec. **C:** Same patient after one modeling. **D:** Same patient after three modelings.

dular numbness has not been seen. The patient should be advised that his penis will still have curvature with flaccidity. The erection, however, will be fairly straight and usable for intercourse.

CORPORAL FIBROSIS

The implantation of an inflatable three-piece prosthesis in a patient with severe corporal fibrosis represents one of the most difficult cases in prosthetic urology. Fibrosis of the corpora occurs idiopathically, after priapism, with Peyronie's disease or after intracavernosal pharmacotherapy.[24] After removal of infected penile prosthesis corporal fibrosis is particularly severe and usually results in replacement of erectile tissue with scar and significant penile shortening. Reimplantation in these patients has been described as often difficult, if not impossible. Dilatation of the scar tissue sufficient to place a prosthesis is a formidable challenge. The occasional implanter would be wise to refer these "trainwrecks" to a tertiary referral center for prosthetics. A variety of techniques have been offered for dealing with the fibrotic corpora. They have included coring out the corpora with thin-walled brass tubing, making proximal and distal incisions in the corpora, and extensively dissecting the penis.[4]

Implantation in patients with corporal fibrosis has been extensively discussed in the literature. Accepted technique involves choosing an incision location that allows access to the corpora, if possible, through previously unoperated tissue planes. In other words, if the initial implant was placed penoscrotal, the new attempt should be made infrapubically. After the initial corporotomies are made, dilatation should be attempted with Metzenbaum scissors, Hegar & Brooks dilators, or the Dilamez insertion tool. Due to severe fibrosis, extensive corporotomies are usually necessary. This pervasive fibrosis frequently necessitates excising the fibrotic corporal tissue sharply to create sufficient space for the cylinder. If possible, the tunica albuginea should be closed over the prosthesis. If the corporotomy cannot be closed, a synthetic patch of Gor-Tex (polytetrafluroethylene) should be used to bridge the gaps. This traditional technique usually fails for three reasons. The urethra may be lacerated distally during the difficult dilatation or it may not be possible to dilate the stenotic proximal corpora enough to permit implantation of the prosthesis base. In addition, the synthetic grafting material may result in infection.[4] Recent reports utilizing these techniques showed only a 50% 1-yr implant survival.[26]

Improved implant results in these difficult cases can be achieved by the addition of specialized tools to traditional techniques. A combination of a high transverse scrotal incision, the novel Carrion-Rossello Cavernotomes and down-sized prostheses in conjunction with more traditional methods have improved 1-yr implant survival to over 80%.[27] The transverse scrotal incision gives superior exposure to the proximal corpora.[22] With this incision it is possible to incise the corpora under direct vision to the crus of the corporal body. Proper placement of the Lonestar "Scott" retractor facilitates this exposure (Fig. 14.3A, 14.8A).

The Carrion-Rossello Cavernotomes are novel dilators with cutting "woodrasp" surfaces which permit passage through the scarred corpora (Fig. 14.3B). The Cavernotomes are sized 9–12 mm. After making the initial 2–3 cm vertical corporotomy on the ventral surface of the corpora, it usually is necessary to resect a small amount of fibrotic tissue with a scalpel to create a space for introduction of the cavernotomes. Cruciate incisions with a #15 blade to a depth of 2 cm proximally and distally through the cross-sectional surface of the corpora allow the cavernotome to engage its roughened surface (Fig. 14.8A). The cavernotmes are advanced with an oscillating motion alternately pronating and supinating the wrist, allowing the rasplike surface to advance the dilator through the fibrotic tissue (Fig. 14.8B). The teeth permit the dilator to "walk" through the fibrotic tissue. Withdrawal of the cavernotome with its cutting projections resects a channel (Fig. 14.8C, 14.8D). In effect, a channel is drilled through the fibrosis. Minimal dilatation to 11 mm distally and 10 mm proximally will allow the downsized AMS 700 CXM or the Mentor Alpha 1 NB to be placed. These prostheses have smaller diameter bases (10 mm versus 12–13 mm for standard sized CX and Alpha) which facilitate insertion into the stenotic proximal corpora. Liberal use of rear tip extenders is recommended to avoid running the input tubing alongside the cylinder within the corpora. If the tubing exits the corporotomy directly, it is not necessary to dilate larger than size 11 mm. If the tubing is allowed to run alongside the cylinder, dilatation must be carried as high as 14 mm. The downsized prostheses also have smaller diameter cylinders which obviate the use of grafting material to close corporal defects. The erection

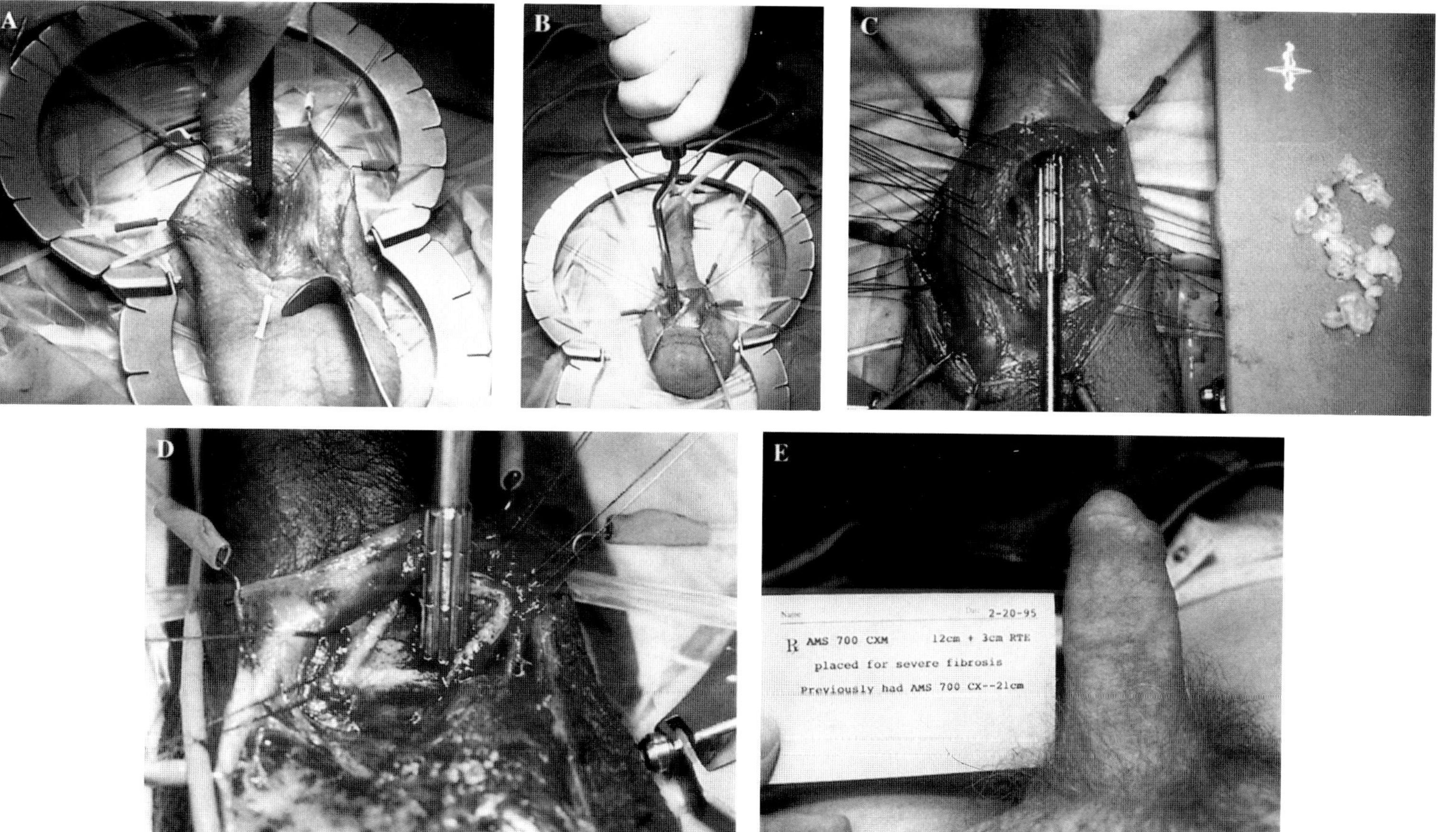

Fig. 14.8. **A:** Use of #15 knife blade to make cruciate incisions in fibrotic corpora. **B:** Oscillating motion to advance engaged cavernotomes. **C:** Cavernotome advanced distally. Note resected fibrosis to engage instrument. **D:** Cavernotome advanced proximally; note "teeth". **E:** Post implant erection; note smaller length prosthesis.

quality with these downsized cylinders is surprisingly good. The Carrion-Rossello Cavernotomes have drilled a channel through the fibrotic corpora and rigidity is aided by the fibrotic rim. The erection with these smaller diameter cylinders seems firmer than that created in patients with standard sized cylinders who have required extensive corporal resection. Figure 14.8E illustrates the erect penis with downsized cylinders. This photograph also documents the penile shortening which accompanies corporal fibrosis.

REFERENCES

1. Wilson SK: Current treatment of impotence with inflatable penile prostheses examined: *AUA Today* Sept 1992.

2. Wilson SK, Delk JR II: Inflatable penile implant infection: predisposing factors and treatment suggestions. *J Urol* 153:659–661, 1994.

3. Brant MD, Ludlow JK, Mulcahy JJ: The prosthesis salvage operation: immediate replacement of the infected penile prosthesis. *J Urol* 155:155–157, 1996.

4. Knoll LD, Furlow WL, Benson RC, et al: Management of nondilatable cavernous fibrosis with the use of a downsized inflatable penile prosthesis. *J Urol* 153:366–368, 1995.

5. Wilson SK, Wahman GE, Lange JL: Eleven years experience with inflatable penile prostheses. *J Urol* 139:951–953, 1988.

6. Randrup E, Wilson S, Mobley D, et al: Clinical experience with Mentor Alpha I inflatable penile prosthesis. *Urology* 42:305–308, 1993.

7. Wilson SK, Cleves M, Delk JR II: Long term results with Hydroflex and Dynaflex penile prostheses: device survival comparison to multi-component inflatables. *J Urol* 155:1621–1623, 1996.

8. Lewis RW: Long-term results of penile prosthetic implants. In Melman A: *Impotence. Urol Clin North Am* 22:847–855, 1995.

9. Parulkar BG, Lamontagne DP, Vickers MA: Detection of leakage in inflatable genitourinary devices. *Urology* 47:97–101, 1996.

10. Williams CB: Out-patient implantation of Mentor Alpha I inflatable penile prosthesis: results of 647 single surgeon cases. *Int J Impot Res* 6:A59, 1995.

11. Baum N, Rhodes D: A practical approach to the evaluation and treatment of erectile dysfunction. In Melman A: *Impotence. Urol Clin North Am* 22:865–877, 1995.

12. Mulcahy JJ: Prevention and correction of penile implant problems. *AUA Update* 13:214–218, 1994.

13. Wilson SK, Delk JR II: Excessive periprosthetic capsule formation of the penile prosthesis reservoir: incidence in various prosthesis and a simple surgical solution. *J Urol* 153:359A, 1995.

14. Stefani SD, Simonato A, M. Caponi et al: The benefit of glans fixation in prosthetic penile surgery. *J Urol* 152:1533–1554, 1994.

15. Ball TP: Surgical repair of penile "SST" deformity. *Urology* 15:603, 1980.

16. Furlow WL, Goldwasser B: Salvage of the eroded inflatable penile prosthesis: a new concept. *J Urol* 138:312–315, 1987.

17. Teloken C, Souto JC, Da Ros C, et al: Prosthetic penile infection: "rescue procedure: with rifamycin. *J Urol* 148:1905–1907, 1992.

18. Fishman JJ, Scott FB, Selim AM: Rescue procedure: an alternative to complete removal for treatment of infected penile prosthesis. *J Urol* 137:202A, 1987.

19. Wilson SK, Delk JR II: Scrotal hematoma prevention following penile prosthesis implantation: to drain or not to drain. *J Urol* 155:634A, 1996.

20. Eigner EB, Kabalin JN, Dessler R: Penile implants in the treatment of Peyronie's disease. *J Urol* 145:69–71, 1991.

21. Montague DK, Lakin MM: Penile prosthesis implantation in men with Peyronie's disease. *J Urol* 151:355A, 1994.

22. Wilson SK, Delk JR II: A new treatment for Peyronie's disease: modeling the penis over an inflatable penile prosthesis. *J Urol* 152:1121–1123, 1994.

23. Wilson SK, Cleves MA, Delk JR II: Ultrex cylinders: problems with uncontrolled lengthening (the S-shaped deformity). *J Urol* 155:135–137, 1996.

24. Montague DK, Lakin MM: Penile prostheses. In Bennet AH: *Impotence* Philadelphia, WB Saunders, 1994, pp 257–295.

25. Knoll LD: Use of penile prosthetic implants in patients with penile fibrosis. In Melman A: *Impotence. Urol Clin North Am* 22:847–863, 1995.

26. Boyd SD, Martins FE: Simultaneous Ultrex penile prosthesis reimplantation and Gore-Tex grafting corporoplasty: functional outcomes of a surgical challenge. *J Urol* 153:359A, 1995.

27. Wilson SK, Delk JR II, Terry T: Improved implant survival in patients with severe corporal fibrosis: a new technique without necessity of grafting. *J Urol* 153:359A, 1995.

INDEX

ISBN 0-89640-322-X

FIFTH EDITION

Optimization Modeling with

LINDO

Linus Schrage

Graduate School of Business
University of Chicago

Duxbury Press
An Imprint of Brooks/Cole Publishing Company
I(T)P® An International Thomson Publishing Company

Pacific Grove • Albany • Belmont • Bonn • Boston • Cincinnati • Detroit • Johannesburg • London
Madrid • Melbourne • Mexico City • New York • Paris • Singapore • Tokyo • Toronto • Washington

Sponsoring Editor: Curt Hinrichs
Assistant Editor: Cynthia Mazow
Marketing Team: Carolyn Crockett, Romy Taormina
Editorial Assistants: Martha O'Connor,
    Rita Jaramillo

Production Editor: Keith Faivre
Interior Design: TBH/Typecast, Inc.
Cover Design: Kelly Shoemaker
Typesetting: TBH/Typecast, Inc.
Printing and Binding: Courier Westford, Inc.

*For more information, contact Duxbury Press at
Brooks/Cole Publishing Company:*

BROOKS/COLE PUBLISHING COMPANY
511 Forest Lodge Road
Pacific Grove, CA 93950
USA

International Thomson Publishing Europe
Berkshire House 168–173
High Holborn
London WC1V 7AA
England

Thomas Nelson Australia
102 Dodds Street
South Melbourne, 3205
Victoria, Australia

Nelson Canada
1120 Birchmount Road
Scarborough, Ontario
Canada M1K 5G4

International Thomson Editores
Seneca 53
Col. Polanco
11560 México, D.F., México

International Thomson Publishing GmbH
Königswinterer Strasse 418
53227 Bonn
Germany

International Thomson Publishing Asia
221 Henderson Road
#05–10 Henderson Building
Singapore 0315

International Thomson Publishing Japan
Hirakawacho Kyowa Building, 3F
2-2-1 Hirakawacho
Chiyoda-ku, Tokyo 102
Japan

Printed in the United States of America.
10 9 8 7 6 5 4 3 2 1

Library of Congress Cataloging-in-Publication Data

Schrage, Linus E.
    Optimization modeling with LINDO / Linus Schrage. — 5th ed.
        p.   cm.
    Rev. ed. of: LINDO. 4th ed.
    Includes bibliographical references and index.
    ISBN 0-534-34857-2 (alk. paper)
    1. Industrial management—Mathematical models—Case studies.
    2. Industrial management—Linear programming—Case studies.
    3. Business mathematics—Linear programming—Case studies.
    4. Industrial management—Linear programming—Computer programs.
    5. Schrage, Linus E.   LINDO.   I. Schrage, Linus E.   LINDO.
    II. Title.
HD30.25.S36   1997
658.4'033—dc21   96-49946
                                                                 CIP

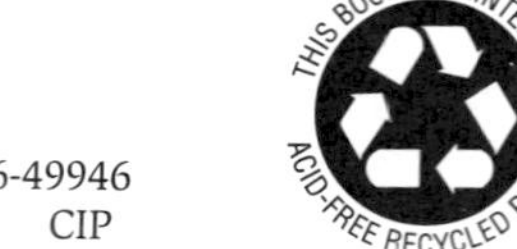

Contents

Preface

The respected mathematician Paul Halmos, in a discussion of how to do technical writing, gave this advice: "Never write a second edition." He never said anything about fifth editions, so we have naively proceeded with this project.

As with the first edition back in 1981, this book is about applying the power of optimization models to problems of business and industry. The intended audience is students of business, managers, and engineers.

Changes to the Fifth Edition

The most obvious change is that the text has been updated to reflect the availability of the Windows version of LINDO. Even more than in previous editions, the emphasis is on how to use the power of optimization models on real problems.

More numerical examples have been added to almost every chapter. All but the smallest examples in the text are included on the distribution disks so that readers need not reenter the examples if they wish to "play around" with the examples.

More problem exercises have been added to the end of every chapter. The examples and exercises are typically based on actual applications of optimization to real industrial problems.

Substantial new material has been added to the chapters on:

Networks and their variations.   Special cases such as the assignment problem are presented, as are generalizations such as multicommodity flow, generalized networks, and activity-resource diagrams.

Goal programming, multicriteria, data envelopment analysis and other methods for measuring efficiency.   A very comprehensive treatment is given, with numerical examples, of methods for measuring efficiency of organizations.

Financial portfolio models and quadratic programming.   A comprehensive sequence of numerical examples illustrates the simple Markowitz portfolio model, the effect of a risk-free investment, the factor model, scenario approach, managing a portfolio in the face of transaction costs, hedging, and matching benchmark portfolios.

Decision making under uncertainty.   Examples illustrate the scenario approach and concepts such as the value of information, the value of modeling uncertainty, utility functions and downside risk, and certainty equivalence.

Integer programming.   More examples are given, there is an emphasis on the great importance of proper formulation when solving integer programs, and tricks for solving difficult problems are presented.

More material has been added related to some of the more recent commands in LINDO, such as the goal programming command GLEX and the DEBUG command. Illustrations are given showing how the DEBUG command can help locate formulation errors when the model is either infeasible or unbounded.

All of the above help make this text one of the most comprehensive expositions available on how to apply optimization/mathematical programming to industrial problems.

Organization and Prerequisites

There are essentially four kinds of chapters in the book:

1. introduction to modeling (chapters 1, 3 and 4)
2. solving models on the computer (chapter 2)
3. application-specific illustrations of the use of LINDO (chapters 5–17)
4. parametric analysis and solution algorithms (chapters 18 and 19)

The major technical prerequisite to understanding and using the book is to be comfortable with the idea of using a symbol to represent an unknown quantity. Most readers should find the first four chapters useful. Instructors should be able to select topics relatively freely from chapters 5 through 17, depending upon the applications they choose to emphasize in their course. Most of the examples in the text were developed and used with MBA students. Except for chapters 18 and 19, all of the chapters should be understandable to MBA students with modest technical ability. Chapters 18 and 19 are of interest to readers who are curious about what is "under the hood" with regard to solving optimization problems. Given the availability on the distribution disks of most of the examples, the best way for most readers to learn the ideas in the book is to immediately sit down at a computer and try them.

Acknowledgments

We are most grateful to Curt Hinrichs, our editor at Duxbury Press, for helping put the fifth edition on the street and into the bookstores. We are more grateful than ever to Paul Kelly of Scientific Press for giving us our first opportunity with the first edition way back in 1981. A variety of people have contributed in a variety of ways to this edition. This edition has benefited from comments by Egon Balas, Kipp Martin, Saul Gass, Zonghao Gu, Tom Knowles, Rick Rosenthal, Paul Schweitzer, Shuichi Shinmura, and Mark Wiley. The outstanding software expertise and sage advice of Kevin Cunningham was crucial. The text has benefited from the text processing skills of Cassandra Baymon and Gloria Aclaro. The expert, yet patient, editorial skills of Keith Faivre and the lovely MLE are much appreciated.

Linus Schrage

What Is Linear Programming?

1.1 Introduction

Linear Programming (LP) is a mathematical procedure for determining optimal allocation of scarce resources. LP is a procedure that has found practical application in almost all facets of business, from advertising to production planning. Transportation and aggregate production planning problems are the most typical objects of LP analysis. The petroleum industry seems to be the most intensive user of LP. A data processing manager at a large oil company recently estimated that from 5% to 10% of the firm's computer time was devoted to the processing of LP and LP-like models.

It is important for the reader to appreciate at the outset that the "programming" in Linear Programming is of a different flavor than the "programming" in Computer Programming. In the former case it means to plan and organize (as in "Get with the program!"), whereas in the latter case it means to write instructions for performing calculations. Training in the one kind of programming has very little direct relevance to the other.

For most LP problems, one can think of there being *two important classes of objects:* first, limited *resources* such as land, plant capacity, and sales force size, and second, *activities* such as "produce low carbon steel," "produce stainless steel," and "produce high carbon steel." *Each activity consumes* or possibly *contributes* additional amounts of the *resources.* The problem is to determine the best combination of activity levels that does not use more resources than are actually available. We can best gain the flavor of LP by using a simple example.

1.2 A Simple Product Mix Problem

The Enginola Television Company produces two types of TV sets, the "Astro" and the "Cosmo." There are two production lines, one for each set. The capacity of the Astro production line is 60 sets per day, whereas the capacity of the Cosmo line is 50 sets per day. The Astro set requires 1 work-hour of labor, whereas the Cosmo set requires 2 work-hours. At most, 120 work-hours of labor per day are available to be assigned to production of the two types of sets. If the profit contributions are \$20 and \$30, respectively, for each Astro and Cosmo set, what should be the daily production?

A structured but still verbal description of what we want to do is:

Maximize   Profit contribution

subject to   Astro production less than or equal to Astro capacity,
             Cosmo production less than or equal to Cosmo capacity,
             Labor used less than or equal to labor availability.

Until there is a significant improvement in artificial intelligence/expert system software, we will need to be more precise if we wish to get some help in solving our problem. We can be more precise if we define:

A = units of Astros to be produced per day,
C = units of Cosmos to be produced per day.

Further, we decide to measure:

Profit contribution in dollars,
Astro usage in units of Astros produced,
Cosmo usage in units of Cosmos produced, and
Labor in hours.

Then a precise statement of our verbal description above is:

Maximize $20A + 30C$ (Dollars)

subject to $A \quad\quad\ \ \leq 60$ (Astro capacity)
             $C \leq 50$ (Cosmo capacity)
             $A + 2C \leq 120$ (Labor in hours)

The basic idea of a constraint is illustrated by the labor hours constraint. The left-hand side, given values for A and C, is a formula for computing the amount of labor used. The right-hand side is the amount of labor available. Given sufficient imagination, you can always interpret a constraint as saying: "amount used of a certain commodity is less than (or equal to) amount available of that commodity."

The first line ("Maximize $20A + 30C$") is known as the *objective function*, whereas the remaining three lines are known as *constraints*. Most LP computer programs assume that all variables are constrained to be nonnegative, so stating the constraints $A \geq 0$, $C \geq 0$ is unnecessary.

Using the terminology of resources and activities, there are three resources: Astro capacity, Cosmo capacity, and labor capacity. The activities are Astro and Cosmo production. It is generally true that with each constraint in an LP one can associate some resource, whereas for each decision variable there is a corresponding activity.

1.2.1 Graphical Analysis

The Enginola problem is represented graphically in Figure 1.1. A set of values for our decision variables, A and C in this case, is said to be *feasible* if the values satisfy all the constraints. The feasible production combinations are the points in the lower left

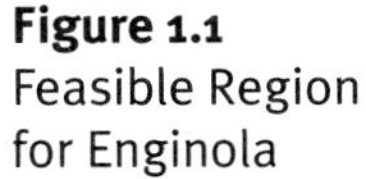
Figure 1.1
Feasible Region
for Enginola

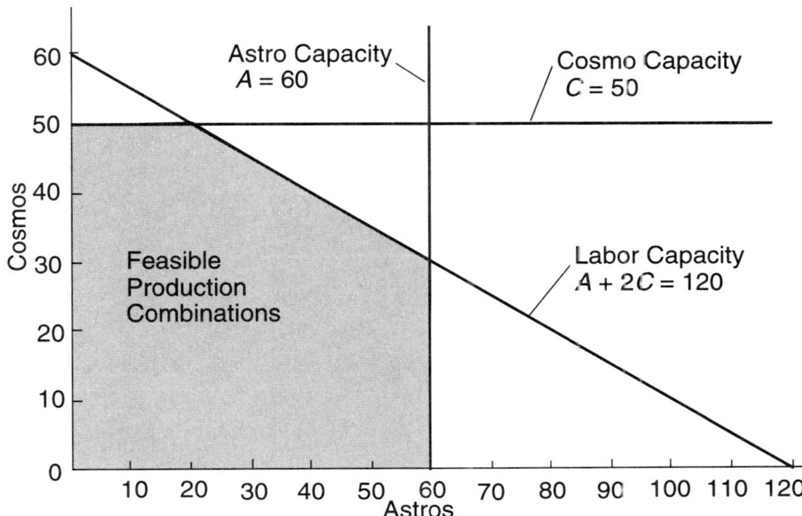

enclosed by the five solid lines. We want to find the point in the feasible region that gives the highest profit.

To gain some idea of where the maximum profit point lies, let's consider some possibilities. Producing no Astros and no Cosmos corresponds to $A = C = 0$. This point in the lower left corner is feasible but it does not help much with respect to profits. If we spoke with the manager of the Cosmo line, the response might be: "The Cosmo is our more profitable product; therefore, we should make as many of it as possible, namely 50, and be satisfied with the profit contribution of $30 \times 50 = \$1500$."

You, the thoughtful reader, might observe that there are many combinations of A and C, other than just $A = 0$ and $C = 50$, that achieve $\$1500$ of profit. Indeed, if you plot the line $20A + 30C = 1500$ and add it to the graph, you get Figure 1.2. Any point on the dotted line segment achieves a profit of $\$1500$.

If we next talk with the manager of the Astro line, the response might be: "If you produce 50 Cosmos, you still have enough labor to produce 20 Astros. This corresponds to $A = 20$ and $C = 50$ and would give a profit of $30 \times 50 + 20 \times 20 = \$1900$. That is certainly a respectable profit; why don't we call it a day and go home?"

Our ever alert reader might again observe that there are many ways of making $\$1900$ of profit. If you plot the line $20A + 30C = 1900$ and add it to the graph, you get Figure 1.3. Any feasible point on the higher rightmost dotted line segment achieves a profit of $\$1900$.

Now our ever perceptive reader makes a leap of insight: As we increase our profit aspirations, the dotted line representing all points that achieve a given profit simply shifts in a parallel fashion. Why not shift it as far as possible as long as the

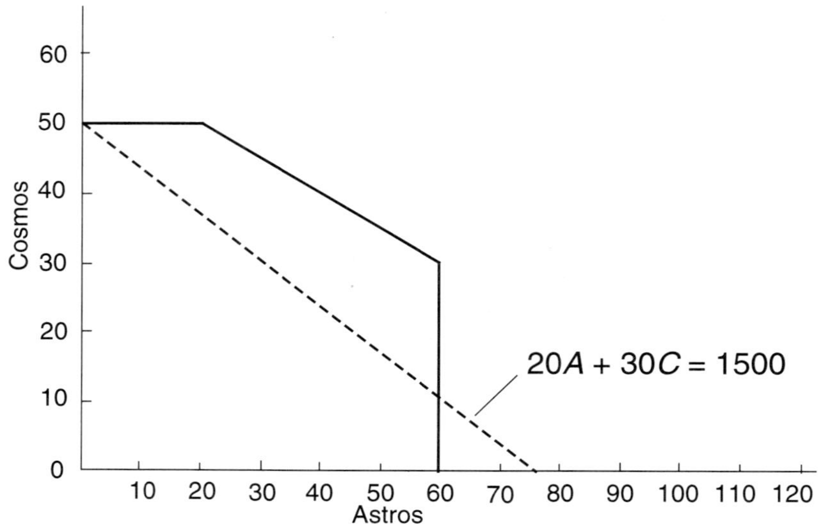

Figure 1.2
Enginola with
"Profit = 1500"

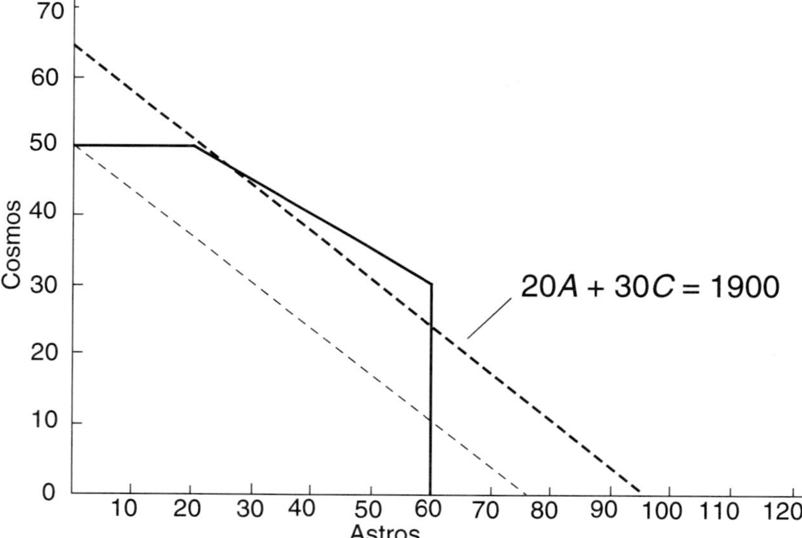

Figure 1.3
Enginola with
"Profit = 1900"

line contains a feasible point? This last and best feasible point is $A = 60$, $C = 30$. It lies on the line $20A + 30C = 2100$. This is illustrated in Figure 1.4. Notice that even though the profit contribution per unit is higher for Cosmo, we did not make as many (30) as we feasibly could have made (50). Intuitively, this is an optimal solution, and in fact it is. This graphical analysis of this small problem will help us understand what is going on when we analyze larger problems.

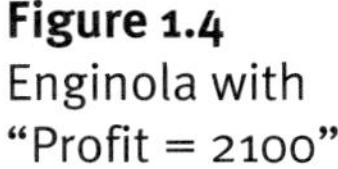

Figure 1.4
Enginola with
"Profit = 2100"

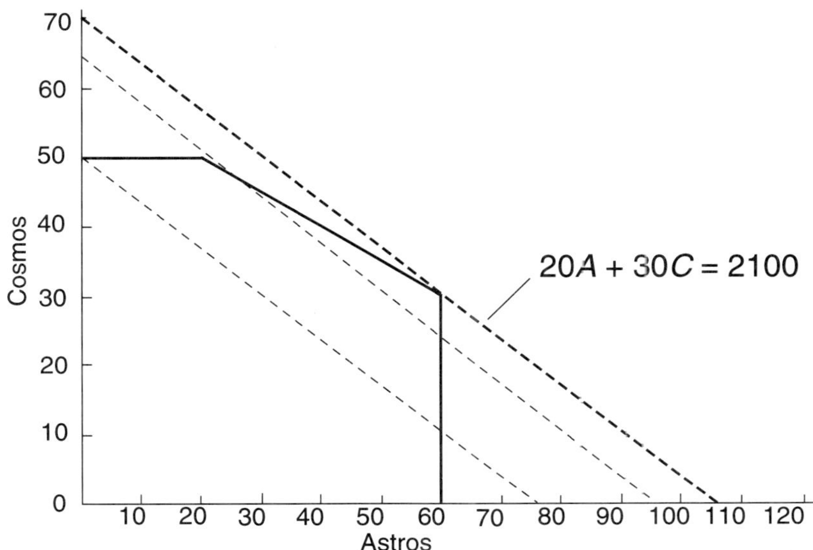

1.3 Linearity

We have now seen one example. We will return to it regularly. The possible formulations to which LP is applicable are substantially more general than that suggested by the example. The objective function may be minimized rather than maximized; the direction of the constraints may be $\geq$ rather than $\leq$, or even $=$; any or all of the parameters, e.g., the 20, 30, 60, 50, 120, 2, 1, etc., may be negative instead of positive. The principal restriction on the class of problems that can be analyzed results from the linearity restriction.

Linear programming applies *directly* only to situations in which the effects of the different activities in which we can engage are linear. For practical purposes we can think of the linearity requirement as consisting of three features:

1. *Proportionality.* The effects of a single variable or activity by itself are proportional; e.g., doubling the amount of steel purchased will double the dollar cost of steel purchased.
2. *Additivity.* The interactions among variables must be additive; e.g., the dollar amount of sales is the sum of the steel dollar sales, the aluminum dollar sales, etc., whereas the amount of electricity used is the sum of that used to produce steel, aluminum, etc.
3. *Continuity.* The variables must be continuous; i.e., fractional values for the decision variables, such as 6.38, must be allowed.

A model that included the two decision variables "price per unit sold" and "quantity of units sold" is probably not linear. The proportionality requirement is

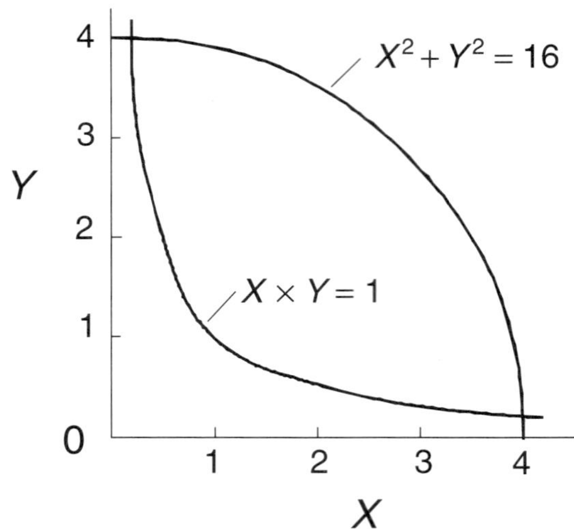

Figure 1.5
Nonlinear
Relations

satisfied; however, the interaction between the two decision variables is multiplicative rather than additive; i.e., dollar sales = price × quantity, not price + quantity.

If a supplier gives you quantity discounts on your purchases, then the cost of purchases will not satisfy the proportionality requirement; e.g., the total cost of the stainless steel purchased may be less than proportional to the amount purchased.

A model that includes the decision variable "number of floors to build" might satisfy the proportionality and additivity requirements but violate the continuity conditions. The recommendation to build 6.38 floors might be difficult to implement unless one had a designer who was ingenious with split-level designs; nevertheless, the solution of an LP might recommend such fractional answers.

Fortunately, as we will see later in the chapters on integer programming and quadratic programming, there are other ways of accommodating these violations of linearity.

Figure 1.5 illustrates some nonlinear functions. For example, the expression $X \times Y$ satisfies the proportionality requirement but the effects of X and Y are not additive. In the expression $X^2 + Y^2$, the effects of X and Y are additive, but the effects of each individual variable are not proportional.

1.4 Analysis of LP Solutions

When you direct the computer to solve an LP, the possible outcomes are indicated in Figure 1.6. For a properly formulated LP, the leftmost path will be taken. The solution procedure will first attempt to find a feasible solution, i.e., a solution that simultaneously satisfies all constraints but does not necessarily maximize the objec-

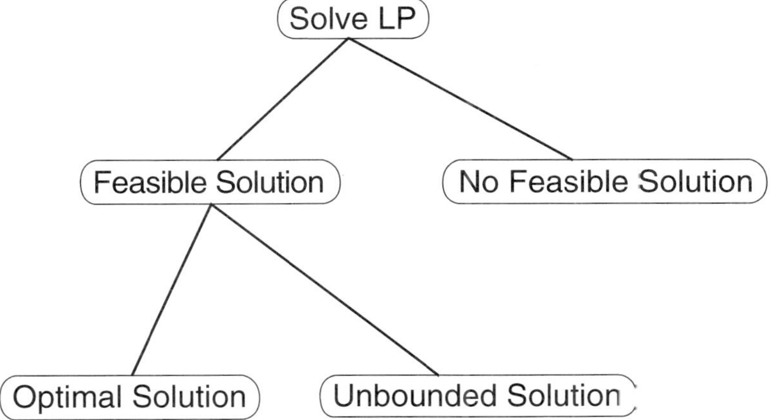

Figure 1.6
Solution
Outcomes

tive function. The rightmost, "No Feasible Solution," path will be taken if the formulator has been too demanding; that is, two or more constraints are specified that cannot be simultaneously satisfied. A simple example is the pair of constraints $x \leq 2$ and $x \geq 3$. The nonexistence of a feasible solution does not depend upon the objective function. It depends solely upon the constraints. In practice, the "No Feasible Solution" outcome might occur in a large complicated problem in which an upper limit was specified on the number of productive hours available and an unrealistically high demand was placed on the number of units to be produced. An alternative message to "No Feasible Solution" is "You Can't Have Your Cake and Eat It Too." If a feasible solution has been found, the procedure attempts to find an optimal solution. If the "Unbounded Solution" termination occurs, it implies that the formulation admits the unrealistic result that an infinite amount of profit can be made. A more realistic conclusion is that an important constraint has been omitted or the formulation contains a critical typographical error.

When the Enginola problem is solved with the LINDO computer program, the following solution report is produced:

```
OBJECTIVE FUNCTION VALUE

  1)         2100.000

  VARIABLE        VALUE           REDUCED COST
     A          60.000000            0.000000
     C          30.000000            0.000000

  ROW             SLACK           DUAL PRICES
    2)            0.000000            5.000000
    3)           20.000000            0.000000
    4)            0.000000           15.000000

  NO. ITERATIONS =    3
```

The output has two sections, a "variables" section and a "rows" section. The first two columns in each section are straightforward. The maximum profit solution is to produce 60 Astros and 30 Cosmos for a profit contribution of 2100. The *slack* in a row is defined as the amount by which the amount used of a commodity (e.g., Astro line capacity, Cosmo line capacity, or labor) falls short of the amount available of that commodity. The report shows that there is zero slack in row 2 (the constraint $A \leq 60$), a slack of 20 in row 3 (the constraint $C \leq 50$), and no slack in row 4 (the constraint $A + 2C \leq 120$). Note that $60 + 2 \times 30 = 120$.

Useful by-products of the computations are a number of opportunity or marginal cost figures that appear in the third column. The interpretation of these "reduced costs" and "dual prices" is discussed in the next section.

1.5 Sensitivity Analysis, Reduced Costs, and Dual Prices

Realistic LPs require large amounts of data. Accurate data are expensive to collect and so we will generally be forced to use data in which we have less than complete confidence. A time-honored adage in data processing circles is "garbage in, garbage out." A user of a model should be concerned with how the recommendations of the model are altered by changes in the input data. *Sensitivity analysis* is the term applied to the process of answering this question. Fortunately, an LP solution report provides supplemental information that is useful in sensitivity analysis. This information falls under two headings, reduced costs and dual prices.

Sensitivity analysis can reveal which pieces of information should be estimated most carefully. For example, if it is blatantly obvious that a certain product is unprofitable, little effort need be expended in accurately estimating its costs. The first law of modeling is: do not waste time accurately estimating a parameter if a modest error in the parameter has little effect on the recommended decision.

1.5.1 Reduced Costs

Associated with each variable in any solution is a quantity known as the *reduced cost*. If the units of the objective function are dollars and the units of the variable are gallons, the units of the reduced cost are dollars per gallon. The reduced cost of a variable is the amount by which the profit contribution of the variable must be improved before the variable in question would have a positive value in an optimal solution. Obviously, a variable that already appears in the optimal solution will have a zero reduced cost.

It follows that a second, correct interpretation of the reduced cost is that it is the rate at which the objective function value will be hurt if a variable currently at zero is arbitrarily forced to increase a small amount. Suppose the reduced cost of x is \$2/gallon. This means that if the profitability of x could be increased by \$2/gallon (e.g., by some combination of raising its selling price/unit and decreasing its cost/unit), increasing the amount produced of x by one unit (if 1 unit is a "small change") would not change the total profit. Clearly, if we did not alter the original profit contribution of x, the total profit would be reduced by \$2 if x is arbitrarily increased by 1.0.

1.5.2 Dual Prices

Associated with each constraint is a quantity known as the *dual price*. If the units of the objective function are cruzeiros and the units of the constraint in question are kilograms, the units of the dual price are cruzeiros per kilogram. The dual price of a constraint is the rate at which the objective function value will improve as the right-hand side or constant term of the constraint is increased a small amount.

Different LP packages may use different sign conventions with regard to the dual prices. LINDO uses the convention that a positive dual price means that increasing the right-hand side in question will improve the objective function value, whereas a negative dual price means increasing the right-hand side will cause the objective function value to deteriorate. A zero dual price means that changing the right-hand side a small amount will have no effect on the solution value.

It follows that under this convention, $\leq$ constraints will have nonnegative dual prices, $\geq$ constraints will have nonpositive dual prices, and $=$ constraints can have dual prices of any sign. Why?

Understanding Dual Prices. It is instructive to analyze the dual prices in the solution to the Enginola problem. The dual price on the constraint $A \leq 60$ is \$5/unit. At first, one might suspect that this quantity should be \$20/unit, because if one more Astro is produced, the simple profit contribution of this unit is \$20. An additional Astro unit will require sacrifices elsewhere, however. Because all of the labor supply is being used, producing more Astros would require the production of Cosmos to be reduced in order to free up labor. The labor tradeoff rate for Astros and Cosmos is 1/2; that is, producing one more Astro implies reducing Cosmo production by 1/2 of a unit. Because Cosmos have a profit contribution of \$30 per unit, the net increase in profits is $\$20 - \frac{1}{2} \times \$30 = \$5$.

Now consider the dual price of \$15/hour on the labor constraint. If we have 1 more hour of labor, it will be used solely to produce more Cosmos. One Cosmo has a profit contribution of \$30/unit. Because 1 hour of labor is only sufficient for 1/2 of a Cosmo, the value of the additional hour of labor is \$15.

1.6 Unbounded Formulations

If we forget to include the labor constraint and the constraint on the production of Cosmos, an unlimited amount of profit is possible by producing a large number of Cosmos. This is illustrated here:

```
LOOK  ALL

MAX        20 A + 30 C
SUBJECT  TO
     2)        A <=     60
END
```

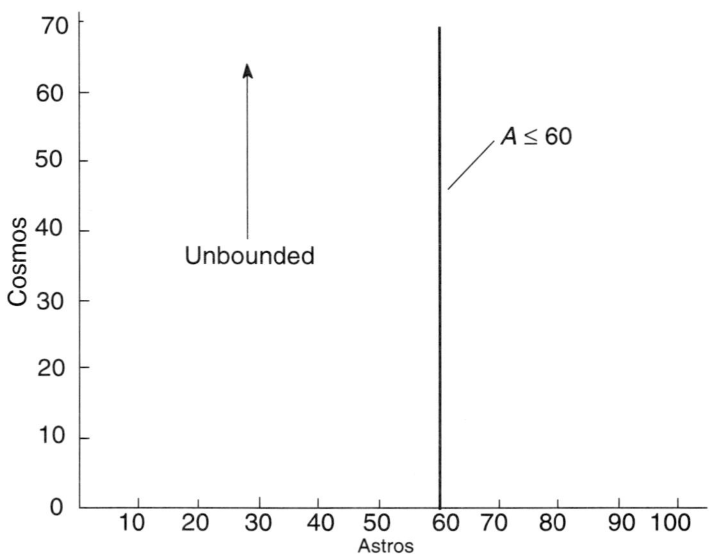

Figure 1.7
Graph of
Unbounded
Formulation


```
:GO

        UNBOUNDED  SOLUTION
        UNBOUNDED  VARIABLES  ARE:

            C
```

There is nothing to prevent C from being infinitely large. The feasible region is illustrated in Figure 1.7. In larger problems, there are typically several variables that are unbounded, and it is not as easy to identify the manner in which the unboundedness arises.

1.7 Infeasible Formulations

An example of an infeasible formulation is obtained if the right-hand side of the labor constraint is made 190 and its direction is, inadvertently, say, reversed. In this case, the most labor that can be used is to produce 60 Astros and 50 Cosmos for a total labor consumption of $60 + 2 \times 50 = 160$ hours. The formulation and attempted solution are:

```
MAX       20 A + 30 C
SUBJECT TO
    2)       A <=      60
    3)       C <=      50
    4)       A + 2 C >=   190
END
```

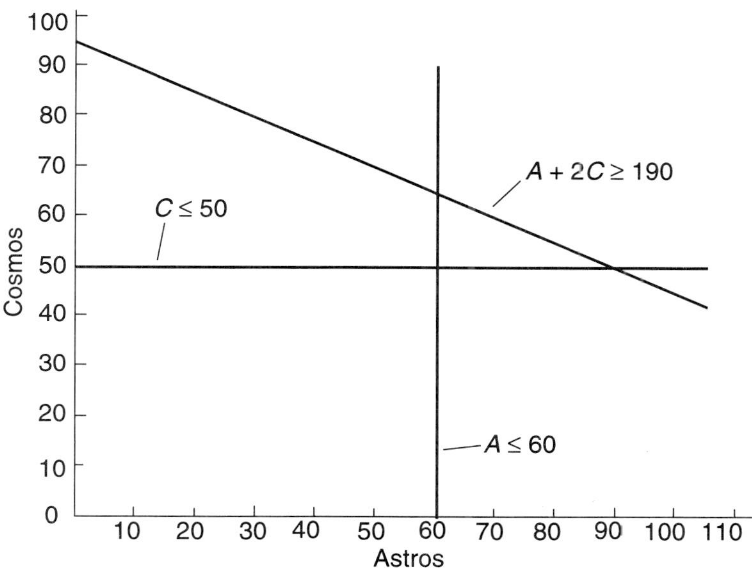

Figure 1.8
Graph of
Infeasible
Formulation

```
:GO
        NO FEASIBLE SOLUTION.
   VIOLATED ROWS HAVE NEGATIVE SLACK.
   OR (EQUALITY ROWS) NONZERO SLACKS.
   ROWS CONTRIBUTING TO INFEASIBILITY HAVE
   NONZERO DUAL PRICE.

              OBJECTIVE FUNCTION VALUE

   1)              3300.000

   VARIABLE            VALUE           REDUCED COST
      A             90.000000             0.000000
      C             50.000000             0.000000

   ROW                 SLACK           DUAL PRICES
    2)             -30.000000             1.000000
    3)               0.000000             2.000000
    4)               0.000000            -1.000000
```

The dual prices in this case give information helpful in determining how the infeasibility arose. For example, the +1 associated with row 2 indicates that increasing its right-hand side by 1 will decrease the infeasibility by 1. The +2 with row 3 means that if we allowed 1 more unit of Cosmo production, the infeasibility would be decreased by 2 units, because each Cosmo uses 2 hours of labor. The −1 associated with row 4 means that if the right-hand side of the labor constraint were decreased by 1, the infeasibility would be reduced by 1. Figure 1.8 illustrates the constraints for this formulation.

1.8 Multiple Optimal Solutions and Degeneracy

For a given LP formulation having a bounded optimal solution, there will be a unique optimum objective function value. Sometimes, however, there may be several different combinations of decision variable values and dual prices, all of which produce the same total profit. Such solutions are said to be *degenerate* in some sense. Let us illustrate with the Enginola problem. Suppose the profit contribution/unit of A is \$15 rather than \$20. The model and a solution are:

```
MAX        15 A + 30 C
SUBJECT TO
     2)        A <=      60
     3)        C <=      50
     4)        A + 2 C <= 120
END

 :GO
                OBJECTIVE FUNCTION VALUE

     1)                 1800.000

     VARIABLE               VALUE          REDUCED COST
     A                   60.000000             0.000000
     C                   30.000000             0.000000

     ROW                    SLACK          DUAL PRICES
     2)                  0.000000             0.000000
     3)                 20.000000             0.000000
     4)                  0.000000            15.000000
```

The feasible region as well as a "profit = 1500" line are shown in Figure 1.9. Notice that the lines $A + 2C = 120$ and $15A + 30C = 1500$ are parallel. It should be apparent that any feasible point on the line $A + 2C = 120$ is optimal. For example, the point $A = 40$, $C = 40$ and the point $A = 20$, $C = 50$ both give a profit of 1800 and use 120 hours of labor.

The particularly observant may have noted in the solution report that the constraint, $A \le 60$, i.e., row 2 has both zero slack and a zero dual price. This suggests that the production of Astros could be decreased a small amount without any effect on total profits. Of course, there would have to be a compensatory increase in the production of Cosmos. We conclude that there must be an alternate optimum solution that produces fewer Astros but more Cosmos. We can discover this solution by increasing the profitability of Cosmos ever so slightly. Observe:

```
MAX        15 A + 30.0001 C
SUBJECT TO
     2)        A <=      60
     3)        C <=      50
     4)        A + 2 C <= 120
END
```

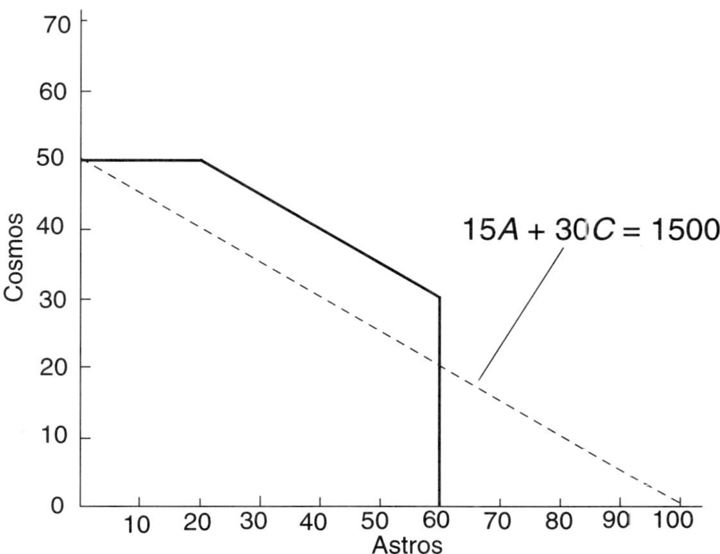

Figure 1.9
Model with
Alternate
Optima


```
  :GO
    LP OPTIMUM FOUND   AT STEP   1

           OBJECTIVE FUNCTION VALUE

     1)            1800.001

   VARIABLE          VALUE           REDUCED COST
      A            20.000000             0.000000
      C            50.000000             0.000000

   ROW               SLACK           DUAL PRICES
     2)            40.000000             0.000000
     3)             0.000000             0.000010
     4)             0.000000            15.000000
```

As predicted, the profit is still about \$1800; however, the production of Cosmos has been increased to 50 from 30, whereas the production of Astros has been decreased to 20 from 60.

1.8.1 The "Snake Eyes" Condition

Alternate optima may exist only if some row in the solution report has zeroes in both the second and third columns of the report, a configuration that some applied statisticians call "snake eyes." That is, alternate optima may exist only if some variable has both zero value and zero reduced cost or some constraint has both zero slack and zero dual price. Mathematicians, with no intent of moral judgment, refer to such solutions as degenerate.

If there are alternate optima, you may find that your computer gives a different solution from that in the text. You should, however, always get the same objective function value.

There are in fact two ways in which multiple optimal solutions can occur. For the example in Figure 1.9, the two optimal solution reports differ only in the values of the so-called primal variables, i.e., our original decision variables A, C, and the slack variables in the constraint. There can also be situations where there are multiple optimal solutions in which only the dual variables differ. Consider this variation of the Enginola problem wherein the capacity of the Cosmo line has been reduced to 30. The formulation is:

```
MAX        20 A + 30 C
SUBJECT TO
    2)   A           <=    60
    3)           C <=    30
    4)    A + 2 C <=   120
END
```

The corresponding graph of this problem appears in Figure 1.10. An optimal solution is:

```
              OBJECTIVE FUNCTION VALUE

    1)              2100.0000

    VARIABLE        VALUE           REDUCED COST
    A               60.000000          0.000000
    C               30.000000          0.000000

    ROW         SLACK OR SURPLUS      DUAL PRICES
    2)              0.000000           5.000000
    3)              0.000000           0.000000
    4)              0.000000          15.000000
```

Again notice the "snake eyes" in the solution, i.e., the pair of zeroes in a row of the solution report. This suggests that the capacity of the Cosmo line (the RHS of row 3) could be changed without changing the objective value. Figure 1.10 illustrates the situation. Three constraints pass through the point $A = 60$, $C = 30$. Any two of the constraints determine the point. In fact, the constraint $A + 2C \leq 120$ is mathematically redundant; i.e., it could be dropped without changing the feasible region.

If you decrease the RHS of row 3 very slightly, you will get essentially the following solution.

```
              OBJECTIVE FUNCTION VALUE
    1)              2100.0000

    VARIABLE        VALUE           REDUCED COST
    A               60.000000          0.000000
    C               30.000000          0.000000
```

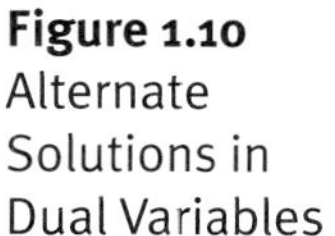

Figure 1.10
Alternate
Solutions in
Dual Variables

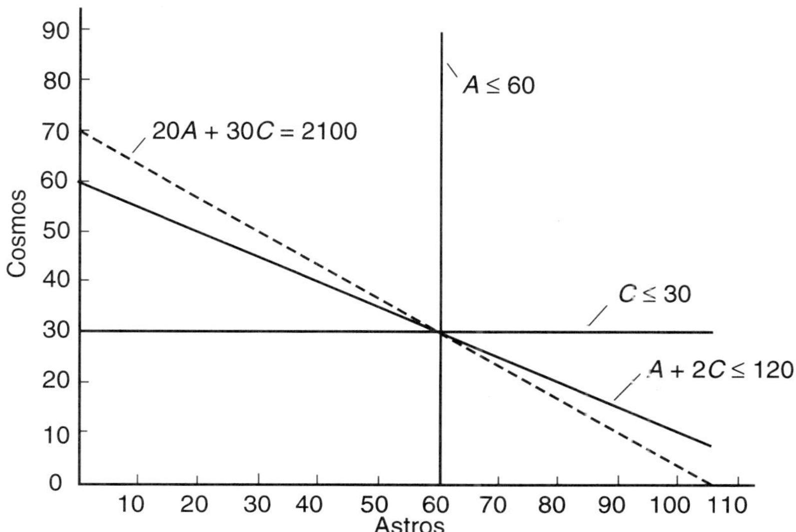


```
ROW           SLACK OR SURPLUS       DUAL PRICES
 2)              0.000000            20.000000
 3)              0.000000            30.000000
 4)              0.000000             0.000000
```

Notice that this solution differs from the previous one only in the dual values.

We can now state the following rule: If a solution report has the "snake eyes" feature, i.e., a pair of zeroes in any row of the report, there is another alternate optimal solution that differs either in the primal variables or the dual variables or both.

If a solution report exhibits the "snake eyes" configuration, a natural question to ask is: can we determine from the solution report alone whether the alternate optima are in the primal variables or the dual variables? The answer is "no," as the following two related problems illustrate.

Problem D	**Problem P**

```
MAX   X + Y                     MAX   X + Y
SUBJECT TO                      SUBJECT TO
 2) X + Y + Z ≤ 1                2) X + Y + Z  ≤ 1
 3) X + 2Y     ≤ 1               3) X      + 2Z ≤ 1
END                             END
```

Both problems possess multiple optimal solutions. The ones that can be identified by standard solution methods are:

Solution 1

Problem D			Problem P		
OBJECTIVE FUNCTION VALUE			OBJECTIVE FUNCTION VALUE		
1)	1.00000000		1)	1.00000000	
VARIABLE	VALUE	REDUCED COST	VARIABLE	VALUE	REDUCED COST
X	1.000000	0 000000	X	1.000000	0.000000
Y	0.000000	0.000000	Y	0.000000	0.000000
Z	0.000000	1.000000	Z	0.000000	1.000000
ROW	SLACK OR SURPLUS	DUAL PRICES	ROW	SLACK OR SURPLUS	DUAL PRICES
2)	0.000000	1.000000	2)	0.000000	1.000000
3)	0.000000	0.000000	3)	0.000000	0.000000

Solution 2

Problem D			Problem P		
OBJECTIVE FUNCTION VALUE			OBJECTIVE FUNCTION VALUE		
1)	1.00000000		1)	1.00000000	
VARIABLE	VALUE	REDUCED COST	VARIABLE	VALUE	REDUCED COST
X	1.000000	0.000000	X	0.000000	0.000000
Y	0.000000	1.000000	Y	1.000000	0.000000
Z	0.000000	0.000000	Z	0.000000	1.000000
ROW	SLACK OR SURPLUS	DUAL PRICES	ROW	SLACK OR SURPLUS	DUAL PRICES
2)	0.000000	0.000000	2)	0.000000	1.000000
3)	0.000000	1.000000	3)	1.000000	0.000000

Notice that:

- *Solution 1* is exactly the same for both problems.
- *Problem D* has multiple optimal solutions in the dual variables (only), whereas
- *Problem P* has multiple optimal solutions in the primal variables (only).

Thus, one cannot determine from the solution report alone the kind of alternate optima that might exist. You can generate Solution 1 by setting the RHS of row 3 and the coefficient of X in the objective to slightly larger than 1, e.g., 1.001, and Solution 2 by setting the RHS of row 3 and the coefficient of X in the objective to slightly less than 1, e.g., 0.9999.

Some authors refer to a problem that has multiple solutions to the primal variables as *dual degenerate* and a problem with multiple solutions in the dual variables as *primal degenerate*. Other authors say a problem has multiple optima only if there are multiple optimal solutions for the primal variables.

1.8.2 Degeneracy and Redundant Constraints

In small examples, degeneracy usually means there are redundant constraints. In general, however, especially in large problems, degeneracy does not imply that there

Figure 1.11
Degeneracy but
No Redundancy

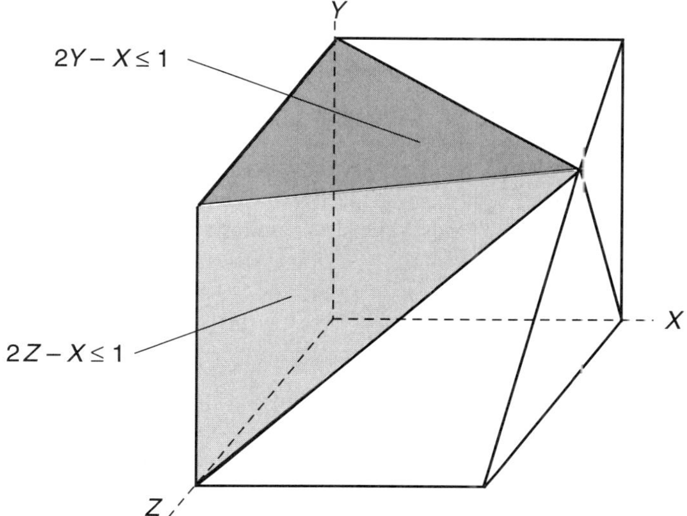

are redundant constraints. The constraint set below and the corresponding Figure
1.11 illustrate.

$$2x - y \leq 1 \qquad 2y - x \leq 1 \qquad 2z - x \leq 1$$
$$2x - z \leq 1 \qquad 2y - z \leq 1 \qquad 2z - y \leq 1$$

These constraints define a cone with apex or point at $x = y = z = 1$, having six sides.
The point $x = y = z = 1$ is degenerate because it has more than three constraints pass-
ing through it. Nevertheless, none of the constraints is redundant. Notice the point
$x = 0.6$, $y = 0$, $z = 0.5$ violates the first constraint but satisfies all the others. There-
fore, the first constraint is nonredundant. By trying all six permutations of 0.6, 0,
0.5, you can verify that each of the six constraints is nonredundant.

1.9 PROBLEMS

Problem 1

Your firm produces two products, Thyristors (T) and Lozenges (L), which compete
for the scarce resources of your distribution system. For the next planning period,
your distribution system has available 6,000 person-hours. Proper distribution of
each T requires 3 hours and each L requires 2 hours. The profit contributions per
unit are 40 and 30 for Ts and Ls. Product line considerations dictate that at least 1 T
be sold for each 2 Ls.

    (a) Draw the feasible region and draw the profit line that passes through the op-
timum point.

    (b) By simple commonsense arguments, what is the optimal solution?

Problem 2

Graph the following LP problem:

$$\text{Minimize} \quad 4X + 6Y$$

$$\text{subject to} \quad 5X + 2Y \geq 12$$
$$3X + 7Y \geq 13$$

In addition, plot the line $4X + 6Y = 18$. Show an iso-cost line and indicate the optimum point.

Problem 3

The Volkswagen Company produces two products, the Bug and the SuperBug, which share production facilities. Raw materials costs are $600 per car for the Bug and $750 per car for the SuperBug. The Bug requires 4 hours in the foundry/forge area per car, whereas the Superbug, because it uses newer, more advanced dies, requires only 2 hours in the foundry/forge. The Bug requires 2 hours per car in the assembly plant, whereas the SuperBug, because it is a more complicated car, requires 3 hours per car in the assembly plant. The available daily capacities in the two areas are 160 hours in the foundry/forge and 180 hours in the assembly plant. The selling price of the Bug at the factory door is $4800, whereas for the SuperBug it is $5250. It is safe to assume that whatever number of cars are produced by this factory can be sold.

(a) Write the linear program formulation of this problem.
(b) The above description implies that the capacities of the two departments, foundry/forge and assembly, are sunk costs. Reformulate the LP under the conditions that each hour of foundry/forge time costs $90, whereas each hour of assembly time costs $60. The capacities remain as before. Unused capacity has no charge.

Problem 4

The Keyesport Quarry has two different pits from which it obtains rock. The rock is run through a crusher to produce two products: concrete grade stone and road surface chat. Each ton of rock from the South pit converts into 0.75 tons of stone and 0.25 tons of chat when crushed. Rock from the North pit is of different quality. When it is crushed it produces a "50-50" split of stone and chat. The Quarry has contracts for 60 tons of stone and 40 tons of chat this planning period. The cost per ton of extracting and crushing rock for the South pit is 1.6 times as large as that from the North pit.

(a) What are the decision variables in the problem?
(b) There are two constraints for this problem. State them in words.
(c) Graph the feasible region for this problem.
(d) Draw an appropriate objective function line on the graph and indicate graphically and numerically the optimal solution.

(e) Suppose all the information given in the problem description is accurate. What additional information might you nevertheless wish to know before having confidence in this model?

Problem 5

A problem faced by railroads is that of assembling engine sets for particular trains. There are three important characteristics associated with each engine type, namely, operating cost per hour, horsepower, and tractive power. Associated with each train, e.g., the Super Chief run from Chicago to Los Angeles, is a required horsepower and a required tractive power. The horsepower required depends largely upon the speed required by the run, whereas the tractive power required depends largely upon the weight of the train and the steepness of the grades encountered on the run. For a particular train, the problem is to find the combination of engines that satisfies the horsepower and tractive power requirements at lowest cost.

In particular, consider the Cimarron Special, the train that runs from Omaha to Santa Fe. This train requires 12,000 horsepower and 50,000 tractive power units. Two engine types, the GM-I and the GM-II, are available for pulling this train. The GM-I has 2,000 horsepower, 10,000 tractive power units, and its variable operating costs are $150 per hour. The GM-II has 3,000 horsepower, 10,000 tractive power units, and its variable operating costs are $180 per hour. The engine set may be mixed, e.g., use two GM-Is and three GM-IIs.

(a) Write the linear program formulation of this problem.

Problem 6

Graph the constraint lines and the objective function line passing through the optimum point and indicate the feasible region for the Enginola problem when:

(a) All parameters are as given except that the labor supply is 70 rather than 120.
(b) All parameters are as given originally except that the variable profit contribution of a Cosmo is $40 instead of $30.

Problem 7

Consider the problem:

$$\text{Minimize} \quad 4x_1 + 3x_2$$

$$\text{Subject to} \quad \begin{aligned} 2x_1 + x_2 &\geq 10 \\ -3x_1 + 2x_2 &\leq 6 \\ x_1 + x_2 &\geq 6 \end{aligned} \qquad x_1 \geq 0, x_2 \geq 0$$

Solve the problem graphically.

Problem 8

The surgical unit of a small hospital is becoming more concerned about finances. The hospital cannot control or set many of the important factors that determine its financial health. For example, the length of stay in the hospital for a given type of surgery is determined in large part by government regulation. The amount that can be charged for a given type of surgical procedure is controlled largely by the combination of the market and government regulation. Most of the hospital's surgical procedures are elective, so the hospital has considerable control over which patients and associated procedures are attracted and admitted to the hospital. The surgical unit has effectively two scarce resources, the hospital beds available to it (70 in a typical week), and the surgical suite hours available (165 hours in a typical week). Patients admitted to this surgical unit can be classified into the following three categories:

Patient Type	Days of Stay	Surgical Suite Hours Needed	Financial Contribution
A	3	2	$240
B	5	1.5	$225
C	6	3	$425

For example, each type B patient admitted will use 5 days of the $7 \times 70 = 490$ bed days available each week, and 1.5 hours of the 165 surgical suite hours available each week. One doctor has argued that the surgical unit should try to admit more type A patients. Her argument is that, "in terms of $/days of stay, type A is clearly the best, whereas in terms of $/(surgical suite hour), it is not much worse than B and C."

Suppose the surgical unit can in fact control the number of each type of patient admitted each week; i.e., they are decision variables. How many of each type should be admitted each week?

Can you formulate it as an LP?

Solving LPs on the Computer: The LINDO Program

2.1 Introduction

The process of solving an LP requires a large number of calculations and is therefore best performed by a computer program. The computer program we will use is called LINDO. The acronym stands for <u>L</u>inear, <u>I</u>nteractive, <u>D</u>iscrete <u>O</u>ptimizer. The main purpose of LINDO is to allow a user to quickly input an LP formulation, solve it, assess the correctness or appropriateness of the formulation based on the solution, and then quickly make minor modifications to the formulation and repeat the process. LINDO features a wide range of commands, any of which may be invoked at any time. LINDO checks whether a particular command makes sense in a particular context.

LINDO is available in two versions: a Windows version and a generic text-based version. The text-based version runs under most popular operating systems, including Unix, MS-DOS, and Macintosh. For either version, additional information is available to the user under the Help menu item or Help command. We will cover the Windows commands first, followed by the Unix/text-based commands.

2.2 LINDO for Windows®

2.2.1 Installing LINDO for Windows

To install a PC Windows version of LINDO under Windows 3.1 and Windows NT, simply insert the LINDO system diskette in floppy drive A: and from the File Menu in the Program Manager select the Run command. In the dialog box enter:

```
A:SETUP
```

and then respond to the prompts presented by the LINDO Setup program.

Windows 95 users should press the Windows Start button, select the Run command, and then enter A:SETUP as above.

To start Windows versions of LINDO, double click on the LINDO icon on your desktop.

Now let's illustrate how to get started using LINDO by entering a small model.

2.2.2 Getting Started on a Small Problem

When you start LINDO for Windows, the program opens an <untitled> window for you. Your screen should resemble the following:

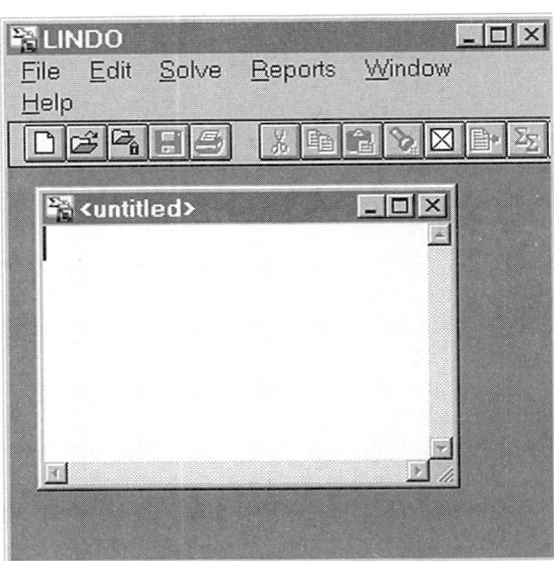

The outer window labeled "LINDO" is the main frame window. All other windows will be contained within this window. The frame window also contains all the command menus and the command toolbar. The smaller window labeled "<untitled>" is a new, blank model window. We will type our sample model directly into this window.

For purposes of introduction, let's enter the Enginola problem we looked at in the previous chapter:

```
MAX      20 A + 30 C
SUBJECT TO
A <   60
C <   50
A + 2 C <    120
END
```

A LINDO model has a minimum requirement of three things. It needs an objective, it needs variables, and it needs constraints. The objective function must always be at the start of the model and is initiated with either MAX (for maximize) or MIN (for minimize). In LINDO, the minute you use a variable in your model, it exists. You don't have to do anything other than enter it in a formula. The end of the objective function and the beginning of the constraints is signified with any of the following:

```
SUBJECT TO
SUCH THAT
S.T.
ST
```

The end of the constraints is signified with the word END.

Note that even though the strict inequality, "<", was entered above, LINDO interprets it as the loose inequality, "≤". The reason is that typical keyboards have only the strict inequalities, "<" and ">".

After entering the above, your screen should look like this:

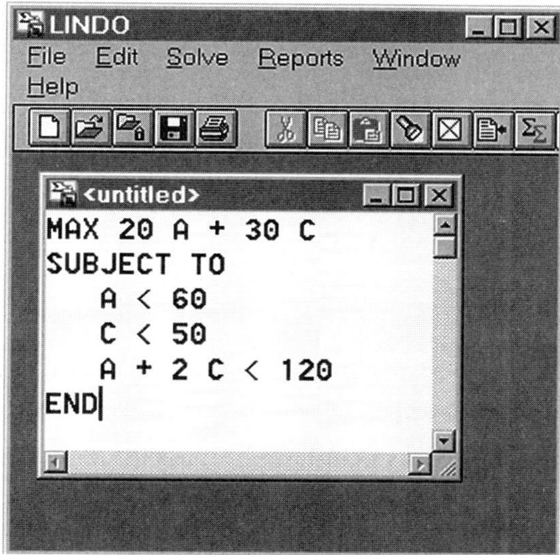

Your model has now been entered and it's ready to be solved. Click on the Solve button, use the Solve command from the Solve menu, or press F2 to solve the model. LINDO will begin by trying to compile the model. This means LINDO will determine whether the model makes mathematical sense and whether it conforms to syntactical requirements. If the model doesn't pass these tests, you'll be informed with the following error message:

```
An error occurred during compilation on line: n
```

LINDO will then jump to the line where the error occurred. You should examine this line for any syntax errors and correct them.

If there are no formulation errors during the compilation phase, LINDO will then begin to actually solve the model. While solving, LINDO will show the Solver Status Window on your screen that looks like the following:

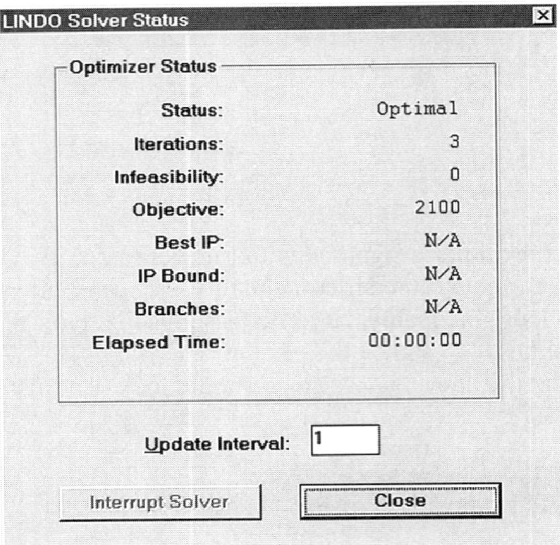

This Status Window shows information about the model and the solution process. The various fields and controls within the Status Window are described in Table 2.1.

At this point you'll be asked whether you wish to do sensitivity or range analysis. Unless you are already familiar with these concepts, you should answer no to this question. Then click on the "Close" button to close the Solver Status Window.

There will now be a new window on your screen titled "Reports Window." The Reports Window is where LINDO sends all text-based reporting output. The window can hold up to 64,000 characters of information. If you have a lengthy solution report that you need to examine in its entirety, you can log all information sent to the Reports Window in a disk file using the File|Log Output command. This file can then be examined using an external editor or the File|View command. The Reports Window now contains the solution to our model and should resemble the following:

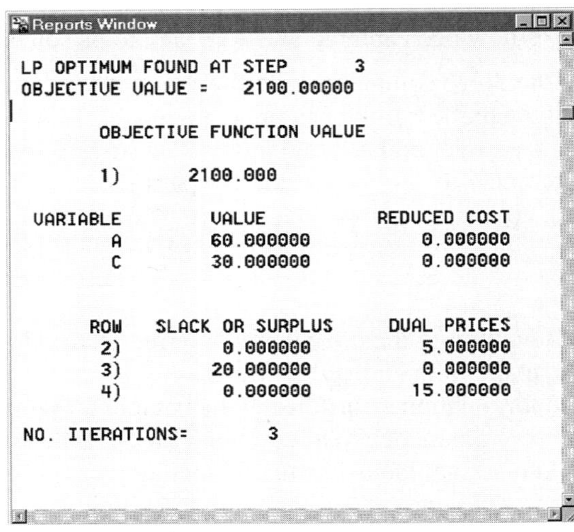

Table 2.1	Field/Control	Description
Description of the LINDO Solver Status Window	Status	Gives status of current solution Possible values include: Optimal, Feasible, Infeasible, Unbounded.
	Iterations	Number of solver iterations.
	Infeasibility	Amount by which constraints are violated.
	Objective	Current value of the objective function.
	Best IP	Objective value of best integer solution found. Only relevant in integer programming (IP) models.
	IP Bound	Theoretical bound on the objective for IP models.
	Branches	The number of integer variables "branched" on by LINDO's IP solver.
	Elapsed Time	Elapsed time since the solver was invoked.
	Update Interval	The frequency (in seconds) that the Status Window is updated. You can set this to any nonnegative value desired. Setting the interval to zero will tend to increase solution times.
	Interrupt Solver	Press this button to interrupt the solver at any point and have it return the current best solution found.
	Close	Press this button to close the Status Window. Optimization will continue. The Status Window may be reopened by selecting the Status Window command from the Window menu.

Taken in order, this tells you, first, that LINDO took 3 iterations to solve the model; second, that the maximum profit attainable from the two variables as they are constrained is 2100; third, the variables A and C take on the values 60 and 30, respectively; fourth, there are no reduced costs for either variable; fifth, there is a surplus of 20 for the constraint in row 3; and, sixth, there are dual prices of 5 and 15 for the constraints in rows 2 and 4, respectively.

Editing the model is simply a matter of finding and changing the variable, coefficient, or direction you want to change. Any changes you make will be taken into account the next time you solve the model.

Click on the 🖫 button, use the Save command from the File menu, or press CONTROL + S to save your work.

2.2.3 Integer Programming with LINDO

Fairly shortly after you start looking at problems for which LP might be applicable, you discover the need to restrict certain variables to integer values, i.e., 0, 1, 2, etc. Even though this violates the linearity requirement, LINDO allows you to identify such variables. We give an introductory treatment here. It is discussed more thoroughly in Chapter 14.

Integer variables in LINDO can be either 0/1 or general. Variables that are restricted to the values 0 or 1 are identified with the INTEGER specification. It is used in one of two forms, examples of which are:

```
INTEGER x   or   INTEGER 8.
```

The first (and recommended) form identifies variable x as being 0/1. The second form identifies the first 8 variables in the current formulation as being 0/1. The order of the variables is determined by their order encountered in the input. This order can be verified by observing the order of variables in the solution report.

The second form is more powerful but requires the user to be aware of the exact order of the variables. This may be confusing if not all variables appear in the objective.

To use the first form, enter the model as follows:

```
max 4 tom + 3 dick + 2 harry
st
2.5 tom + 3.1 harry < 5
.2 tom + .7 dick + .4 harry < 1
end
```

After the END statement, enter the INTEGER (abbreviating to INT is acceptable) specification as follows:

```
int tom
int dick
int harry
```

Your model window should now appear as follows:

```
<untitled>
MAX 4 TOM + 3 DICK + 2 HARRY
ST
  2.5 TOM + 3.1 HARRY < 5
  .2 TOM + .7 DICK + .4 HARRY < 1
END
INT TOM
INT DICK
INT HARRY
```

Solving the model results in the following output to the Reports Window:

```
Reports Window

LP OPTIMUM FOUND AT STEP     4
OBJECTIVE VALUE =   7.65898609

NEW INTEGER SOLUTION OF   7.00000000     AT BRANCH     0 PIVOT      6
BOUND ON OPTIMUM:  7.000000
ENUMERATION COMPLETE. BRANCHES=     0 PIVOTS=     6

LAST INTEGER SOLUTION IS THE BEST FOUND
REINSTALLING BEST SOLUTION ...

        OBJECTIVE FUNCTION VALUE

    1)      7.000000

  VARIABLE        VALUE          REDUCED COST
       TOM        1.000000          -4.000000
      DICK        1.000000          -3.000000
     HARRY        0.000000          -2.000000


       ROW   SLACK OR SURPLUS      DUAL PRICES
        2)        2.500000          0.000000
        3)        0.100000          0.000000

NO. ITERATIONS=      7
BRANCHES=     0 DETERM.=  1.000E     0
```

General integers, which can be 0, 1, 2, etc., are identified in analogous fashion by using `GIN` instead of `INT`, for example:

```
GIN TONIC    or    GIN 8.
```

The first restricts variable TONIC to 0, 1, 2, 3, etc. The second restricts the first eight variables to 0, 1, 2, 3, etc.

The solution method used is branch and bound. It is an intelligent enumeration process that will find a sequence of better and better solutions. As each one is found, a short message will be displayed, giving the objective value and a bound on how good a solution might still remain. After the enumeration is complete, the Solution . . . or Peruse . . . command from the Reports menu can be used to reveal information about the best solution found.

Let's look at a slightly modified version of the original Enginola problem and see how the `GIN` specification might help.

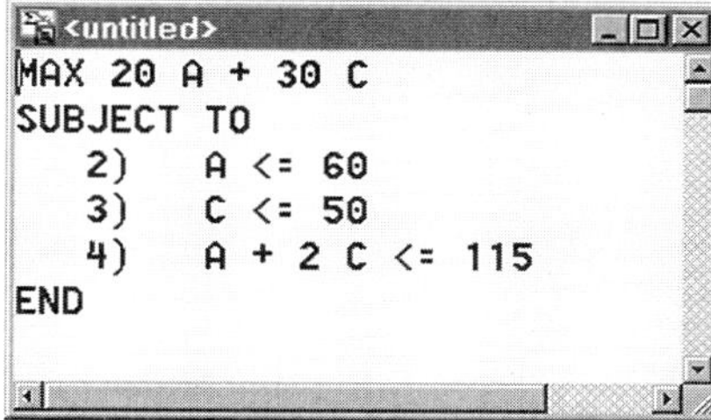

Notice the capacity of 115 on the labor constraint (Row 4).

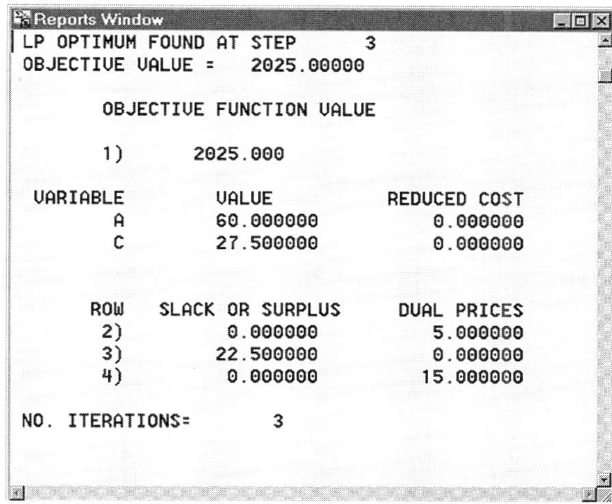

Note that a fractional quantity is recommended for C. If fractional quantities are undesirable, declare A and C as general integer variables:

Solving results in the following:

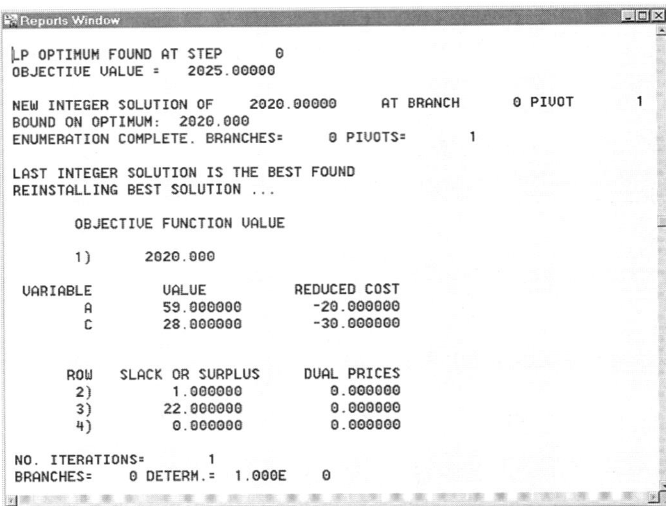

Although the integer programming (IP) capability is very powerful, it requires skill to use effectively. It is very easy to prepare a bad formulation for an essentially easy problem. A bad formulation may require intolerable amounts of computer time to solve. Good formulations of integer programs are discussed further in Chapter 14.

2.2.4 Scaling and Other Numerical Considerations

You should avoid using extremely small or extremely large numbers in a formulation; e.g., you should not measure weight in ounces one place and volume in cubic miles someplace else in the same problem. A rule of thumb is that there should be no nonzero coefficient whose absolute value is greater than 100,000 or less than 0.0001. If LINDO feels that the matrix is poorly scaled, it will print a warning.

2.2.5 Windows Menu Commands

Following are all the commands available in the Windows version of LINDO by menu. For our purposes here, we merely give a brief description of each command.

For a more in-depth discussion, refer to the LINDO Users Manual and/or LINDO's internal Help system.

File Menu

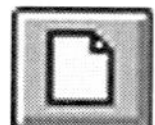

NEW   F2
Use the NEW command from the File menu, press F2, or use the button to create a new Model window. In the Model window, you can enter your model or use the Edit|Paste command to import a model from other applications.

OPEN   F3
Use the OPEN command from the File menu, press F3, or use the button to open an existing file. Files opened with this command are limited to roughly 64,000 characters of data.

VIEW   F4
Use the VIEW command from the File menu, press F4, or use the button to open an existing file in a View Window. These windows do not have all the editing commands found in normal windows, but they are limited in size only by available memory. Therefore, they are useful to look at large models.

TAKE COMMANDS   F11
Use the TAKE COMMANDS . . . command from the File menu or press F11 to "Take" a LINDO batch file with commands and model text for automated operation.

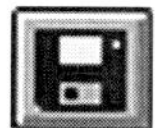

SAVE   F5
Use the SAVE command from the File menu, press F5, or use the button to save the active (frontmost) window as text. You can save any window—Model, Reports, or Command—in this way. Whether the window is a new Model window called <untitled> or a Reports or Command window, SAVE opens the Save As . . . dialog.

SAVE AS...   F6
Use the SAVE AS . . . command from the File menu or press F6 to save the active (frontmost) window as a text file under the name you enter in the dialog box.

CLOSE   F7
Use the CLOSE command from the File menu or press F7 to close the active (frontmost) window. If the window is a new Model window called <untitled>, or if you have changed the file, you'll be asked whether you want to save the changes.

PRINT   F8
Use the PRINT command from the File menu, press F8, or use the button to send the active window to your printer.

PRINTER SETUP...   F9
Use the PRINTER SETUP . . . command from the File menu or press F9 to select the printer to which you want output to go.

LOG OUTPUT... F10
Use the LOG OUTPUT . . . command from the File menu or press F10 to send all subsequent screen activity, which would be sent to the Reports Window, to a text file.

BASIS READ F12
Use the BASIS READ command from the File menu or press F12 to install a previously saved basis (see BASIS SAVE below) as a starting point for solving the current model.

BASIS SAVE Shift+F2
Use the BASIS SAVE command from the File menu or press SHIFT + F2 to save the basis of the current model.

DATE Shift+F4
Use the DATE command from the File menu or press SHIFT + F4 to display the current date and time in the Reports window.

ELAPSED TIME Shift+F5
Use the ELAPSED TIME command from the File menu or press SHIFT + F5 to display the elapsed time of the current LINDO session.

TITLE Shift+F3
Use the TITLE command from the File menu or press SHIFT + F3 to display the title of the active model.

EXIT Shift+F6
Use the EXIT command from the File menu or press SHIFT + F6 to exit LINDO and return to the operating system.

Edit Menu

UNDO Ctrl+Z
Use the UNDO command from the Edit menu or type CONTROL + Z to undo the last action.

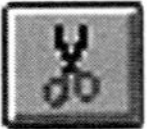

CUT Ctrl+X
Use the CUT command from the Edit menu, click the button, or type CONTROL + X to clear the selected text and place it on the clipboard for pasting.

COPY Ctrl+C
Use the COPY command from the Edit menu, click the button, or type CONTROL + C to copy the selected text to the clipboard for pasting.

PASTE Ctrl+V
Use the PASTE command from the Edit menu, click the button, or type CONTROL + V to paste clipboard contents at the insertion point.

CLEAR Del
Use the CLEAR command from the Edit menu or press the DELETE key to clear the selected text without placing it in the clipboard.

FIND/REPLACE... Ctrl+F
Use the FIND/REPLACE command from the Edit menu, click the button, or type CONTROL+F to search in the active window for the text entered in the "Find What:" box. Click the "Find next" button in the FIND/REPLACE dialog box to find the next instance of the text.

OPTIONS... Alt+O
Use the OPTIONS . . . command from the Edit menu, press ALT+O, or click on the button to change a number of parameters that affect the way LINDO solves your model. These parameters remain as you set them for the extent of the current LINDO session; they are not model-specific and may be saved for use in subsequent sessions by using the Save button in the Options dialog box.

GO TO LINE... Ctrl+T
Use the GO TO LINE command from the Edit menu, click on the button, or type CONTROL+G to enter a line number of the active window to which you want to go.

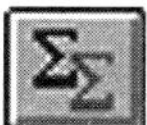

PASTE SYMBOL Ctrl+P
Use the PASTE SYMBOL command from the Edit menu, press CONTROL+P, or click on the button to paste any of LINDO's symbols at the current insertion point. Choose from a listing of available symbols in the dialog box that may then be pasted into your model window at the insertion point.

SELECT ALL Ctrl+A
Use the SELECT ALL command from the Edit menu or press CONTROL+A to select all of the active window.

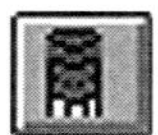

CLEAR ALL
Use the CLEAR ALL command from the Edit menu or click on the button to clear all of the active window.

CHOOSE NEW FONT
Use the CHOOSE NEW FONT command from the Edit menu to reset the font in the active window.

Solve Menu

COMPILE MODEL Ctrl+E
Use the COMPILE MODEL command from the Solve menu, press CONTROL+E, or click on the button to compile the model in the active window; this must be done before any analytical or solution-related commands can be performed. Compiling also clears any current solution from memory, so there is no solution for the active model until the Solve command is given again.

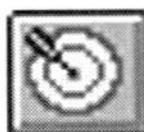

```
SOLVE  Ctrl+S
```
Use the SOLVE command from the Solve menu, press CONTROL + S, or click on the button to send a model to the LINDO solver. If you have more than one model open, the frontmost (or active) window is the one that will be passed to the solver.

```
PIVOT  Ctrl+N
```
Use the PIVOT command from the Solve menu or press CONTROL + N to perform one pivot—i.e., one iteration—on the current model.

```
DEBUG  Ctrl+D
```
Use the DEBUG command from the Solve menu or press CONTROL + D to analyze an unbounded or infeasible model. LINDO will report the sources of the problem and suggest alterations to the formulation. This command may only be applied to linear models and is ineffective on integer and quadratic models.

```
PREEMPTIVE GOAL  Ctrl+G
```
Use the PREEMPTIVE GOAL command from the Solve menu or press CONTROL + G to solve the current model using Preemptive Goal programming. If properly formulated, a model can be solved for more than one objective with this command.

Reports Menu

```
SOLUTION...  Alt+0
```
Use the SOLUTION command from the Reports menu, press ALT + 0, or click the button to open the Solution Report Options dialog box. Here you can specify the way you want a report of the solution currently in memory to appear.

```
RANGE  Alt+1
```
Use the RANGE command from the Reports menu or press ALT + 1 to see a standard range report.

```
PARAMETRICS...  Alt+2
```
Use the PARAMETRICS command from the Reports menu or press ALT + 2 to see a graphical or text representation of the result of changes to the right-hand side of a specified row.

```
STATISTICS...  Alt+3
```
Use the STATISTICS command from the Reports menu or press ALT + 3 to see useful information about the current model.

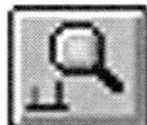

```
PERUSE...  Alt+4
```
Use the PERUSE command from the Reports menu, press ALT + 4, or click on the button to see a graphical or text representation of rows or columns selected according to the criteria you choose.

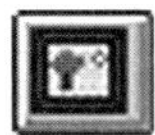

```
PICTURE...  Alt+5
```
Use the PICTURE command from the Reports menu, press ALT + 5, or click on the button to see a graphical or text representation of the nonzero picture of the current model in normal or lower triangulated form.

BASIS PICTURE Alt+6
Use the BASIS PICTURE command from the Reports menu or press ALT + 6 to create a text-based "picture" of the nonzero structure of the current model.

TABLEAU Alt+7
Use the TABLEAU command from the Reports menu or press ALT + 7 to see the tableau of the current model.

FORMULATION... Alt+8
Use the FORMULATION command from the Reports menu or press ALT + 8 to see all or a selected portion of the current model.

SHOW COLUMN... Alt+9
Use the SHOW COLUMN command from the Reports menu or press ALT + 9 to display information on a column. Choose the column from a list in the dialog box.

POSITIVE DEFINITE
Use the POSITIVE DEFINITE command from the Reports menu to analyze a quadratic formulation.

Windows Menu

OPEN COMMAND WINDOW Alt+C
Use the OPEN COMMAND WINDOW command from the Windows menu or press ALT + C to open LINDO's Command Window. The Command Window gives you access to LINDO's command line interface.

OPEN STATUS WINDOW
Use the OPEN STATUS WINDOW command from the Windows menu to open LINDO's Solver Status window.

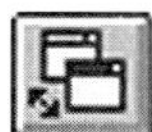

SEND TO BACK Ctrl+B
Use the SEND TO BACK command from the Windows menu, press CONTROL + B, or click on the button to send the frontmost window to the back. This command is very useful for switching between a Model window and the Reports Window.

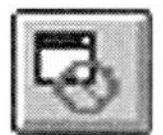

CLOSE ALL Alt+X
Use the CLOSE ALL command from the Windows menu, press ALT + X, or click on the button to close all open model windows and dialog boxes.

CASCADE Alt+A
Use the CASCADE command from the Windows menu or press ALT + A to arrange all open windows in a cascade from upper left to lower right, with the currently active window on top.

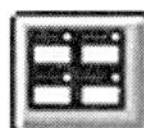

TILE Alt+T
Use the TILE command from the Windows menu, press ALT + T, or click on the button to arrange all open windows so that they each occupy the same amount of space within the LINDO program window.

```
ARRANGE ICONS  Alt+I
```
Use the ARRANGE ICONS command from the Windows menu or press ALT+I to move icons representing any minimized windows so that they are arranged across the bottom of the screen.

```
(LIST OF WINDOWS)
```
A list of all open windows appears at the bottom of the Windows menu, with the currently active window checked. Select a window from the list to bring it to the front.

Help Menu

```
CONTENTS  F1
```
Use the CONTENTS command from the Help menu, press F1, or click the first help button to go to the Contents section of LINDO Help. Press the second button (with the question mark) to invoke context-sensitive help. Once the cursor has changed to the question mark, selecting any menu command or toolbar button will take you to help for that command.

```
SEARCH FOR HELP ON...  Alt+F1
```
Use the SEARCH FOR HELP ON . . . command from the Help menu or press ALT + F1 to search the LINDO help file for a word or topic.

```
HOW TO USE HELP  Ctrl+F1
```
Use the HOW TO USE HELP command from the Help menu or press CONTROL + F1 to learn about using the Windows on-line help system.

```
About LINDO...
```
Use the About LINDO . . . command from the Help menu to display specific information about the version of LINDO being used.

2.3 LINDO for Command Line Environments

2.3.1 Getting Started on a Small Problem

The following input is valid for describing a small problem:

```
MAX 2X + 3Y
ST
4X + 3Y < 10
3X + 5Y < 12
END
```

Typing GO will cause this problem to be solved.

If LOOK is typed, LINDO asks for a row specification. Typical responses might be 3, or 1, 2, or ALL, causing, respectively, row 3, or rows 1 through 2, or all the rows to be printed.

If ALTER is typed, LINDO will ask for a row, a variable, and a new coefficient. Responding 2, X, and 6, respectively, to these queries would change the 4X in the above formulation to 6X. At this point, GO could again be typed to solve the new problem.

After solving a problem, LINDO will ask if you wish to do sensitivity or range analysis. Unless you are already familiar with these concepts you should answer no to this question.

The following is an example session illustrating how the above commands might be used in analyzing the Enginola problem. User input appears in lower case.

```
:! Some comments:
:! Comments can be inserted by prefacing with a "!".
:! When LINDO is awaiting a command,
:!  it prompts with a "!".
:! When expecting input other than a command,
:!  it prompts with a "?"
:max 20A + ! Notice that you can (and should) split long
?30C       ! rows over several input lines by typing a
?          ! carriage return
?st        !  or 'enter' at a convenient split point.
?A < 60
?C < 50
?A + 2 C < 120
?end

:look

ROW:
?all

MAX      20 A + 30 C
SUBJECT TO
   2)      A <=   60
   3)      C <=   50
   4)      A + 2 C <=    120
END
```

Notice how LINDO interprets the strict inequalities that we typed in, "<", as loose inequalities, "<=".

```
:go
   LP OPTIMUM FOUND AT STEP     3
       OBJECTIVE FUNCTION VALUE
1)             2100.00000

VARIABLE        VALUE        REDUCED COST
   A          60.000000          .000000
   C          30.000000          .000000

ROW       SLACK OR SURPLUS    DUAL PRICES
   2)              .000000        5.000000
   3)            20.000000         .000000
   4)              .000000       15.000000
```

```
NO. ITERATIONS=    3

DO RANGE (SENSITIVITY) ANALYSIS?
?no
```

2.3.2 Altering and Editing a Model

Depending upon which version of LINDO you have, there are two ways of modifying or editing a model: (a) use the ALTER command, (b) use the EDIT command. All versions of LINDO have the ALTER command. DOS versions of LINDO have the EDIT command.

2.3.3 Using the ALTER Command

This section illustrates the use of the ALTER command to do simple editing. The ALTER command is available in all versions of LINDO. Continuing where we left off, we might use the ALTER command as follows:

```
:alter
ROW:
1
VAR:
a
NEW COEFFICIENT:
?15

:look 1

MAX        15 A + 30 C

:go

   LP OPTIMUM FOUND AT STEP    2
        OBJECTIVE FUNCTION VALUE
   1)          1800.00000

VARIABLE            VALUE            REDUCED COST
    A            20.000000             .000000
    C            50.000000             .000000

ROW          SLACK OR SURPLUS        DUAL PRICES
   2)            40.000000             .000000
   3)              .000000             .000000
   4)              .000000           15.000000

NO. ITERATIONS=            2
```

Here is how you change a right-hand-side value:

```
:alter 3 rhs
NEW COEFFICIENT:
?30
:look 3

   3)    C <=   30
```

```
:go
   LP OPTIMUM FOUND AT STEP        0
       OBJECTIVE FUNCTION VALUE

    1)          1800.00000

VARIABLE        VALUE            REDUCED COST
   A          60.000000              .000000
   C          30.000000              .000000

ROW        SLACK OR SURPLUS        DUAL PRICES
   2)             .000000            5.000000
   3)             .000000             .000000
   4)             .000000           15.000000

NO.  ITERATIONS=              0

DO RANGE (SENSITIVITY) ANALYSIS?
?n
```

2.3.4 Using the EDIT Command

A full screen editor is available in the DOS version of LINDO. The full screen editor allows you to use the "arrow" keys to move the cursor about the screen. For most other keys, pressing that key will cause the character associated with that key to be inserted at the cursor position.

You access the editor by typing the command EDIT. The effects of special keys within the editor are summarized in the table below.

Key	Effect
→	Moves cursor right one character
←	Moves cursor left one character
↑	Moves cursor up one line
↓	Moves cursor down one line
Home	Moves cursor to beginning
End	Moves cursor to end
PageUp	Moves cursor up one screen
PageDown	Moves cursor down one screen
Ctrl S	Moves cursor to start of current line
Ctrl E	Moves cursor to end of current line
Ctrl →	Moves cursor to end of current word
Ctrl ←	Moves cursor to beginning of current word
Del	Deletes character at current cursor position
Enter	Inserts a carriage return at current cursor position
Ins	Inserts a carriage return at current cursor position
Backspace	Deletes character to the left of cursor
Esc	Exit the editor and try to interpret the edited model
Ctrl Break	Exit the editor without interpreting the edited model

2.3.5 Saving, Retrieving, and Printing Your Work

As you become more sophisticated, you may wish to save your work for future reference cr you may wish to print some of your results. The commands useful in this regard are:

Command	Use
SAVE	Save a problem onto disk (long term) storage
RETR	Retrieve a SAVE(d) problem
DIVERT	Divert output to disk or printer

We discuss these commands further in the following sections.

2.3.6 SAVE and RETRIEVE Commands

When we left off in our example session, things looked as follows:

```
:look all

MAX       15 A + 30 C
SUBJECT TO
    2)     A <=    60
    3)     C <=    30
    4)     A + 2 C <=     120
ENC
```

Suppose we are interested in saving this version of the problem. First, let's look at the HELP SAVE command:

```
:help save

SAVE COMMAND:

SAVES CURRENT MODEL IN A FILE IN CONDENSED LINDO FORMAT.
THE MODEL MAY BE RETRIEVED USING "RETR".
```

So let's try it . . .

```
:save
FILE NAME:
engins.lpk
```

(We arbitrarily use the suffix ".lpk" to identify files containing LINDO problems.) Let's alter the RHS back to the original version:

```
:alter 3 rhs
NEW COEFFICIENT
?5C
```

Now to check what we have done:

```
:look all

MAX       15 A + 30 C
SUBJECT TO
    2)    A <=    60
    3)    C <=    50
    4)    A + 2 C <=    120
END
```

Suppose we change our mind again and wish to retrieve the previous version. First, let's look at the HELP RETR command:

```
:help retr

RETRIEVE COMMAND

FETCHES A MODEL FROM DISK. LINDO WILL PROMPT YOU FOR A
SPECIFIC FILE NAME OR UNIT NUMBER. THE MODEL BEING
RETRIEVED MUST HAVE BEEN PREVIOUSLY SAVED VIA THE "SAVE"
COMMAND.

IF YOU HAVE A PC DOS VERSION OF LINDO YOU MAY INCLUDE THE
DOS WILDCARD CHARACTERS '*' AND '?' IN THE FILENAME TO BE
PRESENTED WITH A MENU OF FILES MATCHING THE SPECIFICATION.
```

If we type:

```
:retr *.lpk
```

we see a screen showing all files with the extension .LPK. If we highlight ENGINS. LPK with the cursor and press [ENTER], that's the file we get. To check . . .

```
:look all

MAX       15 A + 30 C
SUBJECT TO
    2)    A <=    60
    3)    C <=    30
    4)    A + 2 C <=    120
END
```

2.3.7 Diverting Output to a File or Printer

The DIVERT command allows us to send output to a file or printer. If we continue our example session:

```
:help divert

DIVERT COMMAND
```

```
YOU WILL BE ASKED FOR A FILE. ALL SUBSEQUENT HIGH VOLUME
OUTPUT, E.G. SOLUTION REPORTS, WILL BE DIVERTED TO THIS FILE
UNTIL A RVRT (REVERT) COMMAND IS GIVEN.

:dive
FILE NAME:
engins.lot
```

We arbitrarily use the suffix ".lot" to identify LINDO output files. Now, notice that the solution report seems to have disappeared!

```
:go

   LP OPTIMUM FOUND AT STEP      2
        OBJECTIVE FUNCTION VALUE

  1)           1800.00000

DO RANGE (SENSITIVITY) ANALYSIS?
?n
```

It was not displayed! Where did it go? It was sent to the file ENGINS.LOT. The RVRT (revert) command returns subsequent output to the screen.

```
:help rvrt

RVRT COMMAND:

CAUSES ALL SUBSEQUENT OUTPUT TO REVERT TO THE TERMINAL. IT
UNDOES THE EFFECT OF THE "DIVERT" COMMAND.

:rvrt
```

Alternatively on DOS machines, output can be sent directly to the printer by using a file name of PRN.

```
:dive
FILE NAME:
prn

:look all

:GO

   LP OPTIMUM FOUND AT STEP      2

        OBJECTIVE FUNCTION VALUE

  1)           1800.00000

DO RANGE (SENSITIVITY) ANALYSIS?
?n
:rvrt
```

Notice that neither the model formulation nor the solution appeared on the screen. Guess where they went. The following, however, would have appeared on the printer (if you had one attached).

```
MAX        15 A + 30 C
SUBJECT TO
    2)     A <=     60
    3)     C <=     30
    4)     A + 2 C <=      120
END
   LP OPTIMUM FOUND AT STEP    2

        OBJECTIVE FUNCTION VALUE

    1)          1800.00000

VARIABLE        VALUE           REDUCED COST
    A           60.000000            .000000
    C           30.000000            .000000

ROW        SLACK OR SURPLUS     DUAL PRICES
    2)              .000000         5.000000
    3)              .000000          .000000
    4)              .000000        15.000000

NO. ITERATIONS=         2
```

Once out of LINDO, you could discover that the file ENGINS.LOT contains the following.

```
       LP OPTIMUM FOUND AT STEP    2

        OBJECTIVE FUNCTION VALUE

    1)          1800.00000

VARIABLE        VALUE           REDUCED COST
    A           60.000000            .000000
    C           30.000000            .000000

ROW        SLACK OR SURPLUS     DUAL PRICES
    2)              .000000         5.000000
    3)              .000000          .000000
    4)              .000000        15.000000

NO. ITERATIONS=         2
```

On PC-DOS machines, you could display this file on the screen by typing:

```
type engins.lot
```

You could print the file by typing:

```
print engins.lot
```

Alternatively, on most computers you could incorporate the file contents into a document you are preparing with your favorite word processor. LINDO Divert files are in standard text format that can be imported into most word processors with commands such as "TEXT IN".

2.3.8 Integer Programming with LINDO

Fairly shortly after you start looking at problems for which LP might be applicable, you discover the need to restrict certain variables to integer values, i.e., 0, 1, 2, etc. Even though this violates the linearity requirement, LINDO allows you to identify such variables. We give an introductory treatment here. It is discussed more thoroughly in Chapter 14.

Integer variables in LINDO can be either 0/1 or general. Variables that are restricted to the values 0 or 1 are identified with the INTEGER command. It is used in one of two forms, examples of which are:

```
INTEGER x   or   INTEGER 8
```

The first (and recommended) form identifies variable x as being 0/1. The second form identifies the first 8 variables in the current formulation as being 0/1. The order of the variables is determined by their order encountered in the input. This order can be verified by observing the order of variables in the solution report.

The second form is more powerful, but it requires the user to be aware of the exact order of the variables. This may be confusing if not all variables appear in the objective.

The following example session illustrates the INT command:

```
:max 4 tom + 3 dick + 2 harry
?st
?2.5 tom + 3.1 harry < 5
?.2 tom + .7 dick + .4 harry < 1
?end

:int tom
:int dick
:int harry

:go

   LP OPTIMUM FOUND AT STEP 4

        OBJECTIVE FUNCTION VALUE

    1)              7.65898620

SET HARRY TO  <= 0  AT  1 BND=  7.0000000   TWIN= 7.4285715
NEW INTEGER SOLUTION AT BRANCH    1 PIVOT     6

        OBJECTIVE FUNCTION VALUE

    1)              7.0000000

BEST REMAINING SOLUTION NO BETTER THAN  7.428571

DELETE HARRY AT LEVEL        1
    ENUMERATION COMPLETE.   BRANCHES=  1   PIVOTS=     6
LAST INTEGER SOLUTION IS THE BEST FOUND

:solution

        OBJECTIVE FUNCTION VALUE

    1)              7.000000
```

```
VARIABLE         VALUE          REDUCED COST
   TOM           1.00000          -4.00000
   DICK          1.00000          -3.00000
   HARRY         0.00000          -2.00000

ROW         SLACK OR SURPLUS    DUAL PRICE
  2)            2.500000          0.00000
  3)            0.100000          0.00000
```

General integers, which can be 0, 1, 2, etc., are identified in analogous fashion by using `GIN` instead of `INT`, for example:

```
GIN TONIC    or    GIN 8
```

The first restricts variable TONIC to 0, 1, 2, 3, ... The second restricts the first eight variables to 0, 1, 2, 3, ...

The solution method used is branch and bound. It is an intelligent enumeration process that will find a sequence of better and better solutions. As each one is found, a short message will be displayed, giving the objective value and a bound on how good a solution might still remain. After the enumeration is complete, the `SOLUTION` (or the `NONZEROES`, `CPRI` or `RPRI`) command can be used to reveal information about the best solution found.

Let's look at a slightly modified version of the original Enginola problem and see how the `GIN` command might help.

```
:look all

MAX      20 A + 30 C
SUBJECT TO
    2)    A <=    60
    3)    C <=    50
    4)    A + 2 C <=     115
END
```

Notice the capacity of 115 on the labor constraint (Row 4).

```
:go

    LP OPTIMUM FOUND AT STEP      3

         OBJECTIVE FUNCTION VALUE
    1)        2025.00000

VARIABLE        VALUE          REDUCED COST
   A          60.000000          .000000
   C          27.500000          .000000

ROW        SLACK OR SURPLUS     DUAL PRICES
  2)            .000000          5.000000
  3)          22.500000           .000000
  4)            .000000         15.000000

NO. ITERATIONS=          3

DO RANGE (SENSITIVITY ANALYSIS)?
?n
```

Note that a fractional quantity is recommended for C. If fractional quantities are undesirable, declare A and C as general integer variables:

```
:gin a
:gin c

:look all

MAX       20 A + 30 C
SUBJECT TO
   2)    A <=  60
   3)    C <=  50
   4)    A + 2 C <=    115
END

GIN        2
```

The GIN 2 means the first two variables, A and C, are to be integer.

```
:GO

LP OPTIMUM FOUND AT STEP    0
OBJECTIVE VALUE =   2025.00000

SET        C TO    >=  28 AT    1, BND= 2020.   TWIN= 2010.    3

NEW INTEGER SOLUTION OF 2020.00000   AT BRANCH 1   PIVOT  3

           OBJECTIVE FUNCTION VALUE

   1)         2020.00000

VARIABLE      VALUE          REDUCED COST
   A          59.000000          .000000
   C          28.000000        10.000000

ROW      SLACK OR SURPLUS    DUAL PRICES
   2)          1.000000          .000000
   3)         22.000000          .000000
   4)           .000000        20.000000

NO. ITERATIONS=            3
BRANCHES=    1 DETERM.=   1.000E    0
BOUND ON OPTIMUM:   2020.000

DELETE          C AT LEVEL    1

ENUMERATION COMPLETE. BRANCHES=    1 PIVOTS=    3
LAST INTEGER SOLUTION IS THE BEST FOUND
RE-INSTALLING BEST SOLUTION . . .
```

The SOLUTION command can be used whenever we need to see the current solution.

```
:help solution

SOLUTION COMMAND:

PRINTS STANDARD SOLUTION REPORT. TO SEND IT TO DISK, SEE
THE "DIVERT" COMMAND. TO GET AN ABBREVIATED REPORT SEE
```

```
THE "NONZ", "CPRI" AND "RPRI" COMMANDS.
:solution
         OBJECTIVE FUNCTION VALUE
   1)         2020.00000
   VARIABLE        VALUE           REDUCED COST
     A          59.000000           20.000000
     C          28.000000           30.000000
   ROW        SLACK OR SURPLUS      DUAL PRICES
    2)             1.000000           .000000
    3)            22.000000           .000000
    4)              .000000           .000000
   NO. ITERATIONS=        4
   BRANCHES=     1 DETERM.= 1.000E      0
```

Although the integer programming (IP) capability is very powerful, it requires skill to use effectively. It is very easy to prepare a bad formulation for an essentially easy problem. A bad formulation may require intolerable amounts of computer time to solve. Therefore you should have access to someone who is experienced in IP formulations if you plan to make use of the IP capability. LINDO, however, will cut short the IP solution process if it appears to be taking too long. Thus, the novice is protected somewhat against the cost of solving a poor formulation. Good formulations of integer programs are discussed further in Chapter 14.

2.3.9 Scaling and Other Numerical Considerations

You should avoid using extremely small or extremely large numbers in a formulation; e.g., you should not measure weight in ounces one place and volume in cubic miles someplace else in the same problem. A rule of thumb is that there should be no nonzero coefficient whose absolute value is greater than 100,000 or less than 0.0001. If LINDO feels that the matrix is poorly scaled, it will print a warning.

2.3.10 Getting Help

There are three Command line commands for helping the user get more information on LINDO: HELP, CATEGORIES (or CAT for short), and COMMANDS (or COM). COM will simply list all the commands available, grouped into categories according to use, e.g., input, output, etc. HELP followed by a command name will describe the specified command. HELP by itself gives general information. CAT will list only the categories and then allow one to list the commands in a specific category. The following illustrates:

```
:cat

LINDO  COMMANDS BY CATEGORY.  FOR INFORMATION
ON A SPECIFIC COMMAND, TYPE:  HELP FOLLOWED BY
```

```
THE COMMAND NAME.
  1) INFORMATION
  2) INPUT
  3) DISPLAY
  4) FILE OUTPUT
  5) SOLUTION
  6) PROBLEM EDITING
  7) QUIT
  8) INTEGER, QUADRATIC, AND PARAMETRIC PROGRAMS
  9) CONVERSATIONAL PARAMETERS
 10) USER SUPPLIED ROUTINES
 11) MISCELLANEOUS

WHICH CATEGORY IS OF INTEREST (1 TO 11)?
?5

THE COMMANDS IN THIS CATEGORY ARE:
     GO      PIV

WHICH CATEGORY IS OF INTEREST (1 TO 11)?
?0

:help go

GO COMMAND

USE: SOLVES THE CURRENT MODEL. THE MODEL REMAINS INTACT THROUGH
THE SOLUTION PROCESS. A POSITIVE INTEGER TYPED AFTER GO IS
INTERPRETED AS AN UPPER LIMIT ON THE NUMBER OF PIVOTS.
```

2.3.11 Command Line Commands

The commands available from the command line in LINDO (for Unix and DOS versions) are as follows, by category:

1. *Information*

CAT	Lists categories of commands
COM	Lists commands by category
DATE	Display current date and time
HELP	Gives help in various situations
LOCAL	Gives info specific to your local installation
TIME	Display compute time used

2. *Input*

FBR	Retrieve a basis saved with FBS command
FINS	Retrieve a basis saved with FPUN command
LEAVE	Undo the previous TAKE
MAX	Start natural input
MIN	Start natural input
RDBC	Retrieve old solution from file
RETR	Retrieve old problem from file
RMPS	Retrieve an MPS format file
TAKE	Take terminal input from a file

3. *Display*

BPICTURE	Print logical PICTURE of basis
CPRI	Print column information
DMPS	Create a detailed MPS format solution report
LOOK	Print (part of) problem in natural format
NONZEROES	Print nonzero variables solution report
PICTURE	Print logical PICTURE of matrix
RANGE	Print RANGE analysis report
RPRI	Print row information
SHOCOLUMN	Display a column of the problem
SOLUTION	Print standard solution report
TABLEAU	Print current tableau

4. *File output*

DIVERT	Divert output to file
RVRT	Revert output to terminal
SAVE	Save current problem to file
SDBC	Save solution in database format
SMPS	Save current problem in MPS format

5. *Solution*

GLEX	Solve the problem for multiple objectives
GO	Go solve the problem
PIVOT	Do the next simplex pivot

6. *Problem editing*

ALTER	Alter an element of current problem with prompts from LINDO
APPC	Append a new column to the formulation
DEL	Delete a specified constraint
EDIT	Full screen editor with cursor keys controlling the cursor (DOS versions only)
EXT	Extend problem by adding constraints
FREE	Declare a variable unconstrained in sign
SLB	Enter a simple lower bound for a variable
SUB	Enter a simple upper bound for a variable

7. *Integer, quadratic, and parametric programs*

BIP	Set IP bound on optimal solution
GIN	Identify general integer variables
INT	Identify integer variables
IPTOL	Set IP tolerance on optimal solution
PARA	Parametric programming
POSD	Check positive definiteness
QCP	Quadratic programming
TITAN	Tighten an IP

8. *Conversational parameters*

!	Insert a comment
BATCH	Tell LINDO that this is a batch run

PAGE	Set page/screen size
PAUSE	Pause for keyboard action
TERSE	Set conversational style to terse
VERBOSE	Set conversational style to verbose (default)
WIDTH	Set terminal width

9. *User supplied subroutines*

| USER | Call user written subroutine |

10. *Miscellaneous*

BUG	What to do if you find a bug
DEBUG	Help debug an infeasible model
INVERT	Invert current basis to get more accurate answers
SET	Set solution parameters
STAT	Print matrix summary statistics
TITLE	Display or change problem title

11. *Quit*

| QUIT | Quit |

2.4 PROBLEMS

Problem 1

Recall the Enginola problem of the previous chapter. Suppose we add the restriction that only an even number, 0, 2, 4, . . . , of Cosmos are allowed. Show how to exploit the GIN command to represent this feature.

Problem 2

Using your favorite text editor, enter the Enginola formulation. Save it as a simple, unformatted text file. Start up LINDO and use the TAKE command to read in the model prepared with your text editor.

Problem 3

Continuing from (2), use LINDO to prepare an output file containing both the formulation and the solution.

Sensitivity Analysis of LP Solutions

3.1 Economic Analysis of Solution Reports

A substantial amount of interesting economic information can be gleaned from the solution report of a model. In addition, optional reports such as range analysis can provide further information. The usual use of this information is to do quick "what if" analysis. The typical kinds of what if questions are:

(a) What would be the effect of increasing a capacity or demand?

(b) What if a new opportunity becomes available? Is it a worthwhile opportunity?

3.2 Economic Relationship Between Dual Prices and Reduced Costs

The reader hungering for unity in systems may convince himself or herself that a reduced cost is really a dual price born under the wrong sign. Under our convention, the reduced cost of a variable x is really the dual price with the sign reversed on the constraint $x \geq 0$. Recall that the reduced cost of the variable x measures the rate at which the solution value deteriorates as x is increased from zero. The dual price on $x \geq 0$ measures the rate at which the solution value improves as the right-hand side (and thus x) is increased from zero.

Our knowledge about reduced costs and dual prices can be restated as follows:

Reduced cost of an (unused) activity: amount by which profits will decrease if one unit of this activity is forced into the solution.

Dual price of a constraint: amount by which profits will decrease if the availability of the resource associated with this constraint is reduced by one unit.

We shall argue and illustrate that the reduced cost of an activity is really its net opportunity cost if we "cost out" the activity using the dual prices as charges for resource usage. This sounds like good economic sense. If one unit of an activity is forced into the solution, it effectively reduces the availability of the resources it uses. These resources have an imputed value by way of the dual prices; therefore, the activity should be charged for the value used. Let's look at an example and check if the argument works.

3.2.1 The Costing Out Operation: An Illustration

Suppose that Enginola is considering adding a video recorder to its product line. Market Research and Engineering estimate the direct profit contribution of a video recorder as $47 per unit. It would be manufactured on the Astro line and would require 3 hours of labor. If it is produced, it will force the reduction of both Astro production (because it competes for a production line) and Cosmo production (because it competes for labor). Is this tradeoff worthwhile? It looks promising. It makes more dollars per hour of labor than a Cosmo, and it makes more efficient use of Astro capacity than Astros. Recall that the dual prices on the Astro capacity and the labor capacity in the original solution were $5 and $15. If we add this variable to the model, it would have a +47 in the objective function, a +1 in row 2 (the Astro capacity constraint), and a +3 in row 4 (the labor capacity constraint). We can "cost out" an activity or decision variable by charging it for the use of scarce resources. What prices should be charged? The obvious prices to use are the dual prices. The +47 profit contribution can be thought of as a negative cost. The costing out calculations can be arrayed as in the little table below:

Row	Coefficient	Dual Price	Charge
1	47	−47	−47
2	1	+5	+5
3	0	0	0
4	3	45	+45

Total opportunity cost = +3

Thus, a video recorder has an opportunity cost of $3. A −1 is applied to the 47 profit contribution because a profit contribution is effectively a negative cost. The video recorder's net cost is positive, so it is apparently not worth producing.

The analysis could be stopped at this point, but out of curiosity we'll formulate the relevant LP and solve it. If V = number of video recorders to produce, then we wish to solve:

```
MAX        20 A + 30 C + 47 V
SUBJECT TO
    2)      A +             V <=   60
    3)              C             <=   50
    4)      A + 2 C + 3 V <= 120
```

The solution is:

```
          OBJECTIVE FUNCTION VALUE
    1)           2100.000
```

```
VARIABLE        VALUE              REDUCED COST
    A          60.000000              0.000000
    C          30.000000              0.000000
    V           0.000000              3.000000

  ROW           SLACK              DUAL PRICES
    2)           0.000000              5.000000
    3)          20.000000              0.000000
    4)           0.000000             15.000000
```

Video recorders are not produced, and notice that the reduced cost of *V* is $3, the value we computed when we "costed out" *V*. This is an illustration of the following relationship:

> *The reduced cost of an activity equals the weighted sum of its resource usage rates minus its profit contribution rate, where the weights applied are the dual prices. A "min" objective is treated as having a dual price of +1, and a "max" objective is treated as having a dual price of −1 in the costing-out process.*

3.3 Range of Validity of Reduced Costs and Dual Prices

In describing reduced costs and dual prices, we have been careful to limit the changes to "small" changes; e.g., if the dual price of a constraint is $3/hour, increasing the number of hours available will improve profits by $3 for each of the first few hours (possibly less than one) added. In general, however, this improvement rate will not hold forever. We might expect that as we make more hours of capacity available, the value (i.e., the dual price) of these hours would not increase and might decrease. This might not be true for all situations, but for LPs it is true that increasing the right-hand side of a constraint cannot cause the constraint's dual price to increase. The dual price can only stay the same or decrease.

As we change the right-hand side of an LP, the optimal values of the decision variables may change; however, the dual prices and reduced costs will not change as long as the "character" of the optimal solution does not change. We will say that the character changes (mathematicians say the basis changes) when either the set of nonzero variables or the set of binding constraints (i.e., having zero slack) changes. In summary, as we alter the right-hand side, the same dual prices apply as long as the "character" or "basis" does not change.

Most LP programs will optionally supplement the solution report with a range or sensitivity analysis report, which indicates the amounts by which individual right-hand side or objective function coefficients can be changed unilaterally without affecting the character or "basis" of the optimal solution. Recall the previous model:

```
MAX        20 A + 30 C + 47 V
SUBJECT TO
          A +        V <=   60
               C       <=   50
          A + 2C + 3V <=  120
END
```

The sensitivity report for this problem appears below:

```
DO RANGE (SENSITIVITY) ANALYSIS?
>y
            RANGES IN WHICH THE BASIS IS UNCHANGED
                 OBJ COEFFICIENT RANGES
     VARIABLE        CURRENT       ALLOWABLE       ALLOWABLE
                      COEF         INCREASE        DECREASE
        A           20.00000       INFINITY        5.000000
        C           30.00000       10.000000       30.000000
        V           47.00000       3.000000        INFINITY

                 RIGHTHAND SIDE RANGES
       ROW          CURRENT        ALLOWABLE       ALLOWABLE
                      RHS          INCREASE        DECREASE
        2           60.00000       60.000000       40.00000
        3           50.00000       INFINITY        20.00000
        4          120.00000       40.000000       60.00000
```

Again, we find two sections, one for variables and the second for rows or constraints. The 5 in the A row of the report means that the profit contribution of A could be decreased by up to \$5/unit without affecting the optimal amount of A and C to produce. This is plausible because Astros currently make more efficient use of labor, \$20 per 1 hour vs. \$30 per 2 hours for Cosmos. If the profit contribution of an Astro were reduced by \$5, to \$15 per unit, the two would make equally efficient use of labor and one would be willing to increase Cosmo production at the expense of Astros until the slack of row 3 (the constraint $C \geq 50$) went to zero (or "departed"). The INFINITY in the same section of the report means that increasing the profitability of A by any positive amount would have no effect on the optimal amount of A and C to produce. This is intuitive because we are already producing As to their upper limit.

The "allowable decrease" of 30 for variable C means that the profitability of C could be reduced by \$30/unit (i.e., to zero) without changing the optimal solution. This makes sense because at the moment Cosmo production is made simply to make profitable use of any labor left over from Astro production. The 10 in the C's row means that the profitability of C would have to be increased by at least \$10/unit (thus to \$40/unit) before we would consider changing the values of A and C. Notice that at \$40/unit for Cs, the profit per hour of labor is the same for both A and C.

In general, *if the objective function coefficient* of a single variable *is changed within the range* specified in the first section of the range report, *the optimal values of the decision variables, A, C, and V in this case, will not change.* The dual prices, reduced cost and profitability of the solution, however, may change.

In a complementary sense, *if the right-hand side* of a single constraint *is changed within the range* specified in the second section of the range report, *the optimal values of the dual prices and reduced costs will not change.* The values of the decision variables and the profitability of the solution, however, may change.

For example, the second section tells us that if the right-hand side of row 3 (the constraint $C \geq 50$) is decreased by more than 20, the dual prices and reduced costs will change. The constraint will then be $C \geq 30$ and the character of the solution changes in that the labor constraint will no longer be binding. The right-hand side of this constraint ($C \geq 50$) could be increased, according to the range report, an infinite amount without affecting the optimal dual prices and reduced costs. This makes sense because there already is excess capacity on the Cosmo line, so adding more capacity should have no effect.

Let us illustrate some of these concepts by resolving our three-variable problem with the amount of labor reduced by 61 hours down to 59 hours. The formulation and the solution are:

```
MAX       20 A + 30 C + 47 V
SUBJECT TO
    2)        A +            V  <=  60
    3)             C              <=  50
    4)        A  + 2 C  + 3 V  <=  59
END

:GO

     LP OPTIMUM FOUND AT STEP     1
          OBJECTIVE FUNCTION VALUE

     1)        1180.000
VARIABLE        VALUE           REDUCED COST
   A          59.000000             0.000000
   C           0.000000            10.000000
   V           0.000000            13.000000

ROW            SLACK            DUAL  PRICES
   2)         1.000000             0.000000
   3)        50.000000             0.000000
   4)         0.000000            20.000000

        RANGES  IN  WHICH  THE  BASIS  IS  UNCHANGED
              OBJ  COEFFICIENT  RANGES
VARIABLE        CURRENT          ALLOWABLE         ALLOWABLE
                COEF             INCREASE          DECREASE
   A          20.000000          INFINITY          5.000000
   C          30.000000          10.000000         INFINITY
   V          47.000000          13.000000         INFINITY

              RIGHTHAND  SIDE  RANGES
ROW             CURRENT          ALLOWABLE         ALLOWABLE
                RHS              INCREASE          DECREASE
   2          60.00000           INFINITY          1.00000
   3          50.00000           INFINITY          50.00000
   4          59.00000           1.000000          59.00000
```

First of all, note that with the reduced labor supply we no longer produce any Cosmos. Their reduced cost is now $10/unit, which means that if their profitability were increased by $10 to $40/unit, we would start considering their production again. At $40/unit for Cosmos, both products make equally efficient use of labor.

Also notice that, because the right-hand side of the labor constraint has been reduced by more than 60, most of the dual prices and reduced costs have changed. In particular, the dual price or marginal value of labor is now $20 per hour. This is because an additional hour of labor would be used to produce one more $20 Astro. You should be able to convince yourself that the marginal value of labor behaves as follows:

Labor Available	Dual Price	Reason
0 tc 60 hours	$20/hour	Each additional hour will be used to produce one $20 Astro.
60 to 160 hours	$15/hour	Each additional hour will be used to produce half a $30 Cosmo.
160 to 280 hours	$13.5/hour	Give up half an Astro and add half of a V for profit of 0.5 (−20 + 47).
More than 280 hours	$0	No use for additional labor.

In general, the dual price on any constraint will behave in the above stepwise decreasing fashion.

Figures 3.1 and 3.2 give a global view of how total profit is affected by changing either a single objective coefficient or a single right-hand side. The artists in the audience may wish to note that for a maximization problem:

(a) Optimal total profit as a function of a single objective coefficient always has a bowl shape. Mathematicians say it is a convex function.
(b) Optimal total profit as a function of a single right-hand-side value always has an inverted bowl shape. Mathematicians say it is a concave function.

For some problems, as in Figures 3.1 and 3.2, we only see half of the bowl. For minimization problems, the orientation of the bowl in (a) and (b) is simply reversed. When we solve a problem for a particular objective coefficient or right-hand-side value, we obtain a single point on one of these curves. A range report gives us the endpoints of the line segment on which this one point lies.

3.3.1 Predicting the Effect of Simultaneous Changes in Parameters—The 100% Rule

The information in the range analysis report tells us the effect of changing a single cost or resource parameter. For example, here is the range report for the Enginola problem:

```
          RANGES IN WHICH THE BASIS IS UNCHANGED
                    OBJ COEFFICIENT RANGES
  VARIABLE        CURRENT        ALLOWABLE        ALLOWABLE
                    COEF          INCREASE         DECREASE
    A           20.000000        INFINITY          5.00000
    C           30.000000        60.00000         30.00000

                    RIGHTHAND SIDE RANGES
   RCW            CURRENT        ALLOWABLE        ALLOWABLE
                    RHS           INCREASE         DECREASE
    2            60.00000        60.000000        40.000000
    3            50.00000        INFINITY         20.000000
    4           120.00000        40.000000        60.000000
```

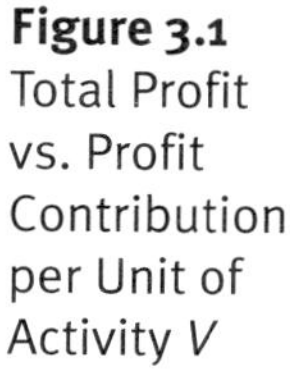

Figure 3.1
Total Profit
vs. Profit
Contribution
per Unit of
Activity *V*

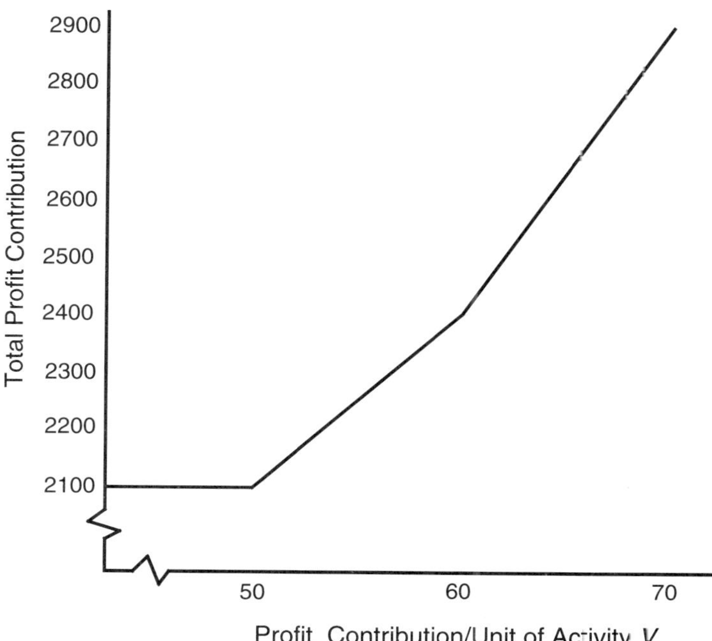

Figure 3.2
Profit as Labor
Available
Increases

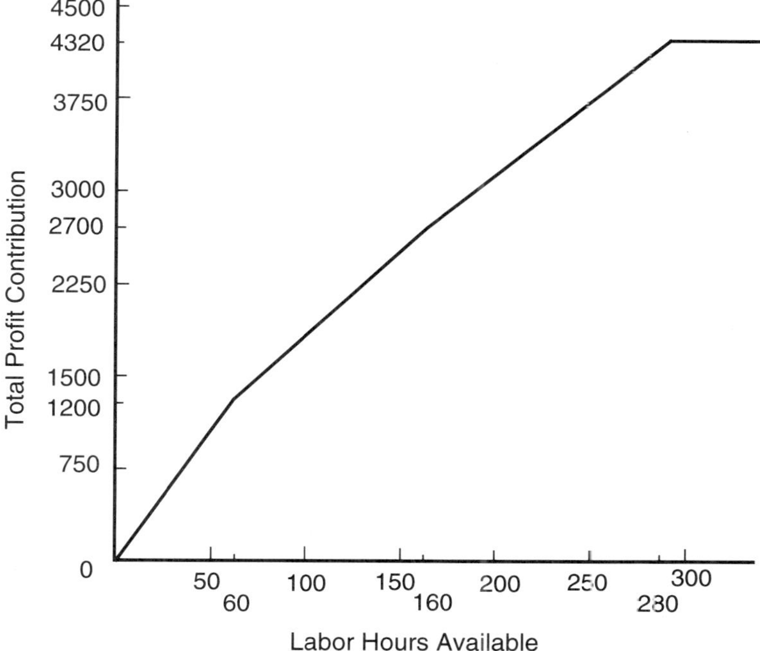

The report indicates that the profit contribution of an Astro could be decreased by as much as $5/unit without changing the basis. In this case, this means that the optimal solution would still recommend producing 60 Astros and 30 Cosmos.

Now suppose that in order to meet competition, we're considering lowering the price of an Astro by $3/unit and the price of a Cosmo by $10/unit. Will it still be profitable to produce the same mix? Individually, each of these changes would not change the solution because $3 < 5$ and $10 < 30$.

But it is not clear that these two changes can be made simultaneously. What does your intuition suggest as a rule describing the simultaneous changes which don't change the basis (mix)?

The 100% Rule. You can think of the allowable ranges as slack that may be used up in changing parameters. It is a fact that any combination of changes will not change the basis if the sum of percentages of slack used sums to less than 100%. For the simultaneous changes we are contemplating, we have:

$$\left(\frac{3}{5}\right) \times 100 + \left(\frac{10}{30}\right) \times 100 = 60\% + 33.3\% = 93.3\% < 100\%$$

This satisfies the condition, so the changes can be made without changing the basis. Bradley, Hax, and Magnanti (1977) have dubbed this rule the 100% rule. Because the value of A and C do not change, we can calculate the effect on profits of these changes as $-3 \times 60 - 10 \times 30 = -480$. So the new profit will be $2100 - 480 = 1620$.

The altered formulation and its solution are:

```
MAX        17 A + 20 C
SUBJECT TO
    2)      A           <=   60
    3)              C <=   50
    4)      A + 2 C <= 120
END
            OBJECTIVE FUNCTION VALUE

    1)          1620.000

VARIABLE        VALUE           REDUCED COST
    A           60.000000           0.000000
    C           30.000000           0.000000

ROW             SLACK           DUAL PRICES
    2)           0.000000           7.000000
    3)          20.000000           0.000000
    4)           0.000000          10.000000
```

3.4 Sensitivity Analysis of the Constraint Coefficients

Sensitivity analysis of the right-hand-side and objective function coefficients is somewhat easy to understand, because the objective function value changes linearly with modest changes in these coefficients. Unfortunately, the objective function value may change nonlinearly with changes in constraint coefficients. There is, however, a very simple formula for approximating the effect of small changes in constraint coefficients. Suppose we wish to examine the effect of decreasing by a small amount e the coefficient of variable j in row i of the LP. The formula is:

$$(\text{improvement in objective value}) = (\text{value of variable } j) \times (\text{dual price of row } i) \times e$$

Example: Consider the problem:

```
MAX        20 A + 30 C
SUBJECT TO
     2)      A          <=    65
     3)            C <=    50
     4)      A + 2 C <= 115
END
```

With solution:

```
     LP OPTIMUM FOUND

          OBJECTIVE FUNCTION VALUE
     1)            2050.000

     VARIABLE       VALUE           REDUCED COST
     A              65.000000           0.000000
     C              25.000000           0.000000

     ROW            SLACK           DUAL PRICES
     2)              0.000000           5.000000
     3)             25.000000           0.000000
     4)              0.000000          15.000000
```

Now suppose that it is discovered that the coefficient of C in row 4 should have been 2.01 rather than 2. The formula implies that the objective value should be decreased by approximately $25 \times 15 \times .01 = 3.75$.

The actual objective value when this altered problem is solved is 2046.269, so the actual decrease in objective value is 3.731.

The formula for the effect of a small change in constraint coefficient makes sense. If the change in coefficient is small, the values of all the variables and dual prices should remain essentially unchanged. So the net effect of changing the 2 to a 2.01 in our problem is to effectively try to use $25 \times .01$ additional hours of labor. So there is effectively $25 \times .01$ fewer hours available. But we've seen that labor is worth $15 per hour, so the change in profits should be about $25 \times .01 \times 15$, which is in agreement with the original formula.

This type of sensitivity analysis gives some guidance in identifying which coefficient should be accurately estimated. If the product of variable j's value and row i's dual price is relatively large, the coefficient in row i for variable j should be accurately estimated if an accurate estimate of total profit is desired.

3.5 The Dual LP Problem, or the Landlord and the Renter

You will probably discover as you formulate models for various problems that there are several rather different looking formulations for the same problem. Each formulation may be correct and may be based on taking a different perspective on the problem. An interesting mathematical fact is that for LP problems, there are always two formulations (more accurately, a multiple of two) to a problem. One formulation is arbitrarily called the primal, and the other is referred to as the dual. The two different formulations arise from two different perspectives that one can take toward a problem. One can think of these two perspectives as the landlord's and the renter's perspectives.

In order to motivate things, consider the following situations. Some textile "manufacturers" in Italy own no manufacturing facilities but simply rent time as needed from firms that own the appropriate equipment. In the U.S., a similar situation exists in the recycling of some products. Firms that recycle old telephone cable may simply rent time on the stripping machines that are needed to separate the copper from the insulation. This rental process is sometimes called "tolling." In the perfume industry, many of the owners of well-known brands of perfume own no manufacturing facilities, but simply rent time from certain chemical formulation companies to have the perfumes produced as needed. The basic feature of this form of industrial organization is that the owner of the manufacturing resources never owns either the raw materials or the finished product.

Now suppose you want to produce a product that can use the manufacturing resources of the famous Enginola company, manufacturer of Astros, Cosmos, and Video Recorders. You would thus like to rent production capacity from Enginola. You need to deduce initial reasonable hourly rates to offer to Enginola for each of its three resources, Astro line capacity, Cosmo line capacity, and labor. These three hourly rates are your decision variables. You in fact would like to rent all the capacity on each of the three resources; thus you want to minimize the total charge from renting the entire capacities (60, 50, and 120). If your offer is to succeed, you know that your hourly rates must be sufficiently high so that none of Enginola's products are worth producing; e.g., the rental fees foregone by producing an Astro should be greater than 20. These "it's better to rent" conditions constitute the constraints.

We will formulate a model for this problem as follows. Define:

PA = price per unit to be offered for Astro line capacity,

PC = price per unit to be offered for Cosmo line capacity,

PL = price per unit to be offered for labor capacity.

Then the appropriate model is:

The Dual Problem

```
MIN     60 PA + 50 PC  + 120 PL
  ASTRO)    PA              +      PL >= 20;
  COSMO)             PC  +    2 PL >= 30;
  VR)       PA +     PC  +    3 PL >= 47;
END
```

The three constraints force the prices to be high enough so that it is not profitable for Enginola to produce any of its products.

The solution is:

```
             OBJECTIVE FUNCTION VALUE

    1)               2100.000              1.000000

    VARIABLE          VALUE            REDUCED COST
      PA            5.000000              0.000000
      PC            0.000000             20.000000
      PL           15.000000              0.000000

    ROW          SLACK OR SURPLUS        DUAL PRICES
     ASTRO)         0.000000            -60.00000
     COSMO)         0.000000            -30.00000
     VR)            3.000000              0.00000
```

Recall that the original, three-product Enginola problem was:

The Primal Problem

```
MAX        20 A + 30 C + 47 V
SUBJECT TO
    2)        A +           V <=    60
    3)              C             <=    50
    4)        A + 2 C + 3 V <= 120
```

with solution:

```
             OBJECTIVE FUNCTION VALUE

    1)               2100.000

    VARIABLE          VALUE            REDUCED COST
      A            60.000000              0.000000
      C            30.000000              0.000000
      V             0.000000              3.000000

    ROW             SLACK               DUAL PRICES
     2)             0.000000              5.000000
     3)            20.000000              0.000000
     4)             0.000000             15.000000
```

Notice that the two solutions are essentially the same, except that prices and decision variables are reversed. In particular, note that the price the renter should pay is exactly the same as Enginola's original profit contribution. This "Minimize the rental cost of the resources, subject to all activities being unprofitable" model is said to be the dual problem of the original "Maximize the total profit, subject to not exceeding any resource availabilities" model. The equivalence between the two solutions shown above always holds. Upon closer scrutiny, you should also notice that the dual formulation is essentially the primal formulation "stood on its ear," or its transpose, in fancier terminology.

Why might the dual model be of interest? The computational difficulty of an LP is approximately proportional to m^2n, where m = number of rows and n = number of columns. If the number of rows in the dual is substantially smaller than the number of rows in the primal, then one may prefer to solve the dual.

Additionally, certain constraints, such as simple upper bounds, e.g., $x \leq 1$, are computationally less expensive than arbitrary constraints. If the dual contains only a small number of arbitrary constraints, it may be easier to solve the dual even though it may have a large number of simple constraints.

The term *dual price* arose because the marginal price information to which this term is applied is a decision variable value in the dual problem.

We can summarize the idea of dual problems as follows. If the original or primal problem has a Maximize objective with $\leq$ constraints, its dual has a Minimize objective with $\geq$ constraints. The dual has one variable for each constraint in the primal and one constraint for each variable in the primal. The objective coefficient of the kth variable of the dual is the right-hand side of the kth constraint in the primal. The right-hand side of constraint k in the dual is equal to the objective coefficient of variable k in the primal. Similarly, the coefficient in row i of variable j in the dual is equal to the coefficient in row j of variable i in the primal.

In order to convert all constraints in a problem to the same type so that one can apply the above, note the following two transformations:

1. The constraint $2x + 3y = 5$ is equivalent to the two constraints $2x + 3y \geq 5$ and $2x + 3y \leq 5$;
2. The constraint $2x + 3y \geq 5$ is equivalent to $-2x - 3y \leq -5$.

Example

Write the dual of the following problem:

$$
\begin{array}{lll}
\text{Maximize} & 4x - 2y \\
\text{subject to} & 2x + 6y \leq 12 \\
& 3x - 2y = 1 \\
& 4x + 2y \geq 5.
\end{array}
$$

Using transformations (1) and (2) above we can rewrite this as

$$
\begin{array}{lll}
\text{Maximize} & 4x - 2y \\
\text{subject to} & 2x + 6y \leq 12 \\
& 3x - 2y \leq 1 \\
& -3x + 2y \leq -1 \\
& -4x - 2y \leq -5.
\end{array}
$$

Introducing the dual variables r, s, t, and u, corresponding to the four constraints, we can write the dual as

$$
\begin{array}{lll}
\text{Minimize} & 12r + s - t - 5u \\
\text{subject to} & 2r + 3s - 3t - 4u \geq 4 \\
& 6r - 2s + 2t - 2u \geq -2.
\end{array}
$$

3.6 PROBLEMS

Problem 1

The Enginola Company is considering introducing a new TV set, the Quasi. The expected profit contribution is $25 per unit. This unit is produced on the Astro line. Production of one Quasi requires 1.6 hours of labor. Using only the original solution below, determine whether it is worthwhile to produce any Quasis, assuming no change in labor and Astro line capacity.

The original Enginola problem with solution is below.

```
MAX       20 A + 30 C
SUBJECT TO
    2)        A          <=   60
    3)             C <=   50
    4)        A + 2 C <=   120
END

:go
   LP OPTIMUM FOUND AT STEP       3

         OBJECTIVE FUNCTION VALUE

  1)            2100.000

VARIABLE        VALUE          REDUCED COST
   A          60.000000          0.000000
   C          30.000000          0.000000

ROW             SLACK          DUAL PRICES
   2)          0.000000          5.000000
   3)         20.000000          0.000000
   4)          0.000000         15.000000
```

Problem 2

The Judson Corporation has acquired 100 lots on which it is about to build homes. Two styles of homes are to be built, the "Cape Cod" and the "Ranch Home." Judson wishes to build these 100 homes over the next nine months. During this time, Judson will have available 13,000 person-hours of bricklayer labor and 12,000 hours of carpenter labor. Each Cape Cod house requires 200 person-hours of carpentry labor and 50 person-hours of bricklayer labor. Each Ranch Home requires 120 hours of bricklayer labor and 100 person-hours of carpentry. The profit contribution of a Cape Cod is projected to be $5,100, while that of a Ranch Home is projected at $5,000. The problem when formulated as an LP and solved is as follows:

```
MAX       5100 C + 5000 R
SUBJECT TO
    2)        C +       R <=    100
    3)    200 C + 100 R <= 12000
    4)     50 C + 120 R <= 13000
END
```

```
LP OPTIMUM FOUND

        OBJECTIVE FUNCTION VALUE

  1)           502000.000

      VARIABLE          VALUE          REDUCED COST
         C            20.000000          0.000000
         R            80.000000          0.000000

      ROW               SLACK          DUAL PRICES
       2)             0.000000        4900.000000
       3)             0.000000           1.000000
       4)          2400.000000           0.000000


     RANGES IN WHICH THE BASIS IS UNCHANGED
          OBJ COEFFICIENT RANGES

   VARIABLE        CURRENT         ALLOWABLE        ALLOWABLE
                    COEF           INCREASE         DECREASE
      C          5100.000000     4900.000000      100.000000
      R          5000.000000      100.000000     2450.000000

          RIGHTHAND SIDE RANGES
   ROW            CURRENT         ALLOWABLE        ALLOWABLE
                   RHS            INCREASE         DECREASE
    2           100.00000         12.631579       40.000000
    3         12000.00000       8000.00000      2000.000000
    4         13000.00000         INFINITY      2400.000000
```

(a) A gentleman who owns 15 vacant lots adjacent to Judson's 100 lots needs
some money quickly and offers to sell his 15 lots for $60,000. Should Jud-
son buy? What assumptions are you making?

(b) One of Judson's salesmen who is a native of Massachusetts feels certain
that he could sell the Cape Cods for $2,000 more each than Judson is cur-
rently projecting. Should Judson change its planned mix of homes? What
assumptions are inherent in your recommendation?

Problem 3

Jack Mazzola, an industrial engineer with the Enginola Company, has discovered a
way of reducing the amount of labor used in the manufacture of a Cosmo TV set
from 2 hours per set to 1.92 hours per set by replacing one of the assembled portions
of the set with an integrated circuit chip. It is not clear at the moment what this chip
will cost. Based solely on the solution report below (i.e., do not solve another LP),
answer the following questions:

(a) Assuming that labor supply is fixed in the short run, what is the approxi-
mate value of one of these chips in the short run?

(b) Give an estimate of the approximate increase in profit contribution per day
of this change, exclusive of chip cost.

```
MAX        20 A + 30 C
SUBJECT TO
    2)     A          <=   60
    3)              C <=   50
    4)     A + 2 C <= 120
            OBJECTIVE FUNCTION VALUE
  1)            2100.000000

     VARIABLE          VALUE           REDUCED COST
        A            60.000000            0.000000
        C            30.000000            0.000000

       ROW            SLACK            DUAL PRICES
        2)            0.000000            5.000000
        3)           20.000000            0.000000
        4)            0.000000           15.000000

                RIGHTHAND SIDE RANGES
       ROW          CURRENT         ALLOWABLE         ALLOWABLE
                      RHS           INCREASE          DECREASE
        2           60.00000        60.000000         40.00000
        3           50.00000        INFINITY          20.00000
        4          120.00000        40.000000         60.00000
```

Problem 4

The Bug product has a profit contribution of $4100 per unit, requires 4 hours in the foundry department and 2 hours in the assembly department. The Superbug has a profit contribution of $5900 per unit, requires 2 hours in the foundry and 3 hours in assembly. The availabilities in foundry and assembly are 160 hours and 180 hours, respectively. Each hour used in each of foundry and assembly costs $90 and $60, respectively. The following is an LP formulation for maximizing profit contribution in this situation.

```
MAX      4100 B + 5900 S − 90 F − 60 A
SUBJECT TO
    2)     4 B + 2 S − F      =      0
    3)     2 B + 3 S     − A =      0
    4)                   F    <=   160
    5)                   A <=   180
END
```

Following is the solution report printed on a typewriter that skipped some sections of the report.

```
        OBJECTIVE FUNCTION VALUE
               332400.000

     VARIABLE        VALUE           REDUCED COST
        B           0.000000
        S          60.000000           0.000000
        F         120.000000
        A         180.000000           0.000000
```

```
ROW                 SLACK              DUAL PRICES
 2)              0.000000               90.000000
 3)              0.000000             1906.666700
 4)             40.000000
 5)              0.000000             1846.666700
```

Fill in the missing parts, using just the available information, i.e., without resolving the LP.

Problem 5

Suppose the capacities in the Enginola problem were: Astro line capacity $= 45$; Labor capacity $= 100$.

    (a) Allow the labor capacity to vary from 0 to 200 and plot:
- Dual price of labor as a function of labor capacity.
- Total profit as a function of labor capacity.

    (b) Allow the profit contribution/unit of Astros to vary from 0 to 50 and plot:
- Number of Astros to produce as a function of profit/unit.
- Total profit as a function of profit/unit.

Problem 6

Write the dual problem of the following problem:

$$
\begin{array}{ll}
\text{Minimize} & 12q + 5r + 3s \\
\text{subject to} & q + 2r + 4s \geq 6 \\
& 5q + 6r - 7s \leq 5 \\
& 8q - 9r + 11s = 10.
\end{array}
$$

Problem 7

The energetic folks at Enginola, Inc., have not been idle. The R & D department has given some more attention to the proposed digital recorder product (code name R) and enhanced it so much that everyone agrees that it could be sold for a profit contribution of $79 per unit. Unfortunately, its production still requires one unit of capacity on both the A(stro) and C(osmo) lines. Even worse, it now requires 4 hours of labor. The Marketing folks have spread the good word about the Astro and Cosmo products so that a price increase has been made possible. Industrial Engineering has been able to increase the capacity of the two lines. The new ex-marine heading Human Resources has been able to hire a few more good people so that the labor capacity has increased to 135 hours. The net result is that the relevant model is now:

```
MAX =  23 A +  38   C +  79   R
           A                + R <  75
                      C      + R <  65
           A +  2 *  C +  4  * R < 135
    END
```

Without resorting to a computer, answer the following questions, supporting each answer with a one- or two-sentence economic argument that might be understandable to your spouse or "significant other."

(a) How many As should be produced?
(b) How many Cs should be produced?
(c) How many Rs should be produced?
(d) What is the marginal value of an additional hour of labor?
(e) What is the marginal value/unit of additional capacity on the A line?
(f) What is the marginal value per unit of additional capacity on the C line?

The Model Formulation Process

4.1 The Overall Process

In using any kind of analytical or modeling approach for attacking a problem there are five major steps:

1. Understanding the real problem;
2. Formulating a model of the problem;
3. Gathering and generating the input data for the model, e.g., per unit costs to be used, etc.;
4. Solving or running the model;
5. Implementing the solution.

In general there is a certain amount of iteration over the five; e.g., one does not develop the most appropriate model the first time around. Of the above, the easiest is the solving of the model on the computer. This is not because it is intrinsically easiest, but because it is the most susceptible to mathematical analysis. Steps 1, 3, and 5 are, if not the most difficult, at least the most time consuming. Success with these steps depends to a large extent upon being very familiar with the organization involved, e.g., knowing who knows what the real production rate is on the punch press machine. Step 2 requires the most skill.

Formulating good LP models is an art bordering on a science. It is an art because it always involves approximation of the real world. The artistic ability is to develop simple models that are nevertheless good approximations to reality. We shall see that there are a number of classes of problems that are well approximated by LP models.

With all of the above comments in mind, we will devote most of the discussion to formulation of LP models; stating what universal truths seem to apply for steps (3) and (5); and giving an introduction to the mechanics of step (4).

4.2 Approaches to Model Formulation

We take two approaches to formulating models:

1. Constructive approach,
2. Template approach.

The constructive approach is the more fundamental and general; however, students with less analytic skill may prefer the template approach. The latter is essentially a "model in a can" approach. In this approach, examples of standard applications are illustrated in substantial detail. If you have a problem that closely resembles one of these "template" models, you may be able to make modest changes to the template model to adjust it to your situation. The advantage of this approach is that the user may not need much technical background if there is a template model that closely fits the real situation. However, the odds are low that you will find a template model that exactly matches your real situation. Thus, it helps if one has some skill at "constructing a model from the ground up."

4.3 Constructive Approach to Model Formulation

The constructive approach is a set of guidelines for constructing a model from the most basic building blocks. This approach requires somewhat more analytical skill, but the rules apply to any situation you are trying to model. In practice, it is combinations of these two approaches that get used.

In order to illustrate this approach, consider the following situation.

4.3.1 Example

Deglo Toys have been manufacturing a line of precision building blocks for children for a number of years. Deglo is about to introduce a new line of glow-in-the-dark building blocks and thus would like to deplete its old-technology inventories before introducing the new line. The old inventories consist of 19,900 4-dimple blocks and 29,700 8-dimple blocks. These inventories can be sold off in the form of two different kits: the Master Builder and the Empire Builder. The objective is to maximize the revenue from the sale of these two kits. The Master kit sells for $16.95, whereas the Empire kit sells for $24.95. The Master kit is composed of thirty 4-dimple blocks plus forty 8-dimple blocks. The Empire kit is composed of forty 4-dimple blocks plus eighty-five 8-dimple blocks. What is an appropriate model of this problem?

We suggest the following three-step approach in constructing a model:

1. Identify and define the decision variables. Defining a decision variable includes specifying the units in which it is measured, e.g., tons, hours, etc.
2. Specify and define the objective function, including the units in which it is measured.
3. Specify the constraints, including the units in which each is measured.

It is useful to do each of the above in words first.

4.3.2 Defining Decision Variables

The following questions are often helpful in identifying the decision variables (the answers are even more helpful):

(a) What should be the format of a report that gives a solution to this problem? (For example, the numbers that constitute an answer are: the amount to produce of each product; and the amount to use of each ingredient.) The cells in this report are the decision variables.

(b) What is the *objective?* Among useable solutions, how would I measure preference/goodness, e.g., profit?

(c) What are the *constraints?* A way to think about constraints is as follows: given a purported solution to a problem, what numeric checks would you perform to check the validity of the solution?

The majority of the constraints in most problems can be thought of as *sources-equals-uses* constraints. Another common kind of constraint is the *definitional* or *accounting* constraint. Sometimes the distinction between the two is arbitrary. Consider a production setting where we: (a) start with some beginning inventory of some commodity, (b) produce some of that commodity, (c) sell some of the commodity, and (d) some commodity is left in ending inventory. From the sources-equals-uses perspective we might write:

beginning inventory + production = sales + ending inventory.

From the definitional perspective, if we are thinking of how ending inventory is defined, we would write:

ending inventory = (beginning inventory + production) − sales.

The two perspectives are in fact mathematically equivalent.

4.3.3 Formulating Our Example Problem

This process for our example problem would be as follows:

(a) The essential decision variables are:
M = number of master builder kits to assemble and
E = number of empire builder kits to assemble.

(b) The objective function is to maximize sales revenue, i.e.,
Maximize $16.95M + 24.95E$.

(c) If someone gave us a proposed solution, i.e., values for M and E, we would check its feasibility by checking that
(i) number of 4-dimple blocks used $\leq 19{,}900$, and
(ii) number of 8-dimple blocks used $\leq 29{,}700$.

Symbolically, this is:
$$30M + 40E \leq 19{,}900$$
$$40M + 85E \leq 29{,}700$$

In LINDO form the formulation is:

```
MAX        16.95 M + 24.95 E
SUBJECT TO
    2)   30 M + 40 E <=       19900
    3)   40 M + 85 E <=       29700
END
```

with solution:

```
              OBJECTIVE FUNCTION VALUE

      1)          11478.5000

   VARIABLE        VALUE           REDUCED COST
      M           530.000000          0.000000
      E           100.000000          0.000000

   ROW      SLACK OR SURPLUS      DUAL PRICES
    2)             .000000          0.466053
    3)             .000000          0.074210
```

Thus, we should produce 530 Master Builders and 100 Empire Builders.

4.4 The Template Approach to Model Formulation

You may feel more comfortable and confident in your ability to structure problems if you have a classification of "template" problems to which you can relate new problems that you encounter. For LP problems, we will present a classification of about a half-dozen different categories of problems. In practice, a large real problem that you encounter will not fit exactly a single template model but might require a combination of two or more of the categories. The classification is not exhaustive, so you may encounter or develop LP models that seem to fit none of these templates. Subsequent chapters will provide examples of these "templates" for a wide range of problem areas.

4.4.1 Product Mix Problems

These are the problem types typically encountered in introductory LP texts. There are a collection of products that can be sold and a finite set of resources from which these products are made. Associated with each product is a profit contribution rate and a set of resource usage rates. The objective is to find the mix of products (amount of each product) that maximizes profit, subject to not using more resources than are available.

These problems are always of the form "Maximize profit subject to less than or equal to constraints."

4.4.2 Covering, Staffing, and Cutting Stock Problems

These problems are complementary (in the jargon they're called dual) to product mix problems in that their form is "Minimize cost subject to greater than or equal to constraints." The variables in this case might correspond to the number of people hired for various shifts during the day. The constraints arise from the fact that the mix of variables chosen must "cover" the requirements during each hour of the day.

4.4.3 Blending Problems

Problems of this type arise in the food, feed, metals, and oil refining industries. The problem is to mix or blend a collection of raw materials (e.g., different types of meats, cereal grains, crude oils, etc.) into a finished product (e.g., sausage, dog food, or gasoline) so that the cost per unit of the finished product is minimized, subject to satisfying certain quality constraints; e.g., percent protein ≥ 15 percent.

4.4.4 Multiperiod Planning Problems

This is perhaps the most important class of models. These models take into account the fact that the decisions made in this period partially determine which decisions are allowable in future periods. The submodel that is used each period may be a product mix problem, a blending problem, or some other type. These submodels are usually tied together by means of inventory variables (e.g., the inventory of raw materials, finished goods, cash, loans outstanding, etc.) that are carried from one period to the next.

4.4.5 Network, Distribution, and PERT/CPM Models

Network LP models warrant specific attention for two reasons: (a) they have a particularly simple form that makes them easy to describe as a graph or network, and (b) specialized and efficient solution procedures exist for solving them. They therefore tend to be easier to explain and comprehend. Network LPs frequently arise from problems of product distribution. Any enterprise producing a product at several locations and distributing it to many customers may find a network LP relevant. Large problems of this type may be solved rapidly by the specialized procedures.

One of the simplest network problems is that of finding the shortest route from one point in a network to another. A slight variation on this problem, that of finding the longest route, happens to be an important component of the project management tools PERT (Program Evaluation and Review Technique) and CPM (Critical Path Method).

Close cousins of network models are input/output and vertically integrated models. General Motors, for example, makes engines in certain plants; these engines might be sold directly to customers such as industrial equipment manufacturers or the engines may be used in GM's own cars and trucks. Such a company is said to be vertically integrated. In a vertically integrated model, there is usually one constraint for each type of intermediate product; the constraint mathematically enforces the basic law of physics that the amount used of an intermediate product by various processes cannot exceed the amount of this product produced by other processes. There is usually one decision variable for each type of process available.

If one expands one's perspective to the entire economy, the models considered tend to be similar to the input/output model popularized by Wassily Leontief (1951).

Each industry is described by the input products required and the output products produced. These outputs may in turn be inputs to other industries. The problem is to determine appropriate levels at which each industry should be operated in order to satisfy specific consumption requirements.

4.4.6 Multiperiod Planning Problems with Random Elements

One of the fundamental assumptions of LP is that all input data are known with certainty. There are situations, however, where certain key data are highly random. For example, when an oil company makes its fuel oil production decisions for the coming winter, the demand for that fuel oil is very much a random variable. If, however, the distribution probabilities for all the random variables are known, there is a modeling technique for converting a problem that is an LP except for the random elements into an equivalent, although possibly larger, deterministic LP.

4.4.7 Game Theory Models

Game Theory is concerned with the analysis of competitive situations. In its simplest form, a game consists of two players, each of whom has available to him or her a set of possible decisions. Each player must choose a strategy for making a decision in ignorance of the other player's choice. Some time after a decision is made, each player receives a payoff that depends on which combination of decisions was made. The problem of determining each player's optimal strategy can be formulated as a linear program.

4.4.8 Applications in Statistical Estimation

Much of statistical theory is concerned with making a prediction based on a set of data. Usually the prediction is chosen so that the prediction in some sense minimizes the squared forecast error. Very roughly speaking, a datum that is twice as far from the mean gets four times the weight in constructing the prediction. If one wishes to use other measures of goodness, such as mean absolute error or maximum absolute error instead of squared error in determining the prediction, then LP provides a powerful tool.

Not all problems you encounter will fit into one of the above categories. Many problems will be combinations of the above types. For example, in a multiperiod planning problem, the single period subproblems may be product mix or blending problems.

4.5 Common Errors in Formulating Models

When you develop a first formulation of some real problem, the formulation may contain errors or bugs. These errors will fall into the following categories:

1. Simple typographical errors;
2. Fundamental errors of formulation;
3. Errors of approximation.

The first two types of errors are easy to correct once they are identified. In principle, Type 1 errors are easy to identify because they are clerical in nature. In a large model, however, tracking them down may be a difficult search problem. Type 2 errors are more fundamental because they involve a misunderstanding of either the real problem or of the nature of LP models. Type 3 errors are more subtle. Generally, an LP model of a real situation involves some approximation; e.g., many products are aggregated together into a single macro-product, or the days of a week are lumped together, or costs that are not quite proportional to volume are nevertheless treated as linear. Avoiding Type 3 errors requires a skill of identifying which approximations can be tolerated.

Let us first discuss Type 1 errors. The major problem is detecting them. Many LP codes contain facilities for aiding detection of such gross errors. One of these facilities is the PICTURE command. It prints out an abbreviated picture of the coefficients in the formulation in table form. To illustrate its use, study the following formulation. It contains a typographical error that can be identified without understanding the formulation.

```
MIN    5 A0 + 6 A1 + 2 A2 + 4 B0 + 3 B1 + 7 B2
     + 2 C0 + 9 C1 + 8 C2
SUBJECT TO   2 )     A0 + A1 + A2 <=        8
     3)       B0 + B1 + B2 <=       9
     4)       C0 + C1 + C2 <=       6
     5)       A0 + B0 + C0 =        6
     6)       A1 + B2 + C1 =        5
     7)       A2 + B2 + C2 =        9
  END
```

The PICTURE command in LINDO allows us to display a "picture" of the coefficients in the model as follows (the variable names are printed vertically across the top):

```
        A A A B B B C C C
        0 1 2 0 1 2 0 1 2 0
   1: 5 6 2 4 3 7 2 9 8       MIN
   2: 1 1 1                   <= 8
   3:       1 1 1             <= 9
   4:             1 1 1       <= 6
   5: 1       1           1   = 6
   6:   1       1       1     = 5
   7:     1       1       1   = 9
```

Just from observing the pattern of 1's in the constraints, one can detect an aberration. The 1 appearing in the last column seems out of place. It should be in the fourth from last column. What seems to have happened is that the variable name C0 (zero) was misspelled as CO (letter O) in row 5. The computer is very literal and considers these as two separate variables. When the error is corrected, the picture looks as follows:

```
     A A A B B B C C C
     0 1 2 0 1 2 0 1 2
1:  5 6 2 4 3 7 2 9 8    MIN
2:  1 1 1                <= 8
3:        1 1 1          <= 9
4:              1 1 1    <= 6
5:  1       1       1    = 6
6:    1       1       1  = 5
7:      1       1       1  = 9
```

Additionally, if the user is fortunate, Type 1 errors will manifest themselves by caus-
ing solutions that are obviously incorrect.

Errors of formulation are more difficult to discuss because they are of many
forms. The kinds of errors made by a novice can frequently be exposed by doing what
we call dimensional analysis. Anyone who has taken a physics or chemistry course
would know it as "checking your units." Let us illustrate by considering an example.

A distributor of toys is analyzing his strategy for assembling Tinkertoy sets for
the upcoming holiday season. He assembles two kinds of sets. The "Big" set is com-
posed of 60 sticks and 30 connectors, whereas the "Tot" set is composed of 30 sticks
and 20 connectors. An important factor is that for this season he has a supply of only
60,000 connectors and 93,000 sticks. He will be able to sell all that he assembles of
either set. The profit contributions are \$5.5 and \$3.5 per set, respectively, for Big and
Tot. How much should he sell of each set to maximize profit?

He developed the following formulation. Define:

B = number of Big sets to assemble;

T = number of Tot sets to assemble;

S = number of sticks actually used;

C = number of connectors actually used.

```
MAX    5.5 B + 3.5 T
SUBJECT TO
          B - 30C - 60S = 0
          T - 20C - 30S = 0
          C         <=    60,000
          S         <=    93,000
```

Notice that the first two constraints are equivalent to:

$$B = 30C + 60S \qquad T = 20C + 30S$$

Do you agree with the formulation? If so, you should analyze its solution below:

```
              OBJECTIVE FUNCTION VALUE

     1)           54555000.

     VARIABLE            VALUE              REDUCED COST
        B           7380000.000000           0.000000
        T           3990000.000000           0.000000
        C             60000.000000           0.000000
        S             93000.000000           0.000000
```

```
ROW                    SLACK              DUAL PRICES
  2)              0.0000000                 5.500000
  3)              0.0000000                 3.500000
  4)              0.0000000               235.000000
  5)              0.0000000               435.000000
```

There is a hint that the formulation is incorrect because the solution is able to magically produce almost four million Tot sets from only 100,000 sticks.

The mistake that was made is a very common one for newcomers to LP, namely, trying to describe the features of an activity by a constraint. A constraint can always be thought of as a statement that the usages of some item must be less than or equal to the sources of the item. The last two constraints have this characteristic, but the first two do not.

If one analyzes the dimensions of the components of the first two constraints, one can see that there is trouble. The dimensions (or "units") for the first constraint are:

Term	Units
B	Big sets
30 C	30 [connectors/(Big set)] $\times$ connectors
60 S	60 [sticks/(Big set)] $\times$ sticks

Clearly, they have different units, but if you are adding items together, they must have the same units. Everyone is born with the knowledge that you cannot add apples and oranges. The units of all components of a constraint must be the same.

If one first formulates a problem in words and then converts it to the algebraic form in LINDO, one frequently avoids the above kind of error. In words, we wish to:

Maximize profit contribution
Subject to: Usage of connectors $\leq$ sources of connectors
Usage of sticks $\leq$ sources of sticks

Converted to algebraic form in LINDO, it is:

```
MAX       5.5 B + 3.5 T
SUBJECT TO
     2)     30 B + 20 T <=   60000
     3)     60 B + 30 T <=   93000
END
```

The units of the components of the constraint $30\ B + 20\ T <= 60,000$ are:

Term	Units
30 B	30 [connectors/(Big set)] $\times$ (Big set) = 30 connectors
20 T	20 [connectors/(Tot set)] $\times$ (Tot set) = 20 connectors
60,000	60,000 connectors available

Thus, all the terms have the same units of "connectors." Solving the problem, we obtain the sensible solution:

```
            OBJECTIVE FUNCTION VALUE

        1)        10550.00

    VARIABLE        VALUE          REDUCED COST
        B         200.000000         0.000000
        T        2700.000000         0.000000

    ROW             SLACK          DUAL PRICES
        2)          0.000000         0.150000
        3)          0.000000         0.016667
```

4.6 The Nonsimultaneity Error

It must be stressed that all the constraints in an LP formulation apply simultaneously. A combination of activity levels must be found that simultaneously satisfies all the constraints. The constraints do not apply in an either/or fashion, even though we might like them to be so interpreted. As an example, suppose that we denote by B the batch size for a production run of footwear. A reasonable policy might be that, if a production run is made, at least two dozen units should be made. Thus, B will be either zero or some number greater than or equal to 24. There might be a temptation to state this policy by writing the two constraints:

$$B \leq 0$$

$$B \geq 24.$$

The desire is that exactly one of these constraints be satisfied. If these two constraints are part of an LP formulation, the computer will reject such a formulation with a curt remark to the effect that no feasible solution exists. There is not a unique value for B that is simultaneously less than or equal to zero and greater than or equal to 24.

If such either/or constraints are important, one must resort to integer programming. Such formulations will be discussed in a later section.

4.7 Debugging Models

When you get the message "No Feasible Solution" or "Unbounded Solution," it usually means there is a bug in your model. On large models, finding the bug or bugs can be just as challenging as finding a bug in a large computer program. What you would probably like is some help narrowing down the search. Fortunately, LINDO has a command, appropriately named DEBUG, for doing just that.

First consider the case of an infeasible model. The DEBUG command will identify a subset of the constraints that must contain at least one bug. The feature of this subset is that as long as this set of constraints is present in the model (and no bounds on variables are changed), the model will be infeasible. This subset, called a "necessary set," is a minimal set in that, if all other constraints are dropped and any one of this subset is dropped, the model will become feasible. It is necessary to drop (or repair) at least one constraint in the necessary set to make the model feasible. If this subset is small, this is very helpful. If, however, this set is large, the search might still be tedious. LINDO tries to help a bit more. It will try to identify single constraints, which if dropped, make the model feasible. Such a constraint is labeled as "sufficient"; that is, it is sufficient for this constraint to be dropped to make the model feasible. The following little model illustrates:

```
! Test the DEBUG command on an infeasible model
  MAX      X
  SUBJECT TO
        2)    X <=    1
        3)    X >=    2
        4)    X >=    3
  END

  : terse
  : go

NO FEASIBLE SOLUTION AT STEP      1
SUM OF INFEASIBILITIES=  3.00000
  : solu

WARNING, SOLUTION MAY BE NONOPTIMAL/NONFEASIBLE

        OBJECTIVE FUNCTION VALUE

        1)          1.000000

  VARIABLE            VALUE          REDUCED COST
        X           1.000000            0.000000

        ROW    SLACK OR SURPLUS       DUAL PRICES
        2)          0.000000            2.000000
        3)         -1.000000           -1.000000
        4)         -2.000000           -1.000000

NO. ITERATIONS=           1
  : debug
SUFFICIENT SET (ROWS), CORRECT ONE OF:
            2
NECESSARY SET (ROWS), CORRECT ONE OF:
            4
```

Row 2 and 4 together constitute a necessary set. As long as both constraints are in the model, it will be infeasible. Row 2 seems a more likely candidate for the bug. In fact, if there is an error in only one row, it must be in row 2. Even though row 4 is in conflict with row 2, dropping, or otherwise repairing, row 4 is not sufficient to make the model feasible.

To summarize, first check the sufficient set, if there is one. If you are lucky, the mistake is in the sufficient set, the correction of which makes the model feasible. Otherwise, check the necessary set. You should discover a mistake that it is necessary to correct; however, there may still be other mistakes that keep the model infeasible.

The same sort of ideas apply for unbounded models. The following illustrates:

```
! Test DEBUG on an unbounded model
  MAX       5 Y1 + 4 Y2 - 16 Y3 - 9 Y4
  SUBJECT TO
        2)    Y1 - 3 Y3 - Y4 <=   1
        3)    Y2 - Y3 - 2 Y4 <=   1
  END

  : terse   ! Turn off the verbose messages . . .
  : go

  UNBOUNDED SOLUTION AT STEP      3 REDUCED COST=  -3.00000
  USE THE "DEBUG" COMMAND FOR MORE INFORMATION.
  UNBOUNDED VARIABLES ARE:
        Y3
        Y1
        Y2

  : debug
  SUFFICIENT SET (COLS), CORRECT ONE OF:
         Y1           Y2
  NECESSARY SET (COLS), CORRECT ONE OF:
         Y4
```

Variables $Y1$, $Y2$, and $Y4$ together constitute a necessary set. As long as all three variables are in the model, it will be unbounded. Variables $Y1$ and $Y2$ seem more likely candidates for the bug. In fact, if there is an error in only one variable's coefficients, it must be in the coefficients of either $Y1$ or $Y2$. Notice that if we constrain variable $Y4$ to be finite, the model is still unbounded. Infinite profit is still possible by making $Y1$, $Y2$, and $Y3$ arbitrarily large.

4.8 PROBLEMS

Problem 1

The Tiny Timber Company wants to best utilize the wood resources in one of its forest regions. Within this region, there is a sawmill and a plywood mill; thus timber can be converted to lumber or plywood.

Producing a marketable mix of 1000 board feet of lumber products requires 1000 board feet of spruce and 4000 board feet of Douglas fir. Producing 1000 square feet of plywood requires 2000 board feet of spruce and 4000 board feet of Douglas fir. This region has available 32,000 board feet of spruce and 72,000 board feet of Douglas fir.

Sales commitments require that at least 5000 board feet of lumber and 12,000 square feet of plywood be produced during the planning period. The profit contributions are $45 per 1000 board feet of lumber products and $60 per 1000 square feet of plywood. Let L be the amount (in 1000 board feet) of lumber produced and P be the amount (in 1000 square feet) of plywood produced. Express the problem as a linear programming model.

Problem 2

Shmuzzles, Inc., is a struggling toy company that hopes to make it big this year. It makes three fundamental toys: the Shmacrobat, the Shlameleon, and the Jig Saw Shmuzzle. Shmuzzles is trying to unload its current inventories through airline in-flight magazines by packaging these three toys in two different size kits, the Dilettante Shmuzzler kit and the Advanced Shmuzzler kit. The Dilettante sells for $29.95, whereas the Advanced sells for $39.95. The compositions of these two kits are:

Dilettante = 6 Shmacrobats plus 10 Shlameleons plus 1 Jig Saw

Advanced = 8 Shmacrobats plus 18 Shlameleons plus 2 Jig Saws

Current inventory levels are: 6,000 Shmacrobats, 15,000 Shlameleons and 1,500 Jig Saws. Formulate a model for helping Shmuzzles, Inc., maximize its profits.

Problem 3

Ely Provisioners produces, packages, and distributes freeze-dried food for the camping and outdoor sportsman market. Ely is ready to introduce a new line of products based on a new drying technology that produces a higher quality, tastier food. The basic ingredients of the current (about to be discontinued) line are dried fruits, dried meat, and dried vegetables. There are two products in the current line: the "Weekender" and the "Expedition Pak." The respective profit contributions per package of these two products are $1.25 and $2.75. The makeup of a "Weekender" package equals 3 ounces of dried fruit, plus 7 ounces of dried meat, plus 2 ounces of dried vegetables. The makeup of the "Expedition" package is 5 ounces of dried fruit, plus 18 ounces of dried meat, plus 5 ounces of dried vegetables. Ely would like to deplete its inventories of "old technology" fruit, meat, and vegetables before introducing the new line. The current inventories of these products are respectively 10,000 ounces, 25,000 ounces, and 12,000 ounces. Because there is as yet no "new technology" food on the market, Ely is confident it can sell its current inventories via the "Weekender" and "Expedition Pak" products without lowering prices. Formulate an LP that should be useful in telling Ely how many "Weekender" and "Expedition Pak" packages should be mixed so as to maximize profits from its current inventories.

Problem 4

Quart Industries produces a variety of bottled food products at its various plants. At its Americus plant it produces two products, peanut butter and apple butter. There are two scarce resources at this plant: packaging capacity and sterilization capacity. Both have a capacity of 40 hours per week. Production of 1000 jars of peanut butter requires 4 hours of sterilizer time and 5 hours of packaging time, whereas 1000 jars of apple butter requires 6 hours of sterilizer time and 4 hours of packaging time. The profit contributions per 1000 jars for the two products are $1100 and $1300, respectively. Apple butter preparation requires a boil-down process that is best done in batches of at least 5000 jars. Thus, apple butter production during the week should be either 0 or 5000 or more jars. How much should be produced this week of each product? Note: You could use integer programming ideas introduced very briefly earlier; however, you should be able to solve this problem with repeated use of simple linear programming.

Problem 5

Type in the model for the Enginola model, but "accidentally" enter the Cosmo line capacity constraint as C >= 70, so that the model is infeasible. Try to solve it. Then use the DEBUG command. Where does it suggest looking for the error?

Product Mix Problems

5.1 Introduction

Product mix problems are conceptually the easiest to comprehend. The Astro/Cosmo problem considered earlier is an example. Although product mix problems are seldom encountered in their simple textbook form in practice, they very frequently constitute important components of larger problems, such as multiperiod planning models.

The features of a product mix problem are that there are a collection of products that compete for a finite set of resources. If there are m resources and n products, the so-called "technology" is characterized by a table with m rows and n columns of technologic coefficients. The coefficient in row i, column j, is the number of units of resource i used by each unit of product j. The numbers in a row of the table are simply the coefficients of a constraint in the LP. In simple product mix problems, these coefficients are nonnegative. Additionally, associated with each product is a profit contribution per unit, and associated with each resource is an availability. The objective is to find how much to produce of each product (i.e., the mix) so as to maximize profits subject to not using more of each resource than is available.

The following product mix example will illustrate not only product mix LP formulations but also: (1) representation of nonlinear profit functions, and (2) the fact that most problems have alternative correct LP formulations. Two people may develop ostensibly different formulations of the same problem, but both may be correct.

5.1.1 Example

A certain plant can manufacture five different products in any combination. Each product requires time on each of three machines in the following manner (figures in minutes/unit):

<table>
<tr><td></td><td colspan="3" align="center">Machine</td></tr>
<tr><td>Product</td><td align="center">1</td><td align="center">2</td><td align="center">3</td></tr>
<tr><td>A</td><td>12</td><td>8</td><td>5</td></tr>
<tr><td>B</td><td>7</td><td>9</td><td>10</td></tr>
<tr><td>C</td><td>8</td><td>4</td><td>7</td></tr>
<tr><td>D</td><td>10</td><td>0</td><td>3</td></tr>
<tr><td>E</td><td>7</td><td>11</td><td>2</td></tr>
</table>

Each machine is available 128 hours per week.

Products A, B, and C are purely competitive, and any amounts made may be sold at respective prices of \$5, \$4, and \$5. The first 20 units of D and E produced per week can be sold at \$4 each, but all made in excess of 20 can only be sold at \$3 each. Variable labor costs are \$4 per hour for machines 1 and 2 and \$3 per hour for machine 3. Material costs are \$2 for products A and C and \$1 for products B, D, and E. You wish to maximize profit to the firm.

The principal complication is that the profit contributions of products D and E are not linear. You may find the following device useful for eliminating this complication. Define two additional products D_2 and E_2 that sell for \$3 per unit. What upper limits must then be placed on the sale of the original products D and E? The decision variables and their profit contributions are as follows:

Decision Variables	Definition	Profit Contribution per Unit
A	Number of units of A produced per week	$5 - 2 = \$3$
B	Number of units of B produced per week	$4 - 1 = \$3$
C	Number of units of C produced per week	$5 - 2 = \$3$
D	Number of units of D not in excess of 20 produced/week	\$3
D_2	Number of units of D produced in excess of 20 per week*	\$2
E	Number of units of E not in excess of 20 produced/week	\$3
E_2	Number of units of E produced in excess of 20	\$2
M_1	Hours of machine 1 used per week	−\$4
M_2	Hours of machine 2 used per week	−\$4
M_3	Hours of machine 3 used per week	−\$3

*Total production of product D is $D + D_2$.

In words, we want to:

Maximize   Revenues minus costs
Subject to   Minutes used equals minutes run on each machine,
At most, 20 units each can be produced of products D and E,
Each machine can be run 128 hours at most.

More precisely, the formulation in LINDO is:

```
OBJECTIVE FUNCTION
! Maximize revenue minus costs;
  MAX    3 A  + 3 B  + 3 C + 3 D + 2 D2 + 3 E + 2 E2
       - 4 M1 - 4 M2 - 3 M3
SUBJECT TO
! Machine time used = machine time made available;
    2)   12 A +   7 B   + 8 C + 10 D + 10 D2
         + 7 E +   7 E2 - 60 M1 = 0
    3)    8 A +   9 B   + 4 C + 11E + 11 E2 - 60 M2 = 0
    4)    5 A + 10 B   + 7 C +  3 D +  3 D2
         + 2 E + 2 E2 - 60 M3 = 0
! Product limits;
    5)   D <= 20
    6)   E <= 20
END
Machine availability;
    7)   M1 <= 128
    8)   M2 <= 128
    9)   M3 <= 128
END
```

The first three *constraints* have the units of "minutes" and specify the hours of machine time as a function of the number of units produced. The next two constraints (5 and 6) place upper limits on the number of high profit units of D and E that may be sold. The final three constraints put upper limits on the amount of machine time that may be used, and have the units of "hours."

Constraint 2 can be first written as:

$$\frac{12A + 7B + 8C + 10D + 10D_2 + 7E + 7E_2}{60} = M_1$$

Multiplying by 60 and bringing M_1 to the left gives Constraint 2. The solution is:

```
              OBJECTIVE FUNCTION VALUE
     1)            1777.62

   VARIABLE          VALUE              REDUCED COST
      A             0.00000               1.35833
      B             0.00000               0.18542
      C           942.49999               0.00000
      D             0.00000               0.12917
      D2            0.00000               1.12917
      E            20.00000               0.00000
      E2            0.00000               0.91875
      M1          128.00000               0.00000
      M2           66.49998               0 00000
      M3          110.62501               0.00000

   ROW              SLACK               DUAL PRICES
    2)             0.00000               0.297917
    3)             0.00000               0.0666667
    4)             0.00000               0.05000
    5)            20.00000               0.00000
    6)             0.00000               0.0812497
```

```
 7)              0.00000            13.87500
 8)             61.50000             0.00000
 9)             17.37500             0.00000
```

The solution is really quite simple. The units of E that can be sold at the higher price are the most profitable, and we make as many as possible (20). After that, product C is most profitable. We make as much as possible until we run out of capacity on machine 1.

This problem is a good example of one for which it is very easy to develop alternative formulations of the same problem. These alternative formulations are all correct but may have more or fewer constraints and variables. For example, the constraint

$$8A + 9B + 4C + 11E + 11E_2 - 60M_2 = 0$$

can be rewritten as

$$M_2 = (8A + 9B + 4C + 11E + 11E_2)/60.$$

The expression on the right can be substituted for M_2 wherever M_2 appears in the formulation. Because the expression on the right will always be nonnegative, the nonnegativity constraint on M_2 will automatically be satisfied. Thus, M_2 and the above constraint can be eliminated from the problem if we are willing to do a bit of arithmetic. When similar arguments are applied to M_1 and M_3 and the implied divisions are performed, one obtains the formulation:

```
MAX      1.416667 A +  1.433333 B + 1.85 C + 2.183334 D
      + 1.183333 D2      + 1.7 E  + .7 E2
SUBJECT TO
! Machine time used = machine time made available;
 2) 12 A +   7 B + 8 C + 10 D + 10 D2 + 7 E +   7 E2 <= 7680
 3)  8 A +   9 B + 4 C +                11 E + 11 E2 <= 7680
 4)  5 A + 10 B + 7 C +  3 D +  3 D2 + 2 E +   2 E2 <= 7680
! Product limits;
 5)  D <= 20
 6)  E <= 20
END
```

This looks more like a standard product mix formulation. All the constraints are capacity constraints of some sort. Notice that the solution to this formulation is really the same as that of the previous formulation.

```
               OBJECTIVE FUNCTION VALUE

      1)              1777.62

    VARIABLE          VALUE           REDUCED COST
       A              0.00000            1.35833
       B              0.00000            0.18542
       C            942.49999            0.00000
       D              0.00000            0.12917
       D2             0.00000            1.12917
       E             20.00000            0.00000
       E2             0.00000            0.91875
```

```
ROW                 SLACK              DUAL PRICE
 2)               0.00000               0.23125
 3)            3690.00000               0.00000
 4)            1042.50000               0.00000
 5)              20.00000               0.00000
 6)               0.00000               0.08125
```

The lazy formulator might give the first formulation, whereas the person who enjoys doing arithmetic might give the second formulation.

5.1.2 Process Selection Product Mix Problems

A not uncommon feature of product mix models is that two or more distinct variables in the LP formulation may actually correspond to alternate methods for producing the same product. In this case, the LP is being used not only to discover how much should be produced of a product but also to select the best process for producing each product.

A second feature that almost always appears with product mix problems is a requirement that a certain amount of a product be produced. This condition takes the problem out of the realm of simple product mix, but let us nevertheless consider a problem with the above two features.

The American Metal Fabricating Company (AMFC) produces various products from steel bars. One of the initial steps is a shaping operation that is performed by rolling machines. There are three machines available for this purpose, the B_3, B_4, and B_5. Their features are given by the following table:

Machine	Speed in Feet per Minute	Allowable Raw Material Thickness in Inches	Available Hours per Week	Labor Cost per Hour Operating
B_3	150	3/16 to 3/8	35	$10
B_4	100	5/16 to 1/2	35	$15
B_5	75	3/8 to 3/4	35	$17

This kind of combination of capabilities is not uncommon; machines that process larger material operate at slower speed.

This week there are three products that must be produced. AMFC must produce at least 218,000 feet of ¼″ material, 114,000 feet of ⅜″ material, and 111,000 feet of ½″ material. The profit contributions per foot excluding labor for these three products are 0.017, 0.019, and 0.02. These prices apply to all production, e.g., any in excess of the required production. The shipping department has a capacity limit of 600,000 feet per week, regardless of the thickness.

What are the decision variables and constraints for this problem? The decision variables require some thought. There is only one way of producing ¼″ material, three ways of producing ⅜″, and two ways of producing ½″. Thus, you will want to have at least the following decision variables. For numerical convenience, we measure length in thousands of feet.

$$B_{34} = 1{,}000\text{s of feet of } \tfrac{1}{4}'' \text{ produced on } B_3,$$

$$B_{38} = 1{,}000\text{s of feet of } \tfrac{3}{8}'' \text{ produced on } B_3,$$

$$B_{48} = 1{,}000\text{s of feet of } \tfrac{3}{8}'' \text{ produced on } B_4,$$

$$B_{58} = 1{,}000\text{s of feet of } \tfrac{3}{8}'' \text{ produced on } B_5,$$

$$B_{42} = 1{,}000\text{s of feet of } \tfrac{1}{2}'' \text{ produced on } B_4,$$

$$B_{52} = 1{,}000\text{s of feet of } \tfrac{1}{2}'' \text{ produced on } B_5.$$

For the objective function, we must have the profit contribution including labor costs. When this is done we obtain:

Variable	Profit Contribution per Foot
B_{34}	0.01589
B_{38}	0.01789
B_{48}	0.01650
B_{58}	0.01522
B_{42}	0.01750
B_{52}	0.01622

Clearly, there will be four constraints corresponding to AMFC's three scarce machine resources and its shipping department capacity. There should be three more constraints due to the production requirements in the three products. For the machine capacity constraints, we want the number of hours required for 1,000 feet processed. For machine B_3 this figure is $1{,}000/(60 \text{ min./hr.}) \times (150 \text{ ft./min.}) = 0.111111$ hours per 1,000 ft. Similar figures for B_4 and B_5 are 0.16667 hours per 1,000 ft. and 0.22222 hours per 1,000 feet.

The formulation can now be written:

Maximize $15.89B_{34} + 17.89B_{38} + 16.5B_{48} + 15.22B_{58} + 17.5B_{42} + 16.22B_{52}$

subject to

$$0.11111B_{34} + 0.11111B_{38} \le 35$$
$$0.16667B_{48} + 0.16667B_{42} \le 35 \qquad \left\} \begin{array}{l} \textit{Machine capacities} \\ \textit{in hours} \end{array} \right.$$
$$0.22222B_{58} + 0.22222B_{52} \le 35$$

$$B_{34} + B_{38} + B_{48} + B_{58} + B_{42} + B_{52} \le 600 \qquad \left\{ \begin{array}{l} \textit{Shipping capacity} \\ \textit{in 1,000s of feet} \end{array} \right.$$

$$B_{34} \ge 218$$
$$B_{38} + B_{48} + B_{58} \ge 114 \qquad \left\{ \begin{array}{l} \textit{Production requirements} \\ \textit{in 1,000s of feet} \end{array} \right.$$
$$B_{42} + B_{52} \ge 111$$

Without the last three constraints the problem is a simple product mix problem.

It is a worthwhile exercise to attempt to deduce the optimal solution just from cost arguments. The $\tfrac{1}{4}''$ product can be produced on only machine B_3, so that we know that B_{34} is at least 218. The $\tfrac{3}{8}''$ product is more profitable than the $\tfrac{1}{4}''$ on machine B_3; therefore, we can conclude that $B_{34} = 218$ and B_{38} will take up the slack.

The $\frac{1}{2}''$ and the $\frac{3}{8}''$ product can be produced on either B_4 or B_5. In either case, the $\frac{1}{2}''$ is more profitable per foot, so we know that B_{48} and B_{58} will be no greater than absolutely necessary. The question is: What is "absolutely necessary"? The $\frac{3}{8}''$ is more profitably run on B_3 than on B_4 or B_5, so it follows that we will satisfy the $\frac{3}{8}''$ demand from B_3 and, if sufficient, the remainder from B_4 and then from B_5. Specifically, we proceed as follows:

Set $B_{34} = 218$.

This leaves a slack of $35 - 218 \times 0.11111 = 10.78$ hours on B_3. This is sufficient to produce 97,000 feet of $\frac{3}{8}''$, so we conclude that

$B_{38} = 97$.

The remainder of the $\frac{3}{8}''$ demand must be made up from either machine B_4 or B_5. It would appear that it should be done on machine B_4 because the profit contribution for $\frac{3}{8}''$ is higher on B_4 than B_5. Note, however, that $\frac{1}{2}''$ is also more profitable on B_4 than B_5 by exactly the same amount. Thus, we are indifferent. Let us arbitrarily use machine B_4 to fill the rest of $\frac{3}{8}''$ demand, thus

$B_{48} = 17$.

Now any remaining capacity will be used to produce $\frac{3}{8}''$ product. There are $35 - 17 \times 0.16667 = 32.16667$ hours of capacity on B_4. At this point, we should worry about shipping capacity. We still have capacity for $600 - 218 - 97 - 17 = 268$ in 1,000's of feet. B_{42} is more profitable than B_{52}, so we will make it as large as possible, namely, $32.16667/0.16667 = 193$, so

$B_{42} = 193$.

The remaining shipping capacity is $268 - 193 = 75$, so

$B_{52} = 75$.

Any LP is in theory solvable by similar manual economic arguments, but the calculations could be very tedious and prone to errors of both arithmetic and logic. If we take the lazy route and solve it with LINDO, we get the same solution as our manual one:

```
             OBJECTIVE FUNCTION VALUE

        1)           10073.85

     VARIABLE          VALUE          REDUCED COST
       B34          218.000000          0.000000
       B38           97.000000          0.000000
       B48           17.000000          0.000000
       B58            0.000000          0.000000
       B42          193.000000          0.000000
       B52           75.000000          0.000000

       ROW            SLACK           DUAL PRICES
        2)            0.000000         24.029995
        3)            0.000000          7.680000
        4)           18.333338          0 000000
        5)            0.000000         16.220000
```

6)	0.000000	−2.999999
7)	0.000000	−1.000000
8)	157.000000	0.000000

RANGES IN WHICH THE BASIS IS UNCHANGED

COST COEFFICIENT RANGES

VARIABLE	CURRENT COEF	ALLOWABLE INCREASE	ALLOWABLE DECREASE
B34	15.890000	2.999999	INFINITY
B38	17.890000	INFINITY	2.669999
B48	16.500000	1.000000	0.000000
B58	15.220000	0.000000	INFINITY
B42	17.500000	0.000000	1.000000
B52	16.220000	1.280000	0.000000

RIGHTHAND SIDE RANGES

ROW	CURRENT RHS	ALLOWABLE INCREASE	ALLOWABLE DECREASE
2	35.000000	1.883888	9.166672
3	35.000000	12.499996	13.750003
4	35.000000	INFINITY	18.333338
5	600.000000	82.500023	74.999978
6	218.000000	97.000006	16.999994
7	114.000000	157.000055	16.999994
8	111.000000	157.000000	INFINITY

Notice that the B58 is zero but its reduced cost is also zero, meaning that B58 could be increased (and B48 decreased) without affecting profits. This is consistent with our earlier statement that we were indifferent between using B48 and B58 to satisfy the 3/8″ demand.

5.2 PROBLEMS

Problem 1

Consider a manufacturer that produces two products, Widgets and Frisbees. Each product is made from the two raw materials, Polyester and Polypropylene. The amounts required by each of the two products are given by the following table:

Widgets	Frisbees	Raw Material
3	5	Polyester
6	2	Polypropylene

Because of import quotas, the company is able to obtain only 12 units and 10 units of Polyester and Polypropylene, respectively, this month. The company is interested in planning its production for the next month. For this purpose it is important to know the profit contribution of each product. These contributions have been found to be $3 and $4 for Widgets and Frisbees, respectively. What should be the amounts of Widgets and Frisbees produced next month?

Problem 2

The Otto Maddick Machine Tool Company produces two products, muffler bearings and torque amplifiers. One muffler bearing requires $\frac{1}{8}$ hour of assembly labor, 0.25 hours in the stamping department, and 9 square feet of sheet steel. Each torque amplifier requires $\frac{1}{3}$ hour in both assembly and stamping and uses 6 square feet of sheet steel. Current weekly capacities in the two departments are 400 hours of assembly labor and 350 hours of stamping capacity. Sheet steel costs 15 cents per square foot. Muffler bearings can be sold for $8 each. Torque amplifiers can be sold for $7 each. Unused capacity in either department cannot be laid off or otherwise fruitfully used.

(a) Formulate the LP useful in maximizing the weekly profit contribution.
(b) It has just been discovered that two important considerations had not been included.
  (i) Up to 100 hours of overtime assembly labor can be scheduled at a cost of $5 per hour.
  (ii) The sheet metal supplier only charges 12 cents per square foot for weekly usage in excess of 5000 square feet.

Which of the above considerations could easily be incorporated in the LP model and how? If one or both cannot be easily incorporated, indicate how you might nevertheless solve the problem.

Problem 3

Review the solution to the 5-product, 3-machine product mix problem introduced at the beginning of the chapter.

(a) What is the marginal value of an additional hour of capacity on each of the machines?
(b) The current selling price of product A is $5. What would the price have to be before we would produce any A?
(c) It would be profitable to sell more product E at $4 if you could, but it is not profitable to sell E at $3 per unit even though you can. What is the break-even price at which you would be indifferent about selling any more E?
(d) It is possible to gain additional capacity by renting by the hour automatic versions of each of the three machines; that is, they require no labor. What is the maximum hourly rate you would be willing to pay to rent each of the three types of automatic machines?

Problem 4

The Aviston Electronics company manufactures motors for toys and small appliances. The marketing department is predicting sales of 6,100 units of the Dynamonster motor in the next quarter. This is a new high, and meeting this demand will test Aviston's production capacities. A Dynamonster is assembled from three components: a shaft, base, and cage. It is clear that some of these components will have to be purchased from outside suppliers because of limited in-house capacity. The variable in-house production cost per unit is compared with the outside purchase cost in the table below:

Component	Outside Cost	Inside Cost
Shaft	1.21	0.81
Base	2.50	2.30
Cage	1.95	1.45

Aviston's plant has three departments. Time requirements in hours of each component in each department if manufactured in-house are summarized in the following table. Hours available for Dynamonster production are listed in the last row.

Component	Cutting Department	Shaping Department	Fabrication Department
Shaft	0.04	0.06	0.04
Base	0.08	0.02	0.05
Cage	0.07	0.09	0.06
Capacity	820	820	820

(a) What are the decision variables?
(b) Formulate the appropriate LP.
(c) How many units of each component should be purchased outside?

Problem 5

Buster Sod's younger brother, Marky Dee, operates three ranches in Texas. The acreage and irrigation water available for the three farms are shown below:

Farm	Acreage	Water Available (acre feet)
1	400	1500
2	600	2000
3	300	900

Three crops can be grown; however, the maximum acreage which can be grown of each crop is limited by the amount of appropriate harvesting equipment available. The three crops are described below:

Crop	Total Harvesting Capacity (in acres)	Water Requirements (in acre-feet/acre)	Expected Profit (in $/acre)
Milo	700	6	400
Cotton	800	4	300
Wheat	300	2	100

Any combination of crops may be grown on a farm.

> (a) What are the decision variables?
> (b) Formulate the LP.

Problem 6

Review the formulation and solution of the American Metal Fabricating process selection/product mix problem in this chapter. Based on the solution report:

> (a) What is the value of an additional hour of capacity on the B_4 machine?
> (b) What is the value of an additional 2 hours of capacity on the B_3 machine?
> (c) By how much would one have to raise the profit contribution/1,000 ft. of $\frac{1}{4}''$ material before it would be worth producing more of it?
> (d) If the speed of machine B_5 could be doubled without changing the labor cost, what would it be worth per week? (Note that labor on B_5 is \$17/hour.)

Problem 7

A coupon recently appeared in an advertisement in the weekend edition of a newspaper. The coupon provided \$1 off the price of any size jar of Ocean Spray cranberry juice. The cost of the weekend paper was more than \$1.

Upon checking at a local store, we found two sizes available as follows:

Size in oz.	Price	Price/oz. w/o Coupon	Price/oz. with Coupon
32	2.09	.0653125	.0340625
48	2.89	.0602083	.039375

What questions, if any, should we ask in deciding which size to purchase? What should be our overall objective in analyzing a purchasing decision such as this?

Covering, Staffing, and Cutting Stock Models

6.1 Introduction

Covering problems tend to arise in service industries. The crucial feature is that there is a set of requirements to be covered. We have available to us various activities, each of which helps cover some but not all the requirements. The qualitative form of a covering problem is:

Choose a minimum cost set of activities

Subject to
The chosen activities cover all of our requirements.

Some examples of activities and requirement types for various problems are listed below:

Problem	Requirements	Activities
Staff scheduling	Number of people required on duty each period of the day or week.	Work or shift patterns. Each pattern covers some but not all periods.
Routing	Each customer must be visited.	Various feasible trips, each of which covers some but not all customers.
Cutting of bulk raw material stock, e.g., paper, wood, steel, textiles	Units required of each finished good size.	Cutting patterns for cutting raw material into various finished good size. Each pattern produces some but not every finished good.

In the next sections we look at several of these problems in more detail.

6.2 Staffing Problems

One part of the management of most service facilities is the scheduling or staffing of personnel, that is, deciding how many people to use on what shifts. This problem exists in the staffing of a telephone company information operators department, a toll plaza, a large hospital, and in general, any facility that must provide service to the public.

The solution process consists of at least three parts: (1) Develop good forecasts of the number of personnel required during each hour of the day or each day of the week during the scheduling period; (2) Identify the possible shift patterns that can be worked based on the personnel available and work agreements and regulations. A particular shift pattern might be to work Tuesday through Saturday and then be off two days; (3) Determine how many people should work each shift pattern so that costs are minimized and the total number of people on duty during each time period satisfies the requirements determined in (1). All three of these steps are difficult. LP can help in solving step 3.

We will illustrate a staff covering LP with a problem that is based on an approach first developed at the New York Port Authority by Edie (1954) for analyzing the staffing of toll booths. Though over forty years old, Edie's discussion is still very pertinent and thorough. His thoroughness is illustrated by his summary:

> *A trial was conducted at the Lincoln Tunnel. . . . Each toll collector was given a slip showing his booth assignments and relief periods and instructed to follow the schedule strictly. . . . At no times did excessive backups occur. . . . The movement of collectors and the opening and closing of booths took place without the attention of the toll sergeant. At times the number of booths were slightly excessive, but not to the extent previously. . . . Needless to say, there is a good deal of satisfaction. . . .(p. 138)*

6.2.1 Northeast Tollway Staffing Problems

The Northeast Tollway out of Chicago has a toll plaza with the following staffing demands during each 24-hour period:

Hours	Collectors Needed
12 A.M. to 6 A.M.	2
6 A.M. to 10 A.M.	8
10 A.M. to Noon	4
Noon to 4 P.M.	3
4 P.M. to 6 P.M.	6
6 P.M. to 10 P.M.	5
10 P.M. to 12 Midnight	3

Each collector works four hours, is off one hour, and then works another four hours. A collector can be started at any hour. Assuming the objective is to minimize the number of collectors hired, formulate the appropriate LP.

6.2.2 Formulation and Solution

Define the decision variables:

x_1 = number of collectors to start work at 12 Midnight
x_2 = number of collectors to start work at 1 A.M.
$\vdots$
x_{24} = number of collectors to start work at 11 P.M.

There will be one constraint for each hour of the day, stating that the number of collectors on at that hour be the number required for that hour. The objective will be to minimize the number of collectors hired for the 24-hour period. More formally:

Minimize $x_1 + x_2 + x_3 + \ldots + x_{24}$
subject to

$$x_1 + x_{24} + x_{23} + x_{22} + x_{20} + x_{19} + x_{18} + x_{17} \geq 2 \quad \text{(12 Midnight to 1 A.M.)}.$$
$$x_2 + x_1 + x_{24} + x_{23} + x_{21} + x_{20} + x_{19} + x_{18} \geq 2 \quad \text{(1 A.M. to 2 A.M.)}$$
$$\vdots$$
$$x_7 + x_6 + x_5 + x_4 + x_2 + x_1 + x_{24} + x_{23} \geq 8 \quad \text{(6 A.M. to 7 A.M.)}$$
$$\vdots$$
$$x_{24} + x_{23} + x_{22} + x_{21} + x_{19} + x_{18} + x_{17} + x_{16} \geq 3 \quad \text{(11 P.M. to 12 Midnight)}$$

It may help to see the effect of the one hour off in the middle of the shift by looking at the PICTURE of equation coefficients:

Constraint Row	x_1	x_2	x_3	x_4	x_5	x_6	x_7	x_8	x_9	$\cdots$	x_{17}	x_{18}	x_{19}	x_{20}	x_{21}	x_{22}	x_{23}	x_{24}	RHS
12 M. to 1 A.M.	1										1	1	1	1		1	1	1	≥2
1 A.M. to 2 A.M.	1	1										1	1	1	1		1	1	≥2
2 A.M. to 3 A.M.	1	1	1										1	1	1	1		1	≥2
3 A.M. to 4 A.M.	1	1	1	1										1	1	1	1		≥2
4 A.M. to 5 A.M.		1	1	1	1										1	1	1	1	≥2
5 A.M. to 6 A.M.	1		1	1	1	1										1	1	1	≥2
6 A.M. to 7 A.M.	1	1		1	1	1	1										1	1	≥8
7 A.M. to 8 A.M.	1	1	1		1	1	1	1										1	≥8
8 A.M. to 9 A.M.	1	1	1	1		1	1	1	1										≥8
9 A.M. to 10 A.M.		1	1	1	1		1	1	1										≥8
10 A.M. to 11 A.M.			1	1	1	1		1	1										≥4
11 A.M. to 12 P.M.				1	1	1	1		1										≥4
12 P.M. to 1 P.M.					1	1	1	1											≥3
1 P.M. to 2 P.M.						1	1	1	1										≥3
2 P.M. to 3 P.M.							1	1	1										≥3
								1	1										≥3

etc.   etc.

When it is solved, we get an objective value of 15.75 with the following variables nonzero.

$$x_2 = 5 \qquad x_5 = 0.75 \qquad x_{11} = 1 \qquad x_{16} = 1$$
$$x_3 = 0.75 \qquad x_6 = 0.75 \qquad x_{14} = 1 \qquad x_{17} = 1$$
$$x_4 = 0.75 \qquad x_7 = 0.75 \qquad x_{15} = 2 \qquad x_{18} = 1$$

The answer is not directly useful because some of the numbers are fractional. The value of 15.75 implies that we must hire at least 16 collectors. It is very easy to round this solution so that we get an integer answer that hires 16, namely, set $x_3 = x_4 = x_6 = x_7 = 1$ and $x_5 = 0$.

If the shifts or duty periods contain no or very few breaks, the LP solution will tend to be integer without resorting to integer programming. For a discussion of how to solve large staffing problems with multiple breaks in a shift, see Aykin (1996).

6.3 Cutting Stock and Pattern Selection

In industries such as paper and textiles, a product is manufactured in large economically produced sizes at the outset. These sizes are cut into a variety of smaller, more usable sizes as the product nears the consumer. The determination of how to cut the larger sizes into smaller sizes at minimal cost is known as the cutting stock problem. As an example of the so-called one-dimensional cutting stock problem, suppose that machine design dictates that material be manufactured in 72-inch widths. There are a variety of ways of cutting these smaller widths from the 72-inch width, two of which are shown in Figure 6.1.

Pattern 1 has 2 inches of edge waste ($72 - 2 \times 35 = 2$), whereas pattern 2 has only 1 inch of edge waste ($72 - 2 \times 18 - 35 = 1$). Pattern 2, however, is not very useful unless the number of linear feet of 18-inch material required is about twice the number of linear feet of 35-inch material required. Thus, a compromise must be struck between edge waste and end waste.

The solution of a cutting stock problem can be partitioned into the 3-step procedure discussed earlier: (1) Forecast the needs for the final widths; (2) Construct a large collection of possible patterns for cutting the large manufactured width(s) into the smaller widths; (3) Determine how much of each pattern should be run of each of the patterns in (2) so that the requirements in (1) are satisfied at minimum cost. LP can be used in performing step (3).

Many large paper manufacturing firms have LP-based procedures for solving the cutting stock problem. Actual cutting stock problems may involve a variety of cost factors in addition to the edge waste/end waste compromise. The usefulness of the LP-based procedure depends upon the importance of these other factors. The following example illustrates the fundamental features of the cutting stock problem with no complicating cost factors.

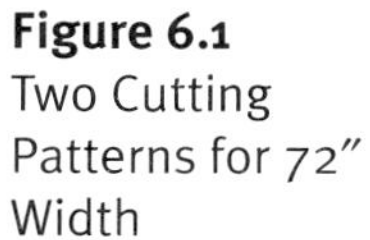

Figure 6.1
Two Cutting Patterns for 72″ Width

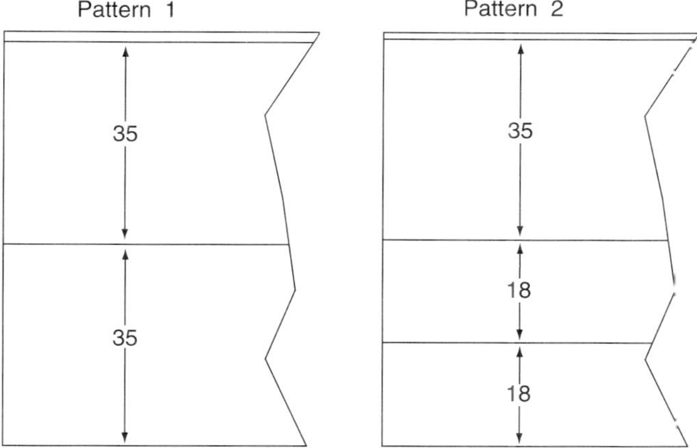

6.3.1 Example: Cooldot Cutting Stock Problem

The Cooldot Appliance Company produces a wide range of large household appliances such as refrigerators and stoves. A significant portion of the raw material cost is due to the purchase of sheet steel. Currently, sheet steel is purchased in coils in three different widths: 72 inches, 48 inches, and 36 inches. In the manufacturing process eight different widths of sheet steel are required: 60, 56, 42, 38, 34, 24, 15, and 10 inches. All uses require the same quality and thickness of steel.

A continuing problem is trim waste. For example, one way of cutting a 72-inch-width coil is to slit it into one 38-inch-width coil and two 15-inch-width coils. There will then be a 4-inch coil of trim waste that must be scrapped.

The prices per linear foot of the three different raw material widths are 15 cents for the 36-inch width, 19 cents for the 48-inch width, and 28 cents for the 72-inch width. Simple arithmetic reveals that the costs per inch × foot of the three widths are $15/36 = 0.416667$ cents/(inch × foot), 0.395833 cents/(inch × foot), and 0.388889 cents/(inch × foot) for the 36″, 48″ and 72″ widths, respectively.

The coils may be slit in any feasible solution. The possible efficient ways of slitting the three raw material widths are tabulated in Table 6.1.

For example, pattern C_4 corresponds to cutting a 72-inch-width coil into one 24-inch width and four 10-inch widths with 8 inches left over as trim waste. The lengths of the various widths required in this planning period are:

Width	60″	56″	42″	38″	34″	24″	15″	10″
Number of feet required	500	400	300	450	350	100	800	1000

The raw material availabilities this planning period are 1600 ft. of the 72-inch coils and 10,000 ft. each of the 48-inch and 36-inch widths.

Formulate a model for determining the number of feet of each pattern that should be cut so as to minimize costs while satisfying the requirements or the various widths. Can you predict beforehand the amount of 36-inch material used?

Table 6.1
Cutting Patterns
for Raw Material

Pattern Designation	Number to Cut of the Required Width								Waste in Inches
	60″	56″	42″	38″	34″	24″	15″	10″	
72-Inch Raw Material									
A_1	1	0	0	0	0	0	0	1	2
A_2	0	1	0	0	0	0	1	0	1
A_3	0	1	0	0	0	0	0	1	6
A_4	0	0	1	0	0	1	0	0	6
A_5	0	0	1	0	0	0	2	0	0
A_6	0	0	1	0	0	0	1	1	5
A_7	0	0	1	0	0	0	0	3	0
A_8	0	0	0	1	1	0	0	0	0
A_9	0	0	0	1	0	1	0	1	0
B_0	0	0	0	1	0	0	2	0	4
B_1	0	0	0	1	0	0	1	1	9
B_2	0	0	0	1	0	0	0	3	4
B_3	0	0	0	0	2	0	0	0	4
B_4	0	0	0	0	1	1	0	1	4
B_5	0	0	0	0	1	0	2	0	8
B_6	0	0	0	0	1	0	1	2	3
B_7	0	0	0	0	1	0	0	3	8
B_8	0	0	0	0	0	3	0	0	0
B_9	0	0	0	0	0	2	1	0	9
C_0	0	0	0	0	0	2	0	2	4
C_1	0	0	0	0	0	1	3	0	3
C_2	0	0	0	0	0	1	2	1	8
C_3	0	0	0	0	0	1	1	3	3
C_4	0	0	0	0	0	1	0	4	8
C_5	0	0	0	0	0	0	4	1	2
C_6	0	0	0	0	0	0	3	2	7
C_7	0	0	0	0	0	0	2	4	2
C_8	0	0	0	0	0	0	1	5	7
C_9	0	0	0	0	0	0	0	7	2
48-Inch Raw Material									
D_0	0	0	1	0	0	0	0	0	6
D_1	0	0	0	1	0	0	0	1	0
D_2	0	0	0	0	1	0	0	1	4
D_3	0	0	0	0	0	2	0	0	0
D_4	0	0	0	0	0	1	1	0	9
D_5	0	0	0	0	0	1	0	2	4
D_6	0	0	0	0	0	0	3	0	3
D_7	0	0	0	0	0	0	2	1	8
D_8	0	0	0	0	0	0	1	3	3
D_9	0	0	0	0	0	0	0	4	8
36-Inch Raw Material									
E_0	0	0	0	0	1	0	0	0	2
E_1	0	0	0	0	0	1	0	1	2
E_2	0	0	0	0	0	0	2	0	6
E_3	0	0	0	0	0	0	1	2	1
E_4	0	0	0	0	0	0	0	3	6

6.3.2 Formulation and Solution of Cooldot

Let the symbols $A_1, A_2, \ldots, E_4$ appearing in the cutting patterns in Table 6.1 denote the number of feet to cut of the corresponding pattern.

For accounting purposes it is useful to additionally define:

T_2 = number feet cut of 48-inch patterns,
T_3 = number feet cut of 36-inch patterns,
W_1 = inch $\times$ feet of trim waste from 72-inch patterns,
W_2 = inch $\times$ feet of trim waste from 48-inch patterns,
W_3 = inch $\times$ feet of trim waste from 36-inch patterns,
X_1 = number of feet of excess cut of the 60-inch width,
X_2 = number of feet of excess cut of the 56-inch width,
$\vdots$
X_8 = number of feet of excess cut of the 10-inch width.

It may not be immediately clear what the objective function should be. One might be tempted to calculate a cost of trim waste per foot for each pattern cut and then minimize the total trim waste cost, i.e.,

$$\text{Minimize } 0.3888891 W_1 + 0.395833 W_2 + 0.416667 W_3.$$

However, such an objective can easily lead to solutions that have very little trim waste but very high cost. This is possible in particular when the cost per square inch is not the same for all raw material widths. A more reasonable objective is to minimize the total cost, that is,

$$\text{Minimize } 28T_1 + 19T_2 + 15T_3.$$

The constraints in either case are:

```
          ! The supply constraints;
S72)  T1 <= 1600
S48)  T2 <= 10000
S36)  T3 <= 10000
          ! Totaling up usage of each of the 3 raw materials;
U72)  T1 - A1 - A2 - A3 - A4 - A5 - A6 - A7 - A8 - A9
        - B0 - B1 - B2 - B3 - B4 - B5 - B6 - B7 - B8 - B9
        - C0 - C1 - C2 - C3 - C4 - C5 - C6 - C7 - C8 - C9 = 0
U48)  T2 - D0 - D1 - D2 -D3 - D4 - D5 - D6 - D7 - D8 - D9
        = 0
U36)  T3 - E0 - E1 - E2-E3 - E4 = 0
          ! Compute edge waste for each raw material
W72)  - 2A1 - A2 - 6A3 - 6A4 - 5A6 - 4B0 - 9B1 - 4B2
        - 4B3 - 4B4 - 8B5 - 3B6 - 8B7 - 9B9 -4C0 - 3C1
        - 8C2 - 3C3 - 8C4 - 2C5 - 7C6 - 2C7 - 7C8 - 2C9
        + W1 = 0
W48)  - 6D0 - 4D2 - 9D4 - 4D5 - 3D6 - 8D7 - 3D8 - 8D9
        + W2 = 0
W36)  - 2E0 - 2E1 - 6E2 - E3 - 6E4 + W3 = 0
          ! The demand requirements
D60)  A1 - X1= 500
D56)  A2 + A3 - X2 = 400
```

```
D42)  A4 + A5 + A6 + A7 + D0 - X3= 300
D38)  A8 + A9 + B0 + B1 + B2 + D1 - X4 = 450
D34)  A8 + 2B3 + B4 + B5 + B6 + B7 + D2 + E0 - X5= 350
D24)  A4 + A9 + B4 + 3B8 + 2B9 + 2C0 + C1 + C2 + C3 + C4
      + 2D3 + D4 + D5 + E1 - X6 = 100
D15)  A2 + 2A5 + A6 + 2B0 + B1 + 2B5 + B6 + B9 + 3C1 + 2C2
      + C3 + 4C5 + 3C6 + 2C7 + C8 + D4 + 3D6 + 2D7 + D8
      + 2E2 + E3 - X7 = 800
D10)  A1 + A3 + A6 + 3A7 + A9 + B1 + 3B2 + B4  + 2B6 + 3B7
      + 2C0 + C2 + 3C3 + 4C4 + C5 + 2C6 + 4C7 + 5C8 + 7C9
      + D1 + D2 + 2D5 + D7 + 3D8 + 4D9
      + E1 + 2E3 + 3E4 - X8 = 1000
```

Constraints (S72), (S48), and (S36) enforce the availability limits of the three raw material widths. Constraints (U72), (U48), and (U36) define variables T_1, T_2, and T_3. Constraints (D60) through (D10) force the eight demand requirements to be fulfilled. For example, (D60) forces the amount of 60-inch width produced to equal at least 500 feet, whereas (D10) enforces a similar requirement for the 10-inch width.

The two different solutions obtained under the two different objectives are compared in Table 6.2.

The key difference in the solutions is that the "Min trim waste" solution uses more of the 48-inch-width raw material and cuts it in a way so that the edge waste is minimized. More material of the 42-inch width and the 34-inch width is cut than is needed, however, because the objective function does not count this as waste.

Table 6.2
Cutting Stock
Solutions

	Feet to Cut	
Nonzero Patterns	**Trim Waste Minimizing Solution**	**Total Cost Minimizing Solution**
A_1	500	500
A_2	400	400
A_5	200	171.42865
A_7	135.5	128.57135
A_8	362.5	350
A_9	0	3.57139
B_8	0	32.1429
C_5	0	14.286
D_1	87.5	96.4286
D_3	50	0
Trim Waste Cost	$5.44	$5.55
Total Cost	$474.13	$466.32
X_3	37.5	0
X_5	12.5	0
T_1	1600	1600
T_2	137.5	96.429
T_3	0	0

Both solutions involve fractional answers, but the fractional parts are so small relative to the run lengths that in a practical problem most people would be willing to disregard this fact, e.g., by rounding up to the nearest integer, if possible.

6.3.3 Generalizations of the Cutting Stock Problem

In large cutting stock problems, it may be unrealistic to generate all possible patterns. There is an efficient method for generating only the patterns that have a very high probability of appearing in the optimal solution. It is beyond the scope of this section to discuss this procedure; however, it does become important in large problems (see Chapter 16 for details). Dyckhoff (1981) describes another formulation that avoids the need to generate patterns; however, that formulation may have a very large number of rows.

In complex cutting stock problems, the following additional cost considerations may be important:

1. *Fixed cost of setting up a particular pattern*. This cost consists of lost machine time, labor, etc. This motivates solutions with few patterns.
2. *Value of overage or end waste*. For example, there may be some demand next period for the excess cut this period.
3. *Underage cost*. In some industries you may supply plus or minus, say 5%, of a specified quantity. The cost of producing the least allowable amount is measured in foregone profits.
4. *Machine usage cost*. The cost of operating a machine is usually fairly independent of the material being run. This motivates solutions that cut up wide raw material widths.
5. *Material specific products*. It may be impossible to run two different products in the same pattern if they require different materials, e.g., different thickness, quality, surface finish, or type.
6. *Upgrading costs*. It may be possible to reduce setup, edge waste, and end waste costs by substituting a higher grade material than required for a particular demand width.
7. *Order splitting costs*. If a demand width is produced from several patterns, there will be consolidation costs due to bringing the different lots of the output together for shipment.
8. *Stock width change costs*. A setup involving only a pattern change usually takes less time than one involving both a pattern change and a raw material width change. This motivates solutions that use few raw material widths.
9. *Minimum allowable edge waste*. For some materials, a very narrow ribbon of edge waste may be very difficult to handle. Therefore, one may wish to restrict attention to patterns that have either zero edge waste or edge waste that exceeds some minimum such as two centimeters.
10. *Due dates and sequencing*. Some of the demands need to be satisfied immediately, whereas others are less urgent. The patterns containing the urgent or high priority products should be run first. If the urgent demands appear in the same patterns as low priority demands, it is more difficult to satisfy the high priority demands quickly.

11. *Inventory restrictions*. Typically, a customer's order will not be shipped until all the demands for the customer can be shipped. Thus, one is motivated to distribute a given customer's demands over as few patterns as possible. If every customer has product in every pattern, no customer's order can be shipped until every pattern has been run. Thus, there will be substantial work in process inventory until all patterns have been run.

12. *Limit on 1-set patterns*. In some industries, such as paper, there is no explicit cost associated with setting up a pattern, but there is a limit on the rate at which pattern changes can be made. It may take about 15 minutes to do a pattern change, much of this work being done off-line without shutting down the main machine. The run time to produce one roll set might take 10 minutes. Thus, if too many 1-set patterns are run, the main machine will have to wait for pattern changes to be completed.

13. *Pattern restrictions*. In some applications there may be a limit on the total number of final product widths that may appear in a pattern, and/or a limit on the number of "small" widths in a pattern. The first restriction would apply, for example, if there are a limited number of take-up reels for winding the slit goods. The second restriction might occur in the paper industry where rolls of narrow product width have a tendency to fall over, so one does not want to have too many of them to handle in a single pattern. Some demanding customers may request that their product be cut from a particular position (e.g., the center of a pattern) because they feel the quality of the material is higher in that position.

The most troublesome complications are high fixed setup costs, order-splitting costs, and stock width change costs. If they are important, one will usually be forced to use some ad hoc, manual solution procedure. An LP solution may provide some insight into which solutions are likely to be good, but other methods must be used to determine a final workable solution.

6.3.4 Two-Dimensional Cutting Stock Problems

The one-dimensional cutting stock problem is concerned with the cutting of a raw material that is in coils. The basic idea still applies if the raw material comes in sheets and the problem is to cut these sheets into smaller sheets. For example, suppose that plywood is supplied in 48- by 96-inch rectangular sheets and the end-product demand is for sheets with dimensions in inches of 36×50, 24×36, 20×60, and 18×30. Once you have enumerated all possible patterns for cutting a 48×96 sheet into combinations of the 4 smaller sheets, the problem is exactly as before.

Enumerating all possible two-dimensional patterns may be a daunting task. Two features of practical two-dimensional cutting problems can reduce the size of this task: (a) orientation requirements, and (b) "guillotine" cut requirements. Applications in which (a) is important are in the cutting of wood and fabric. For reasons of strength or appearance, a demand unit may be limited in how it is positioned on the raw material. (Imagine a plaid suit for which the manufacturer randomly oriented the pattern on the raw material.) Any good baseball player knows that the grain of the bat must face the ball when hitting. Attention must be paid to the grain of the wood if the resulting wood product is to be used for structural or aesthetic purposes. Glass is an example of a raw material for which orientation is not important. A pattern is said to be cuttable with guillotine cuts if each cut must be made by a shear across the full width of the item being cut.

6.4 Crew Scheduling Problems

Managing the aircraft and crews of a large airline involves complex scheduling problems. Paying special attention to these scheduling problems can be rewarding. The yearly cost of operating an airliner far exceeds the onetime cost of a respectable computer, so devoting some computing resources to make more efficient use of airplanes is attractive. One small part of an airline's scheduling problems is discussed below.

Large airlines face a staffing problem known as the crew scheduling problem. The requirements to be covered are the crew requirements of the flights that the line is committed to fly during the next scheduling period, e.g., one month. A specific crew during its working day flies a number of flights usually, but not necessarily, on the same aircraft. The problem is to determine which flights should comprise the day's work of a crew.

The approach taken by a number of airlines is similar to the approach described for staffing problems: (1) Identify the demand requirements, i.e., the flights to be covered; (2) Generate a large number of feasible collections of flights that one crew could cover in a work period; (3) Select a minimum cost subset of the collections generated in (2) so that the cost is minimized and every flight is contained in exactly one of the selected collections.

LP can be used for step (3). Until 1985 most large airlines used computerized ad hoc or heuristic procedures for solving (3), because the resulting LP tends to be large and difficult to solve. Marsten, Muller, and Killion (1979), however, describe an LP-based solution procedure that was used very successfully by Flying Tiger Airlines. Flying Tiger had a smaller fleet than the big passenger carriers, so the resulting LP could be economically solved and gave markedly lower cost solutions than the ad hoc, heuristic methods. These optimizing methods are now being extended to large airlines.

A drastically simplified version of the crew scheduling problem is given in the following example. This example has only ten flights to be covered. By contrast, in 1990 United Airlines had close to 2000 flights per day to be covered.

6.4.1 Example: Sayre-Priors Crew Scheduling

The Sayre-Priors Airline and Stormdoor Company is a small diversified company that operates the following set of scheduled flights:

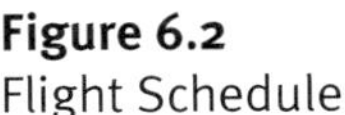

Figure 6.2
Flight Schedule

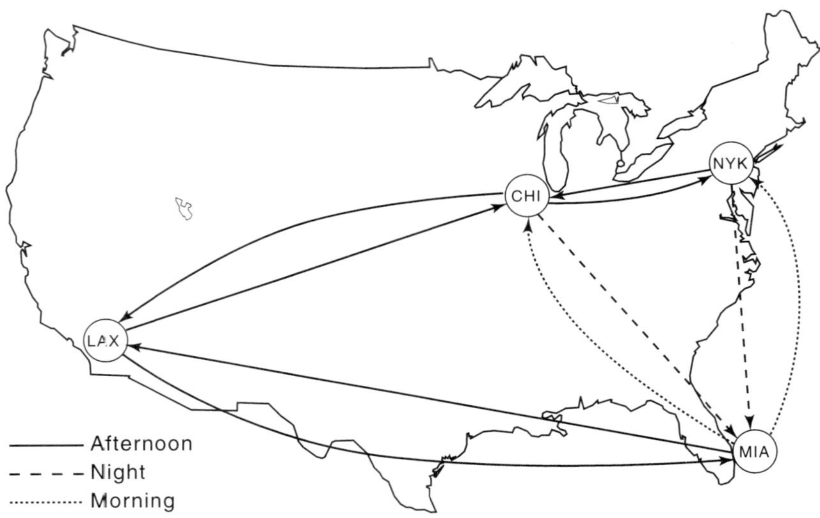

Flights

Flight Number	Origin	Destination	Time of Day
101	Chicago	Los Angeles	Afternoon
410	New York	Chicago	Afternoon
220	New York	Miami	Night
17	Miami	Chicago	Morning
7	Los Angeles	Chicago	Afternoon
13	Chicago	New York	Night
11	Miami	New York	Morning
19	Chicago	Miami	Night
23	Los Angeles	Miami	Night
3	Miami	Los Angeles	Afternoon

The flight schedule is illustrated graphically in Figure 6.2.

The Flight Operations Staff would like to set up a low-cost crew assignment schedule. The basic problem is to determine the next flight, if any, that a crew operates after it completes one flight. A basic concept needed in understanding this problem is that of a tour. The characteristics of a tour are as follows:

- A tour consists of from 1 to 3 connecting flights.
- A tour has a cost of $2,000 if it terminates in its city of origin.
- A tour that requires "deadheading," i.e., terminates in a city other than the origin city, costs $3,000.

In airline parlance, a tour is frequently called a "pairing" or a "rotation." The following are examples of acceptable tours:

Tour	Cost
17, 101, 23	$2,000
220, 17, 101	$3,000
410, 13	$2,000

In practice, the calculation of the cost of a tour is substantially more complicated than above. For example, a pilot may be paid one rate while flying, another rate while in uniform waiting between flights, and a per diem stipend while away from the home base.

6.4.2 Solving the Sayre-Priors Crew Scheduling Problem

The first thing to do for this small problem is to enumerate all feasible tours. We do not consider a collection of flights that involves an intermediate layover a tour. There are 10 one-flight tours, 14 two-flight tours, and either 37 or 41 three-flight tours, depending upon whether one distinguishes the origin city on a non-deadheading tour. These tours are indicated in Table 6.3 on page 104.

Define the decision variables:

$$T_i = 1 \text{ if tour } i \text{ is used}, = 0 \text{ if not used; for } i = 1, 2, \ldots, 37.$$

We do not distinguish the city of origin on non-deadheading three-flight tours. The formulation, with cost measured in $1000s, is:

```
MIN    3 T1 + 3 T2 + 3 T3 + 3 T4 + 3 T5 + 3 T6 + 3 T7 + 3 T8 + 3 T9
       + 3 T10 + 3 T11 + 2 T12 + 3 T13 + 3 T14 + 2 T15 + 3 T16 + 3 T17
       + 3 T18 + 3 T19 + 2 T20 + 3 T21 + 3 T22 + 3 T23 + 2 T24 + 2 T25
       + 3 T26 + 2 T27 + 2 T28 + 3 T29 + 3 T30 + 3 T31 + 3 T32 + 3 T33
       + 3 T34 + 3 T35 + 3 T36 + 3 T37
SUBJECT TO
F101)    T1 +   T11 +   T16 +   T25 +   T26 +   T29 +   T34 =    1
F410)    T2 +   T12 +   T13 +   T19 +   T27 +   T23 +   T30 +   T33
     +   T35 =    1
F220)    T3 +   T14 +   T15 +   T29 +   T30 =    1
 F17)    T4 +   T16 +   T20 +   T22 +   T25 +   T27 +   T29 +   T31
     +   T34 +   T36 =    1
  F7)    T5 +   T17 +   T18 +   T31 +   T32 =    1
 F13)    T6 +   T12 +   T17 +   T33 =    1
 F11)    T7 +   T15 +   T19 +   T21 +   T23 +   T25 +   T28 +   T30
     +   T32 +   T33 +   T35 +   T37 =    1
 F19)    T8 +   T13 +   T18 +   T20 +   T21 +   T27 +   T28 +   T31
     +   T32 +   T34 =    1
 F23)    T9 +   T11 +   T22 +   T23 +   T24 +   T25 +   T26 +   T35
     +   T36 +   T37 =    1
  F3)    T10 +   T24 +   T36 +   T37 =    1
END
```

A PICTURE of the coefficients gives a better feel for the structure of the problem and is given below. The first constraint, for example, forces exactly one of the tours that includes flight 101 to be chosen.

Table 6.3
List of Tours

One-Flight Tours	Cost	Two-Flight Tours	Cost	Three-Flight Tours	Cost
1. 101	$3,000	11. 101, 23	$3,000	25. 101, 23, 17	$2,000
2. 410	$3,000	12. 410, 13	$2,000	26. 101, 23, 11	$3,000
3. 220	$3,000	13. 410, 19	$3,000	27. 410, 19, 17	$3,000
4. 17	$3,000	14. 220, 17	$3,000	28. 410, 19, 11	$2,000
5. 7	$3,000	15. 220, 11	$2,000	29. 220, 27, 101	$3,000
6. 13	$3,000	16. 17, 101	$3,000	30. 220, 11, 410	$3,000
7. 11	$3,000	17. 7, 13	$3,000	25. 17, 101, 23	$2,000
8. 19	$3,000	18. 7, 19	$3,000	31. 7, 19, 17	$3,000
9. 23	$3,000	19. 11, 410	$3,000	32. 7, 19, 11	$3,000
10. 3	$3,000	20. 19, 17	$2,000	33. 11, 417, 13	$3,000
		21. 19, 11	$3,000	28. 11, 410, 19	$2,000
		22. 23, 17	$3,000	34. 19, 17, 101	$3,000
		23. 23, 11	$3,000	28. 19, 11, 410	$2,000
		24. 3, 23	$2,000	25. 23, 17, 101	$2,000
				35. 23, 11, 410	$3,000
				36. 3, 23, 17	$3,000
				37. 3, 23, 11	$3,000

```
?:PICTURE
                         T T T T T T T T T T T T T T T T T T T T T T T T T T T T
     T T T T T T T T T 1 1 1 1 1 1 1 1 1 1 2 2 2 2 2 2 2 2 2 2 3 3 3 3 3 3 3 3
     1 2 3 4 5 6 7 8 9 0 1 2 3 4 5 6 7 8 9 0 1 2 3 4 5 6 7 8 9 0 1 2 3 4 5 6 7
  1: 3 3 3 3 3 3 3 3 3 3 3 2 3 3 2 3 3 3 3 2 3 3 3 2 2 3 3 2 3 3 3 3 3 3 3 3 3 MIN
  2: 1                   1         1                 1 1     1         1       = 1
  3:     1                   1 1           1               1 1   1     1   1     = 1
  4:         1                   1 1                           1 1               = 1
  5:             1                   1     1       1   1     1   1   1   1     1   1   = 1
  6:                 1                       1 1                             1 1           = 1
  7:                     1       1               1                             1         = 1
  8:                         1               1       1   1   1     1   1   1   1 1   1   1 = 1
  9:                             1         1               1     1 1           1 1       1 1   1 1       1         = 1
 10:                                 1   1                     1 1 1 1 1                 1 1 1 = 1
 11:                                     1                                               1 1 = 1
```

When solved as an LP, the solution is conveniently integer, with the tours selected being:

Tour	Flights
T17	7, 13
T24	3, 23
T23	410, 19, 11
T29	220, 17, 101

The cost of this solution is \$10,000. There may be alternative optima with the same cost.

The dual prices on the constraints are:

ROW	SLACK	DUAL PRICES	Flight
2)	0.000000	-2.000000	(101)
3)	0.000000	0.000000	(410)
4)	0.000000	-2.000000	(220)
5)	0.000000	1.000000	(17)
6)	0.000000	-1.000000	(7)
7)	0.000000	-2.000000	(13)
8)	0.000000	0.000000	(11)
9)	0.000000	-2.000000	(19)
10)	0.000000	-1.000000	(23)
11)	0.000000	-1.000000	(3)

The dual prices suggest that flight 101, 220, 13, and 19 are the most expensive to cover, whereas crew costs could actually be reduced by adding another flight 17, because of the reduced deadheading.

The kind of LP that results from the crew scheduling problem is surprisingly difficult to solve. LPs of this type with more than 500 constraints have proven very difficult to solve. An additional detail sometimes added to the above formulation in practice is crewing basing constraints. Associated with each tour is a home base. Given the number of pilots living near each home base, one may wish to add a constraint for each home base limiting the number of tours selected for that home base. A simplification in practice is that a given pilot is typically qualified for only one type of aircraft. Thus, a separate crew scheduling problem can be solved for aircraft fleet, e.g., Boeing 747, Lockheed 1011, etc. Similarly, cabin attendant crews can be scheduled independently of flight (pilot) crews.

6.5 PROBLEMS

Problem 1

Certain types of facilities operate seven days each week and face the problem of allocating person power during the week as staffing requirements change as a function of the day of the week. This kind of problem is commonly encountered in public service and transportation organizations. Perhaps the most fundamental staffing problem involves the assignment of days off to full-time employees. In particular, it is regularly the case that each employee is entitled to two consecutive days off per week. If the number of employees required on each of the seven days of the week is given, the problem is to find the minimum workforce size that will allow these demands to be met, and then to determine the days off for the people in this workforce.

To be specific, let us study the problem faced by the Festus City Bus Company. The number of drivers required for each day of the week is as follows:

Monday	Tuesday	Wednesday	Thursday	Friday	Saturday	Sunday
18	16	15	16	19	14	12

How many drivers should be scheduled to start a five-day stint on each day of the week? Formulate this problem as a linear program. What is the optimal solution to it?

Problem 2

Completely unintentionally, several important details were omitted from the Festus City Staffing Problem (see previous question):

(a) Daily pay is $50 per person on weekdays, $75 on Saturday, and $90 on Sunday.
(b) There are up to three people that can be hired who will work part-time, specifically a 3-day week consisting of Friday, Sunday, and Monday. Their pay for this 3-day stint is $200.

Modify the formulation appropriately. Is it obvious whether the part-time people will be used?

Problem 3

A political organization, Uncommon Result, wants to make a mass mailing to solicit funds. It has identified six "audiences" that it wishes to reach. There are eight mailing lists that it can purchase in order to get the names of the people in each audience. Each mailing list covers only a portion of the audiences. This coverage is indicated in the table below:

Mailing List				Audience			
	M.D.	LL.D.	D.D.S.	Business Executive	Brick Layers	Plumbers	Cost
1	Y	N	N	Y	N	N	$5000
2	N	Y	Y	N	N	N	$4000
3	N	Y	N	N	N	Y	$6000
4	Y	N	N	N	N	Y	$4750
5	N	N	N	Y	N	Y	$5500
6	N	N	Y	N	N	N	$3000
7	N	Y	N	N	Y	N	$5750
8	Y	N	N	N	Y	N	$5250

A "Y" indicates that the mailing list contains essentially all the names in the audience. An "N" indicates that essentially no names in the audience are contained in the mailing list. The costs associated with purchasing and processing a mailing list are given in the far right column. No change in total costs is incurred if an audience is contained in several mailing lists.

Formulate a model that will minimize total costs while ensuring that all audiences are reached. Which mailing lists should be purchased?

Problem 4

The Pap-Iris Company prints various types of advertising brochures for a wide range of customers. The raw material for these brochures is a special finish paper that comes in 50-inch-width rolls. The 50-inch width costs $10 per inch-roll (i.e., $500/roll). A roll is 1,000 feet long. Currently Pap-Iris has three orders. Order number 1 is a brochure that is 16 inches wide with a run length of 400,000 feet. Order number 2 is a brochure that is 30 inches wide and has a run length of 80,000 feet. Order number 3 is a brochure that is 24 inches wide and has a run length of 120,000 feet. The major question is how to slit the larger raw material rolls into widths suitable for the brochures. With the paper and energy shortages, Pap-Iris wants to be as efficient as possible in its use of paper. Formulate an appropriate LP.

Problem 5

Postal Optimality Analysis (Due to Gene Moore). As part of a modernization effort, the U.S. Postal Service decided to improve the handling and distribution of bulk mail (second-, third-, and fourth-class nonpreferential) in the Chicago area. As part of this goal, a new processing facility was proposed for the Chicago area. One part of this proposal was development of a low-cost operational plan for the staffing of this facility. The plan would recognize the widely fluctuating hourly volume that is characteristic of such a facility and would suggest a staffing pattern or patterns that would accomplish the dual objectives of processing all mail received in a day's time while having no idle time.

A bulk mailing processing facility, as the name implies, performs the function of receiving, unpacking, weighing, sorting by destination, and shipping of mail designated as nonpreferential, including second-class (bulk rate), third-class (parcel post), and fourth-class (books). It is frequently designed as a single-purpose structure and is typically located in or adjacent to the large metropolitan areas that produce this type of mail in significant volume. Although the trend in such facilities has been increased utilization of automated equipment (including highly sophisticated handling and sorting devices), paid manpower continues to account for a substantial portion of total operating expense.

Mail is received by the facility in mail bags and in containers, both of which are shipped in trucks. It is also received in tied and wrapped packages, which are sent directly to the facility on railroad flatcars. Receipts of mail by the facility tend to be cyclical on a predictable basis throughout the 24-hour working day, resulting in the build-up of an "inventory" of mail during busy hours, which inventory must be processed during less busy hours. A policy decision to have "no idle time" imposes a constraint on the optimal level of staffing.

Once the facility is ready for operations, it will be necessary to implement an operating plan that will include staffing requirements. A number of assumptions regarding such a plan are necessary at the outset. Some of them are based upon existing Postal Service policy whereas others evolve from functional constraints. These assumptions are as follows:

i. Pieces of mail are homogeneous in terms of processing effort.

ii. Each employee can process 1800 pieces per hour.

iii. Only full shifts are worked; i.e., it is impossible to introduce additional labor inputs or reduce existing labor inputs at times other than shift changes.

iv. Shift changes occur at midnight, 8:00 A.M. and 4:00 P.M., which are the ends of the first, second, and third shifts, respectively.

v. All mail arrivals occur on the hour.

vi. All mail must be processed the same day it is received; i.e., there may be no "inventory" carryover from the third shift to the following day's first shift.

vii. Labor rates, including shift differential, are given in the following table:

Shift	$/Hour	Daily Rate
1st (Midnight–8 A.M.)	3.90	31.20
2nd (8 A.M.–4 P.M.)	3.60	28.80
3rd (4 P.M.–Midnight)	3.80	30.40

viii. Hourly mail arrival is predictable and is given in the following table.

	Cumulative Mail Arrival				
1st Shift		2nd Shift		3rd Shift	
Hour	Pieces	Hour	Pieces	Hour	Pieces
0100	56,350	0900	242,550	1700	578,100
0200	83,300	1000	245,000	1800	592,800
0300	147,000	1100	249,900	1900	597,700
0400	171,500	1200	259,700	2000	901,500
0500	188,650	1300	323,400	2100	908,850
0600	193,550	1400	369,950	2200	928,450
0700	210,700	1500	421,400	2300	950,500
0800	220,500	1600	485,100	2400	974,000

(a) Formulate the appropriate LP under the no idle time requirement. Can you predict beforehand the number to staff on the first shift? Will there always be a feasible solution to this problem for arbitrary arrival patterns?

(b) Suppose we allow idle time to occur. What is the appropriate formulation? Do you expect this solution to incur higher cost because it has idle time?

Problem 6

In the famous Northeast Tollway staffing problem, it was implied that at least a certain specified number of collectors were needed each period of the day. No extra benefit was assumed from having more collectors on duty than specified. You may recall that because of the fluctuations in requirements over the course of the day, the optimal solution did have more collectors than required on duty during certain periods.

In reality, if more collectors are on duty than specified, the extra collectors are not completely valueless. The presence of the extra collectors results in less waiting for the motorists. Similarly, if less than the specified number of collectors are on duty, the situation is not necessarily intolerable. Motorists will still be processed, but they may have to wait longer.

After much soul searching and economic analysis, you have concluded that one full-time collector costs $100/shift. An extra collector on duty for 1 hour results in $10 worth of benefits to motorists. Further, having one less collector on duty than required during a 1-hour period results in a waiting cost to motorists of $50.

Assuming that you wish to minimize total costs (motorists and collectors), show how you would modify the LP formulation. You only need illustrate for one constraint.

Problem 7

Some cities have analyzed their street cleaning and snow removal scheduling by methods somewhat analogous to those described for the Sayre-Priors airline problem. After a snowfall, each of specified streets must be swept by at least one truck.

(a) What are the analogs of the flight legs in Sayre-Priors?
(b) What might be the decision variables corresponding to the tours in Sayre-Priors?
(c) Should the constraints be equality or inequality in this case and why?

Problem 8

The St. Libory Quarry Company (SLQC) sells the rock that it quarries in four grades: limestone, chat, Redi-Mix-Grade, and coarse. A situation that it regularly encounters is one in which it has large inventories of the grades that it does not need and very little inventory in the grades that are needed at the moment. The four grades are produced by processing through a crusher the large rocks removed from the earth. For example, this week it appears that the demand is for 50 tons of limestone, 60 tons of chat, 70 tons of Redi-Mix and 30 tons of coarse. Its on-hand inventories for these same grades are, respectively, 5, 40, 30, and 40 tons. For practical purposes, one can think of the crusher as having three operating modes: close, medium, and coarse. SLQC has done some data gathering and has concluded that one ton of quarried rock gets converted into the following output grades according to the crusher setting as follows:

Crusher Operating Mode	Tons Output per Ton Input				Operating Cost/Ton
	Limestone	Chat	Redi-Mix	Coarse	
Close	0.50	0.30	0.20	0.00	$8
Medium	0.20	0.40	0.30	0.10	$5
Coarse	0.05	0.20	0.35	0.40	$3

SLQC would like to know how to operate its crusher so as to bring inventories up to the equivalent of at least two weeks' worth of demand. Provide whatever help that your current circumstances permit.

Problem 9

A certain optical instrument is being designed to selectively provide radiation over the spectrum from about 3500 to 6400 Angstrom units. To cover this optical range, a range of chemicals must be incorporated into the design. Each chemical provides coverage of a certain range. A list of the available chemicals, the range each covers, and its relative cost is provided below.

Chemical	Range Covered in Angstroms		Relative Cost
	Lower Limit	Upper Limit	
PBD	3500	3655	4
PPO	3520	3905	3
PPF	3600	3658	1
PBO	3650	4075	4
PPD	3660	3915	1
POPOP	3900	4449	6
A-NPO	3910	4095	2
NASAL	3950	4160	3
AMINOB	3995	4065	1
BBO	4000	4195	2
D-STILB	4000	4200	2
D-POPOP	4210	4405	2
A-NOPON	4320	4451	2
D-ANTH	4350	4500	2
4-METHYL-V	4420	5400	9
7-D-4-M	4450	4800	3
ESCULIN	4450	4570	1
NA-FLUOR	5200	6000	9
RHODAMINE-6G	5600	6200	8
RHODAMINE-B	6010	6400	8
ACRIDINE-RED	6015	6250	2

What subset of the available chemicals should be chosen to provide uninterrupted coverage from 3500 to 6400 Angstroms?

Problem 10

A manufacturer has the following orders in hand:

Order	Units	Selling Price/Unit
X	60,000	.45
Y	90,000	.24
Z	300,000	.17

Each order is for a single distinct type of product. The manufacturer has four different production processes available for satisfying these orders. Each process produces a different combination of the three products. Each process costs $0.50 per unit. The manufacturer must satisfy the volumes specified in the above table. The manufacturer formulated the following LP:

```
Min   .5 A  +   .5 B  +   .5 C  + .5 D
s.t.
         A                            >= 60000
              2 B  +   C              >= 90000
         A          + C     +  3 D    >= 300000
```

(a) Which products does process C produce?
(b) Suppose the agreements with customers are such that for each product the manufacturer is said to have filled the order if the manufacturer delivers an amount within + or − 10% of the "nominal" volume in the above table. The customer pays for whatever is delivered. Modify the formulation to incorporate this more flexible arrangement.

Problem 11

The formulation and solution of a certain staff scheduling problem are shown below:

```
        MIN M + T + W + R + F + S + N
              T + W + R + F + S          >= 14
                  W + R + F + S + N      >= 9
          M           + R + F + S + N    >= 8
          M + T           + F + S + N    >= 6
          M + T + W           + S + N    >= 17
          M + T + W + R           + N    >= 15
          M + T + W + R + F            >= 18
        END


        LP OPTIMUM FOUND AT STEP        4
        OBJECTIVE VALUE =    19.0000000

            VARIABLE          VALUE           REDUCED COST
               M            5.000000            .0000000
               T             .0000000            .0000000
               W           11.00000             .0000000
               R             .0000000            .0000000
               F            2.000000            .0000000
               S            1.000000            .0000000
               N             .0000000            .3333333
```

```
ROW        SLACK OR SURPLUS        DUAL PRICE
 2            .0000000            -.3333333
 3           5.000000             .0000000
 4            .0000000            -.3333333
 5           2.000000             .0000000
 6            .0000000            -.3333333
 7           1.000000             .0000000
 8            .0000000            -.3333333
```

M, T, W, R, F, S, N = number of people starting their five-day workweek on Monday, Tuesday, Wednesday, Thursday, Friday, Saturday, and Sunday, respectively.

(a) How many people are required on duty on Thursday?

(b) Suppose part-time help is available for the three-day pattern Thursday, Friday, and Saturday. That is, if you hire one of them, they will work all three days. These people cost 20% more per day than the ordinary folk who work a five-day week. Let P denote the number of part-timers to hire. Show how to modify the formulation to incorporate this option.

(c) Using information from the solution report, what can you say about the (economic) attractiveness of the part-time help?

Problem 12

Acie Knielson runs a small survey research company out of a little office on the Northwest side. He has recently been contracted to do a telephone survey of the head-of-household of at least 220 households. The demographics of the survey must satisfy the following profile:

Age of head-of-household:	18–25	26–35	36–60	61 or more
Households in survey (min):	30	50	100	40

When Acie makes a phone call, he knows only on average what kind of head-of-household he will find (if any). Acie can make either daytime or nighttime phone calls. Calls at night have a higher probability of success; however, they cost more because a higher wage rate must be paid. Being a surveyor, Acie has good statistics on all this, specifically, from past experience he knows that he can expect:

Percent of Calls Finding
Head-of-Household of Given Type

Call Type	18–25	26–35	36–60	61 or More	Not at Home	Cost/ Call
Day:	2%	2%	8%	15%	73%	$2.50
Night:	4%	14%	28%	18%	36%	$5.50

In words, what are the decision variables? What are the constraints?

What is your recommendation? How much do you estimate this project will cost Acie?

Problem 13

A political candidate wants to make a mass mailing of some literature to counteract some nasty remarks that his opponent has recently made. Our candidate has identified five mailing lists that contain names and addresses of voters that our candidate might like to reach. Each list may be purchased for a price. A partial list cannot be purchased. The number of names that each list contains in each of four professions are listed below.

Names on Each List (in 1000s) by Profession

Mailing List	Law	Health	Business Executives	Craft Professionals	Cost of List
1	28	4	7	2	$41,000
2	9	29	11	3	$52,000
3	6	3	34	18	$61,000
4	2	4	6	20	$32,000
5	8	9	12	14	$43,000
Desired Coverage:	20	18	22	20	

Our candidate has estimated how many voters he wants to reach in each profession. This is listed in the row "Desired Coverage." Our candidate has a more limited budget than his opponent. Therefore, our candidate does not want to spend any more than he has to in order to "do the job."

- (a) How many decision variables would you need to model this problem?
- (b) How many constraints would you need to model this problem?
- (c) Define the decision variables you would use and write the objective function.
- (d) Write a complete model formulation.

Problem 14

Your agency provides telephone consultation to the public from 7 A.M. to 8 P.M., five days a week. The telephone load on your agency is heaviest in the months around April 15 of each year. You would like to set up staffing procedures for handling this load during these busy months. Each telephone consultant that you hire starts work each day at either 7, 8, 9, 10, or 11 A.M., works for 4 hours, is off for 1 hour, and then works for another 4 hours. In recent years, however, an increasing fraction of the calls handled by your agency are from Spanish-speaking clients; therefore you must have some consultants who speak Spanish. You are able to hire two kinds of consultants: English speaking only, and bilingual (i.e., both English and Spanish speaking). A bilingual consultant can handle English and Spanish calls equally well. It should not be surprising that a bilingual consultant costs 1.1 times that of an English-only consultant. You have collected some data on the call load by hour of the day and language type, measured in consultants required, for one of your more important offices. These data are summarized below:

Hour of the Day:	7	8	9	10	11	12	1	2	3	4	5	6	7
English load:	4	4	5	6	6	8	5	4	4	5	5	5	3
Spanish load:	5	5	4	3	2	3	4	3	2	1	3	4	4

For example, during the hour from 10 A.M. to 11 A.M., you must have working at least three Spanish-speaking consultants plus at least six more who can speak English.

How many consultants of each type would you start at each hour of the day?

Problem 15

The well-known mail-order company R. R. Bean staffs its order-taking phone lines seven days per week. Each staffer costs $100 per day and can work five consecutive days per week. An important question is: which five-day interval should each staffer work? One of the staffers is pursuing an MBA degree part-time and as part of her course work developed the following model specific to R. R. Bean's staffing requirements.

```
MIN   500 M + 500 T + 500 W + 500 R + 500 F + 500 S + 500 N
  R1)  M                       + R      + F      + S       + N   >= 6
  R2)  M      + T                       + F      + S       + N   >= 7
  R3)  M      + T    + W                         + S       + N   >= 11
  R4)  M      + T    + W    + R                            + N   >= 9
  R5)  M      + T    + W    + R    + F                          >= 11
  R6)         T      + W    + R    + F    + S                   >= 9
  R7)                  W    + R    + F    + S       + N   >= 10
END
```

Note: M denotes the number of staffers starting on Monday, T the number starting on Tuesday, etc. R1, R2, etc., simply serve as row identifiers.

(a) What is the required staffing level on Wednesday (not the number to hire starting on Wednesday; that is a harder question)?

(b) Suppose you can hire people on a three-day-per-week part-time schedule to work the pattern consisting of the three consecutive days Wednesday–Thursday–Friday. Because of training, turnover, and productivity considerations of part-timers, you figure that the daily cost of these part-timers will be $105/day. Show how this additional option would be added to the model above.

(c) Do you think the part-time option above might be worth using?

(d) When the above staffing requirements are met, there will nevertheless be some customer calls that are lost because all staffers may be busy just by chance when a prospective customer calls. A fellow from marketing who is an expert on customer behavior and knows a bit of queuing theory estimates that having an additional staffer on duty on any given day beyond the minimum specified in the model above is worth $75. More than one above the minimum is of no additional value. For example, if the minimum staffers required on a day is 8 but there are actually 10 on duty, the better service will generate $75 of additional revenue. A third fellow, who is working on an economics degree part-time at Freeport Community College, argues that because the $75 per day benefit is less than the $100/day cost of a staffer, the solution will be unaffected by the $75 consideration. Is this fellow's argument correct?

(e) To double check your answer to (b), you decide to generalize the formulation to incorporate the $75 benefit of one-person overstaffing. Define any additional decision variables needed and show (a) modifications to the objective function and to existing constraints and (b) any additional constraints. You need only illustrate for one day of the week.

Networks, Distribution, and PERT/CPM

7.1 What's Special About Network Models

A subclass of LP models called network LPs warrants special attention for three reasons:

1. They can be completely described by simple, easily understood graphical figures;
2. Under typical conditions, they have naturally integer answers; and
3. They are easier to solve than general LPs.

Physical examples that come to mind are pipeline or electrical transmission line networks. Any enterprise producing a product at several locations and distributing it to many warehouses and/or customers may find a network LP a useful device for describing and analyzing the various shipment strategies.

Although not essential, efficient specialized solution procedures may be used to solve network LPs. These procedures may be as much as 100 times faster than the general simplex method. Bradley, Brown, and Graves (1977) give a detailed description. Some of these specialized procedures were developed several years before the simplex method was developed for general LPs.

Figure 7.1 illustrates the network representing the distribution system of a firm using intermediate warehouses to distribute a product. The firm has two plants, denoted by A and B, three warehouses, denoted by X, Y, and Z, and four customer areas, denoted by 1, 2, 3, 4. The numbers adjacent to each node denote the availability of material at that node. Plant A, for example, has 9 units available to be shipped. Customer 3, on the other hand, has −4 units, which means it requires 4 units to be shipped in.

The number above each arc is the cost per unit shipped along that arc. For example, if 5 of plant A's 9 units are shipped to warehouse Y, a cost of $5 \times 2 = 10$ will be incurred as a direct result. The problem is to determine the amount shipped along each arc so that total costs are minimized and every customer has his requirements satisfied.

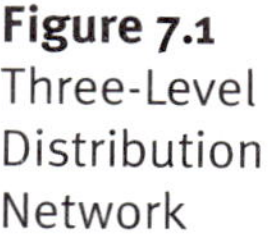

Figure 7.1
Three-Level
Distribution
Network

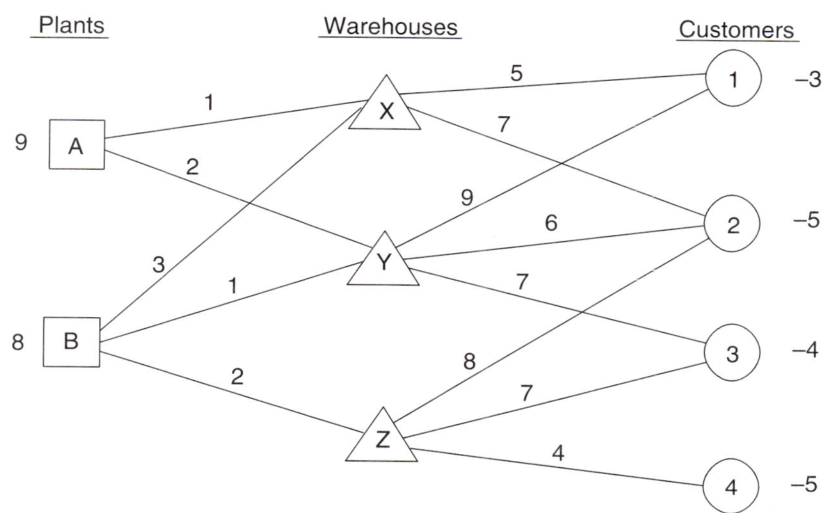

The essential condition on an LP for it to be a network problem is that it be representable as a network. There can be more than three levels of nodes; there can be any number of arcs between any two nodes; and there may be upper and lower limits on the amount shipped along a given arc.

Defining variables in an obvious way, the general LP describing this problem is:

```
MIN       AX + 2 AY + 3 BX + BY + 2 BZ + 5 X1 + 7 X2
      + 9 Y1 + 6 Y2 + 7 Y3 + 8 Z2 + 7 Z3 + 4 Z4
SUBJECT TO
      2)        AX + AY = 9
      3)        BX + BY + BZ = 8
      4)      - AX - BX + X1 + X2 = 0
      5)      - AY - BY + Y1 + Y2 + Y3 = 0
      6)      - BZ + Z2 + Z3 + Z4 = 0
      7)      - X1 - Y1 = -3
      8)      - X2 - Y2 - Z2 = -5
      9)      - Y3 - Z3 = -4
     10)      - Z4 = -5
      END
```

There is one constraint for each node that is of a "sources = uses" form. Constraint 5, for example, is associated with warehouse Y and states that the amount shipped out minus the amount shipped in must equal 0.

A different view of the structure of a network problem is possible by using the PICTURE command of LINDO to display the coefficients of the model in table form. (Note that the apostrophes are placed every third row and column in the picture only to help see the details in the big PICTURE):

118 Chapter 7 Networks, Distribution, and PERT/CPM

```
: PICTURE
              A   A   B   B   B   X   X   Y   Y   Y   Z   Z   Z
              X   Y   X   Y   Z   1   2   1   2   3   2   3   4
                                  '               '               '
      1:      1   2   3   1   2   5   7   9   6   7   8   7   4   MIN
      2:      1   1   '               '               '               =9
      3:      '   '   1   1   1   '   '   '   '   '   '   '   '   =8
      4:     -1      -1               1   1       '               '   =
      5:         -1   '  -1           '       1   1   1           '   =
      6:      '   '   '   '  -1   '   '   '   '   '   1   1   1   =
      7:              '              -1      -1   '               '   =-3
      8:              '               '  -1      -1      -1   '   =-5
      9:      '   '   '   '   '   '   '   '   '  -1   '  -1   '   =-4
     10:              '               '               '          '  -1   =-5
```

You should notice the key feature of the constraint matrix of a network problem: disregarding any bound constraints on individual variables, each column has exactly two nonzeroes in the constraint matrix, a +1 and a −1. According to the convention we have adopted, the +1 appears in the row of the node from which the arc takes material, whereas the −1 appears in the row of the node to which the arc delivers material. On a problem of this size, you should be able to deduce the optimal solution manually simply from examining Figure 7.1. You may check it with the computer solution below:

```
              OBJECTIVE FUNCTION VALUE

      1)           121.000000

   VARIABLE         VALUE          REDUCED COST
      AX           8.000000           0.000000
      AY           1.000000           0.000000
      BX           0.000000           3.000000
      BY           3.000000           0.000000
      BZ           5.000000           0.000000
      X1           3.000000           0.000000
      X2           5.000000           0.000000
      Y1           0.000000           5.000000
      Y2           0.000000           0.000000
      Y3           4.000000           0.000000
      Z2           0.000000           3.000000
      Z3           0.000000           1.000000
      Z4           5.000000           0.000000

     ROW            SLACK           DUAL PRICES
      2)           0.000000          -7.000000
      3)           0.000000          -6.000000
      4)           0.000000          -6.000000
      5)           0.000000          -5.000000
      6)           0.000000          -4.000000
      7)           0.000000          -1.000000
      8)           0.000000           1.000000
      9)           0.000000           2.000000
     10)           0.000000           0.000000
```

This solution exhibits two pleasing features found in the solution to any network problem:

1. If the right-hand side coefficients (the capacities and requirements) are integer, so will be the variables,
2. If the objective coefficients are integer, so will be the dual prices.

We can summarize network LPs as follows:

1. Associated with each node is a number that specifies the amount of commodity available at that node (negative implies that commodity is required at that node).
2. Associated with each arc are:
   (a) a cost per unit shipped (which may be negative) over the arc,
   (b) a lower bound on the amount shipped over the arc (typically zero),
   (c) an upper bound on the amount shipped over the arc (e.g., infinity in our example).

The problem is to determine the flows that minimize total cost subject to satisfying all the supply, demand, and flow constraints.

7.1.1 Special Cases

There are a number of common applications of LP models that are special cases of the standard network LP. The ones worthy of mention are:

1. *Transportation or distribution problems.* A two-level network problem, where all the nodes at the first level are suppliers, all the nodes at the second level are users, and the only arcs are from suppliers to users, is called a transportation or distribution model.
2. *Shortest and longest path problems.* Suppose that one is given the road network of the U.S. and wishes to find the shortest route from Bangor to San Diego. This is equivalent to a special case of a network or transshipment problem in which one unit of material is available at Bangor and one unit is required at San Diego. The cost of shipping over an arc is the length of the arc. Simple, fast procedures exist for solving this problem. An important first cousin of this problem, the longest route problem, arises in the analysis of PERT/CPM projects.
3. *The assignment problem.* A transportation problem in which the number of suppliers equals the number of customers, and further, each supplier has one unit available and each customer requires one unit, is called an assignment problem. An efficient specialized procedure exists for its solution.
4. *Maximal flow.* Given a directed network with an upper bound on the flow on each arc, one wants to find the maximum that can be shipped through the network from some specified origin or source node to some other destination or sink node. Applications might be to determine the rate at which a building can be evacuated or military material can be shipped to a distant trouble spot.

7.2 PERT/CPM Networks and LP

PERT (Project Evaluation and Review Technique) and CPM (Critical Path Method) are two closely related techniques for monitoring the progress of a large project. A key part of PERT/CPM is calculating the critical path, that is, identifying the subset of the activities which must be performed exactly as planned in order for the project to finish on time.

We will show that the calculation of the critical path is a very simple network LP problem, specifically, a longest path problem. You do not need this fact in order to efficiently calculate the critical path, but it is an interesting observation that becomes useful if you wish to examine a multitude of "crashing" options for accelerating a tardy project.

In the table below, we list the activities involved in the simple but nontrivial project of building a house. An activity cannot be started until all of its predecessors are finished.

Activity	Mnemonic	Activity Time	Predecessors (Mnemonic)
Dig Basement	DIG	3	—
Pour Foundation	FOUND	4	DIG
Pour Basement Floor	POURB	2	FOUND
Install Floor Joists	JOISTS	3	FOUND
Install Walls	WALLS	5	FOUND
Install Rafters	RAFTERS	3	WALLS, POURB
Install Flooring	FLOOR	4	JOISTS
Rough Interior	ROUGH	6	FLOOR
Install Roof	ROOF	7	RAFTERS
Finish Interior	FINISH	5	ROUGH, ROOF
Landscape	SCAPE	2	POURB, WALLS

In Figure 7.2 we show the so-called PERT (or activity-on-arrow) network for this project. We would like to calculate the minimum elapsed time to complete this project. Relative to this figure, the number of interest is simply the longest path from left to right in this figure. The project can be completed no sooner than the sum of the times of the successive activities on this path. Verify for yourself that the critical path consists of activities DIG, FOUND, WALLS, RAFTERS, ROOF, and FINISH and has length 27.

Even though this example can be worked out by hand, almost without pencil and paper, let us derive an LP formulation for solving this problem. Most people attempting this derivation will come up with one of two seemingly unrelated formulations.

The first formulation is motivated as follows. Let variables DIG, FOUND, etc., be either 1 or 0 depending upon whether activities DIG, FOUND, etc., are on or not on the critical path. The variables equal to one will define the critical path. The objective function will be related to the fact that we want to find the maximum length path in the PERT diagram.

Our objective is in fact:

```
MAX   3 DIG + 4 FOUND + 2 POURB + 3 JOISTS + 5 WALLS
+ 3 RAFTERS + 4 FLOOR + 6 ROUGH + 7 ROOF + 5 FINISH + 2 SCAPE
```

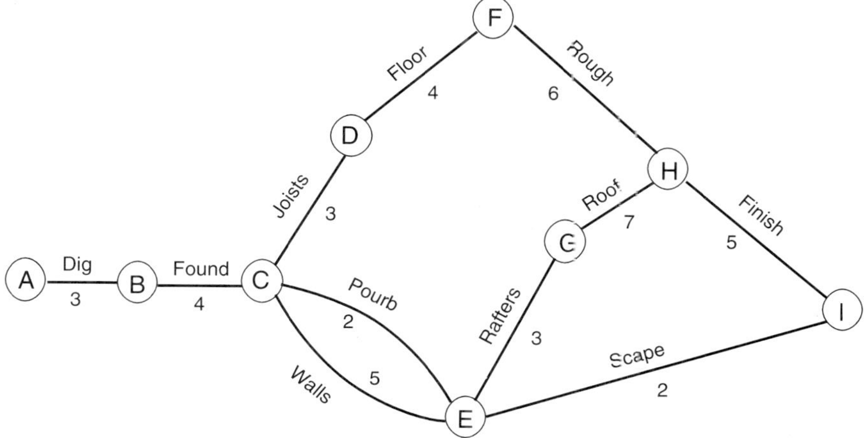

Figure 7.2
Activity-on-Arc
PERT/CPM
Network

By itself, this objective seems to take the wrong point of view. We do not want to maximize the project length. If, however, we specify the proper constraints, we shall see that this objective will seek out the maximum length path in the PERT network. We want to use the constraints to enforce the following:

1. DIG must be on the critical path;
2. An activity can be on the critical path only if one of its predecessors is on the critical path. Further, if an activity is on a critical path, exactly one of its successors must be on the critical path, if it has successors;
3. Exactly one of SCAPE or FINISH must be on the critical path.

Convince yourself that the following set of constraints will enforce the above:

```
- DIG = -1
- FOUND + DIG = 0
- JOISTS - POURB - WALLS + FOUND = 0
- FLOOR + JOISTS = 0
- RAFTERS - SCAPE + POURB + WALLS = 0
- ROUGH + FLOOR = 0
- ROOF + RAFTERS = 0
- FINISH + ROUGH + ROOF = 0
+ FINISH + SCAPE = +1
```

If you interpret the length of each arc in the network as the scenic beauty of the arc, the formulation corresponds to finding the most scenic route by which to ship one unit from A to I.

The solution of the problem is:

```
          OBJECTIVE FUNCTION VALUE
    1)           27.0000000

    VARIABLE          VALUE          REDUCED COST
    DIG            1.000000            0.000000
    FOUND          1.000000            0.000000
    POURB          0.000000            3.000000
    JOISTS         0.000000            0.000000
    WALLS          1.000000            0.000000
    RAFTERS        1.000000            0.000000
    FLOOR          0.000000            0.000000
    ROUGH          0.000000            2.000000
    ROOF           1.000000            0.000000
    FINISH         1.000000            0.000000
    SCAPE          0.000000           13.000000

    ROW              SLACK           DUAL PRICES
    2)            0.000000            0.000000
    3)            0.000000            3.000000
    4)            0.000000            0.000000
    5)            0.000000           10.000000
    6)            0.000000           12.000000
    7)            0.000000           14.000000
    8)            0.000000           15.000000
    9)            0.000000           22.000000
   10)            0.000000           27.000000
```

Notice that the variables corresponding to the activities on the critical path have value 1. What is the solution if the first constraint, -DIG = -1, is deleted?

It is instructive to look at the PICTURE of this problem in the following figure.

```
                            R
                  J         A                   F
            F  P  O  W  F  F  R        I  S
            O  O  I  A  T  L  O  R  N  C
         D  U  U  S  L  E  O  U  O  I  A
         I  N  R  T  L  R  O  G  O  S  P
         G  D  B  S  S  S  R  H  F  H  E
   1:    3  4  2  3  5  3  4  6  7  5  2   MAX
   2:  -1          '           '           '       = -1
   3:   1 -1    '     '     '     '     '     '     '     '     =
   4:       1 -1 -1 -1        '           '           =
   5:             1          -1           '           =
   6:  '  '  '  '  1 -1  '     '     '     '  -1      =
   7:          '           1 -1           '           =
   8:          '        1     '     -1     '           =
   9:  '  '  '  '  '  '     '  1' 1 -1     '           =
  10:          '                 '        1  1   = 1
```

Notice that each variable has at most two coefficients in the constraints. When two, they are +1 and −1. This is the distinguishing feature of a network LP.

Now let us look at the second possible formulation. The motivation for this formulation is to minimize the elapsed time of the project. To do this, realize that each node in the PERT network represents an event, e.g., as follows: *A*, start digging the basement; *C*, complete the foundation; and *I*, complete landscaping and finish interior.

Define variables $A, B, C, \ldots, H, I$ as the time at which these events occur. Our objective function is then:

Minimize $I - A.$

These event times are constrained by the fact that each event has to occur later than each of its preceding events, at least by the amount of any intervening activity. Thus, we get one constraint for each activity:

```
B - A >=  3            ! DIG
C - B >=  4            ! FOUND
E - C >=  2               .
D - C >=  3               .
E - C >=  5               .
F - D >=  4
G - E >=  3
H - F >=  6
H - G >=  7
I - H >=  5
I - E >=  2
```

The solution to this problem is:

```
          OBJECTIVE FUNCTION VALUE
   1)          27.000000
VARIABLE        VALUE              REDUCED COST
   A          0.000000              0 000000
   B          3.000000              0.000000
   C          7.000000              0.000000
   D         10.000000              0.000000
   E         12.000000              0.000000
   F         14.000000              0.000000
   I         27.000000              0.000000

  ROW          SLACK               DUAL PRICES
   2)          0.000000             -1.000000
   3)          0.000000             -1.000000
   4)          3.000000              0.000000
   5)          0.000000              0.000000
   6)          0.000000             -1.000000
   7)          0.000000             -1.000000
   8)          0.000000              0.000000
   9)          2.000000              0.000000
  10)          0.000000             -1.000000
  11)          0.000000             -1.000000
  12)         13.000000              0.000000
```

Notice that the objective function value equals the critical path length. We can indirectly identify the activities on the critical path by noting the constraints with nonzero dual prices. The activities corresponding to these constraints are on the critical path. This correspondence makes sense. The right-hand side of a constraint is the activity time. If we increase the time of an activity on the critical path, it should increase the project length and thus should have a nonzero dual price. What is the solution if the first variable, A, is deleted?

The PICTURE of the coefficient matrix for this problem appears below:

```
        A   B   C   D   E   F   G   H   I
 1:    -1          '           '           1 MIN
 2:    -1   1      '           '             > 3
 3:     '  -1  '1  '       '   '       '     > 4
 4:            -1  '   1           '         > 2
 5:            -1   1               '        > 3
 6:     '      -1  '   1  '         '   '    > 5
 7:               '  -1       1              > 3
 8:            -1           1   '            > 4
 9:     '       '   '      -1   '   1  '     > 6
10:               '           -1   1         > 7
11:               '               '  -1   1  > 5
12:     '       '   '  -1  '       '      '1  > 2
```

Notice that the PICTURE of this formulation is essentially the PICTURE of the previous formulation rotated ninety degrees. Even though these two formulations originally were seemingly unrelated, there is a really close relationship between the two, a relationship that mathematicians refer to as duality.

7.3 Activity-on-Arc vs. Activity-on-Node Network Diagrams

Two conventions are used in practice for displaying project networks: (1) Activity-on-Arc (AOA) and (2) Activity-on-Node (AON). Our previous example used the AOA convention. The characteristics of the two are:

AON

- Each activity is represented by a node in the network.
- A precedence relationship between two activities is represented by an arc or link between the two.
- May be less error prone because it does not need dummy activities or arcs.

AOA

- Each activity is represented by an arc in the network.
- If activity X must precede activity Y, there are X leads into arc Y. The nodes thus represent events or "milestones," e.g., "finished activity X." Dummy activities of zero length may be required to properly represent precedences.
- Historically more popular, perhaps because of its similarity to Gantt charts used in scheduling.

An AON project with six activities is shown in Figure 7.3. The number next to each node is the duration of the activity. By inspection you can discover that the longest path consists of activities 1, 3, 5, and 6. It has a length of 29. The corresponding AOA network for the same project is shown in Figure 7.4. In the AOA network, we have enclosed the activity numbers in circles above the associated arc. The unenclosed numbers below each arc are the activity durations. We have given the nodes,

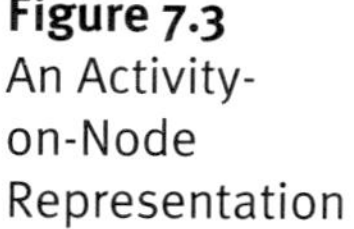

Figure 7.3
An Activity-on-Node Representation

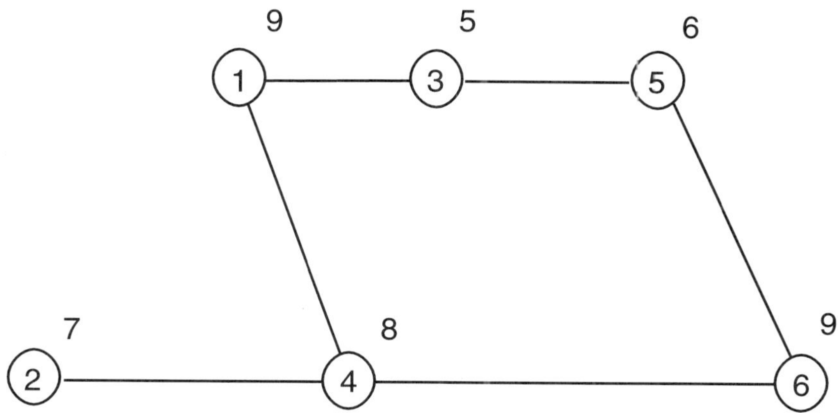

Figure 7.4
An Activity-on-Arc Representation

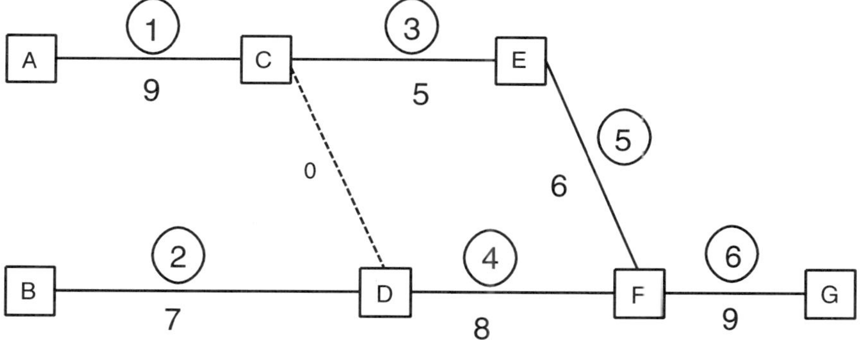

or milestones, arbitrary letter designations, enclosed in squares. Notice the dummy activity (the dotted arc) between nodes C and D. This is because *a dummy activity will be required in an AOA diagram any time that two activities*, e.g., 1 and 2, *share some*, e.g., activity 4, *but not all*, e.g., activity 3, *successor activities.*

7.4 Crashing of Project Networks

Once the critical path length for a project has been identified, the next question that is invariably asked is: can we shorten the project? The process of decreasing the duration of a project or activity is commonly called crashing. For many construction projects, it is common for the customer to pay an incentive to the contractor for finishing the project in a shorter length of time. For example, in highway repair projects it is not unusual to have incentives of from $5,000 to $25,000 per day that the project finishes before a target or benchmark date.

7.4.1 The Cost and Value of Crashing

There is value in crashing a project. In order to crash a project, we must crash one or more activities. Crashing an activity costs money. Deciding to crash an activity requires us to compare the cost of crashing that activity with the value of the resulting reduction in project length. This decision is frequently complicated by the fact that some negotiation may be required between the party that incurs the cost of crashing the activity (e.g., the contractor) and the party that enjoys the value of the crashed project (e.g., the customer).

7.4.2 The Cost of Crashing an Activity

The typical activity is crashed by applying more labor to it, e.g., overtime or a second shift. We might typically expect that using second-shift labor could cost 1.5 times as much per hour as first-shift labor. We might expect third-shift labor to cost twice as much as first-shift labor.

Consider an activity that can be done in six days if only first-shift labor is used and has a labor cost of \$6,000. If we allow the use of second-shift labor and thus work two shifts per day, the activity can be done in three days for a cost of $3 \times 1000 + 3 \times 1000 \times 1.5 = 7,500$. If third-shift labor is allowed, the project can be done in two days by working 3 shifts per day and incurring a total of

$$2 \times 1000 + 2 \times 1000 \times 1.5 + 2 \times 1000 \times 2 = \$9,000.$$

Thus, we get a crashing cost curve for the activity as shown in Figure 7.5.

7.4.3 The Value of Crashing a Project

There are two approaches to deciding upon the amount of project crashing: (a) we simply specify a project duration and crash enough to achieve this duration, or (b) we estimate the value of crashing it for various days. As an example of (a), in 1987 a new stadium was being built for the Montreal Expos baseball team. The obvious completion target was the first home game of the season.

As an example of (b), consider an urban expressway repair. What is the value per day of completing it early? Suppose that 6,000 motorists are affected by the repair project and each is delayed by 10 minutes each day because of the repair work, e.g., by taking alternate routes or by slower traffic. The total daily delay is $6,000 \times 10 = 60,000$ minutes $= 1000$ hours. If we assign an hourly cost of \$5/person $\times$ hours, the social value of reducing the repair project by one day is \$5,000.

7.4.4 Formulation of the Crashing Problem

Suppose we have investigated the crashing possibilities for each activity in our previous project example. These estimates are summarized in the table below:

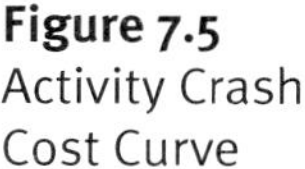

Figure 7.5
Activity Crash
Cost Curve

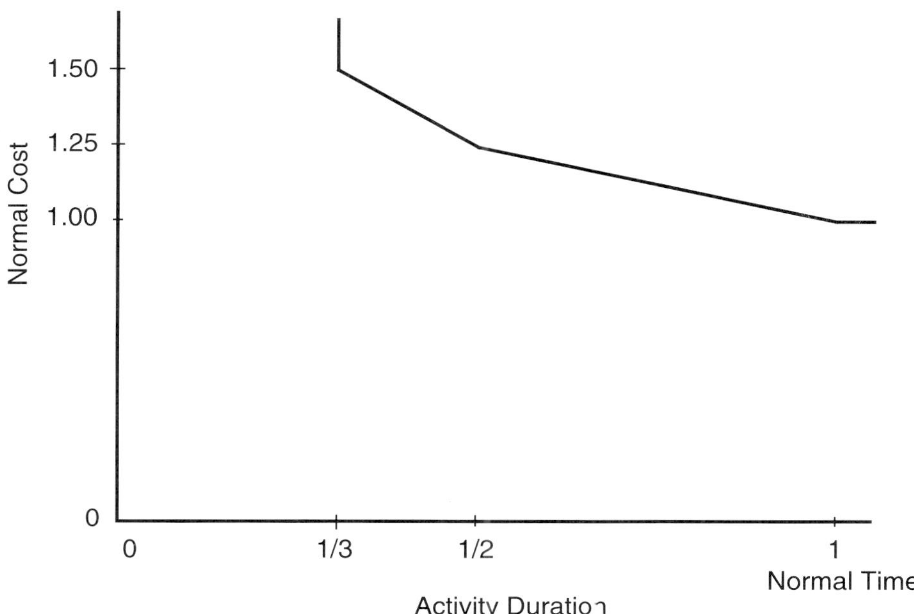

| | | Normal Time | Maximum Crash | |
Activity	Predecessor	(Days)	(Days)	$/Day
1	—	9	5	5000
2	—	7	3	6000
3	1	5	3	4000
4	1,2	8	4	2000
5	3	6	3	3000
6	4,5	9	5	9000

For example, activity 1 could be done in five days rather than nine; however, this would cost us an extra $(9 - 5) \times 5000 = \$20,000$.

First consider the simple case where we have a hard due date by which the project must be done, let us say 22 days in this case. How would we decide which activities to crash? Activity 2 is the cheapest to crash per day, but it is not on the critical path, so its low cost is at best just interesting.

Let us define:

EF_i = earliest finish time of activity i, taking into account any crashing that is done,

C_i = number of days by which activity i is crashed.

In words, the LP model will be:

Minimize   Cost of crashing
Subject to
    For each activity j and each predecessor i:
        earliest finish of $j \geq$ earliest finish of predecessor i
                + duration of j − crashing of j.
    For each activity j:
        crashing of $j \leq$ normal time of j − max crash time allowed for j.

The LINDO formulation is:

```
MIN        5 C1 + 6 C2 + 4 C3 + 2 C4 + 3 C5 + 9 C6
SUBJECT TO
  2)       C1 + EF1              >=   9
  3)       C2 + EF2              >=   7
  4)       C3 - EF1 + EF3        >=   5
  5)       C4 - EF1 + EF4        >=   8
  6)       C4 - EF2 + EF4        >=   8
  7)       C5 - EF3 + EF5        >=   6
  8)       C6 - EF4 + EF6        >=   9
  9)       C6 - EF5 + EF6        >=   9
 10)       EF6                   <=  22
END
SUB        C1        4.00000
SUB        C2        4.00000
SUB        C3        2.00000
SUB        C4        4.00000
SUB        C5        3.00000
SUB        C6        4.00000
```

The SUBs are just compact ways of representing the simple upper bounds, e.g.,
SUB C1 4.0 is equivalent to C1 $\leq$ 4. The solution is:

```
            OBJECTIVE FUNCTION VALUE
     1)           31.0000000

VARIABLE          VALUE              REDUCED COST
   C1            2.000000              0.000000
   C2            0.000000              5.000000
   C3            2.000000              0.000000
   C4            2.000000              0.000000
   C5            3.000000             -1.000000
   C6            0.000000              3.000000
  EF1            7.000000              0.000000
  EF2            7.000000              0.000000
  EF3           10.000000              0.000000
  EF4           13.000000              0.000000
  EF5           13.000000              0.000000
  EF6           22.000000              0.000000

  ROW       SLACK OR SURPLUS         DUAL PRICES
   2)            0.000000             -5.000000
   3)            0.000000             -1.000000
   4)            0.000000             -4.000000
```

```
 5)                   0.000000            -1.000C00
 6)                   0.000000            -1.000C00
 7)                   0.000000            -4.000C00
 8)                   0.000000            -2.000C00
 9)                   0.000000            -4.000C00
10)                   0.000000             6.000C00
```

Thus, for an additional cost of $31,000, we can meet the 22-day deadline.

Now suppose there is no hard project due date but we do receive an incentive payment of $5000 for each day that we reduce the project length. Define PCRASH = number of days that the project is finished before the 29th day. Now the formulation is:

```
MIN     5 C1 + 6 C2 + 4 C3 + 2 C4 + 3 C5 + 9 C6 - 5 PCRASH
SUBJECT TO
  2)        C1 + EF1                    >=    9
  3)        C2 + EF2                    >=    7
  4)        C3 - EF1 + EF3              >=    5
  5)        C4 - EF1 + EF4              >=    8
  6)        C4 - EF2 + EF4              >=    8
  7)        C5 - EF3 + EF5              >=    6
  8)        C6 - EF4 + EF6              >=    9
  9)        C6 - EF5 + EF6              >=    9
 10)        EF6 + PCRASH               =     29
END
SUB        C1            4.00000
SUB        C2            4.00000
SUB        C3            2.00000
SUB        C4            4.00000
SUB        C5            3.00000
SUB        C6            4.00000
```

From the solution, we see that we should crash it by 5 days to give a total project length of 24 days.

```
                 OBJECTIVE FUNCTION VALUE

        1)              -6.000000
        VARIABLE         VALUE            REDUCED COST
        C1             2.000000              0.000000
        C2             0.000000              6.000000
        C3             0.000000              1.000000
        C4             0.000000              0.000000
        C5             3.000000              0.000000
        C6             0.000000              4.000000
        EF1            7.000000              0.000000
        EF2            7.000000              0.000000
        EF3           12.000000              0.000000
        EF4           15.000000              0.000000
        EF5           15.000000              0.000000
        EF6           24.000000              0.000000
        PCRASH         5.000000              0.000000
```

```
ROW        SLACK OR SURPLUS        DUAL PRICES
 2)            0.000000            -5.000000
 3)            0.000000             0.000000
 4)            0.000000            -3.000000
 5)            0.000000            -2.000000
 6)            0.000000             0.000000
 7)            0.000000            -3.000000
 8)            0.000000            -2.000000
 9)            0.000000            -3.000000
10)            0.000000             5.000000
```

The excess of the incentive payments over crash costs is $6,000.

7.5 Path Formulations

In many network problems it is natural to think of a solution in terms of paths that material takes as it flows through the network. For example, in Figure 7.1 and its associated solution, there were 11 paths used (of the 13 possible), namely:

$$A \rightarrow X \rightarrow 1, A \rightarrow X \rightarrow 2, A \rightarrow Y \rightarrow 1, A \rightarrow Y \rightarrow 1, A \rightarrow Y \rightarrow 1,$$
$$B \rightarrow Y \rightarrow 1, B \rightarrow Y \rightarrow 2, B \rightarrow Y \rightarrow 3, B \rightarrow Z \rightarrow 2, B \rightarrow Z \rightarrow 3,$$
$$B \rightarrow Z \rightarrow 4.$$

One can in fact formulate decision variables in terms of complete paths rather than just simple links. The motivations for using the path approach are:

1. More complicated cost structures can be represented; e.g., Geoffrion and Graves (1974) use the path formulation to represent "milling in transit" discount fare structures in shipping food and feed products.
2. Path-related restrictions can be incorporated; e.g., regulations allow a truck driver to be on duty for at most 10 hours; thus, in a truck routing network, one would not consider paths longer than 10 hours.
3. The number of rows in the model may be substantially less.
4. In integer programs where some but not all of the problem has a network structure, the path formulation may be easier to solve.

7.5.1 Example

Let us reconsider the first problem, Figure 7.1. Suppose that shipments from A to X are made by the same carrier as shipments from X to 2. This carrier will give a $1/unit "milling-in-transit" discount for each unit that it handles from both A to X and X to 2. Further, the product is somewhat fragile and cannot tolerate a lot of transportation; in particular, it cannot be shipped both over links $B \rightarrow X$ and $X \rightarrow 2$ or both over links $A \rightarrow Y$ and $Y \rightarrow 1$.

Using the notation AX1 = number of units shipped from A to X to 1, etc., the path formulation is:

```
MIN      6 AX1 + 7 AX2 + 8 AY2 + 9 AY3 + 8 BX1 + 10 BY1
       + 7 BY2 + 8 BY3 + 10 BZ2 + 9 BZ3 + 6 BZ4
```

```
SUBJECT TO
    2)      AX1 + AX2 + AY2 + AY3 =      9
    3)      BX1 + BY1 + BY2 + BY3 + BZ2 + BZ3 + BZ4 =      8
    4)      AX1 + BX1 + BY1 =      3
    5)      AX2 + AY2 + BY2 + BZ2 =      5
    6)      AY3 + BY3 + BZ3 =      4
    7)      BZ4 =      5
END
```

Notice that the cost of path AX2 = 1 + 7 − 1 = 7. Also, paths BX2 and AY1 do not appear. This model has only six constraints as opposed to nine in the original formulation. The reduction in constraints arises from the fact that in path formulations one does not need the "sources = uses" constraints for intermediate nodes.

In general, the path formulation will have fewer rows but more decision variables than the corresponding network LP model.

When solved we get:

```
OBJECTIVE FUNCTION VALUE
        1)        116.000000
   VARIABLE          VALUE
      AX1           3.000000
      AX2           5.000000
      AY3           1.000000
      BY3           3.000000
      BZ4           5.000000
```

This is cheaper than the previous solution, because the five units shipped over path AX2 go for $1/unit less.

A path formulation need not have a naturally integer solution. If the path formulation, however, is equivalent to a network LP, then it will have a naturally integer solution.

The path formulation is popular in long-range forest planning; see, for example, Davis and Johnson (1986), where it is known as the "Model I" approach. The standard network LP based formulation is known as the "Model II" approach. In a forest planning Model II, a link in the network represents a decision to plant an acre of a particular kind of tree in some specified year and harvest it in some future specified year. A node represents a specific harvest and replant decision. A decision variable in Model I is a complete prescription of how to manage (i.e., harvest and replant) a given piece of land over time. Some Model I formulations in forest planning may have just a few hundred constraints but over a million decision variables or paths.

7.6 Path Formulations of Undirected Networks

In many communications networks, the arcs have capacity but are undirected. For example, when you are carrying on a phone conversation with someone in a distant city, the conversation uses capacity on all the links in your connection; however, you cannot speak of a direction of flow of the connection.

A major concern for a long-distance communications company is the management of its communications network. This becomes particularly important during certain holidays, such as Mother's Day, when not only does the volume of calls increase but the pattern of calls also changes dramatically from that of the business-oriented traffic during weekdays of the rest of the year. A communications company faces two problems: (1) the design problem—that is, what capacity should be installed on each link? and (2) the operations problem—that is, given the installed capacity, how are demands best routed? The path formulation is an obvious format for modeling an undirected network. The following illustrates the operational problem.

Consider the case of a phone company with the network structure shown in Figure 7.6. The numbers next to each arc are the number of calls that can be in progress simultaneously along that arc. If someone in MIA tries to call his mother in SEA, the phone company must first find a path from MIA to SEA such that each arc on that path is not at capacity. It is quite easy to inefficiently use the capacity. Suppose there is a demand for 110 calls between CHI and DNV, and 90 calls between ATL and SEA. Further, suppose that all these calls were routed over the ATL, DNV link. Now suppose we wish to make a call between MIA and SEA. Such a connection is impossible because every path between the two contains a saturated link (i.e., either ATL, DNV or CHI, ATL). If, however, some of the 110 calls between CHI and DNV are routed over the CHI, SEA, DNV links, then one could make calls between MIA and SEA. In conventional voice networks, a call cannot be rerouted once it has started. In packet switched data networks and to some extent in cellular phone networks, some rerouting is possible.

7.6.1 Example

Suppose that during a certain time period the demands in the following table occur for connections between pairs of cities.

	DNV	CHI	ATL	MIA
SEA	10	20	38	33
DNV		42	48	23
CHI			90	36
ATL				26

Which demands should be satisfied and via what routes so as to maximize the number of connections satisfied?

Solution. If we use the path formulation, there will be two paths between every pair of cities except ATL and MIA. We will use the notation $P1_{ij}$ for number of calls using the shorter or more northerly path between cities i and j, and $P2_{ij}$ for the other path, if any. There will be two kinds of constraints:

1. for each link, a capacity constraint,
2. for each pair of cities, an upper limit on the calls between that pair.

The complete formulation is:

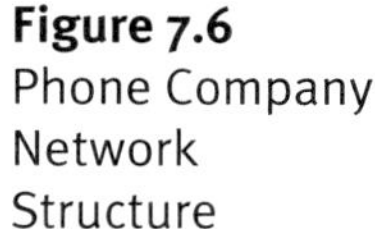

Figure 7.6
Phone Company
Network
Structure

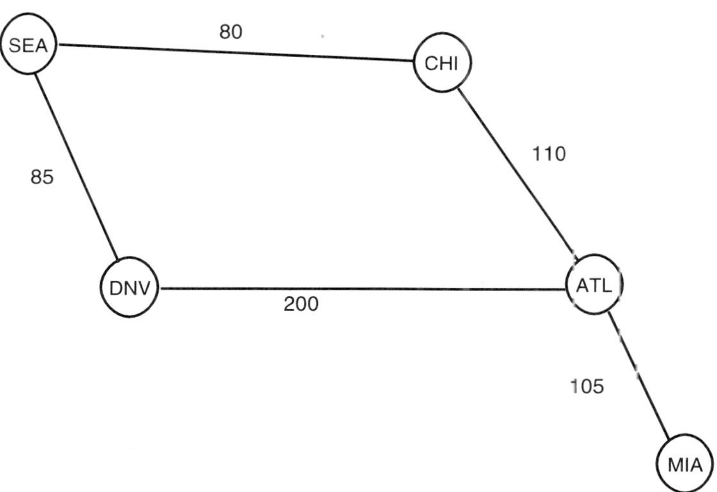


```
MAX       P1SEADNV + P2SEADNV + P1SEACHI - P2SEACHI + P1SEAATL
        + P2SEAATL + P1SEAMIA + P2SEAMIA - P1DNVCHI + P2DNVCHI
        + P1DNVATL + P2DNVATL + P1DNVMIA - P2DNVMIA + P1CHIATL
        + P2CHIATL + P1CHIMIA + P2CHIMIA - P1ATLMIA
SUBJECT TO
! The link capacity constraints;
   LSEADNV)  P1SEADNV + P2SEACHI + P2SEAATL + P2SEAMIA + P1DNVCHI
           + P2DNVATL + P2DNVMIA + P2CHIATL + P2CHIMIA <=    95
   LSEACHI)  P2SEADNV + P1SEACHI + P1SEAATL + P1SEAMIA + P1DNVCHI
           + P2DNVATL + P2DNVMIA + P2CHIATL + P2CHIMIA <=    80
   LDNVATL)  P2SEADNV + P2SEACHI + P2SEAATL + P2SEAMIA + P2DNVCHI
           + P1DNVATL + P1DNVMIA + P2CHIATL + P2CHIMIA <=   200
   LCHIATL)  P2SEADNV + P2SEACHI + P1SEAATL + P1SEAMIA + P2DNVCHI
           + P2DNVATL + P2DNVMIA + P1CHIATL + P1CHIMIA <=   110
   LATLMIA)  P1SEAMIA + P2SEAMIA + P1DNVMIA + P2DNVMIA + P1CHIMIA
           + P2CHIMIA + P1ATLMIA <=   105
! The demand constraints;
   DSEADNV)    P1SEADNV + P2SEADNV <=    10
   DSEACHI)    P1SEACHI + P2SEACHI <=    20
   DSEAATL)    P1SEAATL + P2SEAATL <=    38
   DSEAMIA)    P1SEAMIA + P2SEAMIA <=    33
   DDNVCHI)    P1DNVCHI + P2DNVCHI <=    42
   DDNVATL)    P1DNVATL + P2DNVATL <=    48
   DDNVMIA)    P1DNVMIA + P2DNVMIA <=    23
   DCHIATL)    P1CHIATL + P2CHIATL <=    90
   DCHIMIA)    P1CHIMIA + P2CHIMIA <=    36
   DATLMIA)    P1ATLMIA <=    26
END
```

The structure stands out a little more if it is viewed in PICTURE form:

```
                 P P P P P P P P P P P P P P P P P P P
                 1 2 1 2 1 2 1 2 1 2 1 2 1 2 1 2 1 2 1
                 S S S S S S S S D D D D D C C C C A
                 E E E E E E E E N N N N N H H H H T
                 A A A A A A A A V V V V V I I I I L
                 D D C C A A M M C C A A M A A M M M
                 N N H H T T I I H H T T I T T I I I
                 V V I I L L A A I I L L A A L L A A A
        1:       1 1 1 1 1 1 1 1 1 1 1 1 1 1 1 1 1 1 1 MAX
 LSEADNV:        1     1     1 ' 1 1 '   1 ' 1   1     1 ' < B
 LSEACHI:      ' 1'1 ' 1'  1   '1 '   '1 ' 1'  1   '1 ' < B
 LDNVATL:        1   1     1 ' 1   1 1   1         1   1 ' < C
 LCHIATL:        1   1 1   1       1   1 ' 1 1 ' 1       ' < B
 LATLMIA:      '   '   '   ' 1 1'  '   ' 1 1'  ' 1'1 1 < C
 DSEADNV:      1 1   '         '         '         '       ' < A
 DSEACHI:        1 1         '         '         '       ' < B
 DSEAATL:      '   '   ' 1'1 '   '   '   '   '   '   ' < B
 DSEAMIA:          '     1 1   '         '         '     ' < B
 DDNVCHI:          '         '   1 1     '         '     ' < B
 DDNVATL:      '   '   '   '   '   ' 1'1 '   '   '   ' < B
 DDNVMIA:          '         '         1 1   '         ' < B
 DCHIATL:          '         '         '   1 1       ' < B
 DCHIMIA:      '   '   '   '   '   '   '   ' 1'1 ' < B
 DATLMIA:          '         '         '         '       1 < B
```

When solved, we see that we can handle 322 out of the total demand of 366 calls:

```
                OBJECTIVE FUNCTION VALUE

        1)             322.000000

        VARIABLE           VALUE          REDUCED COST
        P1SEADNV           0.000000          0.000000
        P2SEADNV           0.000000          0.000000
        P1SEACHI          20.000000          0.000000
        P2SEACHI           0.000000          2.000000
        P1SEAATL           0.000000          0.000000
        P2SEAATL          38.000000          0.000000
        P1SEAMIA           0.000000          0.000000
        P2SEAMIA           0.000000          0.000000
        P1DNVCHI          42.000000          0.000000
        P2DNVCHI           0.000000          0.000000
        P1DNVATL          48.000000          0.000000
        P2DNVATL           0.000000          2.000000
        P1DNVMIA          23.000000          0.000000
        P2DNVMIA           0.000000          2.000000
        P1CHIATL          75.000000          0.000000
        P2CHIATL          15.000000          0.000000
        P1CHIMIA          35.000000          0.000000
        P2CHIMIA           0.000000          0.000000
        P1ATLMIA          26.000000          0.000000

        ROW        SLACK OR SURPLUS        DUAL PRICES
        LSEADNV)           0.000000          1.000000
        LSEACHI)           3.000000          0.000000
```

```
LDNVATL)        76.000000         0.000000
LCHIATL)         0.000000         1.000000
LATLMIA)        21.000000         0.000000
DSEADNV)        10.000000         0.000000
DSEACHI)         0.000000         1.000000
DSEAATL)         0.000000         0.000000
DSEAMIA)        33.000000         0.000000
DDNVCHI)         0.000000         0.000000
DDNVATL)         0.000000         1.000000
DDNVMIA)         0.000000         1.000000
DCHIATL)         0.000000         0.000000
DCHIMIA)         1.000000         0.000000
DATLMIA)         0.000000         1.000000
```

Apparently there are a number of alternate optima. The demand not carried is SEA-DNV: 10, SEA-MIA: 33, and CHI-MIA: 1. One may prefer some of the other optima with the same total number of calls but which spread the service a bit more.

7.7 Double Entry Bookkeeping: A Network Model of the Firm

Authors frequently like to identify who was the first to use a given methodology. A contender for the distinction of formulating the first network model is Fra Luca Pacioli. In 1594, while director of a Franciscan monastery in Italy, he published a description of the accounting convention that has come to be known as double entry bookkeeping. From the perspective of networks, each double entry is an arc in a network.

To illustrate, suppose you start up a small dry goods business. During the first two weeks, the following transactions occur:

CAP 1) You invest $50,000 of capital in cash to start the business.
PUR 2) You purchase $27,000 of product on credit from supplier S.
PAY 3) You pay $13,000 of your accounts payable to supplier S.
SEL 4) You sell on credit product costing $5,000 to customer C for $8,000.
REC 5) Customer C pays you $2500 of his debt to you.

In our convention, liabilities and equities will typically have negative balances. So, for example, the initial infusion of cash corresponds to a transfer (an arc) from the equity account (node) to the cash account with a flow of $50,000. The purchase of product on credit corresponds to an arc from the accounts payable account node to the raw materials inventory account with a flow of $27,000. Paying $13,000 to the supplier corresponds to an arc from the cash account to the accounts payable account with a flow of $13,000. Figure 7.7 illustrates.

7.8 Extensions of Network LP Models

There are several generalizations of network models that are important in practice. These extensions share two features in common with true network LP models, namely:

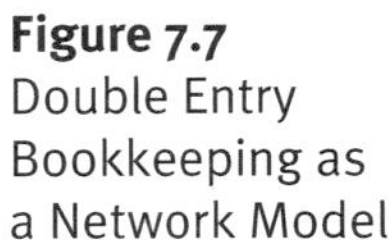

Figure 7.7
Double Entry
Bookkeeping as
a Network Model

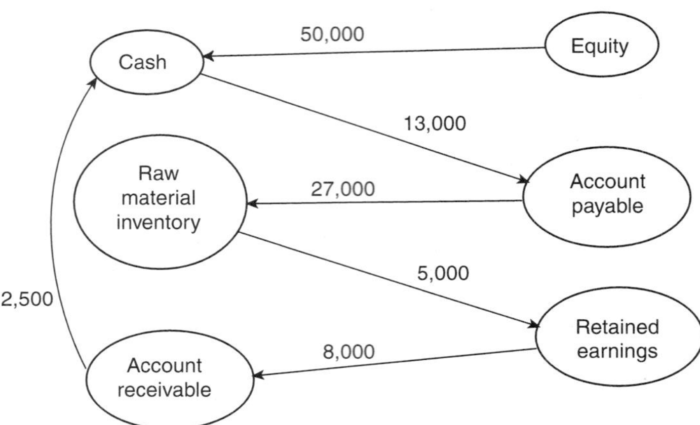

- They can be represented graphically.
- Specialized, fast solution procedures exist for several of these generalizations.

The one feature that is generally not found with these generalizations is:

- Solutions are generally not naturally integer, even if the input data are integers.

The important generalizations we will consider are:

1. *Networks with Gains.* Sometimes called generalized networks, this generalization allows a specified gain or loss of material as it is shipped from one node to another. Structurally, these problems are such that every column has at most two nonzeroes in the constraint matrix; however, the requirement that these coefficients be +1 and −1 is relaxed. Specialized procedures, which may be 20 times faster than the regular simplex method, exist for solving these problems.

   Examples of "shipments" with such gains or losses are: investment in an interest bearing account, electrical transmission with loss, natural gas pipeline shipments where the pipeline pumps burn natural gas from the pipeline, and workforce attrition.

2. *Undirected Networks.* In communications networks, there is typically no direction of shipment. The arcs are undirected.

3. *Multicommodity Networks.* In many distribution situations, there are multiple commodities moving through the network, all competing for scarce network capacity. Each source may produce only one of the commodities, and each destination or sink may accept only one specific commodity.

4. *Leontief Flow.* In a so-called Leontief input-output model (see Leontief, 1951), each activity uses several commodities, although it produces only one commodity. For example, one unit of automotive production may use a half ton of steel, 300 pounds of plastic, and 100 pounds of glass. Material Requirements Planning (MRP) models have the same feature. If each output required only one input, we would simply have a network with gains.

   Special purpose algorithms exist for solving Leontief flow and MRP models; see Jeroslow, Martin, Rardin, and Wang (1992), for example.

5. *Activity/Resource Diagrams.* If Leontief flow models are extended so that each activity can have not only several inputs but also several outputs, one can in fact represent arbitrary LPs. We call the obvious extension to this case of the network diagrams an activity/resource diagram.

7.8.1 Multicommodity Network Flows

In a network LP, the assumption is that a customer is indifferent, except perhaps for cost to the source from which his product was obtained. The assumption is that there is a single commodity flowing through the network. In many network-like situations, there are multiple distinct commodities flowing through the network. If each link has infinite capacity, then an independent network flow LP could be solved for each commodity. However, if a link has a finite capacity that applies to the sum of all commodities flowing over that link, we have a multicommodity network problem.

The most common setting for multicommodity network problems is in shipping. The network might be a natural gas pipeline network, and the commodities might be different fuels shipped over the network. In other shipping problems, such as traffic assignment, or overnight package delivery, each origin/destination pair constitutes a commodity.

The crucial feature is that identity of the commodities must be maintained throughout the network, e.g., customers care which commodity gets delivered. An example is a metals supply company that ships aluminum bars, stainless steel rings, steel beams, etc., all around the country, using a single limited capacity truck fleet.

In general form, the multicommodity network problem is defined as:

D_{ik} = demand for commodity k at node i, with negative values denoting supply,
C_{ijk} = cost per unit of shipping commodity k from node i to node j,
U_{ij} = capacity of the link from node i to node j.

We want to find:

X_{ijk} = amount of commodity k shipped from node i to node j, so as to:

$$\min \ \sum_i \sum_j \sum_k c_{ijk} x_{ijk}.$$

s.t.

For each commodity k and node t:

$$\sum_i x_{itk} = D_{tk} + \sum_j x_{tjk}.$$

For each link i, j:

$$\sum_i x_{itk} = D_{tk} + \sum_j x_{tjk}.$$

7.8.2 Reducing the Size of Multicommodity Problems

If the multiple commodities correspond to origin destination pairs and the cost of shipping a unit over a link is independent of the final destination, you can aggregate commodities over destinations. That is, you need identify a commodity only by its origin, not by both origin and destination. Thus, you have as many commodities as there are origins, rather than (number of origins) * (number of destinations). For example, in a 100-city problem, using this observation you would have 100 commodities rather than 10,000 commodities.

Among the biggest examples of multicommodity network problems in existence are the Patient Distribution System models developed by the U.S. Air Force for planning for transport of sick or wounded personnel.

7.8.3 Multicommodity Flow Example

You have decided to compete with Federal Express by offering "point to point" shipment of materials. Starting small, you have identified six cities as the ones you will first serve. In the matrix below is tabulated the average number of tons that potential customers need to move between each origin/destination pair per day. For example, people in city 2 need to move 4 tons per day to city 3.

FROM \ TO	Demand in tons, $D(i, j)$, by O/D Pair						Cost/ton Shipped, $C(i, j)$, by Link						Capacity in tons, $U(i, j)$, by Link					
	1	2	3	4	5	6	1	2	3	4	5	6	1	2	3	4	5	6
1	0	5	9	7	0	4	0	4	5	8	9	9	0	2	3	2	1	20
2	0	0	4	0	1	0	3	0	3	2	4	6	0	0	2	8	3	9
3	0	0	0	0	0	0	5	3	0	2	3	5	3	0	0	1	3	9
4	0	0	0	0	0	0	7	3	3	0	5	6	5	4	6	0	5	9
5	0	4	0	2	0	8	8	5	3	6	0	3	1	0	2	7	0	9
6	0	0	0	0	0	0	9	7	4	5	5	0	9	9	9	9	9	0

Rather than use a hub system as Federal Express does, you will ship the materials over a regular directed network. The cost per ton of shipping from any node i to any other node j is denoted by $C(i, j)$. There is an upper limit on the number of tons shipped per day over any link in the network of $U(i, j)$. This capacity restriction applies to the total amount of all goods shipped over that link, regardless of origin or destination. Note that $U(i, j)$ and $C(i, j)$ apply to links in the network, whereas $D(i, j)$ applies to origin/destination pairs. This capacity restriction applies only to the directed flow; e.g., $U(i, j)$ need not equal $U(j, i)$. It may be that none of the goods shipped from origin i to destination j moves over link (i, j). It is important that goods maintain their identity as they move through the network. Notice that city 6 looks like a hub; it has high capacity to and from all other cities.

In order to get a compact formulation, we note that only three cities, 1, 2, and 5 are suppliers. Thus, we need keep track of only three commodities in the network, corresponding to the city of origin of the commodity. Define:

X_{ijk} = tons shipped from city i to city j of commodity k.

The resulting formulation is:

```
MIN    5 X655 + 5 X652 + 5 X651 + 5 X645 + 5 X642 + 5 X641
     + 4 X635 + 4 X632 + 4 X631 + 7 X625 + 7 X622 + 7 X621
     + 9 X615 + 9 X612 + 9 X611 + 3 X565 + 3 X562 + 3 X561
     + 6 X545 + 6 X542 + 6 X541 + 3 X535 + 3 X532 + 3 X531
     + 8 X515 + 8 X512 + 8 X511 + 6 X465 + 6 X462 + 6 X461
     + 5 X455 + 5 X452 + 5 X451 + 3 X435 + 3 X432 + 3 X431
     + 3 X425 + 3 X422 + 3 X421 + 7 X415 + 7 X412 + 7 X411
     + 5 X365 + 5 X362 + 5 X361 + 3 X355 + 3 X352 + 3 X351
     + 2 X345 + 2 X342 + 2 X341 + 5 X315 + 5 X312 + 5 X311
     + 6 X265 + 6 X262 + 6 X261 + 4 X255 + 4 X252 + 4 X251
     + 2 X245 + 2 X242 + 2 X241 + 3 X235 + 3 X232 + 3 X231
     + 9 X165 + 9 X162 + 9 X161 + 9 X155 + 9 X152 + 9 X151
     + 8 X145 + 8 X142 + 8 X141 + 5 X135 + 5 X132 + 5 X131
     + 4 X125 + 4 X122 + 4 X121
SUBJECT TO
! Balance constraints, for each commodity k, city i;
   BAL11)    X611 + X511 + X411 + X311- X161 - X151 - X141
             - X131 - X121 =   -25
   BAL12)    X621 + X421 - X261 - X251 - X241 - X231 + X121 =   5
   BAL13)    X631 + X531 + X431 - X361 - X351 - X341 - X311
             + X231 + X131 =    9
   BAL14)    X641 + X541 - X461 - X451 - X431-X421-X411
             + X341 + X241 + X141 =    7
   BAL15)    X651 - X561 - X541 - X531 - X511 + X451 + X351
             + X251 + X151 =    0
   BAL16) -  X651 - X641 - X631 - X621 - X511 + X561 + X461
             + X361 + X261 + X161 =    4
   BAL21)    X612 + X512 + X412 + X312 - X162 - X152 - X142
             - X132 - X122 =    0
   BAL22)    X622 + X422 - X262 - X252 - X242 - X232 + X122 =  -5
   BAL23)    X632 + X532 + X432 - X362 - X352 - X342 - X312
             + X232 + X132 =    4
   BAL24)    X642 + X542 - X462 - X452 - X432 - X422 - X412
             + X342 + X242 + X142 =    0
   BAL25)    X652 - X562 - X542 - X532 - X512 + X452 + X352
             + X252 + X152 =    1
   BAL26) -  X652 - X642 - X632 - X622 - X612 + X562 + X462
             + X362 + X262 + X162 =    0
   BAL51)    X615 + X515 + X415 + X315 - X165 - X155 - X145
             - X135 - X125 =    0
   BAL52)    X625 + X425 - X265 - X255 - X245 - X235 + X125 =   4
   BAL53)    X635 + X535 + X435 - X365 - X355 - X345 - X315
             + X235 + X135 =    0
   BAL54)    X645 + X545 - X465 - X455 - X435 - X425 - X415
             + X345 + X245 + X145 =    2
   BAL55)    X655 - X565 - X545 - X535 - X515 + X455 + X355
             + X255 + X155 =   -14
   BAL56) -  X655 - X645 - X635 - X625 - X615 + X565 + X465
             + X365 + X265 + X165 =    8
! Capacity constraints, for each link i,j;
   CAP12)    X125 + X122 + X121 <=    2
   CAP13)    X135 + X132 + X131 <=    3
   CAP14)    X145 + X142 + X141 <=    2
   CAP15)    X155 + X152 + X151 <=    1
```

```
CAP16)      X165 + X162 + X161 <=      20
CAP23)      X235 + X232 + X231 <=       2
CAP24)      X245 + X242 + X241 <=       8
CAP25)      X255 + X252 + X251 <=       3
CAP26)      X265 + X262 + X261 <=       9
CAP31)      X315 + X312 + X311 <=       3
CAP34)      X345 + X342 + X341 <=       1
CAP35)      X355 + X352 + X351 <=       3
CAP36)      X365 + X362 + X361 <=       9
CAP41)      X415 + X412 + X411 <=       5
CAP42)      X425 + X422 + X421 <=       4
CAP43)      X435 + X432 + X431 <=       6
CAP45)      X455 + X452 + X451 <=       5
CAP46)      X465 + X462 + X461 <=       9
CAP51)      X515 + X512 + X511 <=       1
CAP53)      X535 + X532 + X531 <=       2
CAP54)      X545 + X542 + X541 <=       7
CAP56)      X565 + X562 + X561 <=       9
CAP61)      X615 + X612 + X611 <=       9
CAP62)      X625 + X622 + X621 <=       9
CAP63)      X635 + X632 + X631 <=       9
CAP64)      X645 + X642 + X641 <=       9
CAP65)      X655 + X652 + X651 <=       9
END
```

Notice that there are 3 (commodities) $\times$ 6 (cities) = 18 balance constraints. If instead we identified goods by origin/destination combination rather than just origin, there would have been $9 \times 6 = 54$ balance constraints. Solving, we get:

```
                OBJECTIVE FUNCTION VALUE
        1)            361.000000

        VARIABLE            VALUE          REDUCED COST
          X641             5.000000           0.000000
          X631             5.000000           0.000000
          X621             3.000000           0.000000
          X565             8.000000           0.000000
          X545             5.000000           0.000000
          X535             1.000000           0.000000
          X531             1.000000           0.000000
          X432             2.000000           0.000000
          X425             4.000000           0.000000
          X345             1.000000           0.000000
          X252             1.000000           0.000000
          X242             2.000000           0.000000
          X232             2.000000           0.000000
          X161            17.000000           0.000000
          X151             1.000000           0.000000
          X141             2.000000           0.000000
          X131             3.000000           0.000000
          X121             2.000000           0.000000

          ROW        SLACK OR SURPLUS      DUAL PRICES
        BAL12)           0.000000         -16.000000
        BAL13)           0.000000         -13.000000
        BAL14)           0.000000         -14.000000
```

```
BAL15)        0.000000         -9.000000
BAL16)        0.000000         -9.000000
BAL23)        0.000000         -5.000000
BAL24)        0.000000         -2.000000
BAL25)        0.000000         -4.000000
BAL26)        0.000000         -1.000000
BAL52)        0.000000         -1.000000
BAL53)        0.000000          4.000000
BAL54)        0.000000          2.000000
BAL55)        0.000000          8.000000
BAL56)        0.000000          5.000000
CAP12)        0.000000         12.000000
CAP13)        0.000000          8.000000
CAP14)        0.000000          6.000000
CAP23)        0.000000          2.000000
CAP53)        0.000000          1.000000
```

Notice that because of capacity limitations on other links, the depot city, 6, is used
for many of the shipments.

7.8.4 Fleet Routing and Assignment

An important problem in the airline and trucking industry is fleet routing and as-
signment. Given a set of shipments or flights to be made, the routing part is con-
cerned with the path that each vehicle takes. The assignment part is of interest if the
firm has several different fleets of vehicles available. The question is, then, what
type of vehicle is assigned to each flight or shipment. We will describe a simplified
version of the approach used by Subramanian et al. (1994) to do fleet assignment at
Delta Airlines.

To motivate things, consider the following set of flights serving Chicago (ORD),
Denver (DEN) and Los Angeles (LAX) that United Airlines offered at one time on a
typical weekday.

Daily Flight Schedule

		City			Time	
	Flight	Depart	Arrive		Depart	Arrive
1	221	ORD	DEN		0800	0934
2	223	ORD	DEN		0900	1039
3	274	LAX	DEN		0800	1116
4	105	ORD	LAX		1100	1314
5	228	DEN	ORD		1100	1423
6	230	DEN	ORD		1200	1521
7	259	ORD	LAX		1400	1609
8	293	DEN	LAX		1400	1510
9	412	LAX	ORD		1400	1959
10	766	LAX	DEN		1600	1912
11	238	DEN	ORD		1800	2121

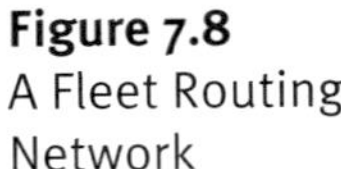

Figure 7.8
A Fleet Routing
Network

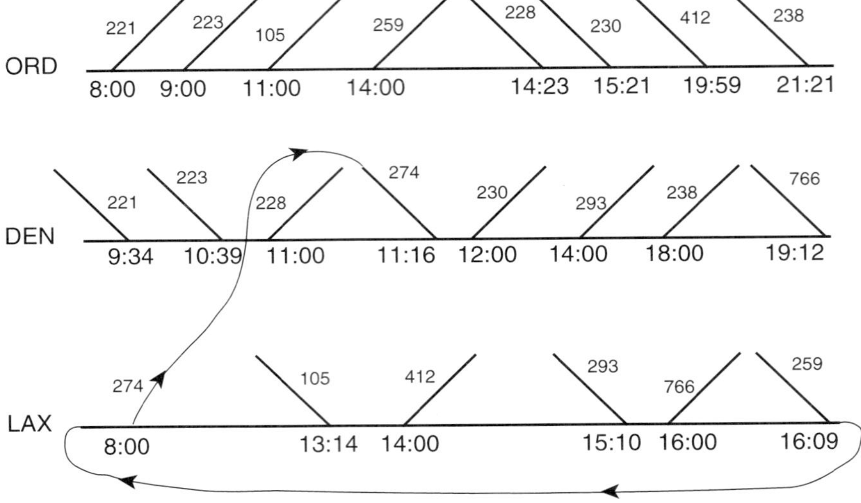

This schedule can be represented by the network in Figure 7.8. The diagonal lines from upper left to lower right represent flight arrivals. The diagonal lines from lower left to upper right represent departures. To complete the diagram, we need to add the lines connecting each flight departure to each flight arrival. The thin line connecting the departure of Flight 274 from LAX to the arrival of Flight 274 in Denver illustrates one of the missing lines. To avoid clutter, these lines have not been added. If the schedule repeats every day, it is reasonable to have the network have a backloop for each city, as illustrated for LAX. To avoid clutter, these lines have not been added.

The (perhaps?) obvious way of interpreting this as a network problem is as follows:

(a) each diagonal line (with the connection to its partner) constitutes a variable, corresponding to a flight;
(b) each horizontal line or backloop corresponds to a decision variable representing the number of aircraft on the ground;
(c) each point of either an arrival or a departure constitutes a node, and the model will have a constraint saying in words:

(number of aircraft on the ground at this city at this instant)
  + (arrivals at this instant)

= (number of departures from this city at this instant)
  + (number of aircraft on the ground after this instant).

With this convention there would be 22 constraints (8 at ORD, 8 at DEN, and 6 at LAX), and 33 variables (11 flight variables and 22 ground variables). The number of constraints and variables can be reduced substant ally if we make the observations that the feasibility of a solution is not affected if, for each city:

(a) each arrival is delayed until the first departure after that arrival,
(b) each departure is advanced (made earlier) to the most recent departure just after an arrival.

Thus, the only nodes required are when a departure immediately follows an arrival.

If we have a fleet of just one type of aircraft, we probably want to know what is the minimum number of aircraft needed to fly this schedule. In words, our model is:

Minimize number of aircraft on the ground overnight
    (That is the only place they can be)
s.t.

    source of aircraft = use of aircraft at each node of the network
and

    each flight must be covered.

Taking all the above observations into account gives the following formulation of a network LP. Note the *G* variables represent the number of aircraft on the ground at a given city just after a specified instant.

```
! Fleet routing with a single plane type;
!  Minimize number of planes on ground overnight;
MIN  GC2400 + GD2400 + GL2400
 ST
! The plane (old) conservation constraints;
! Chicago at 8 am,  sources - uses = 0;
 + GC2400 - F221 - F223 - F105 - F259 - GC1400 = 0
! Chicago at midnight;
 GC1400 + F228 + F230 + F412 + F238 - GC2400 = 0
! Denver at 11 am;
 GD2400 + F221 + F223 - F228-GD1100 = 0
! Denver at high noon;
 GD1100 + F274 - F230 - F293 - F238 - GD1800 = 0
! Denver at midnight;
 GD1800 + F766 - GD2400 = 0
! LA at 8 am;
 GL2400 - F274 - GL0800 = 0
! LA  at 1400;
 GL0800 + F105 - F412 - GL1400 = 0
! LA  at 1600;
 GL1400 + F293 - F766 - GL1600 = 0
! LA  at midnight;
 GL1600 + F259 - GL2400 = 0
! Cover our flights constraints;
 F221 = 1;
 F223 = 1;
 F274 = 1;
 F105 = 1;
 F228 = 1;
 F230 = 1;
 F259 = 1;
```

```
    F293 = 1;
    F412 = 1;
    F766 = 1;
    F238 = 1;
  END
```

This model assumes that no deadheading is to be used; that is, no plane is flown empty from one city to another in order to position it for the next day. The reader probably figured out by simple intuitive arguments that six aircraft are needed. The following solution gives the details:

```
OBJECTIVE FUNCTION VALUE

        1)              6.000000

    VARIABLE            VALUE          REDUCED COST
      GC2400          4.000000          0.000000
      GD2400          1.000000          0.000000
      GL2400          1.000000          0.000000
      F221            1.000000          0.000000
      F223            1.000000          0.000000
      F105            1.000000          0.000000
      F259            1.000000          0.000000
      F228            1.000000          0.000000
      F230            1.000000          0.000000
      F412            1.000000          0.000000
      F238            1.000000          0.000000
      GD1100          2.000000          0.000000
      F274            1.000000          0.000000
      F293            1.000000          0.000000
      F766            1.000000          0.000000
```

Thus, there are four aircraft on the ground overnight at Chicago, one overnight at Denver, and one overnight at Los Angeles.

7.8.5 Fleet Assignment

If we have two or more aircraft types, we have the additional decision of specifying the type of aircraft assigned to each flight. The typical setting is that we have a limited number of new aircraft that are more efficient than previous aircraft. Let us extend our previous example by assuming we have two aircraft of type B. They are more fuel efficient than our original type A aircraft; however, the capacity of type B is slightly less than that of A. We now probably want to maximize the profit contribution. The profit contribution from assigning an aircraft of type i to flight j is:

+ (revenue from satisfying all demand on flight j)

− (spill cost of not being able to serve all demand on j because of the limited capacity of aircraft type i)

− (the operating cost of flying aircraft type i on flight j)

+ (revenue from demand spilled from previous flights captured on this flight).

The spill costs and recoveries are probably the most difficult to estimate. The previous model easily generalizes with the two modifications:

(a) Conservation of flow constraints are needed for each aircraft type.
(b) The flight coverage constraints become more flexible because there are now two ways of covering a flight.

After carefully calculating the profit contribution for each combination of aircraft type and flight, we get the following model:

```
! Fleet routing and assignment with two plane types;
!  Maximize profit contribution from flights covered;
  MAX 105 F221A + 121 F221B + 109 F223A + 108 F223B
    + 110 F274A + 115 F274B + 130 F105A + 140 F105B
    + 106 F228A + 122 F228B + 112 F230A + 115 F230B
    + 132 F259A + 129 F259B + 115 F293A + 123 F293B
    + 133 F412A + 135 F412B + 108 F766A + 117 F766B
    + 116 F238A + 124 F238B
  SUBJECT TO
! Conservation of flow constraints,
!  for type A aircraft,
!   Chicago at 8 am, sources - uses = 0;
   2) - F221A - F223A - F105A - F259A - GC1400A + GC2400A  =  0
!    Chicago at midnight;
   3)   F228A + F230A + F412A + F238A + GC1400A - GC2400A  =  0
! Denver at 11 am;
   4)   F221A + F223A - F228A - GD1100A + GD2400A  =  0
! Denver at high noon;
   5)   F274A - F230A - F293A - F238A + GD1100A - GD1800A  =  0
! Denver at midnight;
   6)   F766A - GD2400A + GD1800A  =  0
! LA at 8 am;
   7) - F274A - GL0800A + GL2400A  =  0
! LA  at 1400;
   8)   F105A - F412A + GL0800A - GL1400A  =  0
! LA  at 1600;
   9)   F293A - F766A + GL1400A - GL1600A  =  0
! LA  at midnight;
   0)   F259A - GL2400A + GL1600A  =  0
!   Aircraft type B, conservation of flow;
! Chicago at 8 am;
   11) - F221B - F223B - F105B - F259B - GC1400B + GC2400B  =  0
! Chicago at midnight;
   12)   F228B + F230B + F412B + F238B + GC1400B - GC2400B  =  0
! Denver at 11 am;
   13)   F221B + F223B - F228B - GD1100B + GD2400B  =  0
! Denver at high noon;
   14)   F274B - F230B - F293B - F238B + GD1100B - GD1800B  =  0
! Denver at midnight;
   15)   F766B - GD2400B + GD1800B  =  0
! LA at 8 am;
   16) - F274B - GL0800B + GL2400B  =  0
! LA  at 1400;
   17)   F105B - F412B + GL0800B - GL1400B  =  0
! LA  at 1600;
```

```
  18)    F293B - F766B + GL1400B - GL1600B  =  0
! LA  at midnight;
  19)    F259B - GL2400B + GL1600B  =  0
! Can put at most one plane on each flight;
  20)    F221A + F221B <=  1
  21)    F223A + F223B <=  1
  22)    F274A + F274B <=  1
  23)    F105A + F105B <=  1
  24)    F228A + F228B <=  1
  25)    F230A + F230B <=  1
  26)    F259A + F259B <=  1
  27)    F293A + F293B <=  1
  28)    F412A + F412B <=  1
  29)    F766A + F766B <=  1
  30)    F238A + F238B <=  1
! Fleet size of type B;
  31)    GC2400B + GD2400B + GL2400B <=  2
  END
```

The not so obvious solution is:

```
OBJECTIVE FUNCTION VALUE

        1)      1325.000000

    VARIABLE           VALUE          REDUCED COST
      F221B          1.000000           0.000000
      F223A          1.000000           0.000000
      F274A          1.000000           0.000000
      F105A          1.000000           0.000000
      F228B          1.000000           0.000000
      F230A          1.000000           0.000000
      F259A          1.000000           0.000000
      F293B          1.000000           0.000000
      F412A          1.000000           0.000000
      F766B          1.000000           0.000000
      F238A          1.000000           0.000000
      GC2400A        3.000000           0.000000
      GD1100A        1.000000           0.000000
      GL2400A        1.000000           0.000000
      GC2400B        1.000000           0.000000
      GD1100B        1.000000           0.000000
      GD2400B        1.000000           0.000000

        ROW    SLACK OR SURPLUS     DUAL PRICES
        4)          0.000000        109.000000
        5)          0.000000        109.000000
        6)          0.000000        109.000000
        7)          0.000000        130.000000
        8)          0.000000        130.000000
        9)          0.000000        130.000000
        0)          0.000000        130.000000
       11)          0.000000        -13.000000
       13)          0.000000         99.000000
       14)          0.000000         99.000000
       15)          0.000000        112.000000
```

```
16)        0.000000        115.000000
17)        0.000000        128.000000
18)        0.000000        128.000000
19)        0.000000        128.000000
20)        0.000000          9.000000
22)        0.000000        131.000000
24)        0.000000        221.000000
25)        0.000000        221.000000
26)        0.000000          2.000000
27)        0.000000         94.000000
28)        0.000000        263.000000
29)        0.000000        133.000000
30)        0.000000        225.000000
31)        0.000000         13.000000
```

Six aircraft are still used. The newer, type B aircraft cover flights 221, 228, 293, and 766. Because there are two vehicle types, this model is a multicommodity network flow model rather than a pure network flow model. Thus, we are not guaranteed to be able to find an optimal solution to the LP that is naturally integer. Nevertheless, such was the case for the example above.

Sometimes, especially in trucking, one has the option to use rented vehicles to cover only selected trips. With regard to the model, the major modification is that rented vehicles do not have to honor the conservation of flow constraints.

7.8.6 Leontief Flow Models

In a Leontief flow model, each activity produces one output; however, it may use 0 or more inputs. The following example illustrates.

7.8.7 Example: Islandia Input-Output Model

The country of Islandia has four major export industries: Steel, Automotive, Electronics, and Plastics. The economic minister of Islandia wants to maximize exports-imports. The unit of exchange in Islandia is the klutz. The prices in klutzes on the world market per unit of Steel, Automotive, Electronics, and Plastics are, respectively, 500, 1500, 300, and 1200. Production of one unit of Steel requires 0.02 units of automotive production, 0.01 units of plastics, 250 klutzes of raw material purchased on the world market, plus 0.5 worker-year of labor. Production of one Automotive unit requires 0.8 units of steel, 0.15 units of electronics, 0.11 units of plastic, one worker-year of labor, and 300 klutzes of imported material. Production of one unit of Electronic equipment requires 0.01 units of steel, 0.01 units of automotive, 0.05 units of plastic, 0.5 worker-year of labor, and 50 klutzes of imported material. Automotive production is limited at 650,000 units. Production of one unit of Plastic requires 0.03 units of automotive production, 0.2 units of steel, 0.05 units of electronics, 2 worker-years of labor, plus 300 klutzes of imported materials. The upper limit on Plastic is 60,000 units. The total labor available in Islandia is 830,000 workers per year. No Steel, Automotive, Electronics, or Plastic products may be imported.

How much should be produced and exported of the various products?

7.8.8 Formulation and Solution of the Islandia Problem

The formulation of an input-output model should follow the same two-step procedure for formulating any LP model, namely: (1) identify the decision variables; and (2) identify the constraints. The key to identifying the decision variables for this problem is to make the distinction between amount of commodity produced and the amount exported. Once this is done, the decision variables can be defined as:

```
S   = units of steel produced,
A   = units of automotive produced,
P   = units of plastic produced,
E   = units of electronics produced,
SEX = units of steel exported,
AEX = units of automotive exported,
PEX = units of plastic exported,
EEX = units of electronics exported.
```

The commodities can be straightforwardly identified as steel, automotive, electronics, plastics, labor, automotive capacity, and plastics capacity. Thus, there will be seven constraints.

The formulation and solution are:

```
MAX                     500 SEX + 1500 AEX + 300 EEX + 1200 PEX
                          - 250 S   - 300 A    - 50 E   - 300 P
SUBJECT TO
   2)  SEX                  - S   + 0.8 A + 0.01 E   + 0.2 P   = 0
   3)      AEX          + 0.02 S       - A + 0.01 E + 0.03 P   = 0
   4)          EEX              + 0.15 A       - E + 0.05 P   = 0
   5)          PEX + 0.01 S + 0.11 A + 0.05 E       - P   = 0
   6)                  0.5 S       + A   + 0.5 E     + 2 P  <= 830000
   7)                            A                        <= 650000
   8)                                               P   <= 60000
END
```

Notice that this model has the Leontief Flow feature; namely, each decision variable has at most one negative constraint coefficient.

The solution is:

```
                OBJECTIVE FUNCTION VALUE

        1)          435431260.0

        VARIABLE           VALUE          REDUCED COST
          SEX           547.914290           0.000000
          AEX        465410.420000           0.000000
          EEX             0.000000         121.874870
          PEX             0.000000        2096.875200
          S          393958.330000           0.000000
          A          475833.340000           0.000000
          E           74375.001000           0.000000
          P           60000.000000           0.000000
```

```
         ROW                    SLACK              DUAL PRICES
          2)               0.000000               500.000000
          3)               0.000000              1500.000000
          4)               0.000000               421.374870
          5)               0.000000              3296.375200
          6)               0.000000               374.062500
          7)          174166.660000                 0.000000
          8)               0.000000              2082.656500
```

The solution indicates that the best way of selling Islandia's steel, automotive, electronics, plastics, and labor resources is in the form of automobiles.

This problem would fit the classical input-output model format of Leontief if, instead of maximizing profits, target levels were set for the exports (or consumption) of steel, automotive, and plastics. The problem would then be to determine the production levels necessary to support the specified export/consumption levels. In this case, the objective function is irrelevant.

A natural generalization is to allow alternative technologies for producing various commodities. These various technologies may correspond to the degree of mechanization or the form of energy consumed, e.g., gas, coal, hydroelectric, etc.

7.8.9 Activity/Resource Diagrams

The graphical approach for depicting a model can be extended to arbitrary LP models. The price one must pay to represent a general LP graphically is that one must introduce an additional component type into the network. There are two component types in such a diagram: (1) activities, which correspond to variables and are denoted by a square, and (2) resources, which correspond to constraints and are denoted by a circle. Each constraint can be thought of as corresponding to some commodity and in words as saying "uses of commodity $\leq$ sources of commodity." The arrows incident to a square correspond to the resources, commodities, or constraints with which that variable has an interaction. The arrows incident to a circle must obviously then correspond to the activities or decision variables with which the constraint has an interaction.

7.8.10 Example: The Vertically Integrated Farmer

A farmer has 120 acres that can be used for growing wheat or corn. The yield is 55 bushels of wheat or 95 bushels of corn per acre per year. Any fraction of the 120 acres can be devoted to growing wheat or corn. Labor requirements are 4 hours per acre per year, plus 0.15 hour per bushel of wheat and 0.70 hour per bushel of corn. Cost of seed, fertilizer, etc., is 20 cents per bushel of wheat produced and 12 cents per bushel of corn produced. Wheat can be sold for $1.75 per bushel, and corn for $0.95 per bushel. Wheat can be bought for $2.50 per bushel, and corn for $1.50 per bushel.

In addition, the farmer may raise pigs and/or poultry. The farmer sells the pigs or poultry when they reach the age of one year. A pig sells for $40. He measures the poultry in terms of coops. (One coop brings in $40 at the time of sale.) One pig requires 25 bushels of wheat or 20 bushels of corn, plus 25 hours of labor, and 25 square feet of floor space. One coop of poultry requires 25 bushels of corn or 10 bushels of wheat, plus 40 hours of labor, and 15 square feet of floor space.

The farmer has 10,000 square feet of floor space. He has available per year 2,000 hours of his own time and another 2,000 hours from his family. He can hire labor at $1.50 per hour. However, for each hour of hired labor, 0.15 hour of the farmer's time is required for supervision. How much land should be devoted to corn and how much to wheat, and in addition, how many pigs and/or poultry should be raised to maximize the farmer's profits? (This problem is based on an example in Hadley, 1962).

You may find it convenient to use the following variables for this problem:

WH	Wheat Harvested (in bushels)
CH	Corn Harvested (in bushels)
PH	Pigs Raised and Sold
HS	Hens Raised and Sold (number of coops)
LB	Labor Hired (in hours)
WS	Wheat Marketed or Sold (in bushels)
CS	Corn Marketed or Sold (in bushels)
CH	Corn Used to Feed Hens (in bushels)
WH	Wheat Used to Feed Hens (in bushels)
CP	Corn Used to Feed Pigs (in bushels)
WP	Wheat Used to Feed Pigs (in bushels)
CB	Corn Bought (in bushels)
WB	Wheat Bought (in bushels)

The activity-resources diagram for the preceding problem is shown in Figure 7.9. Some things to note about an activity-resource diagram are:

- Each rectangle in the diagram corresponds to a decision variable in the formulation.
- Each circle in the diagram corresponds to a constraint or the objective.
- Each arrow in the diagram corresponds to a coefficient in the formulation.
- Associated with each circle or rectangle is a unit of measure, e.g., hr. or bu.
- The units or dimension of each arrow is:

"Units of the circle" per "unit of the rectangle."

7.8.11 Spanning Trees

Another simple yet important network-related problem is the spanning tree problem. It arises, for example, in the installation of cable to provide cable television to homes. Given a set of homes to be connected, we want to find a minimum cost network so that every home is connected to the network. A reasonable approximation to the cost of the network is that it is the sum of the costs of the arcs in the network. If the arcs have positive costs, then a little reflection should convince you that the minimum cost network contains no loops, i.e., for any two nodes (or homes) on the

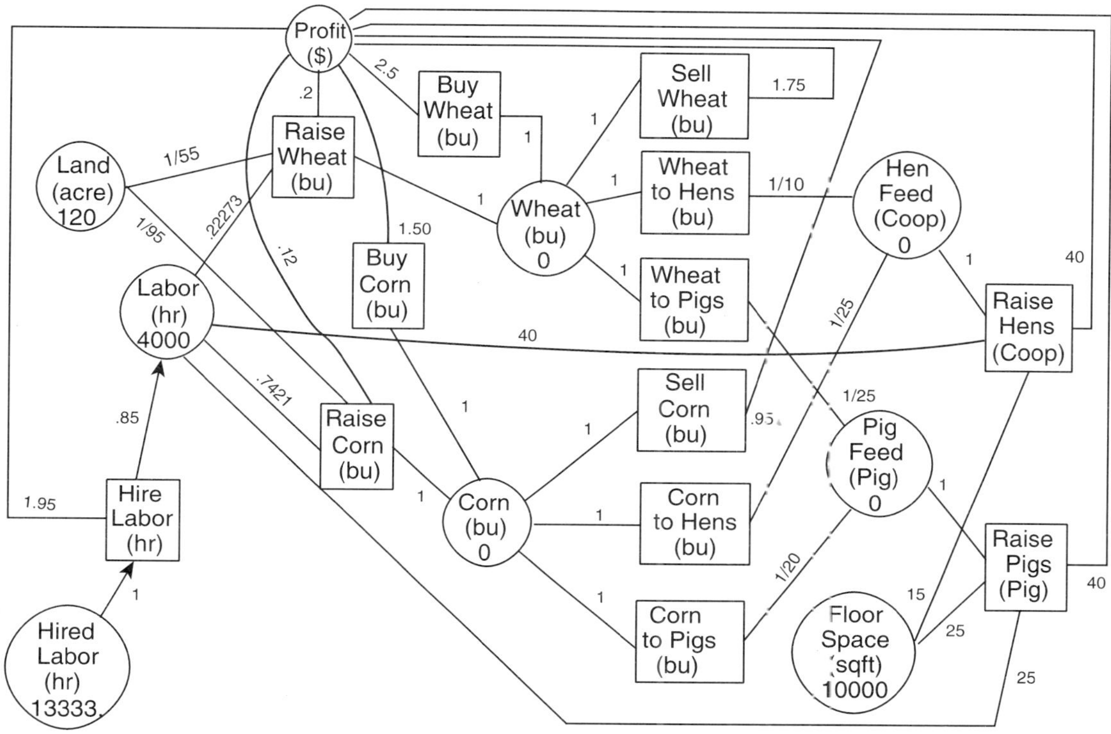

Figure 7.9　An Activity-Resource Diagram

network, there is exactly one path connecting them. Such a network is called a spanning tree.

A delightfully simple algorithm is available for finding a minimum cost spanning tree (see Kruskal, 1956).

(1)　Set　$Y = \{2,3,4 \ldots n\}$, i.e., the set of nodes *yet* to be connected.
　　　　$A = \{1\}$, i.e., the set of *already* connected nodes. We may
　　　　arbitrarily define node 1 as the root of the tree.
(2)　If Y is empty, then we are done,
(3)　else find the shortest arc (i, j) such that i is in A and j is in Y.
(4)　Add arc (i, j) to the network and
　　　set $A = A + j$,
　　　$Y = Y - j$.
(5)　Go to (2).

Because of the above simple and efficient algorithm, LP is not needed to solve the minimum spanning tree problem. In fact, formulating the minimum spanning tree problem as an LP is a bit tedious.

7.9 PROBLEMS

Problem 1

The Slick Oil Company is preparing to make next month's pipeline shipment decisions. The Los Angeles terminal will require 200,000 barrels of oil. This oil can be supplied from either Houston or Casper, Wyoming. Houston can supply oil to L.A. at a transportation cost of $.25/barrel. Casper can supply L.A. at a transportation cost of $.28/barrel. The St. Louis terminal will require 120,000 barrels. St. Louis can be supplied from Houston at a cost of $.18/barrel and from Casper at a cost of $.22/barrel. The terminal at Freshair, Indiana, requires 230,000 barrels. Oil can be shipped to Freshair from Casper at a cost of $.21/barrel, from Houston at a cost of $.19/barrel, and from Titusville, Pa., at a cost of $.17/barrel. Casper will have a total of 250,000 barrels available to be shipped. Houston will have 350,000 barrels available to be shipped. Because of limited pipeline capacity, no more than 180,000 barrels can be shipped from Casper to L.A. next month and no more than 150,000 barrels from Houston to L.A. The Newark, N.J., terminal will require 190,000 barrels next month. It can be supplied only from Titusville at a transportation cost of $.14/barrel. The Atlanta terminal will require 150,000 barrels next month. Atlanta can be supplied from Titusville at a transportation cost of $.16/barrel or from Houston at a cost of $.20/barrel. Titusville will have a total of 300,000 barrels available to be shipped.

Formulate the problem of finding the minimum transportation cost distribution plan as a linear program.

Problem 2

Louis Szathjoseph, proprietor of the Boulangerie Restaurant, knows that he will need 40, 70, and 60 tablecloths on Thursday, Friday, and Saturday, respectively, for scheduled banquets. He can rent tablecloths for three days for $2 each. A tablecloth must be laundered before it can be reused. He can have them cleaned overnight for $1.50 each. He can have them laundered by regular one-day service (e.g., one used on Thursday could be reused on Saturday) for $.80 each. There are currently 20 clean tablecloths on hand, with none dirty or at the laundry. Rented tablecloths need not be cleaned before returning.

(a) What are the decision variables?
(b) Formulate the LP that is appropriate for minimizing the total costs of renting and laundering the tablecloths. For each day you will probably have a constraint requiring the number of clean tablecloths available to at least equal that day's demand. For each of the first two days, you will probably want a constraint requiring the number of tablecloths sent to the laundry not to exceed those that have been made dirty. Is it a network LP?

Problem 3

The Millersburg Supply Company uses a large fleet of vehicles, which it leases from manufacturers. The following pattern of vehicle requirements is forecast for the next 8 months:

Month	Jan.	Feb.	Mar.	Apr.	May	June	July	Aug.
No. of Vehicles Required	430	410	440	390	425	450	465	470

Vehicles can be leased from various manufacturers at various costs and for various lengths of time. The best plans available are: 3-month lease, $1,700; 4-month lease, $2,000; 5-month lease, $2,600. A lease can be started in any month. On January 1, there are 200 cars on lease, all of which go off lease at the end of February.

(a) Formulate an approach for minimizing Millersburg's leasing costs over this 8-month period.

(b) Show that this problem is a network problem.

Problem 4

Several years ago a university in the Westwood section of Los Angeles introduced a bidding system for assigning professors to teach courses in its business school. The table below describes a small, slightly simplified three-professor/two-course version. For the upcoming year, each professor submits a bid for each course and places limits on how many courses he or she wants to teach in each of the school's two semesters. Each professor, however, is expected to teach four courses total per year; at most three per semester.

	Prof. X	Prof. Y	Prof. Z	Sections Needed in the Year Min	Max
Fall Courses	≤ 1	≤ 3	≤ 1		
Spring Courses	≤ 3	≤ 2	≤ 3		
Course A bids	6	3	8	3	7
Course B bids	4	7	2	2	8

From the table, note that professor Z strongly prefers to teach course A, whereas professor X has a slight preference for A, and Professor Y does not want to teach more than two course sections in the spring. Over both semesters, at least three sections of course A must be taught. Can you formulate this problem as a network problem?

Problem 5

Aircraft Fuel Ferrying Problem. A standard problem with any airline is the determination of how much fuel to take on at each stop. Fuel consumption is minimized if just sufficient fuel is taken on at each stop to fly the plane to the next stop. This policy, however, disregards the fact that fuel prices may differ from one airport to the next.

Buying all the fuel at the cheapest stop may not be the cheapest policy either. This might require carrying large fuel loads that would in turn cause large amounts of fuel to be burned.

The stops that a scheduled aircraft must make are numbered in order 1, 2, 3, . . . , N. The parameters of the problem are:

c_t = cost/liter of fuel at stop t,

d_t = liters of fuel burned from t to $t + 1$ if just sufficient fuel is on board at t to get the craft to $t + 1$,

b_t = liters of additional fuel burned per excess liter of fuel delivered to $t + 1$ from t.

The problem is to determine P_t, $t = 1, 2, \ldots , N$, the amount of fuel to purchase at stop t. Formulate an LP model for solving this problem. Is it a network LP?

Problem 6

Show that any LP can be converted to an equivalent LP in which every column (variable) has at most three nonzero constraint coefficients. What does this suggest about the fundamental complexity of a network LP vs. a general LP?

Problem 7

Figure 7.10 is the activity-on-arc diagram showing the precedence relations among the five activities involved in repairing a refinery. The three numbers above each arc represent (from left to right, respectively) the normal time for performing the activity in days, the time to perform the activity if crashed to the maximum extent, and the additional cost in \$1000s for each day that the activity is shortened. An activity can be partially crashed. It is desired that the project be completed in 15 days. Write an LP formulation for determining how much each activity should be crashed.

Problem 8

Given n currencies, the one period currency exchange problem is characterized by a beginning inventory vector, an exchange rate matrix, and an ending inventory requirement vector defined as follows:

n_i = amount of cash on hand in currency i, at the beginning of the period measured in units of currency i, for $i = 1, 2, \ldots , n$.

r_{ij} = units of currency j obtainable per unit of currency i for $i = 1, 2, \ldots , n$, $j = 1, 2, \ldots , n$. Note that $r_{ii} = 1$ and, in general, we can expect that $r_{ij} < 1/r_{ji}$ for $i \neq j$.

e_i = minimum ending inventory requirement for currency i, for $i = 1, 2, \ldots , n$. That is, at the end of the period we must have at least e_i units of currency i on hand.

The decision variables are:

X_{ij} = amount of currency i converted into currency j, for

$$i = 1, 2, \ldots , n; j = 1, 2, \ldots , n.$$

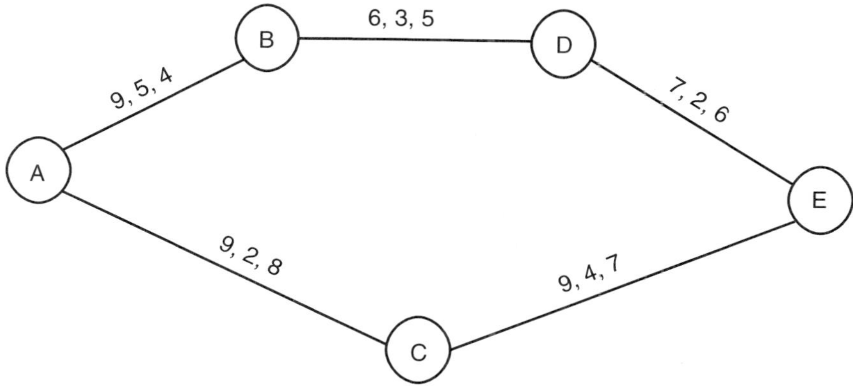

Figure 7.10
PERT Diagram
with Crashing
Allowed

Formulate a model for determining an efficient set of values for the X_{ij}. The formulation should have the following features:

(a) If there is a "money pump" kind of arbitrage opportunity, the model will find it.
(b) It should not be biased against any particular currency; i.e., the solution should be independent of which currency is called 1.
(c) If a currency is worthless, you should buy no more of it than that sufficient to meet the minimum requirement. A currency i is worthless if $r_{ij} = 0$ for all $j \neq i$.

Problem 9

The following linear program happens to be a network LP. Draw the corresponding network. Label the nodes and links.

```
MIN   4 T + 2 U + 3 V + 5 W
    + 6 X + 7 Y + 9 Z
   subject to
   A)  T + Y + Z >= 4
   B)  U - W - X - Z = 0
   C)  - T + W = 1
   D)  V + X - Y = 2
   E)  U + V <= 7
END
```

Problem 10

Consider a set of three flights provided by an airline to serve four cities, A, B, C, and H. The airline uses a two-fare pricing structure and would like to decide upon how many seats to allocate to each fare class on each flight. Node H is a hub for changing planes. The three flights are: from A to H, H to B, and H to C. The respective flight capacities are 120, 100, and 110. Customer demand has the following characteristics:

Itinerary	Class 1 Demand	At a Price of	Class 2 Demand	At a Price of
AH	33	190	56	90
AB (via H)	24	244	43	193
AC (via H)	12	261	67	199
HB	44	140	69	80
HC	16	186	17	103

How many seats should be allocated to each class on each of the three flights? An obvious solution, if it is feasible, is to set aside enough class 1 seats on every flight so that all class 1 travelers can be accommodated. Thus, the leg AH would get 33 + 24 + 12 = 69 class 1 seats, leg HB would get 24 + 44 = 68 class 1 seats, and leg HC would get 12 + 16 = 28 class 1 seats. The total revenue of this solution is $38,854. Is this the most profitable solution?

Problem 11

A common distribution system structure in many parts of the world is the three-level system composed of plants, distribution centers (DC), and outlets. A cost minimization model for a system composed of two plants (A & B), three DCs (X, Y, & Z), and four outlets (1, 2, 3, & 4) is shown below.

```
MIN     AX +  2 AY +  3 BX    +  BY +  2 BZ
   +  5 X1 +  7 X2 +  9 Y1 +  6 Y2 +  7 Y3
   +  8 Z2 +  7 Z3 +  4 Z4
        AX +  AY =   9
        BX +  BY +  BZ =   8
    -  AX -  BX +  X1 +  X2 =   0
    -  AY -  BY +  Y1 +  Y2 +  Y3 =   0
    -  BZ +  Z2 +  Z3 +  Z4 =   0
    -  X1 -  Y1 = -  3
    -  X2 -  Y2 -  Z2 = -  5
    -  Y3 -  Z3 = -  4
    -  Z4 = -  5
   END
```

Part of the solution is shown below.

```
SOLUTION OBJECTIVE VALUE =       121.0

           VARIABLE              VALUE            REDUCED COST
                 AX           3.000000              0.0000000
                 AY           6.000000              0.0000000
                 BX           0.000000              3.0000000
                 BY           3.000000              0.0000000
                 BZ           5.000000              0.0000000
                 X1           3.000000              0.0000000
```

X2	0.0000000	0.0000000
Y1	0.0000000	5.000000
Y2	5.000000	0.0000000
Y3	4.000000	0.0000000
Z2	0.0000000	3.000000
Z3	0.0000000	1.000000
Z4	5.000000	0.0000000

(a) Is there an alternate optimal solution to this distribution problem?

(b) A trucking firm that offers services from city Y to city 1 would like to get more of your business. At what price per unit might you be willing to give them more business according to the above solution?

(c) The demand at city 2 has been decreased to 3 units. Show how the model is changed.

(d) The capacity of plant B has been increased to 13 units. Show how the model is changed.

(e) Distribution center Y is actually in a large city where there is an untapped demand of 3 units that could be served directly from the DC at Y. Show how to include this additional demand at Y.

Problem 12

Labor on the first shift of a day (8 A.M. to 4 P.M.) costs $15 per person/hour. Labor on the second (4 P.M. to midnight) and third (midnight to 8 A.M.) shifts costs $20 per person/hour and $25 per person/hour, respectively. A certain task requires 18 days if done with just first-shift labor and costs $8640. Second- and third-shift labor have the same efficiency as first-shift labor. The only way of accelerating or crashing the task is to add additional shifts for one or more additional days. The total cost of the task consists solely of labor costs.

Complete the following crash cost table for this task.

Task time in whole days:
18   17   16   15   14   13   12   11   10   9   8   7   6   5   4

Total cost:
8640

Problem 13

You are on a camping trip and wish to prepare a recipe for a certain food delight that calls for 4 cups of water. The only containers in your possession are two ungraduated steel vessels, one of 3-cup capacity, the other of 5-cup capacity. Show how you can solve this problem by drawing a certain two-dimensional network, where each node represents a specific combination of contents in your two containers.

Problem 14

Following is part of the schedule for an airline.

	Flight	City		Time		Difference in Profit
		Depart	Arrive	Depart	Arrive	
1	221	ORD	DEN	0800	0934	+$3000
2	223	ORD	DEN	0900	1039	−$4000
3	274	LAX	DEN	0800	1116	−$3000
4	105	ORD	LAX	1100	1314	+$10000
5	228	DEN	ORD	1100	1423	−$2000
6	230	DEN	ORD	1200	1521	−$3000
7	259	ORD	LAX	1400	1609	+$4000
8	293	DEN	LAX	1400	1510	+$1000
9	412	LAX	ORD	1400	1959	+$7000
10	766	LAX	DEN	1600	1912	+$2000
11	238	DEN	ORD	1800	2121	−$4000

The airline currently flies the above schedule using standard Boeing 737 aircraft. Boeing is trying to convince the airline to use a new aircraft, the 737-XX, known affectionately as the Dos Equis. The 737-XX consumes more fuel per kilometer; however, it is sufficiently larger that if it carries enough passengers, it is more efficient per passenger/kilometer. The "Difference in Profitability" column above shows the relative profitability of using the 737-XX instead of the standard 737 on each flight. The airline is considering using at most one 737-XX.

Based on the available information, analyze the wisdom of using the 737-XX in place of one of the standard 737s.

Problem 15

The following linear program happens to be a network LP.

```
MIN    9 S + 4 T + 2 U + 3 V + 5 W + 6 X + 7 Y
       A)  - T + W = 1
       B)  S + T + Y   >= 4
       C)  U - W - X - S = 0
       D)  U + V <= 7
       E)  V + X - Y = 2
       END
```

Draw the corresponding network. Label the nodes and links.

Problem 16

A small but growing long-distance phone company, SBG, Inc., is trying to decide in which markets it should try to expand. It has used the following model to decide how to maximize the calls that it carries per hour.

```
MAX  P1SEADNV + P2SEADNV + P1SEACHI + P2SEACHI + P1SEAATL
    + P2SEAATL + P1SEAMIA + P2SEAMIA + P1DNVCHI + P2DNVCHI
```

```
      + P1DNVATL + P2DNVATL + P1DNVMIA + P2DNVMIA + P1CHIATL
      + P2CHIATL + P1CHIMIA + P2CHIMIA + P1ATLMIA
subject to
  LSEADNV) P1SEADNV + P2SEACHI + P2SEAATL + P2SEAMIA +
           P1DNVCHI + P2DNVATL + P2DNVMIA + P2CHIATL +
           P2CHIMIA <= 95
  LSEACHI) P2SEADNV + P1SEACHI + P1SEAATL + P1SEAMIA +
           P1DNVCHI + P2DNVATL + P2DNVMIA + P2CHIATL +
           P2CHIMIA <= 80
  LDNVATL) P2SEADNV + P2SEACHI + P2SEAATL + P2SEAMIA +
           P2DNVCHI + P1DNVATL + P1DNVMIA + P2CHIATL
          +P2CHIMIA <= 200
  LCHIATL) P2SEADNV + P2SEACHI + P1SEAATL + P1SEAMIA +
           P2DNVCHI + P2DNVALT + P2DNVMIA + P1CHIATL +
           P1CHIMIA <= 110
  LATLMIA) P1SEAMIA + P2SEAMIA + P1DNVMIA + P2DNVMIA +
           P1CHIMIA + P2CHIMIA + P1ATLMIA   <= 105
  DSEADNV) P1SEADNV + P2SEADNV <= 10
  DSEACHI) P1SEACHI + P2SEACHI <= 20
  DSEAATL) P1SEAATL + P2SEAATL <= 38
  DSEAMIA) P1SEAMIA + P2SEAMIA <= 33
  DDNVCHI) P1DNVCHI + P2DNVCHI <= 42
  DDNVATL) P1DNVATL + P2DNVATL <= 48
  DDNVMIA) P1DNVMIA + P2DNVMIA <= 23
  DCHIATL) P1CHIATL + P2CHIATL <= 90
  DCHIMIA) P1CHIMIA + P2CHIMIA <= 36
  DATLMIA) P1ATLMIA            <= 26
```

Now it would like to refine the model so that it takes into account not only revenue per call but also modest variable costs associated with each link for carrying a call. The variable cost per typical call according to link used is shown in the table below:

Variable Cost/Call

	DNV	CHI	ATL	MIA
SEA	.11	.16	X	X
DNV		X	.15	X
CHI			.06	X
ATL				.07

An X means there is no direct link between the two cities. SBG would like to find the combination of calls to accept so as to maximize profit contribution. Suppose the typical revenue per call between ATL and SEA is $1.20. Show how to modify the model just to represent the revenue and cost information for the demand between SEA and ATL.

Problem 17

Below is a four-activity project network presented in activity-on-node form, along with information on crashing opportunities for each activity.

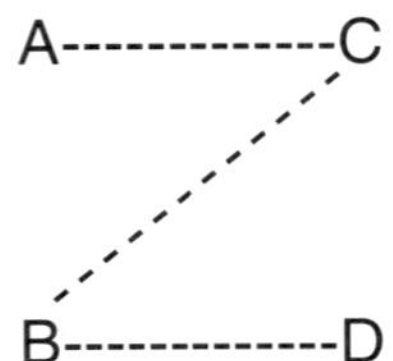

Activity	NORMAL Time (Days)	Crash Cost Per Day	Minimum Possible Time (Days)
A	8	3	4
B	7	4	5
C	6	6	3
D	9	2	5

Complete the following tabulation of crashing cost vs. project length.

Step	Incremental Project Length	Total Crashing Cost/Day	Activities Crashing	Cost to Crash
0	16	0	0	—
1				
2				
3				
4				

Multiperiod Planning Problems

8.1 Introduction

One of the most important uses of LP is in multiperiod planning. Most of the problems we have considered thus far have been essentially one-period problems. The formulations acted as if decisions this period were decoupled from decisions in future periods. Typically, however, if we produce more of a certain product this period than a constraint requires, that extra production will not be worthless but can probably be used next period.

These interactions between periods can be represented very easily within LP models. In fact, most large LPs encountered in practice are multiperiod models. A common synonym for "multiperiod" is "dynamic"; e.g., a multiperiod LP may be referred to as a dynamic model.

In some applications, the need to represent the multiperiod aspects is quite obvious. One setting in which multiperiod LP has been used for a number of years is in the manufacture of cheese. Production decisions must be made monthly or even weekly. The production time for many cheeses, however, may be months. For example, Parmesan cheese may need to be stored in inventory for up to ten months. Swiss cheese may take from two to four months, and the various grades of cheddar obtained depend upon the number of weeks held in storage. Clearly, in this application, it is the multiperiod aspect of the model that is the important feature.

Models for planning over time partition time into a number of periods. The portion of the model corresponding to a single period might be some combination of product mix, blending, etc., models. These single period or static models are linked by:

1. A link or inventory variable for each commodity and period. The linking variable represents the amount of commodity transferred from one period to the next.
2. A "material balance" or "sources = uses" constraint for each commodity and period. The simplest form of this constraint is "beginning inventory + production = ending inventory + goods sold."

Multiperiod models are usually used in a rolling or sliding format. In this format, the model is solved at the beginning of each period. The recommendaticns of the solution for the first period are implemented. As one period elapses and better data and forecasts become available, the model is slid forward one period. The period that had been number 2 becomes number 1, etc.

There is nothing sacred about having all periods of the same length. For example, when a petroleum company plans production for the coming year, it is sensible to have the periods correspond to the seasons of the year. One possible partition is to have the winter period extend from December 1 to March 15; the spring period extend from March 16 to May 15; the summer period extend from May 16 to September 15; and the autumn period extend from September 16 to November 30.

Some companies, such as forest products- or mineral resources-based companies, plan as much as 50 years into the future. In such a case, one might have the first two periods be one year each, the next period be two years, the next two periods three years each, the next two periods five years each, and the final three periods ten years each.

Interperiod interactions are usually accounted for in LPs by the introduction of inventory decision variables. These variables "link" adjacent periods. As an example, suppose we have a single explicit decision to make each period, namely, how much to produce of a single product. Call this decision variable for period j, P_j. Further, suppose we have contracts to sell known amounts of this product, d_j, in period j. Define the decision variable I_j as the amount of inventory left over at the end of period j. By this convention, the beginning inventory in period j is I_{j-1}. The LP formulation will then contain one "sources of product = uses of product" constraint for each period. For period 2 the sources of product are: beginning inventory, I_1, and production in the period, P_2. The uses of product are: demand, d_2, and end-of-period inventory, I_2. For example, if $d_2 = 60$ and $d_3 = 40$, the constraint for period 2 is

$$I_1 + P_2 = 60 + I_2 \quad \text{or} \quad I_1 + P_2 - I_2 = 60.$$

The constraint for period 3 is

$$I_2 + P_3 - I_3 = 40.$$

Notice how I_2 "links," i.e., appears in both the constraints for period 2 and 3.

In some problems the net outflow need not exactly equal the net inflow into the next period. For example, if the product is cash, one of the linking variables may be short-term borrowing or lending. For each dollar that is carried over from period 2 by lending, we will enter period 3 with $1.05 if the interest rate is 5% per period.

On the other hand, if the "product" is workforce and there is a predictable attrition rate of 10% per period, the above two constraints would be modified to

$$.90I_1 + P_2 - I_2 = 60,$$

$$.90I_2 + P_3 - I_3 = 40.$$

In this case, P_i is the number hired in period i.

The following example provides a simplified illustration of a single product, multiperiod planning situation.

8.2 A Dynamic Production Problem

A company produces one product for which the demand for the next four quarters is predicted to be:

Spring	Summer	Autumn	Winter
20	30	50	60

Assuming all the demand is to be met, there are two extreme policies that might be followed:

1. "Track" demand with production and carry no inventory.
2. Produce at a constant rate of 40 units per quarter and allow inventory to absorb the fluctuations in demand.

There are costs associated with carrying inventory and costs associated with varying the production level, so one would expect that the least cost policy is probably a combination of (1) and (2), i.e., carry some inventory but also vary the production level somewhat.

For costing purposes, the company estimates that changing the production level from one period to the next costs $500 per unit. These costs are often called "hiring and firing" costs. It is estimated that inventory costs can be accurately approximated by charging $800 for each unit of inventory at the end of the period. The initial inventory is zero and the current production level is 55 units per quarter. We require that these same levels be achieved or returned to at the end of the winter quarter.

We can now calculate that the cost of the no inventory policy is:

$$\$500 \times (35 + 10 + 20 + 10 + 5) = \$40,000.$$

On the other hand, the cost of the constant production policy is

$$\$800 \times (20 + 30 + 20 + 0) + 500 \times (15 + 15) = \$71,000.$$

We can find the least cost policy by formulating a linear program.

8.2.1 Formulation

The following definitions of variables will be useful:

P_i = number of units produced in period i, for $i = 1, 2, 3,$ and 4,
I_i = units in inventory at the end of period I,
U_i = increase in production level between period $i - 1$ and I,
D_i = decrease in production level between $i - 1$ and I.

The P_i variables are the obvious decision variables. It is useful to define the I_i, U_i and D_i variables so that we can conveniently compute the costs each period. To minimize the cost per year, we want to minimize the sum of inventory costs:

$$\$800 \, I_1 + \$800 \, I_2 + \$800 \, I_3 + \$800 \, I_4$$

plus production change costs:

$$\$500\ U_1 + \$500\ U_2 + \$500\ U_3 + \$500\ U_4 + \$500\ D_1$$
$$+ \$500\ D_2 + \$500\ D_3 + \$500\ D_4.$$

8.2.2 Constraints

Every multiperiod problem will have a "material balance" or "sources = uses" constraint for each product for each period. The usual form of these constraints in words is:

beginning inventory + production − ending inventory = demand.

Algebraically these constraints for the problem at hand are:

$$P_1 - I_1 = 20$$
$$I_1 + P_2 - I_2 = 30$$
$$I_2 + P_3 - I_3 = 50$$
$$I_3 + P_4 = 60.$$

Notice that I_4 and I_0 do not appear in the first and last constraints, because initial and ending inventories are required to be zero.

If the formulation is solved as is, there is nothing to force U_1, D_1, etc., to be greater than zero. Therefore, the solution will be the pure production policy, namely, $P_1 = 20$, $P_2 = 30$, $P_3 = 50$, $P_4 = 60$. This policy implies a production increase at the end of each period but the last. This suggests that a way of forcing U_1, U_2, U_3, U_4 to take the proper values is to append the constraints:

$$U_1 \geq P_1 - 55$$
$$U_2 \geq P_2 - P_1$$
$$U_3 \geq P_3 - P_2$$
$$U_4 \geq P_4 - P_3.$$

Production decreases are still not properly measured. An analogous set of four constraints should take care of this problem, specifically:

$$D_1 \geq 55 - P_1$$
$$D_2 \geq P_1 - P_2$$
$$D_3 \geq P_2 - P_3$$
$$D_4 \geq P_3 - P_4.$$

To incorporate the requirement that the production level be returned to 55 at the end of the winter quarter, we add the variables U_5 and D_5 to measure changes at the end of the last quarter. U_5 and D_5 are forced to take on the right values with the constraints:

$$U_5 \geq 55 - P_4$$
$$D_5 \geq P_4 - 55.$$

This completes the formulation. When it is solved we get the mixed policy:

$$P_1 = P_2 = 25;\ P_3 = P_4 = 55.$$

Before moving on, we will note that the formulation can be simplified from one with 14 constraints to one with 9 constraints. The key observation is that two constraints like

$$U_2 \geq P_2 - P_1$$
$$D_2 \geq P_1 - P_2$$

can be replaced by the single constraint

$$U_2 - D_2 = P_2 - P_1.$$

The argument is more economic than algebraic. The purpose with either formulation is to force $U_2 = P_2 - P_1$ if $P_2 - P_1 \geq 0$ and $D_2 = P_1 - P_2$ if $P_1 - P_2 \geq 0$. From economics you can argue that at the optimal solution you will find at most one of U_2 and D_2 are > 0 under either formulation. If both U_2 and D_2 are > 0 under the second formulation, both can be reduced by an equal amount, thus reducing costs without violating any constraints.

The complete, compact formulation is

```
MIN     800  I1 +  800  I2 +  800  I3 +  500  J1
      +  500  U2 +  500  U3 +  500  U4 +  500  D1
      +  500  D2 +  500  D3 +  500  D4 +  500  J5
      +  500  D5
SUBJECT TO
      2)    -   I1 +  P1 =      20
      3)        I1 -  I2 +   P2 =      30
      4)        I2 -  I3 +   P3 =      50
      5)        I3 +  P4 =      60
      6)        U1 -  D1 -   P1 = -  55
      7)        U2 -  D2 +   P1 -  P2 =      0
      8)        U3 -  D3 +   P2 -  P3 =      0
      9)        U4 -  D4 +   P3 -  P4 =      0
     10)        U5 -  D5 +   P4 =      55
END
```

The solution is

```
                    LP OPTIMUM FOUND

                OBJECTIVE FUNCTION VALUE

        1)           38000.0000

    VARIABLE            VALUE              REDUCED COST
        I1            5.000000               0.000000
        I2            0.000000             700.000000
        I3            5.000000               0.000000
        U1            0.000000            1000.000000
        U2            0.000000             100.000000
        U3           30.000000               0.000000
        U4            0.000000               0.000000
        D1           30.000000               0.000000
        D2            0.000000             900.000000
        D3            0.000000            1000.000000
        D4            0.000000            1000.000000
        P1           25.000000               0.000000
```

```
        P2              25.000000              0.000000
        P3              55.000000              0.000000
        U5               0.000000            800.000000
        D5               0.000000            200.000000
        P4              55.000000              0.000000

       ROW                 SLACK           DUAL PRICES
        2)               0.000000            900.000000
        3)               0.000000            100.000000
        4)               0.000000              0.000000
        5)               0.000000           -800.000000
        6)               0.000000            500.000000
        7)               0.000000           -400.000000
        8)               0.000000           -500.000000
        9)               0.000000           -500.000000
       10)               0.000000            300.000000
```

The mixed policy found by LP is $2,000 cheaper than the best pure policy.

Most realistic multiperiod problems involve more than one product. The next example moves a step in this direction toward realism by considering several products.

8.3 Multiperiod Financial Models

In most multiperiod planning problems, the management of liquid or cash-like assets is an important consideration. If you are willing to consider cash holdings as an inventory just like an inventory of any other commodity, it is a small step to incorporate financial management decisions into a multiperiod model. The key feature is that, for every period, there is a constraint that effectively says "sources of cash − uses of cash = 0." The following simple but realistic example illustrates the major features of such models.

8.3.1 Example: Cash Flow Matching

Suppose that as a result of a careful planning exercise you have concluded that to meet certain commitments you will need the following amounts of cash for the current plus next 14 years:

Year:	0	1	2	3	4	5	6	7	8	9	10	11	12	13	14
Cash (in $1,000s):	10	11	12	14	15	17	19	20	22	24	26	29	31	33	36

A common example where such a projection is made is in a personal injury lawsuit. Both parties may reach an agreement that the injured party should receive a stream of payments such as above or its equivalent. Other examples where the above approach has been used are the design of bond portfolios to satisfy cash needs for a pension fund, or for so-called balance sheet defeasance, where one kind of debt is replaced by another having the same cash flow stream.

For administrative simplicity in the personal injury example, both parties prefer an immediate single lump sum payment that is "equivalent" to the above stream of

15 payments. The party receiving the lump sum will argue that the lump sum payment should equal the present value of the stream using a low interest rate such as that obtained in a very low risk investment, such as a government guaranteed savings account. For example, if an interest rate of 4% is used, the present value of the stream of payments is $230,437. The party that must pay the lump sum, however, would like to argue for a much higher interest rate. To be successful, such an argument must include evidence that such higher interest rate investments are available and are no riskier than savings accounts. The investments usually offered are government securities. Generally, a broad spectrum of such investments are available on a given day. For simplicity, assume that there are just two such investments available with the following features:

Security	Current Cost	Yearly Return	Years to Maturity	Principal Repayment at Maturity
1	$980	$60	5	$1000
2	$965	$65	12	$1000

The paying party will offer a lump sum now with a recommendation of how much should be invested in securities 1, 2, and in savings accounts, such that the yearly cash requirements are met with the minimum lump sum payment.

The following decision variables are useful in solving this problem:

B_1 = amount invested now into security 1, measured in "face value amount,"
B_2 = amount invested now into security 2, measured in "face value amount,"
S_i = amount invested into a savings account in year i,
L = initial lump sum.

The objective function will be to minimize the initial lump sum. There will be a constraint for each year which forces the cash flows to net to zero. If we assume that idle cash is invested at 4% in a savings account and all amounts are measured in $1000s, then the formulation is:

```
MIN      L
SUBJECT TO
    2)    L - 0.98 B1 - 0.965 B2  - S0 =    10
    3)    0.06 B1 + 0.065 B2 + 1.04 S0 - S1 =    11
    4)    0.06 B1 + 0.065 B2 + 1.04 S1 - S2 =    12
    5)    0.06 B1 + 0.065 B2 + 1.04 S2 - S3 =    14
    6)    0.06 B1 + 0.065 B2 + 1.04 S3 - S4 =    15
    7)    1.06 B1 + 0.065 B2 + 1.04 S4 - S5 =    17
    8)    0.065 B2 + 1.04 S5 - S6 =    19
    9)    0.065 B2 + 1.04 S6 - S7 =    20
   10)    0.065 B2 + 1.04 S7 - S8 =    22
   11)    0.065 B2 + 1.04 S8 - S9 =    24
   12)    0.065 B2 + 1.04 S9 - S10 =    26
   13)    0.065 B2 + 1.04 S10 - S11 =    29
   14)    1.065 B2 + 1.04 S11 - S12 =    31
   15)    1.04 S12 -    S13 =    33
   16)    1.04 S13 -    S14 =    36
END
```

Using the PICTURE command of LINDO, the PICTURE of the constraint coefficients gives a better appreciation of the structure of the problem. In order to fit as much information on a page, the PICTURE command represents numbers bigger than 1.0 but less than 10.0 by an A. Numbers less than 1.0 but at least 0.1 are represented by a T. Numbers less than 0.1 but at least 0.01 are represented by a U.

```
                                 S S S S S
               B B S S S S S S S S S S 1 1 1 1 1
             L 1 2 0 1 2 3 4 5 6 7 8 9 0 1 2 3 4
    1:  1                                            MIN
    2:  1-T-T-1                                      = A
    3:     U U A-1                                   = B
    4:     U U   A-1                                 = B
    5:     U U     A-1                               = B
    6:     U U       A-1                             = B
    7:     A U         A-1                           = B
    8:       U           A-1                         = B
    9:       U             A-1                       = B
   10:       U               A-1                     = B
   11:       U                 A-1                   = B
   12:       U                   A-1                 = B
   13:       U                     A-1               = B
   14:       A                       A-1             = B
   15:                                 A-1   = B
   16:                                   A-1 = B
```

Notice that in row 7 B_1 has a coefficient of 1.06. This represents the principal repayment of \$1000 plus the interest payment of \$60 measured in \$1000s. Variable S_{14} (investment of funds in a savings account after the final payment is made) appears in the problem even though at first you might think it useless to allow such an option. S_{14} is effectively a surplus cash variable in the final period. Nevertheless, it is not unusual for the solution that minimizes the lump sum payment to have cash left over at the end of the problem. This is because a bond may be the most economical way of delivering funds to intermediate periods. This may cause the big principal repayment at the end of a bond's life to "overpay" the most distant periods. The solution is:

```
                  OBJECTIVE FUNCTION VALUE

        1)            195.683700

     VARIABLE           VALUE           REDUCED COST
        L             195.683672           0.000000
        B1             95.795770           0.000000
        B2             90.154735           0.000000
        S0              4.804497           0.000000
        S1              5.604481           0.000000
        S2              5.436464           0.000000
        S3              3.261727           0.000000
        S4              0.000000           0.106979
        S5             90.403574           0.000000
        S6             80.879776           0.000000
        S7             69.975025           0.000000
```

```
S8                  56.634084              0.000000
S9                  40.759506              0.000000
S10                 22.249944              0.000000
S11                  0.000000              0.141246
S12                 65.014792              0.000000
S13                 34.615385              0.000000
S14                  0.000000              0.379637

ROW                 SLACK                DUAL PRICES
 2)                  0.000000             -1.000000
 3)                  0.000000             -0.961538
 4)                  0.000000             -0.924556
 5)                  0.000000             -0.888996
 6)                  0.000000             -0.854804
 7)                  0.000000             -0.719063
 8)                  0.000000             -0.691406
 9)                  0.000000             -0.664814
10)                  0.000000             -0.639244
11)                  0.000000             -0.614658
12)                  0.000000             -0.591017
13)                  0.000000             -0.568286
14)                  0.000000             -0.410615
15)                  0.000000             -0.394822
16)                  0.000000             -0.379637
```

Of the \$195,683.70 lump sum payment, \$10,000 goes to immediate requirements, \$4,804.50 goes into a savings account, and $0.98 \times 95,795.77 + 0.965 \times 90,154.74 =$ \$180,879.20 goes into longer term securities. By considering a wide range of investments rather than just savings accounts, the amount of the lump sum payment has been reduced by about \$34,750 or 15%.

In actual solutions, one may find that a major fraction of the lump sum is invested in a single security. For example, limiting the amount invested in security 1 to half the initial lump sum is enforced by appending the constraint:

$$0.98 \, B_1 - 0.5 \, L \le 0.$$

Such constraints are typically called portfolio constraints.

An additional complication may arise due to integrality requirements on the B_1 and B_2 investments. For example, bonds can be bought only in \$1000 increments. Generally, with a modest amount of judgment, the fractional values can be rounded to neighboring integer values with no great increase in lump sum payment. For example, if B_1 and B_2 are set to 96 and 90 in the previous example, the total cost increases to \$195,726.50 from \$195,683.70. When this is done, S_{14} becomes nonzero; specifically, the last period is overpaid by about \$40.

8.4 Financial Planning Models with Tax Considerations

The next example treats a slightly more complicated version of the portfolio selection problem and then illustrates how to include and examine the effect of taxes. Winston-Salem Development Management (WSDM) is trying to complete its investment plans for the next three years. Currently, WSDM has 2 million dollars available for investment. At six-month intervals over the next three years, WSDM expects the following income stream from previous investments: $500,000 (6 months from now); $400,000; $380,000; $360,000; $340,000; and $300,000 (at the end of the third year). There are three development projects in which WSDM is considering participating. The Foster City Development would, if WSDM participated fully, have the following cash flow stream (projected) at six-month intervals over the next three years (negative numbers represent investments, and positive numbers represent income): −$3,000,000; −$1,000,000; −$1,800,000; $400,000; $1,800,000; $1,800,000; $5,500,000. The last figure is its estimated value at the end of three years. A second project involves taking over the operation of some old lower-middle-income housing on the condition that certain initial repairs to it be made and that it be demolished at the end of three years. The cash flow stream for this project, if participated in fully, would be: −$2,000,000; −$500,000; $1,500,000; $1,500,000; $1,500,000; $200,000; −$1,000,000.

The third project, the Disney-Universe Hotel, would have the following cash flow stream (six-month intervals) if WSDM participated fully. Again, the last figure is the estimated value at the end of the three years: −$2,000,000; −$2,000,000; −$1,800,000; $1,000,000; $1,000,000; $1,000,000; $6,000,000. WSDM can borrow money for half-year intervals at 3.5 percent interest per half year. At most, 2 million dollars can be borrowed at one time; i.e., the total outstanding principal can never exceed 2 million. WSDM can invest surplus funds at 3 percent per half-year.

Initially, we will disregard taxes. We will formulate the problem of maximizing WSDM's net worth at the end of three years as a linear program. If WSDM participates in a project at less than 100 percent, all the cash flows of that project are reduced proportionately.

8.4.1 Formulation and Solution of the WSDM Problem

Define:

F = fractional participation in the Foster City project;
M = fractional participation in Lower-Middle;
D = participation in Disney;
B_i = amount borrowed in period i in 1000s of dollars, $i = 1, \ldots, 6$;
L_i = amount lent in period i in 1000s of dollars, $i = 1, \ldots, 6$;
Z = net worth after the six periods in 1000s of dollars.

The problem formally is then (all numbers will be measured in units of 1000):

```
MAX       Z    ! Max worth at end of final period;
SUBJECT TO
      ! Uses - sources = supply of cash in each period;
   2)    3000 F + 2000 M + 2000 D - B1 + L1 =      2000
   3)    1000 F + 500 M + 2000 D + 1.035 B1 - 1.03 L1 - B2 + L2
       =     500
   4)    1800 F - 1500 M + 1800 D + 1.035 B2 - 1.03 L2 - B3 + L3
       =     400
```

```
 5)  -  400 F -  1500 M -  1000 D + 1.035 B3 -  1.03 L3 -  B4 + L4
     =    380
 6)  - 1800 F -  1500 M -  1000 D + 1.035 B4 -  1.03 L4 -  B5 + L5
     =    360
 7)  - 1800 F -   200 M -  1000 D + 1.035 B5 -  1.03 L5 -  B6 + L6
     =    340
 8)     Z -  5500 F +  1000 M-6000 D + 1.035 B6 -  1.03 L6 =   300
     ! Borrowing limits;
 9)      B1 <=    2000
10)      B2 <=    2000
11)      B3 <=    2000
12)      B4 <=    2000
13)      B5 <=    2000
14)      B6 <=    2000
     ! We can invest at most 100% in a project;
15)       F <=    1
16)       M <=    1
17)       D <=    1
```

Constraints 2 through 8 are the cash flow constraints for each of the periods. They enforce the requirement that uses of cash − sources of cash = 0 for each period. In the initial period, for example, L_1 is a use of cash whereas B_1 is a source of cash.

The solution is:

```
                    OBJECTIVE FUNCTION VALUE
 1)                 7665.179

VARIABLE               VALUE              REDUCED COST
   Z               7665.179080             0.000000
   F                  0.714341             0.000000
   M                  0.637210             0.000000
   D                  0.000000           452.381714
   B1              1417.443340             0.000000
   L1                 0.000000             0.008788
   B2              2000.000000             0.000000
   L2                 0.000000             0.334314
   B3              2000.000000             0.000000
   L3                 0.000000             0.250956
   B4               448.449000             0.000000
   L4                 0.000000             0.005305
   B5                 0.000000             0.005150
   L5              2137.484220             0.000000
   B6                 0.000000             0.000000
   L6              3954.865110             0.000000

ROW                  SLACK              DUAL PRICES
 2)                 0.000000             1.819220
 3)                 0.000000             1.757701
 4)                 0.000000             1.381929
 5)                 0.000000             1.098032
 6)                 0.000000             1.060900
 7)                 0.000000             1.030000
 8)                 0.000000             1.000000
```

```
 9)            582.556671            0.000000
10)              0.000000            0.327404
11)              0.000000            0.245466
12)           1551.551010            0.000000
13)           2000.000000            0.000000
14)           2000.000000            0.000000
15)              0.285659            0.000000
16)              0.362790            0.000000
17)              1.000000            0.000000
```

SENSITIVITY ANALYSIS:

  RANGES IN WHICH THE BASIS IS UNCHANGED

                    COST COEFFICIENT RANGES

VARIABLE	CURRENT COEF	ALLOWABLE INCREASE	ALLOWABLE DECREASE
Z	1.000000	INFINITY	1.000000
F	0.000000	3043.722050	454.594936
M	0.000000	644.819443	583.692337
D	0.000000	452.381714	INFINITY
B1	0.000000	0.008822	0.409697
L1	0.000000	0.008788	INFINITY
B2	0.000000	INFINITY	0.327404
L2	0.000000	0.334314	INFINITY
B3	0.000000	INFINITY	0.245466
L3	0.000000	0.250956	INFINITY
B4	0.000000	0.005305	0.162487
L4	0.000000	0.005305	INFINITY
B5	0.000000	0.005150	INFINITY
L5	0.000000	0.005150	0.222112
B6	0.000000	0.005000	INFINITY
L6	0.000000	0.005000	0.227865

                    RIGHTHAND SIDE RANGES

ROW	CURRENT RHS	ALLOWABLE INCREASE	ALLOWABLE DECREASE
2	2000.000000	1415.854160	2526.244390
3	500.000000	775.555534	1887.037060
4	400.000000	1198.599240	942.752693
5	380.000000	448.449009	1551.551030
6	360.000000	INFINITY	2137.484220
7	340.000000	INFINITY	3954.865110
8	300.000000	INFINITY	7665.179080
9	2000.000000	INFINITY	582.556671
10	2000.000000	561.718163	1136.009160
11	2000.000000	1027.054430	296.852333
12	2000.000000	INFINITY	1551.551010
13	2000.000000	INFINITY	2000.000000
14	2000.000000	INFINITY	2000.000000
15	1.000000	INFINITY	0.285659
16	1.000000	INFINITY	0.362790
17	1.000000	INFINITY	1.000000

8.4.2 Interpretation of the Dual Prices

The dual price on each of the first seven constraints is the increase in net worth in the last period resulting from an extra dollar made available in the earliest period. For example, the 1.81922 indicates that an extra dollar available at the start of period 1 would increase the net worth in the last period by about $1.82.

An extra dollar in period 5 is worth $1.0609 at the end, because all that we will do with it is invest it for 2 periods at 3 percent. Thus, it will grow to $1.03 \times 1.03 = 1.0609$ at the end.

An extra dollar in period 4 will save us from borrowing a dollar that period; thus, we will be $1.035 richer in period 5. We have already seen the value per extra dollar in period 5, so the value of an extra dollar in period 4 is $1.035 \times 1.0609 = \$1.09803$.

The dual prices on the borrowing constraints can be reconciled with the rest of the dual prices as follows. Being able to have an additional dollar in period 2 is worth $1.7577. If this dollar were borrowed, we would have to pay out $1.035 in period 3, which would have an effective cost of 1.035×1.38193. Thus, the net value in the last period of being able to borrow an extra dollar in period 2 is $1.7577 - 1.035 \times 1.38193 = 0.3274$, which agrees with the dual price on the borrowing constraint for period 2.

The effective interest rate or cost of capital, i, in any period t, can be found from the dual prices by deriving the rate at which one would be willing to borrow. Borrowing one dollar in period t would give us $1 more in period t but would require us to pay out $1 + i$ dollars in period $t + 1$. We must balance these two considerations. Consider period 1. An extra dollar is worth $1.81922 at the end of period 6. Paying back $1 + i$ in period 2 would cost $(1 + i)$ $1.7577 at the end of period 6. Balancing these two:

$$1.81922 = (1 + i)1.7577.$$

Solving,

$$i = 0.035.$$

This is not surprising because we are already borrowing at that rate in period 1, but not to the limit.

Applying similar analysis to the other periods we get the following effective rates:

Period	i	Period	i
1	0.035	4	0.035
2	0.2719	5	0.03
3	0.25855	6	0.03

8.5 Accounting for Income Taxes

Suppose we take taxes into account. Let us consider the following simplified situation. There is a tax rate of 50 percent on profit for any period. If there is a loss in a period, 80 percent can be carried forward to the next period. (Typically, tax laws put a limit on how many years a loss can be carried forward, but the 80% may be a good approximation.)

Taxable income figures for each of the prospective projects, as well as all existing projects, are given in the table below. Note that because of things like depreciation, actual net cash flow may be rather different from taxable income in a period.

		Project		
Period	Foster City	Lower-Middle Housing	Disney Universe	Existing
1	−100,000	−200,000	−150,000	0
2	−300,000	−400,000	−200,000	100,000
3	−600,000	−200,000	−300,000	80,000
4	−100,000	500,000	−200,000	76,000
5	500,000	1,000,000	500,000	72,000
6	1,000,000	100,000	800,000	68,000
7	4,000,000	−1,000,000	5,000,000	60,000

To formulate a model in this case we need to additionally define:

P_i = profit in period i.
C_i = loss in period i.

The formulation is affected in two ways. First, we must append some equations that force the P_is and C_is to be computed properly; secondly, terms must be added to the cash flow constraints to account for the cash expended in the payment of tax.

In words, one of the tax computation equations is:

Profit − loss = revenue − expense − 0.8 × (last period's loss).

Algebraically this equation for period 2 is:

$$P_2 - C_2 = 100 + 0.03L_1 - 300F - 400M - 200D - 0.035B_1 - 0.8C_1$$

or in standard form:

$$P_2 - C_2 - 0.03L_1 + 300F + 400M + 200D + 0.035B_1 + 0.8C_1 = 100.$$

The entire formulation is:

```
MAX       Z
SUBJECT TO
      ! Cash flow constraints, including the 50% tax usage;
   2)    3000 F + 2000 M + 2000 D - B1 + L1 + 0.5 P1 =     2000
   3)    1000 F + 500 M + 2000 D + 1.035 B1 - 1.03 L1 - B2 + L2
       + 0.5 P2 =     500
   4)    1800 F - 1500 M + 1800 D + 1.035 B2 - 1.03 L2 - B3 + L3
       + 0.5 P3 =     400
   5)  - 400 F - 1500 M - 1000 D + 1.035 B3 - 1.03 L3 - B4 + L4
       + 0.5 P4 =     380
   6)  - 1800 F - 1500 M - 1000 D + 1.035 B4 - 1.03 L4 - B5 + L5
       + 0.5 P5 =     360
```

```
 7)  - 1800 F - 200 M - 1000 D + 1.035 B5 - 1.03 L5 - B6 + L6
     + 0.5 P6 =     340
 8)    Z - 5500 F + 1000 M - 6000 D + 1.035 B6 - 1.03 L6 + 0.5 P7
     =     300
     ! The borrowing limits;
 9)    B1 <=    2000
10)    B2 <=    2000
11)    B3 <=    2000
12)    B4 <=    2000
13)    B5 <=    2000
14)    B6 <=    2000
     ! The investing limits;
15)    F <=    1
16)    M <=    1
17)    D <=    1
     ! Taxable Profit-Loss for each period;
18)    100 F + 200 M + 150 D + P1 - C1 =     C
19)    300 F + 400 M + 200 D + 0.035 B1 - 0.03 L1 + P2 + 0.8 C1
     - C2     =     100
20)    600 F + 200 M + 300 D + 0.035 B2 - 0.03 L2 + P3 + 0.8 C2
     - C3     =     80
21)    100 F - 500 M + 200 D + 0.035 B3 - 0.03 L3 + P4 + 0.8 C3
     - C4     =     76
22)  - 500 F - 1000 M - 500 D + 0.035 B4 - 0.03 L4 + P5 + 0.8 C4
     - C5     =     72
23)  - 1000 F - 100 M - 800 D + 0.035 B5 - 0.03 L5 + P6 + 0.8 C5
     - C6     =     68
24)  - 4000 F + 1000 M - 5000 D + 0.035 B6 - 0.03 L6 + P7 + 0.8 C6
     - C7 =     60
```

The solution is:

```
                 OBJECTIVE FUNCTION VALUE

   1)              5899.976

   VARIABLE           VALUE           REDUCED COST
      Z          5899.975590            0.000000
      F             0.487211            0.000000
      M             1.000000           -0.000019
      D             0.000000          945.007523
      B1         1461.632140            0.000000
      L1            0.000000            0.005112
      B2         2000.000020           -0.000000
      L2            0.000000            0.196093
      B3         1046.979320           -0.000000
      L3            0.000000            0.003158
      B4            0.000000            0.002576
      L4          991.260727            0.000000
      B5            0.000000            0.002537
      L5         3221.649020            0.000000
      B6            0.000000            0.002500
      L6         4359.347720           -0.000000
      P1            0.000000            0.449947
      P2            0.000000            0.379308
```

```
        P3           0.000000              0.204255
        P4           0.000000              0.110749
        P5        1072.657820             -0.000000
        P6         751.860207             -0.000000
        P7        1139.623200              0.000000
        C1         248.721067             -0.000000
        C2         696.297211              0.000000
        C3        1039.364200              0.000000
        C4         340.856709              0.000000
        C5           0.000000              0.109113
        C6           0.000000              0.107500
        C7           0.000000              0.500000

      ROW             SLACK            DUAL  PRICES
       2)           0.000000              1.321874
       3)           0.000000              1.286092
       4)           0.000000              1.067654
       5)           0.000000              1.045678
       6)           0.000000              1.030225
       7)           0.000000              1.015000
       8)           0.000000              1.000000
       9)         538.367844              0.000000
      10)           0.000000              0.192402
      11)         953.020706              0.000000
      12)        2000.000000              0.000000
      13)        2000.000000              0.000000
      14)        2000.000000              0.000000
      15)           0.512789              0.000000
      16)           0.000000            573.561150
      17)           1.000000              0.000000
      18)           0.000000             -0.210990
      19)           0.000000             -0.263738
      20)           0.000000             -0.329672
      21)           0.000000             -0.412090
      22)           0.000000             -0.515113
      23)           0.000000             -0.507500
      24)           0.000000             -0.500000
```

Notice that tax considerations cause a substantial change in the solution. More funds are placed into the lower-middle-income housing project, M, and less funds are invested in the Foster City, F, project. Project M has cash flows which help to smooth out the stream of yearly profits.

8.6 End Effects

Most multiperiod planning models "chop" off the analysis at some finite time in the future. The manner in which this chopping off is done can be important. In general, we care about the state in which things are left at the end of a planning model, e.g., inventory levels, capital investment, etc. If we arbitrarily terminate our planning model at year five in the future, an optimal solution to our model may in reality be an optimal solution to how to go out of business in five years. Grinold (1983), provides a comprehensive discussion of various methods for mitigating end-of-horizon effects. Some of the options for handling the end effect are:

(a) *Truncation.* Simply drop from the model all periods beyond a chosen cutoff point.
(b) *Primal limits.* Place reasonable limits on things such as inventory level at the end of the final period.
(c) *Salvage values/dual prices.* Place reasonable salvage values on things such as inventory level at the end of the final period.
(d) *Infinite final period.* Let the final period of the model represent a period of infinite length for which the same decision applies throughout the period. Net present value discounting is used in the objective function to make the final period comparable to the earlier finite periods. This is the approach used by Carino et al. (1994) in their model of the Yasuda Kasai Company and by Eppen, Martin, and Schrage (1988) in their model of General Motors.

8.7 Nonoptimality of Cyclic Solutions to Cyclic Problems

In some situations, such as when modeling the end of the planning horizon as above, it is reasonable to assume that demand is cyclic; e.g., it repeats forever in a weekly cycle. A natural question to ask is whether an optimal policy will have the same cycle. To motivate things, suppose that our firm needs to regularly make full truckload shipments between three cities: Los Angeles (L), Phoenix (P), and Reno (R). The shipment requirements follow a weekly cycle described in the table below:

	TO CITY	L	P	R
FROM CITY	L	T, W	M, R, F	
	P	W, R		S, N
	R	M, T, N	F, S	

The days of the week, Monday through Sunday, are denoted by M, T, W, R, F, S, N. Thus, according to the above table, a full truck must be shipped from P to L on Wednesday and Thursday; a full truck must be shipped from L to P on Monday, Thursday, and Friday, etc. In one day a truck can move between two cities, but no farther. We would like to find the minimum number of trucks required to serve these shipment requirements. Notice that two full truckloads need to be shipped each day of the week. Thus, one needs at least two trucks. Can we satisfy the requirements with at most two trucks?

Our earlier question, rephrased for this example, is: can we find an optimal solution to this problem so that each truck makes the same sequence of trips each week? The answer is no. That is, even though the fundamental data have a weekly cycle, an optimal solution does not have a weekly cycle. It is easy to formulate the weekly cycle problem as a linear program. Define the decision variables:

T_{ijk} = number of trucks going from city i to city j on day k. The model will have $3 \times 3 \times 7 = 63$ decision variables.

For example, TAP4 is the number of trucks going from A to P on day 4 (Thursday). Variable TLL7 is the number of trucks that remain in L for all of day 7 (Sunday). A formulation for a one week cycle solution follows. A generalization of this model, applied to an aircraft routing problem from Delta Airlines, appears in Hane et al. (1995).

```
! Full truckload routing problem
! Minimize trucks in use on Monday(and thus on Tues., etc.)
 MIN   TLL1 + TPL1 + TRL1
     + TLP1 + TPP1 + TRP1
     + TLR1 + TPR1 + TRR1
ST
!Period 1;
!Trucks into Los Angeles on Monday = trucks out on Tuesday
   2) TLL1 + TPL1 + TRL1 - TLL2 - TLP2 - TLR2 = 0
!Trucks into Phoenix on Monday = trucks out on Tuesday
   3) TLP1 + TPP1 + TRP1 - TPL2 - TPP2 - TPR2 = 0
!Trucks into Reno on Monday = trucks out on Tuesday
   4) TLR1 + TPR1 + TRR1 - TRL2 - TRP2 - TRR2 = 0
!Demand requirements for period 1
   5) TLR1 > 1
   6) TRL1 > 1
!Period 2, etc.;
   7) TLL2 + TPL2 + TRL2 - TLL3 - TLP3 - TLR3 = 0
   8) TLP2 + TPP2 + TRP2 - TPL3 - TPP3 - TPR3 = 0
   9) TLR2 + TPR2 + TRR2 - TRL3 - TRP3 - TRR3 = 0
  10) TLP2 > 2
  11) TRL2 > 1
!Period 3, etc.;
  12) TLL3 + TPL3 + TRL3 - TLL4 - TLP4 - TLR4 = 0
  13) TLP3 + TPP3 + TRP3 - TPL4 - TPP4 - TPR4 = 0
  14) TLR3 + TPR3 + TRR3 - TRL4 - TRP4 - TRR4 = 0
  15) TLP3 > 1
  16) TPL3 > 1
!Period 4, etc.;
  17) TLL4 + TPL4 + TRL4 - TLL5 - TLP5 - TLR5 = 0
  18) TLP4 + TPP4 + TRP4 - TPL5 - TPP5 - TPR5 = 0
  19) TLR4 + TPR4 + TRR4 - TRL5 - TRP5 - TRR5 = 0
  20) TLR4 > 1
  21) TPL4 > 1
!Period 5, etc.;
  22) TLL5 + TPL5 + TRL5 - TLL6 - TLP6 - TLR6 = 0
  23) TLP5 + TPP5 + TRP5 - TPL6 - TPP6 - TPR6 = 0
  24) TLR5 + TPR5 + TRR5 - TRL6 - TRP6 - TRR6 = 0
  25) TLR5 > 1
  26) TRP5 > 1
!Period 6, etc.;
  27) TLL6 + TPL6 + TRL6 - TLL7 - TLP7 - TLR7 = 0
  28) TLP6 + TPP6 + TRP6 - TPL7 - TPP7 - TPR7 = 0
  29) TLR6 + TPR6 + TRR6 - TRL7 - TRP7 - TRR7 = 0
  30) TPR6 > 1
  31) TRP6 > 1
!Period 7, etc.;
  32) TLL7 + TPL7 + TRL7 - TLL1 - TLP1 - TLR1 = 0
  33) TLP7 + TPP7 + TRP7 - TPL1 - TPP1 - TPR1 = 0
  34) TLR7 + TPR7 + TRR7 - TRL1 - TRP1 - TRR1 = 0
```

```
     35) TPR7 > 1
     36) TRL7 > 1
  END
```

The variables with nonzero values can be displayed with the NONZEROES command:

```
   : nonz

           OBJECTIVE FUNCTION VALUE

        1)          3.000000

     VARIABLE           VALUE        REDUCED COST
        TLL1         1.000000          0.000000
        TRL1         1.000000          0.000000
        TLR1         1.000000          0.000000
        TLP2         2.000000          0.000000
        TRL2         1.000000          0.000000
        TLP3         1.000000          0.000000
        TPL3         2.000000          0.000000
        TLR4         2.000000          0.000000
        TPL4         1.000000          0.000000
        TLR5         1.000000          0.000000
        TRP5         2.000000          0.000000
        TPR6         2.000000          0.000000
        TRP6         1.000000          0.000000
        TPR7         1.000000          0.000000
        TRL7         2.000000          0.000000
```

Notice that three trucks are required.

Figure 8.1 is helpful in understanding why a problem with a one-week cycle in the data has a two-week, rather than one-week, cycle in the solution. Notice that the truck following the solid path is not back in the starting city on Monday of the second week. On Monday of the third week, however, it is back in the starting city, so a two-week cycle minimal cost solution is possible.

In order to find a minimal cost solution to this problem, we had to avoid the temptation to assume that the solution had the same cycle length as the demand. This solution can be obtained by a model essentially identical to the one-week cycle model except one needs to make it a 14-day model rather than a 7-day model. A good discussion of how to avoid the temptation to restrict solutions can be found in the book on "conceptual blockbusting" by Adams (1986). Orlin (1982) gives a more detailed analysis of the cyclic vehicle routing problem.

8.8 PROBLEMS

Problem 1

The Izza Steel Company of Tokyo has predicted delivery requirements of 3,000, 6,000, 5,000, and 2,000 tons of steel in the next four periods. Current workforce is at the 4,000 tons per period level. At the moment, there are 500 tons of steel in stock. At the end of the four periods Izza would like its inventory position to be back at 500 tons. Regular time workforce has a variable cost of $100 per ton. Overtime can be hired in any period at a cost of $140 per ton. Regular time workforce size can be

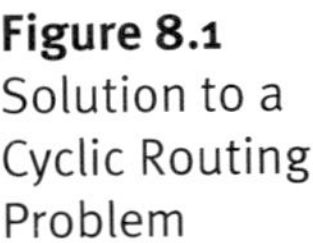

Figure 8.1
Solution to a
Cyclic Routing
Problem

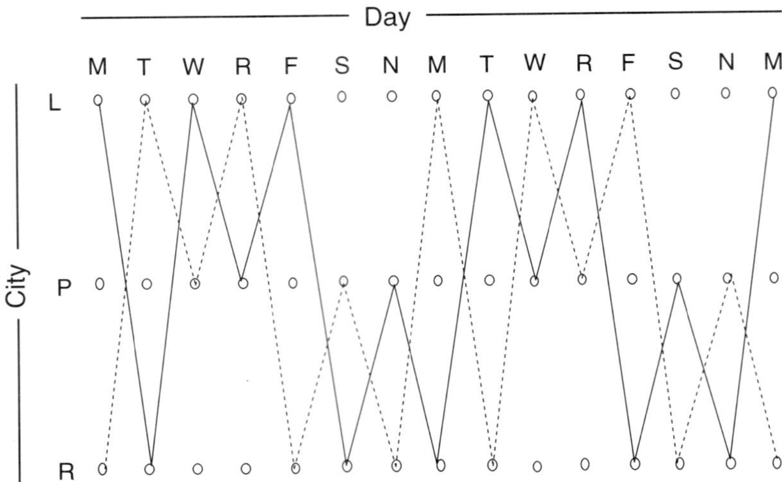

increased from one period to the next at a cost of $300 per ton of change in capacity; it can be decreased at a cost of $80 per ton. There is a charge of $5/ton for inventory at the end of each period. Izza would like the regular time workforce to be at the 3000 ton level at the end of the four periods.

    (a) Formulate Izza's problem as a linear program.
    (b) What assumption does your model make about idle workforce?

Problem 2

An airline predicts the following pilot requirements for the next five quarters: 80, 90, 110, 120, 110. Current staff is 90 pilots. The question of major concern is the number of pilots to hire in each of the next five quarters. A pilot must spend the quarter in which she is hired in training. The line's training facilities limit the number of pilots in training to at most 15. Further, the training of pilots requires the services of experienced pilots at the ratio of 5 to 1; that is, 5 pilots in training require 1 experienced pilot. An experienced pilot so assigned cannot be used to satisfy regular requirements. The cost of hiring and training a pilot is estimated at $20,000 exclusive of the experienced pilot time required. Experienced pilots cost $25,000 per quarter. Company policy does not include firing pilots.

    (a) What are the variables?
    (b) Formulate a model for determining how many pilots to hire in each period.

Problem 3

The Toute de Suite Candy Company includes in its product line a number of different mixed nut products. The Chalet nut mix is required to have no more than 25 percent peanuts and no less than 40 percent almonds.

The nuts available, their prices, and their availabilities this month are as follows:

	Price	Availability
Peanuts	20¢/lb.	400 lbs.
Walnuts	35¢/lb.	no limit
Almonds	50¢/lb.	200 lbs.

The Chalet mix sells for 80 cents per lb. At most, 700 lbs. can be mixed per month in questions (a), (b), and (c).

(a) Formulate the appropriate model for this problem.
(b) Toute de Suite would like to incorporate into the analysis its second major mixed nut line, the Hovel line. The Hovel mix can contain no more than 60 percent peanuts and no less than 20 percent almonds. Hovel sells for 40 cents per lb. Modify your model appropriately.
(c) Toute de Suite would like to incorporate next month's requirements into the analysis. The expected situation next month is:

	Price	Requirement (Availability)
Peanuts	19¢/lb.	500 lbs
Walnuts	36¢/lb.	no limit
Almonds	52¢/lb.	80 lbs.
Chalet	81¢/lb.	
Hovel	39¢/lb.	

It costs 2 cents per lb. to store nuts (plain or mixed) for one month. Because of a contract commitment, at least 200 lbs. of Chalet mix must be sold next month. Modify your model appropriately.

Problem 4

If two parties to a financial agreement, A and B, want the agreement to be treated as a lease for tax purposes, the payment schedule typically must satisfy certain conditions specified by the taxing agency. Suppose that P_i is the payment that A is scheduled to make to B in year i of a seven-year agreement. Parties A and B want to choose at the outset a set of P_is that satisfy a tax regulation that no payment in any given period can be less that 2/3 of the payment in any later period. Show the constraints for period i that enforce this lower bound on P_i. Use as few constraints per period as possible.

Problem 5

One of the options available to a natural gas utility is the renting of a storage facility so that it can buy gas at a cheap rate in the summer and store it until possibly needed in the winter. There is a yearly fee of $80,000 for each year the facility is rented. There is an additional requirement that if the utility starts renting the facility in year t, it must also rent it for at least the next three years. The gas utility has a long range planning model with a variable $x_t = 1$ if the utility rents the storage facility in year t, 0 otherwise, $y_t = 1$ if the utility starts renting in period t, and $z_t = 1$ if the utility stops renting after period t, for $t = 1$ to 25. It is not clear if this facility should be rented. Show how to represent this fee structure in an LP/IP model.

Problem 6

Below is the formulation of a cash flow matching problem, where the B variables represent investments in bonds and the S variables represent investment in savings for one period. The right-hand sides are the cash requirement for the various years.

```
MIN   L
[P00]  L -  .98  B1 -  .965  B2                            -  S0    = 10
[P01]       .06  B1 +  .065  B2 + 1.04  S0   -  S1         = 11
[P02]       .06  B1 +  .065  B2 + 1.04  S1   -  S2         = 12
[P03]       .06  B1 +  .065  B2 + 1.04  S2   -  S3         = 14
[P04]       .06  B1 +  .065  B2 + 1.04  S3   -  S4         = 15
[P05]     1.06   B1 +  .065  B2 + 1.04  S4   -  S5         = 17
[P06]                  .065  B2 + 1.04  S5   -  S6         = 19
[P07]                  .065  B2 + 1.04  S6   -  S7         = 20
[P08]                  .065  B2 + 1.04  S7   -  S8         = 22
[P09]                  .065  B2 + 1.04  S8   -  S9         = 24
[P10]                  .065  B2 + 1.04  S9   -  S10        = 26
[P11]                  .065  B2 + 1.04  S10  -  S11        = 29
[P12]                 1.065  B2 + 1.04  S11  -  S12        = 31
END
```

(a) The option to borrow at 7% per period for a term of one period has become available in every period. Show the modification in the above model for the periods with right-hand sides of 15, 17, and 19. Denote the borrowing variables by M0, M1, etc.

(b) Would this option in fact be attractive in the above model in any period?

(c) Almost all the parties involved were happy with this model until the Internal Revenue Service (IRS) suddenly became interested. The IRS has made the judgment that the initial endowment in the very first period may be tax free; however, thereafter the regular tax laws apply. Upon further inquiry, the IRS responded that regular income is taxed at 37% and capital gains at 15%.

　　We now want to find the initial lump sum such that after taxes have been paid each period, we can still cover the right-hand-side requirements. For simplicity, assume that taxes are paid in the same period as the income being taxed. Show how rows P04 and P05 are altered by this unpleasant new reality. (Disregard (a) and (b) above in answering.)

Blending of Input Materials

9.1 Introduction

In a blending problem there are:

1. Two or more input raw material commodities;
2. One or more qualities associated with each input commodity;
3. One or more output products to be produced by blending the input commodities so that certain output quality requirements are satisfied.

A good approximation is usually that the quality of the finished product is the weighted average of the qualities of the products that went into it.

Some examples are:

Output Commodity	Qualities	Raw Materials
Food, feed	Protein, carbohydrate, fat content	Corn, oats, soybeans
Gasoline	Octane, volatility, vapor pressure	Types of crude oil refinery products
Metals	Carbon, manganese, chrome content	Metal ore, scrap metals
Grain for export	Moisture, % foreign material, % damaged	Grain from various suppliers
Coal for sale	Sulfur, BTU, ash, moisture content	Coal from Illinois, Wyoming, Pennsylvania
Wine	Vintage, variety, region	Pure wines of various regions
Bank balance sheet	Proportion of loans of various types, average duration of loans and investment portfolios	Types of loans and investments available

Blending models are used most frequently in three industries:

1. feed and food, e.g., the blending of cattle feed, hot dogs, etc.;
2. metals industry, e.g., blending of specialty steels and nonferrous alloys, especially where recycled or scrap materials are used;
3. petroleum industry, e.g., for blending gasolines of specified octanes and volatility.

The market price of a typical raw material commodity may change significantly over the period of a month or even a week. The smart buyer will want to be sure to be buying corn, say, from the cheapest supplier. The even smarter buyer will want to exploit the fact that, as the price of corn drops relative to soybeans, the buyer may be able to save some money by switching to a blend that uses more corn.

Fields et al. (1978) describe a feed blending LP for constructing low-cost rations for cattle in a feedlot. This particular model was used at the rate of over 1,000 times/month by feedlot managers.

A recent success story in the steel industry has been the mini-mill. These small mills use mostly recyclable scrap steels to be charged into an electric furnace. The blending problem in this case is to decide what combination of scrap types to use so as to satisfy output quality requirements for specified products, such as reinforcing bars, etc.

The first general LP to appear in print was a blending or diet problem formulated by George Stigler (1945). The problem was to construct a "recipe" from about 80 foods so that the mix satisfied about a dozen nutritional requirements: for example, percent protein greater than 5 percent, percent cellulose less than 40 percent, etc. When Stigler formulated this problem, the Simplex method for solving LPs did not exist, and it was not widely realized that this "diet problem" was just a special case of this wider class of problems. Stigler, realizing its generality, stated: ". . . there does not appear to be any direct method of finding the minimum of a linear function subject to linear conditions." The solution he obtained to his specific problem by ingenious arguments was within a few cents of the least cost solution determined later when the Simplex method was invented. Both the least cost solution and Stigler's solution were not exactly haute cuisine. Both consisted largely of cabbage, flour, and dried navy beans with a touch of spinach for excitement. It is not clear that anyone would want to exist on this diet or even live with someone who was on it. These solutions illustrate the importance of explicitly including in the formulation constraints that are so obvious that they are forgotten, in this case palatability constraints.

9.2 The Structure of Blending Problems

Let us consider a simple feed blending problem. We must produce a batch of cattle feed having a protein content of at least 15%. This feed is produced by mixing corn (which is 6% protein) and soybean meal (which is 35% protein).

If C is the number of bushels of corn in the mix and S is the number of bushels of soybean meal, the protein constraint is:

$$\frac{\text{bushels of protein in mix}}{\text{bushels in mix}} \geq 0.15 \quad \text{(in words)}$$

or

$$\frac{0.06\,C + 0.35\,S}{C + S} \geq 0.15 \qquad \text{(algebraically)}$$

At first glance it looks as if we have trouble. This constraint is not linear. If, however, we multiply both sides by $C + S$, we get

$$0.06\,C + 0.35\,S \geq 0.15\,(C + S)$$

or in standard form finally:

$$-0.09\,C + 0.20\,S \geq 0.$$

Constraints on additional characteristics, such as fat, carbohydrates, and even such slightly nonlinear things as color, taste, and texture, can be handled in similar fashion. For example, if you do not like to have rice and mashed potatoes in the same meal, it is relatively straightforward to add a constraint that at most 30% of the grams in a meal can come from white ingredients.

The distinctive feature of a blending problem is that the crucial constraints, when written in intuitive form, are *ratios* of linear expressions. They can be converted to linear form by multiplying through by the denominator. Ratio constraints may also be found in "balance sheet" financial planning models, where a financial institution may have ratio constraints on the types of loans it makes or on the average duration of its investments.

The formulation is slightly more complicated if the blending aspect is just a small portion of a larger problem in which the batch size is a decision variable. The second example in this section will consider this complication. The first example will consider the situation where the batch size is specified beforehand.

9.2.1 Example: The Pittsburgh Steel Company Blending Problem

The Pittsburgh Steel (PS) Co. has been contracted to produce a new type of steel that has the following tight quality requirements:

	At Least	Not More Than
Carbon Content	3.0%	3.5%
Chrome Content	0.3%	0.45%
Manganese Content	1.35%	1.65%
Silicon Content	2.7%	3.0%

PS has the following materials available for mixing up a batch:

	Cost per Pound	Percent Carbon	Percent Chrome	Percent Manganese	Percent Silicon	Amount Available
Pig Iron 1	0.03	4.0	0	0.9	2.25	unlimited
Pig Iron 2	0.0645	0	10.0	4.5	15.0	unlimited
Ferro-Silicon 1	0.065	0	0	0	45.0	unlimited
Ferro-Silicon 2	0.061	0	0	0	42.0	unlimited
Alloy 1	0.10	0	0	60.0	18.0	unlimited
Alloy 2	0.13	0	20.0	9.0	30.0	unlimited
Alloy 3	0.119	0	8.0	33.0	25.0	unlimited
Carbide (Silicon)	0.08	15.0	0	0	30.0	20 lb.
Steel 1	0.021	0.4	0	0.9	0	200 lb.
Steel 2	0.02	0.1	0	0.3	0	200 lb.
Steel 3	0.0195	0.1	0	0.3	0	200 lb.

A one-ton (2000 lb.) batch must be blended that satisfies the quality requirements stated earlier. The problem now is what amounts of each of the eleven materials should be blended together so as to minimize the cost but satisfy the quality requirements. A steel expert claims that the least cost mix will not use any more than nine of the eleven available raw materials. What is a good blend? Most of the eleven prices and four quality control requirements are negotiable. Which prices and requirements are worth negotiating?

Note that the chemical content of a blend is simply the weighted average of the chemical content of its components. Thus, for example, if we make a blend of 40% Alloy 1 and 60% Alloy 2, the manganese content is $(0.40) \times 60 + (0.60) \times 9 = 29.4$.

9.2.2 Formulation and Structure of the Pittsburgh Steel Blending Problem

The PS blending problem can be formulated as an LP with 11 variables and 13 constraints. The 11 variables correspond to the 11 raw materials from which we can choose. Four constraints are from the upper usage limits on silicon-carbide and steels. Four of the constraints are from the lower quality limits. Another four constraints are from the upper quality limits. The thirteenth constraint is the requirement that the weight of all materials used must sum to 2000 pounds.

If we let P_1 be the number of pounds of Pig Iron 1 to be used, and use similar notation for the remaining materials, the problem of minimizing the cost per ton can be stated as:

```
MIN   0.03 P1 + 0.0645 P2 + 0.065 F1 + 0.061 F2 + 0.1 A1 + 0.13
      A2 + 0.119 A3 + 0.08 CB + 0.021 S1 + 0.02 S2 + C.0195 S3
```

```
SUBJECT TO
  ! Raw material availabilities;
  2)   CB <= 20
  3)   S1 <= 200
  4)   S2 <= 200
  5)   S3 <= 200
   ! Quality requirements on;
    ! Carbon content;
  6)   0.04 P1 + 0.15 CB + 0.004 S1 + 0.001 S2 + 0.001 S3
>= 60
  7)   0.04 P1 + 0.15 CB + 0.004 S1 + 0.001 S2 + 0.001 S3
<= 70
    ! Chrome content;
  8)   0.1 P2 + 0.2 A2 + 0.08 A3 >=    6
  9)   0.1 P2 + 0.2 A2 + 0.08 A3 <=    9
    ! Manganese content;
 10)   0.009 P1 + 0.045 P2 + 0.6 A1 + 0.09 A2 + 0.33 A3 +
       0.009 S1 + 0.003 S2 + 0.003 S3 >=    27
 11)   0.009 P1 + 0.045 P2 + 0.6 A1 + 0.09 A2 + 0.33 A3 +
       0.009 S1 + 0.003 S2 + 0.003 S3 <=    33
    ! Silicon content;
 12)   0.0225 P1 + 0.15 P2 + 0.45 F1 + 0.42 F2 + 0.18 A1 +
       0.3 A2    + 0.25 A3 + 0.3 CB >=    54
 13)   0.0225 P1 + 0.15 P2 + 0.45 F1 + 0.42 F2 + 0.18 A1 +
       0.3 A2    + 0.25 A3 + 0.3 CB <=    60
    ! Finish good requirements;
 14)   P1 + P2 + F1 + F2 + A1 + A2 + A3 + CB + S1 + S2 + S3
= 2000
END
```

The general form of this model is:

Minimize   cost of raw materials
subject to

      (a) Raw material availabilities (rows 2–5)

      (b) Quality requirements (rows 6–13)

      (c) Finish good requirements (row 14).

It is generally good practice to be consistent and group constraints in this fashion.

For this particular example, when writing the quality constraints, we have exploited the knowledge that the batch size is 2000. So, for example, 3% of 2000 is 60, 3.5% of 2000 is 70, etc.

When solved, we get the solution:

```
         OBJECTIVE FUNCTION VALUE

        1)         59.556290
VARIABLE              VALUE           REDUCED COST
      P1         1474.264000            .000000
      P2           60.000000            .000000
      F1             .000000            .001036
      F2           22.062050            .000000
      A1           14.238860            .000000
      A2             .000000            .020503
```

```
        A3            .000000           .019926
        CB            .000000           .003357
        S1         200.000000           .000000
        S2          29.434930           .000000
        S3         200.000000           .000000

       ROW      SLACK OR SURPLUS     DUAL PRICES
        2)         20.000000           .000000
        3)           .000000           .000177
        4)        170.565100           .000000
        5)           .000000           .000500
        6)           .000000          -.183329
        7)         10.000000           .000000
        8)           .000000          -.254731
        9)          3.000000           .000000
       10)           .000000          -.104521
       11)          6.000000           .000000
       12)           .000000          -.098802
       13)          6.000000           .000000
       14)           .000000          -.019503
```

Notice that only 7 of the 11 raw materials were used.

In actual practice, this type of LP was solved on a twice monthly basis. The first solution, including the reduced cost and dual prices, was used by the purchasing agent as a guide in buying materials. The second solution later in the month was mainly for the metallurgist's benefit in making up a blend from the raw materials actually on hand.

Suppose that we can pump oxygen into the furnace. This oxygen combines completely with carbon to produce the gas CO_2, which escapes. The oxygen will burn off carbon at the rate of 12 pounds of carbon burned off for each 32 pounds of oxygen. Oxygen costs two cents a pound. If you reformulated the problem to include this additional option, would it change the decisions? The oxygen injection option to burn off carbon is clearly uninteresting, because in the current solution it is the lower bound constraint rather than the upper bound on carbon that is binding. Thus, burning off carbon, even if by itself it could be done at no expense, would increase the total cost of the solution.

9.3 A Blending Problem within a Product Mix Problem

One additional aspect of blending problem formulation will be illustrated with an example in which the batch size is a decision variable. In the previous example, the batch size was specified. In the following example, the amount of product to be blended depends upon how cheaply the product can be blended. Thus, it appears that the blending decision and the batch size decision must be made simultaneously.

This example is suggestive of gasoline blending problems faced in a petroleum refinery. We wish to blend gasoline from three ingredients: butane, heavy naphtha, and catalytic reformate. Four characteristics of the resultant gasoline and its inputs are important: cost, octane number, vapor pressure, and volatility. These characteristics are summarized in the following table.

		Commodity		
Characteristic	Butane (BT)	Catalytic Reformate (CR)	Heavy Naphtha (HN)	Regular Gasoline (RG)
Cost/Unit	7.3	18.20	12.50	?
Octane	120	100	74	≥ 94
Vapor Pressure	60	2.6	4.1	≤ 11
Volatility	105	3	12	≥ 17

The octane rating is a measure of the gasoline's resistance to "knocking" or "pinging." Vapor pressure and volatility are closely related. Vapor pressure is a measure of susceptibility to stalling, particularly on an unusually warm spring day. Volatility is a measure of how easily the engine starts in cold weather.

In this planning period, there are only 1,000 units of butane available. The production of gasoline competes with heavy fuel (HF) for production facilities. The sum of gasoline plus heavy fuel production this planning period cannot exceed 12,000 units. Any blending problems associated with production of heavy fuel are disregarded. For this example, heavy fuel is treated as a simple product. At the highest level, this is a product mix problem involving the two competing products, gasoline and heavy fuel.

The profit contribution of heavy fuel is $3.6 per unit, *including* the cost of all ingredients. The profit contribution of regular gasoline is $18.40 per unit *exclusive* of the cost of its ingredients.

A slight simplification assumed in this example is that the interaction between ingredients is linear; e.g., if a "fifty/fifty" mixture of BT and CR is made, its octane will be $0.5 \times 120 + 0.5 \times 100 = 110$ and its volatility will be $0.5 \times 105 + 0.5 \times 3 = 54$. In reality, this linearity is violated slightly, especially if gasoline containing tetraethyl lead is blended.

9.3.1 Formulation

The availability and capacity constraints are straightforward, specifically:

$$BT \leq 1,000$$
$$RG + HF \leq 12,000.$$

The quality constraints require a bit of thought. The fractions of the batch consisting of Butane, Catalytic Reformate, and Heavy Naphtha are BT/RG, CR/RG, and HN/RG, respectively. Thus, if the god of linearity smiles upon us, then the octane constraint of the blend should be the expression:

$$(BT/RG) \times 120 + (CR/RG) \times 100 + (HN/RG) \times 74 \geq 94.$$

Your expression, however, may be a frown, because a ratio of variables like BT/RG is definitely not linear. Multiplying through by RG, however, produces the linear constraint:

$$120\ BT + 100\ CR + 74\ HN \geq 94\ RG$$

or in standard form:

$$120 \text{ BT} + 100 \text{ CR} + 74 \text{ HN} - 94 \text{ RG} \geq 0.$$

Similar arguments can be used to develop the vapor and volatility constraints. Finally, a constraint must be appended that states that the whole equals the sum of its parts, specifically:

$$RG = BT + HN + CR.$$

When all constraints are converted to standard form and the expression for profit contribution is written, we obtain the formulation:

```
MAX     18.4 RG + 3.6 HF - 7.3 BT - 12.5 HN - 18.2 CR
SUBJECT TO
        ! Raw material and capacity limits
  2)      BT <=    1000
  3)      RG +   HF <=    12000
        ! Octane requirement
  4)    - 94 RG + 120 BT + 74 HN + 100 CR >=     0
        ! Vapor pressure requirement
  5)    - 11 RG + 60 BT + 4.1 HN + 2.6 CR <=     0
        ! Volatility requirement
  6)    - 17 RG + 105 BT + 12 HN + 3 CR >=     0
          ! Batch size of RG
  7)      RG - BT - HN - CR =    0
END
```

The solution is:

```
                  OBJECTIVE FUNCTION VALUE

    1)              43328.840000

    VARIABLE           VALUE              REDUCED COST
      RG            7270.296450             0.000000
      HF            4729.703550             0.000000
      BT            1000.000000             0.000000
      HN            2446.991390             0.000000
      CR            3823.304840             0.000000

    ROW                SLACK               DUAL PRICES
    2)              0.000000                0.128845
    3)              0.000000                3.600000
    4)              0.000000               -0.204298
    5)              0.000000                0.258835
    6)          22238.774700                0.000000
    7)              0.000000               -1.556829

    NO. ITERATIONS=           5
```

It is not obvious beforehand that the amount of regular gasoline to produce should be 7,270 units. Can you predict how much gasoline should be produced if there were no heavy fuel competing for production capacity?

LP blending models have been a standard operating tool in refineries for years. Recently, there have been some instances where these LP models have been replaced by more sophisticated models that more accurately approximate the nonlinearities in the blending process, although they may not optimize as thoroughly as the Simplex method. See DeWitt, Lasdon et al. (1989) for a discussion of how Texaco does it.

There are a variety of complications as gasoline blending models are made more detailed. For example, in high quality gasoline, the vendor may want the octane to be constant across volatility ranges in the ingredients. The reason is that if you "floor" the accelerator on a non-fuel injected automobile, a shot of raw gas is squirted into the intake. The highly volatile components of the blend will reach the combustion chamber first. If they have low octane you will have knocking, even though the "average" octane rating of the gasoline is high. This may be more important to a station selling gas for city driving than to a station on a cross-country highway in Kansas, where most driving is at a constant speed.

9.4 Proper Choice of Alternate Interpretations of Quality Requirements

Some quality features can be stated either according to some measure of goodness or, alternatively, according to some measure of undesirability. An example is the efficiency of an automobile. It could be stated in miles per gallon or, alternatively, in gallons per mile. When considering the quality of a blend of ingredients (e.g., the efficiency of a fleet of cars), it is important to identify whether it is the goodness or the badness measure that is additive over the components of the blend. The next example illustrates.

A federal regulation required that the average of the miles per gallon computed over all automobiles sold by an automobile company in a specific year be at least 18 miles per gallon. Let us consider a hypothetical case for the Ford Motor Company. Assume that Ford sold only the four car types: Mark V, Ford, Granada, and Fiesta. Various parameters of these cars are listed below:

Car	Miles Per Gallon	Marginal Production Cost	Selling Price
Fiesta	30	13,500	14,000
Granada	18	14,100	15,700
Ford	16	14,500	15,300
Mark V	14	15,700	20,000

There is some flexibility in the production facilities, so capacities may apply to pairs of car types. These limitations are:

Yearly Capacity in Units	Car Types Limited
250,000	Fiesta
2,000,000	Granadas plus Fords
1,500,000	Fords plus Mark Vs

There is a sale capacity limit of 3,000,000 on the total of all cars sold. How many of each car type should Ford plan to sell?

Interpreting the mileage constraint literally results in the following formulation.

```
MAX          500 FIESTA + 1600 GRANADA + 4300 MARKV + 800 FORD
SUBJECT TO
       2)           12 FIESTA - 4 MARKV - 2 FORD >= 0
       3)           FIESTA <= 250
       4)           GRANADA + FORD <= 2000
       5)           MARKV + FORD <= 1500
       6)           FIESTA + GRANADA + MARKV + FORD <= 3000
END
```

Automobiles and dollars are measured in 1000's. Note that row 2 is equivalent to

$$\frac{30 \text{ Fiesta} + 18 \text{ Granada} + 16 \text{ Ford} + 14 \text{ Mark V}}{\text{Fiesta} + \text{Granada} + \text{Ford} + \text{Mark V}} \geq 18$$

The solution is:

```
                  OBJECTIVE FUNCTION VALUE

        1)                   6550000.
           VARIABLE          VALUE          REDUCED COST
            FIESTA        250.000000           0.000000
           GRANADA       2000.000000           0.000000
           MARK  V        750.000000           0.000000
              FORD          0.000000        2950.000000

            ROW             SLACK           DUAL PRICES
             2)           0.000000        -1075.000000
             3)           0.000000        13400.000000
             4)           0.000000         1600.000000
             5)         750.000000            0.000000
             6)           0.000000            0.000000
```

Let's look more closely at this solution. Suppose that each car is driven the same number of miles per year regardless of type. An interesting question is whether the ratio of the total miles driven by the above fleet divided by the number of gallons of gasoline used is at least equal to 18. Without loss, suppose each car is driven one mile. The gasoline used by a car driven one mile is 1/(miles per gallon). Thus, if all the cars are driven the same distance, the ratio of miles to gallons of fuel of the above fleet is $(250 + 2000 + 750)/[(250/30) + (2000/18) + (750/14)] = 17.3$ miles per gallon—which is considerably below the mpg we thought we were getting.

The first formulation is equivalent to allotting each automobile the same number of gallons and then driving each automobile until it exhausts its allotment. Thus, the 18-mpg average is attained by having less efficient cars drive fewer miles. A more sensible way of phrasing things is in terms of gallons per mile. In this case, the mileage constraint is written:

$$\frac{\text{Fiesta}/30 + \text{Granada}/18 + \text{Ford}/16 + \text{Mark V}/14}{\text{Fiesta} + \text{Granada} + \text{Ford} + \text{Mark V}} \leq 1/8.$$

Converted to standard form this becomes:

```
2)   -0.022222 Fiesta + 0.0069444 Ford + 0.015873 MarkV <= 0
```

When this problem is solved with this constraint, we get the solution:

```
        OBJECTIVE FUNCTION VALUE

1)            4830000.

VARIABLE          VALUE            REDUCED COST
   FIESTA      250.000000             0.000000
   GRANADA    2000.000000             0.000000
   MARKV       350.000000             0.000000
   FORD          0.000000          1681.250700
```

Notice that the profit contribution drops noticeably under this second interpretation. The federal regulations could very easily be interpreted to be consistent with the first formulation. Automotive companies, however, wisely implemented the second way of computing fleet mileage rather than leave themselves open to later criticism of implementing what Uncle Sam said rather than what he meant.

9.4.1 Mean Encounters of Three Kinds

The general conclusion is that one should think carefully when one needs to compute an average performance measure for some blend or collection of things. There are at least three ways of computing averages or means when one has N observations, $x_1, x_2, \ldots, x_N$:

1. Arithmetic, i.e., $(x_1 + x_2 \ldots + x_N)/N$
2. Geometric, i.e., $(x_1 * x_2 \ldots * x_N)^{\wedge}(1/N)$
3. Harmonic, i.e., $1/[(1/x_1 + 1/x_2 \ldots + 1/x_N)/N]$.

The arithmetic mean is appropriate for computing the mean return of the assets in a portfolio. If, however, we are interested in the average growth of a portfolio over time, we would probably want to use the geometric mean of the yearly growths rather than the arithmetic average. Consider, for example, an investment that has a growth factor of 1.5 in the first year and 0.67 in the second year (e.g., a rate of return of 50% in the first year and −33% in the second year). Most people would *not* consider the average growth to be $(1.5 + 0.67)/2 = 1.085$. The harmonic mean tends to be appropriate when computing an average rate of something, as in our car fleet example above.

9.5 Interpretation of Dual Prices for Blending Constraints

The dual price for a blending constraint usually requires a slight reinterpretation in order to be useful. As an example, consider the octane constraint of the gasoline blending problem:

$$-94\ RG + 120\ BT + 74\ HN + 100\ CR \geq 0.$$

The dual price of this constraint is the increase in profit if the right-hand side of this constraint is changed from 0 to 1. Unfortunately, this is not a change that we would ordinarily consider. More typical changes that might be entertained would be changing the octane rating from 94 to either 93 or 95. A very approximate rule for estimating the effect of a small change of the coefficient in row i of variable RG is to compute the product of the dual price of row i and the value of variable RG. For variable RG and the octane constraint, this value is $7270.30 \times (-0.204298) = -1485.31$. This suggests that if the octane requirement is reduced to 93 (increased to 95) from 94, the total profit will increase by about 1485, to 44,814 (decrease by about 1485 to 41,843). For small changes, this approximation will generally understate the true profit after the change. When the LP is actually resolved with an octane requirement of 93 (or 95), the actual profit contribution changes to 44,825 (or 43,200).

This approximation can be summarized generally as follows: If we wish to change a certain quality requirement of a blend by a small amount e, the effect on profit of this change is approximately of the magnitude $e \times$ (dual price of the constraint) $\times$ (batch size). For small changes, the approximation tends to understate profit after the change. For large changes, the approximation may err in either direction.

9.6 Fractional or Hyperbolic Programming

In blending problems we have seen that ratio constraints of the form:

$$\frac{\sum_j q_i X_j}{\sum_j X_i} \geq q_0$$

can be converted to linear form, by rewriting:

$$\sum_j q_j X_j \geq q_0 \sum_j X_j \quad \text{or} \quad \sum (q_j - q_0) x_j \geq 0.$$

Can we handle a similar feature in the objective? That is, can a problem of the following form be converted to linear form?

(1) Maximize $\dfrac{u_0 + \sum_j u_j X_j}{v_0 + \sum_j v_j X_j}$

(2) subject to $\sum_j a_{ij} X_j = b_i.$

The a_{ij}, u_0, u_j, v_0, v_j are given constants. For example, we might wish to maximize the fraction of protein in a blend subject to constraints on availability of materials and other quality specifications.

We can make it linear with the following transformations:

Define $\quad r = 1/(v_0 + \sum_j v_j X_j)$
and $\quad y_j = X_j r.$

We assume that $r > 0$. Then our objective is:

(1′) Maximize $u_o r + \sum_j v_j y_j$

subject to $r = 1/(v_o + \sum_j v_j X_j)$

(1.1′) $r v_o + \sum_j v_j y_j = 1.$

Any other constraint i of the form

$$\sum_j a_{ij} X_j = b_i$$

can be written as

$$\sum_j a_{ij} X_j r = b_i r$$

or

(2′) $\sum_j a_{ij} y_i - b_i r = 0.$

9.7 PROBLEMS

Problem 1

The Exxoff Company must decide upon the blends to be used for this week's gasoline production. Two gasolines must be blended, and their characteristics are listed below:

Gasoline	Vapor Pressure	Octane Number	Selling Price (in $/Barrel)
Lo-lead	≤7	≥ 80	$9.80
Premium	≤6	≥100	$12.00

The characteristics of the components from which the gasoline can be blended are shown below:

Component	Vapor Pressure	Octane Number	Available This Week (in Barrels)
Cat-Cracked Gas	8	83	2700
Isopentane	20	109	1350
Straight Gas	4	74	4100

The vapor pressure and octane number of a blend is simply the weighted average of the corresponding characteristics of its components. Components not used can be sold to "independents" for $9 per barrel.

(a) What are the decision variables?
(b) Give the LP formulation.
(c) How much premium should be blended?

Problem 2

The Blendex Oil Company blends a regular and a premium product from two ingredients, Heptane and Octane. Each liter of regular is composed of exactly 50% Heptane and 50% Octane. Each liter of premium is composed of exactly 40% Heptane and 60% Octane. During this planning period, there are exactly 200,000 liters of Heptane and 310,000 liters of Octane available. The profit contributions per liter of the regular and premium product this period are $0.03 and $0.04 per liter, respectively.

(a) Formulate the problem of determining the amounts of the regular and premium products to produce as an LP.
(b) Determine the optimal amounts to produce without the use of a computer.

Problem 3

Hackensack Blended Whiskey Company imports three grades of whiskey: Prime, Choice, and Premium. These unblended grades can be used to make up the following two brands of whiskey with associated characteristics:

Brand	Specifications	Selling Price Per Liter
Scottish Club	Not less than 60% Prime. Not more than 20% Premium.	$6.80
Johnny Gold	Not more than 60% Premium. Not less than 15% Prime.	$5.70

The costs and availabilities of the three raw whiskies are:

Whiskey	Available This Week (Number of Liters)	Cost Per Liter
Prime	2,000	$7.00
Choice	2,500	$5.00
Premium	1,200	$4.00

Hackensack wishes to maximize this week's profit contribution and feels that it can use linear programming to do so. How much should be made of each of the two brands? How should the three raw whiskeys be blended into each of the two brands?

Problem 4

Generic Foods Company has available three ingredients for mixing a certain food product. The ingredients and their percent protein are Corn: 7%, Oats: 9%, and Soybeans: 18%. The following constraint was used in a model for blending this food product:

$$-7 \text{ CORN} - 5 \text{ OATS} + 4 \text{ SOY} < 0.$$

In words, this constraint is:

(a) The mix must be at least 14% protein.
(b) The mix must be at most 7% protein.
(c) The mix must be at least 8% protein.
(d) The mix must be at most 14% protein.
(e) None of the above

Problem 5

The Sebastopol Refinery processes two different kinds of crude oil, Venezuelan and Saudi, to produce two general classes of products, Light and Heavy. Either crude oil can be processed by either of two modes of processing, Short or Regular. The processing cost and amounts of Heavy and Light produced depend upon the mode of processing used and the type of crude oil used. Costs vary, both across crude oils and across processing modes. The relevant characteristics are summarized in the table below. For example, the short process converts each unit of Venezuelan crude to 0.45 units of Light product, 0.52 units of Heavy product, and 0.03 units of waste.

	Short Process		Regular Process	
	Venezuelan	Saudi	Venezuelan	Saudi
Light product fraction	0.45	0.60	0.49	0.68
Heavy product fraction	0.52	0.36	0.50	0.32
Unusable product fraction	0.03	0.04	0.01	0.00

Saudi crude costs $20/unit and Venezuelan crude costs $19/unit. The short process costs $2.50/unit processed, and the regular process costs $2.10/unit. Sebastopol can process 10,000 units of crude per week at the regular rate. When the refinery runs the Short process for the full week, it can process 13,000 units per week. The refinery may run any combination of short and regular processes in a given week.

The respective market values of Light and Heavy products are $27 and $25 per unit. Formulate the problem of deciding how much of which crudes to buy and which processes to run as an LP. What are the optimal purchasing and operating decisions?

Problem 6

There has been a lot of soul searching recently at your company, the Beansoul Coal Company (BCC). Some of its better coal mines have been exhausted, and it is having more difficulty selling its coal from remaining mines. One of BCC's most important customers is the electrical utility, Power to the People Company (PPC). BCC sells coal from its best mine, the Becky mine, to PPC. The Becky mine is currently running at capacity, selling all its 5000 tons/day output to PPC. Delivered to PPC, the Becky coal costs BCC $81/ton, and PPC pays BCC $86/ton. BCC has four other mines, but you have been unable to get PPC to buy coal from these mines; PPC says that coal from these mines does not satisfy its quality requirements. Upon pressing PPC for details, it has agreed that it would consider buying a mix of coal as long as it satisfies the following quality requirements: sulfur $\leq 0.6\%$; ash $\leq 5.9\%$; BTU $\geq$

13,000 per ton; and moisture $\leq 7\%$. You note that your Becky mine satisfies this in that its quality according to the above four measures is: 0.57%, 5.56%, 13,029 BTU, and 6.2%. Your four other mines have the following characteristics:

Mine	BTU Per Ton	Sulfur Percent	Ash Percent	Moisture Percent	Cost Per Ton Delivered to PPC
Lex	14,201	0.88	6.76	5.1	73
Casper	10,630	0.11	4.36	4.6	90
Donora	13,200	0.71	6.66	7.6	74
Rocky	11,990	0.39	4.41	4.5	89

The daily capacities of your Lex, Casper, Donora, and Rocky mines are 4000, 3500, 3000, and 7000 tons, respectively. PPC uses an average of about 13,000 tons per day.

BCC's director of sales was ecstatic upon hearing of your conversation with PPC. His response was "Great! Now we will be able to sell PPC all of the 13,000 tons per day that it needs." Your stock with BCC's newly appointed director of productivity is similarly high. Her reaction to your discussion with PCC was: "Let's see, right now we are making a profit contribution of only $5/ton of coal sold to PPC. I have figured out that we can make a profit contribution of $7/ton if we can sell them a mix. Wow! You are an ingenious negotiator!" What do you recommend to BCC?

Problem 7

The McClendon Company manufactures two products, bird food and dog food. The company has two departments, blending and packaging. The requirements in each department for manufacturing a ton of either product are as follows:

	Time per Unit in Tons	
	Blending	Packaging
Bird food	0.25	0.10
Dog food	0.15	0.30

Each department has 8 hours available per day.

Dog food is made from three ingredients: meat, fish meal, and cereal. Bird food is made from three ingredients: seeds, ground stones, and cereal. Descriptions of these five materials are as follows:

	Descriptions of Materials in Percents				
	Protein	Carbo-hydrates	Trace Minerals	Abrasives	Cost (in $/Ton)
Meat	12	10	1	0	600
Fishmeal	20	8	2	2	900
Cereal	3	30	0	0	200
Seeds	10	10	2	1	700
Stones	0	0	3	100	100

The composition requirements of the two products are as follows:

Composition Requirements of the Products in Percents

	Protein	Carbo- hydrates	Trace Minerals	Abrasives	Seeds
Bird food	5	18	1	2	10
Dog food	11	15	1	0	0

Bird food sells for $750/ton; dog food sells for $980/ton. What should be the composition of bird and dog food, and how much of each should be manufactured each day?

Problem 8

Recent federal regulations strongly encourage the assignment of students to schools in a city so that the racial composition of any school approximates the racial composition of the entire city. Consider the case of the Greenville city schools. The city can be considered as composed of five areas with the following characteristics:

Area	Fraction Minority	Number of Students
1	.20	1,200
2	.10	900
3	.85	1,700
4	.60	2,000
5	.90	2,500

The ruling handed down for Greenville is that a school can have neither more than 75 percent nor less than 30 percent minority enrollment. There are three schools in Greenville with the following capacities:

School	Capacity
Bond	3,900
Pocahontas	3,100
Pierron	2,100

The objective is to design an assignment of students to schools so as to stay within the capacity of each school and satisfy the composition constraints while minimizing the distance traveled by students. The distances in kilometers between areas and schools are:

			Area		
School	1	2	3	4	5
Bond	2.7	1.4	2.4	1.1	0.5
Pocahontas	0.5	0.7	2.9	0.8	1.9
Pierron	1.6	2.0	0.1	1.3	2.2

There is an additional condition that no student can be transported more than 2.6 kilometers. Find the number of students that should be assigned to each school from each area. Assume that any group of students from an area has the same ethnic mix as the whole area.

Problem 9

A farmer is raising pigs for market and wishes to determine the quantity of the available types of feed that should be given to each pig to meet certain nutritional requirements at minimum cost. The units of each type of basic nutritional ingredient contained in a pound of each feed type is given in the following table, along with the daily nutritional requirement and feed costs.

Nutritional Ingredient	Pound of Corn	Pound of Tankage	Pound of Alfalfa	Units Required Per Day
Carbohydrates	9	2	4	20
Proteins	3	8	6	18
Vitamins	1	2	6	15
Cost (cents)/lb.	7	6	5	

Problem 10

Rico-AG is a German fertilizer company that has just received a contract to supply 10,000 tons of 3-12-12 fertilizer. The guaranteed composition of this fertilizer is (by weight) at least 3% nitrogen, 12% phosphorus, and 12% potash. This fertilizer can be mixed from any combination of the raw materials described in the table below.

Raw Material	Percent Nitrogen	Percent Phosphorus	Percent Potash	Current World Price/Ton
AN	50%	0%	0%	190 Dm
SP	1%	40%	5%	180 Dm
CP	2%	4%	35%	196 Dm
BG	1%	15%	17%	215 Dm

Rico-AG has in stock 500 tons of SP that was bought earlier for 220 Dm/ton. Rico-AG has a long-term agreement with Fledermausguano, S.A., which allows it to buy already mixed 3-12-12 at 195 Dm/ton.

(a) Formulate a model for Rico-AG which will allow it to decide how much to buy, mix, and how to mix. State what assumptions you make with regard to goods in inventory.
(b) Can you conclude in advance that no CP and BG will be used because they cost more than 195 Dm/ton?

Problem 11

The Albers Milling Company buys corn and wheat and then grinds and blends them into two final products, Fast-Gro and Quick-Gro. Fast-Gro is required to have at least 2.5% protein, whereas Quick-Gro must have at least 3.2% protein. Corn contains 1.9% protein, whereas wheat contains 3.8% protein. The firm can do the buying and blending at either the Albers (A) plant or the Bartelso (B) plant. The blended products must then be shipped to the firm's two warehouse outlets, one at Carlyle (C) and the other at Damiansville (D). Current costs per bushel at the two plants are:

	A	B
Corn	10.0	14.0
Wheat	12.0	11.0

Transportation costs per bushel between the plants and warehouses are:

		Fast-Gro		Quick-Gro	
To		C	D	C	D
From	A	1.00	2.00	3.00	3.50
	B	3.00	0.75	4.00	1.90

The firm must satisfy the following demand in bushels at the warehouse outlets:

	Product	
Warehouse	Fast-Gro	Quik-Gro
C	1,000	3,000
D	4,000	6,000

Formulate an LP useful in determining the purchasing, blending, and shipping decisions.

Problem 12

A high-quality wine is typically identified by three attributes: (a) its vintage, (b) its variety, and (c) its region. For example, the Optima Winery of Santa Rosa, California, produced a wine with a label that stated: 1984, Cabernet Sauvignon, Sonoma County. Regulations vary from country to country, but generally the wine in the bottle may be a blend of wines, not all of which need be of the vintage, variety, and region specified on the label. For example, suppose that to receive the label 1984, Cabernet Sauvignon, Sonoma County, at least 80% of the contents must be of 1984 vintage, at least 70% of the contents must be Cabernet Sauvignon, and at least 65% must be from Sonoma County. How small might be the fraction of the wine in the bottle that is of 1984 vintage *and* of the Cabernet Sauvignon variety *and* from grapes grown in Sonoma County?

Problem 13

Rogers Foods of Turlock, California, is a producer of high quality dried foods, such as dried onions and garlic. They have regularly received "Supplier of the Year" awards from their customers, retail packaged food manufacturers, such as Pillsbury. A reason for Rogers' quality reputation is that they try to supply their customers with product with quality characteristics that closely match their customer specifications. This is difficult to do, because Rogers does not have complete control over its input. Each food is harvested once per year from a variety of farms, one "lot" per farm. The quality of the crop from each farm is somewhat of a random variable. At harvest time, the crop is dried and each lot placed in the warehouse. Orders throughout the year are then filled from product in the warehouse.

Two of the main quality features of product are its density and its moisture content. Different customers may have different requirements for each quality attribute. If a product is too dense, then a jar that contains five ounces may appear only half full. If a product is not sufficiently dense, it may be impossible to get five ounces into a jar that is labeled as a five-ounce jar.

To illustrate the problem, suppose that you have five lots of product with the following characteristics:

Lot	Fraction Moisture	Density	Kg. Available
1	.03	.80	1000
2	.02	.75	2500
3	.04	.60	3100
4	.01	.60	1500
5	.02	.65	4500

You currently have two prospective customers with the following requirements:

Customer	Fraction Moisture Min	Max	Density Min	Max	Max Kg Desired	Selling Price Per Kg.
P	0.35045	.65	.75	3,000	$5.25	
G	0.103	.60	.70	15,000	$4.25	

What should you do?

Problem 14

The Lexus automobile gets 26 miles per gallon (mpg), the Corolla gets 31 mpg, and the Tercel gets 35 mpg. Let L, C, and T represent the number of automobiles of each type in some fleet. Let F represent the total number in the fleet. We require that in some sense the mpg of the fleet be at least 32 mpg. Fleet mpg is measured by (total miles driven by the fleet)/(total gallons of fuel consumed by the fleet).

(a) Suppose the sense in which mpg is measured is that each auto is given one gallon of fuel, then driven until the fuel is exhausted. Write appropriate constraints to enforce the 32 mpg requirement.

(b) Suppose the sense in which mpg is measured is that each auto is driven one mile and then stopped. Write appropriate constraints to enforce the 32 mpg requirement.

Problem 15

In the financial industry one is often concerned with the "duration" of one's portfolio of various financial instruments. The duration of a portfolio is simply the weighted average of the duration of the instruments in the portfolio, where the weight is simply the number of dollars invested in the instrument. Suppose the Second National Bank is considering revising its portfolio and has denoted by X1, X2, and X3, the number of dollars invested (in millions) in each of three different instruments. The durations of the three instruments are, respectively, 2 years, 4 years, and 5 years. The following constraint appeared in their planning model:

$$X1 - X2 - 2 \ X3 \geq 0x$$

In words, this constraint is:

(a) duration of the portfolio must be at most 10 years,
(b) duration of the portfolio must be at least 3 years,
(c) duration of the portfolio must be at least 2 years,
(d) duration of the portfolio must be at most 3 years
(e) none of the above.

Problem 16

You are manager of a team of ditch diggers, each member of the team characterized by a productivity measure with units of cubic feet per hour. An average productivity measure for the entire team should be based on which of the following:

(a) the arithmetic mean,
(b) the geometric mean,
(c) the harmonic mean.

Problem 17

Generic Foods has three different batches of cashews in its warehouse. The moisture content for batches 1, 2, and 3, respectively, is 8%, 11%, and 13%. In blending a batch of cashews for a particular customer, the following constraint appeared:

$$2 * X1 - X2 - 3 * X3 \geq 0$$

In words, this constraint is:

(a) moisture content must be at most 10%,
(b) moisture content must be at least 3%,

(c) moisture content must be at least 10%,

(d) moisture content must be at most 2%,

(e) none of the above.

Problem 18

The Beanbody Company buys various types of raw coal on the open market and then pulverizes the coal and mixes it to satisfy customer specifications. Last week Beanbody bought 1500 tons of type M coal for $78 per ton that was intended for an order that was canceled at the last minute. Beanbody had to pay an additional $1 per ton to have the coal shipped to its processing facility. Beanbody has no other coal in stock. Type M coal has a BTU content of 13,000 BTU per ton. This week, type M coal can be bought on the open market for $74 per ton. Type W coal, which has a BTU content of 10,000 BTU/ton, can be bought this week for $68 per ton. Both require an additional $1/ton to be shipped into Beanbody's facility. In fact, Beanbody occasionally sells raw coal on the open market and then Beanbody also has to pay $1/ton outbound shipping. Beanbody expects coal prices to continue to drop next week. Right now Beanbody has an order for 2700 tons of pulverized product having a BTU content of at least 11,000 BTU per ton. Clearly, some additional coal must be bought. The president of Beanbody sketched out the following incomplete model for deciding how much of what coal to purchase so as to just satisfy this order.

```
! MH = tons of on-hand type M coal used;
! MP = tons of type M coal purchased;
! WP = tons of type W coal purchased;

MIN _____ MH  +  ____ MP +  _____ WP;
          MH       + MP        + WP  = 2700;
          MH                     <= 1500;
     _____ MH  + _____ MP - _____ WP >= 0;
END
```

What numbers would you place in the _______ places?

Problem 19

A local high school is considering using an outside supplier to provide meals. The big question is: How much will it cost to provide a nutritional meal to a student? Exhibit A reproduces the recommended daily minimums for an adult as recommended by the noted dietitian George Stigler (1945). Because our high school need provide only one meal per day, albeit the main one, it should be sufficient for our meal to satisfy one half of the minimum daily requirements.

With regard to nutritive content of foods, Exhibit B displays nutritional content of various foods available from one of the prospective vendors recommended by a student committee at the high school.

For purposes of preliminary analysis, it is adequate to consider only calories, protein, calcium, iron, and vitamins A, B1, and B2.

(a) Using only the candidate foods and prices in Exhibit B, and allowing fractional portions, what is the minimum cost needed to give a satisfactory meal at our high school?

(b) Suppose we require that only integer portions be served in a meal; e.g., .75 of a Big Mac is not allowed. How is the cost/meal affected?

(c) Suppose that in addition to (b), for meal simplicity we put a limit of at most three food items from Exhibit B in a meal. For example, a meal of hamburger, fries, chicken McNuggets and Garden Salad has one too many items. How is the cost/meal affected?

(d) Suppose that instead of (c), we require that at most one unit/serving of a particular food type may be used. How is the cost/meal affected?

(e) Suppose we modify (a) with the condition that the number of grams of fat in the meal must be less than or equal to 1/20th of the total calories in the meal. How is the cost/meal affected?

(f) How is the answer to (a) affected if you use current prices from your neighborhood MacDonalds? For reference, Stigler claimed to be able to feed an adult in 1944 for $59.88 for a full year.

Exhibit A

Nutrient	Allowance
Calories	3,000 calories
Protein	70 grams
Calcium	.8 grams
Iron	12 milligrams
Vitamin A	5,000 International Units
Thiamine (B1)	1.8 milligrams
Riboflavin (B2 or G)	2.7 milligrams
Niacin (Nicotinic Acid)	18 milligrams
Ascorbic Acid (C)	75 milligrams

Exhibit B

Menu Item	Price	Calories	Protein	Fat	Sodium	Vit A	Vit C	Vit B1	Vit B2	Niacin	Calcium	Iron
Hamburger	.59	255	12	9	490	4	4	20	10	20	10	15
McLean Deluxe	1.79	320	22	10	670	10	10	25	20	35	15	20
Big Mac	1.65	500	25	26	890	6	2	30	25	35	25	20
Small Fr. Fries	0.68	220	3	12	110	0	15	10	0	10	0	2
Chick McNuggets	1.56	270	20	15	580	0	0	8	8	40	0	6
Honey	0.00	45	0	0	0	0	0	0	0	0	0	0
Chef Salad	2.69	170	17	9	400	100	35	20	15	20	15	8
Garden Salad	1.96	50	4	2	70	90	35	6	6	2	4	8
Egg McMuffin	1.36	280	18	11	710	10	0	30	20	20	25	15
Wheaties	1.09	90	2	1	220	20	20	20	20	20	2	20
Van. Yogurt Cone	0.63	105	4	1	80	2	0	2	10	2	10	0

Milk	0.56	110	9	2	130	10	4	8	30	0	30	0
Orange Juice	0.88	80	1	0	0	0	120	10	0	0	0	0
Grapefruit Juice	0.68	80	1	0	0	0	100	4	2	2	0	0
Apple Juice	0.68	90	0	0	5	0	2	2	0	0	0	4

Problem 20

Your firm has just developed two new ingredients code named A and B. They seem to have great potential in the automotive aftermarket. These ingredients are blended in various combinations to produce a variety of products. For these products (and for the ingredients themselves) there are three qualities of interest: (1) viscosity, (2) flashpoint, and (3) friction coefficient. The research lab has provided the following table describing the qualities of various combinations of A and B:

Combination Coef.	Fraction of		Quality of this Combination		
	A	B	Viscosity	Flashpoint	Friction
1	0.0	1.0	10	400	.1
2	0.5	0.5	25	480	.43
3	.75	.25	32.5	533.3	.522
4	1.0	0.0	40	600	.6

For example, the viscosity of B by itself is 10, whereas the flashpoint of A by itself is 600.

(a) For which qualities do the two ingredients appear to interact in a linear fashion?

(b) You wish to prepare a product which, among other considerations, has viscosity of at least 17, a flashpoint of at least 430, and a friction coefficient of no more than .35. Denote by T, A, and B the amount of total product produced, amount of A used, and the amount of B used. Where possible, write the constraints relating T, A, and B to achieve these qualities.

Problem 21

Indiana Flange, Inc., produces a wide variety of formed steel products that it ships to customers all over the country. It uses several different shipping companies to ship these products. The products are shipped in standard size boxes. A shipping company has typically two constraints to worry about in assembling a load: a weight constraint and a volume constraint. One of the shippers, Amarillo Freight, handles this issue by putting a density constraint (kilograms/cubic meter) on all shipments it receives from Indiana Flange. If the shipment has a density greater than a certain threshold (110 kg/m³), Amarillo imposes a surcharge. Currently, Indiana Flange wants to ship the following products to Los Angeles:

Product	Long Tons	Density
A	100	130
B	85	95

Note: there are 1000 kilograms per long ton. Let AY and BY be the number of tons shipped via Amarillo Freight. Although the density of products A and B do not change from week to week, the number of tons that Indiana Flange needs to ship varies considerably from week to week. Indiana Flange does not want to incur the surcharge. Write a constraint enforcing the Amarillo density constraint that is general, i.e., need not be changed from week to week.

Decision Making Under Uncertainty and Stochastic LP

10.1 Introduction

The main reason multiperiod planning is difficult is the presence of uncertainty about the future. Typically, some action or decision must be taken today that somehow strikes a compromise between the actions that would be, in retrospect, best for each of the possible "futures" that might evolve. For example, if next year the demand for your new product proves to be large and the cost of raw material increases markedly, buying a lot of raw material today would win you a lot of respect next year as a wise and perceptive manager. On the other hand, if the market disappears for both your product and your raw material, the company stockholders would probably not be so kind as to call your purchase of lots of raw material bad luck.

10.2 Representing Uncertainty

Typical types of uncertainty we might encounter are:

(a) Weather related, e.g.,
- decisions about how much and where to stockpile supplies of fuel and road salt in preparation for the winter,
- water release decisions in the spring for a river and dam system, taking into account hydroelectric, navigation, and flooding considerations.

(b) Financial uncertainty,
- market price movements, e.g., stock price, interest rate, foreign exchange rate movements,
- defaults by business partner, e.g., bankruptcy of a major customer.

(c) Political events, e.g.,
- changes of government,
- outbreaks of hostilities.

(d) Technology related, e.g.,
- whether a new technology is useable by the time the next version of our product is scheduled to be released.

(e) Market related, e.g.,
- fads or shifts in tastes,
- population shifts.

(f) Competition, e.g.,
- the kinds of strategies used by the competition next year.

(g) Acts of God, e.g.,
- hurricane, tornado, earthquake, fire, equipment failure, etc.

In an analysis of a decision under uncertainty, we would proceed through a list such as the above and identify those items that might interact with our decision. Weather, in particular, can be a big source of uncertainty. Hidroeléctrica Española, for example (see Dembo et al., 1990), reports that available power output per year from one of its hydroelectric facilities varied from 8,350 gwh (gigawatt-hours) to 2,100 gwh over a three-year period simply because of rainfall variation.

Methods very similar to those described here have been used in the automotive industry to make plant opening and closing decisions in the face of uncertainty about future demand, and in the utilities industry to make fuel purchase decisions in the face of uncertainties about weather in the next few years.

10.3 The Scenario Approach

We will start by considering planning problems with two periods. These situations consist of the following sequence of events:

1. We make a first-period decision.
2. Nature (frequently known as the marketplace) makes a random decision.
3. We make a second-period decision that attempts to repair the havoc wrought by nature in (2).

The scenario approach assumes that there are only a finite number of decisions that nature can make. We call each of these possible states of nature a "scenario." For example, in practice, most people are satisfied with classifying demand for a product as being either low, medium, or high; or classifying a winter as being either severe, normal, or mild, rather than requiring a statement of the average daily temperature and total snowfall measured to six decimal places. General Motors has historically used low, medium, and high scenarios to represent demand uncertainty. The type of model that we will describe for representing uncertainty in the context of LPs is called a "stochastic program." For an extensive introduction to stochastic programming ideas, see Kall and Wallace (1994). For a good discussion of some of the issues in applying stochastic programming to financial decisions, see Infanger (1994).

The first example analyzes a situation in which only steps (1) and (2) are important. A farmer can plant his land to either corn, sorghum, or beans. He is willing to classify the growing season as being either wet or dry. For simplicity, assume that the season will be either wet or dry, nothing in between. If it is wet, corn is more profitable; otherwise, beans are more profitable. The specifics are listed in the table below:

Profit per Acre as a Function of Decisions

		Our Decision		
		All Corn	All Sorghum	All Beans
Nature's Decision	Wet	$100	$70	$80
	Dry	−$10	$40	$35

In step (1), the farmer decides upon how much to plant of each crop. In step (2), nature decides if the season is wet or dry. Step (3) is trivial; the farmer simply enjoys his profit or suffers his losses.

There is no scenario in which beans are the best crop. You might be tempted to eliminate beans from further consideration. We shall see, however, that this could be wrong.

A situation in which there are exactly two possible decisions by nature can be fruitfully analyzed by the kind of graph appearing in Figure 10.1.

The three lines specify expected profit for a given pure policy (all corn, all sorghum, or all soybeans) as a function of the probability of a wet season. If the probability of a wet season is p, the expected profit for various crops is:

	Corn	Sorghum	Beans
Expected Profit	$-10 + p \times 110$	$40 + 30p$	$35 + 45p$

We are indifferent between sorghum and beans when $p = 1/3$. We are indifferent between beans and corn when $p = 9/13$. Thus, if the probability of a wet season is judged to be less than $1/3$, all sorghum should be planted. If we feel p is greater than $9/13$, all corn should be planted. If $1/3 < p < 9/13$, all beans should be sown. All of this assumes that the farmer is not risk averse and is interested only in maximizing expected profits. It is important to note that if the farmer is an expected profit maximizer, the optimal strategy is a pure one: He either plants all corn, all beans, or all sorghum.

An approach that one might be tempted to use is to solve for the optimal first-stage decision for each of the possible decisions of nature and then implement a first-stage decision that is a weighted average of the "conditionally optimal" decisions. For this example, the optimal decision, if we know nature's decision is "wet," is to plant all corn, whereas planting all sorghum is optimal if we know beforehand that the season will be dry. Suppose that the probability of a wet season is $3/8$. Then the "weighted" decision is to plant $3/8$ of the acreage in corn and $5/8$ in sorghum. The expected profit per acre is $(3/8)[(3/8)100 + (5/8)70] + (5/8)[(3/8)(-10) + (5/8)40] = \$43.75$.

This should be contrasted with the decision that maximizes the expected profit. For a probability of a wet season equal to $3/8$, the expected profit of planting all soy-

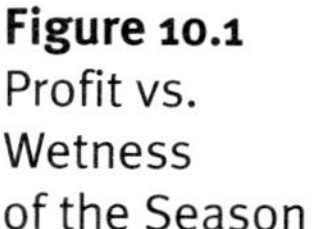

Figure 10.1
Profit vs.
Wetness
of the Season

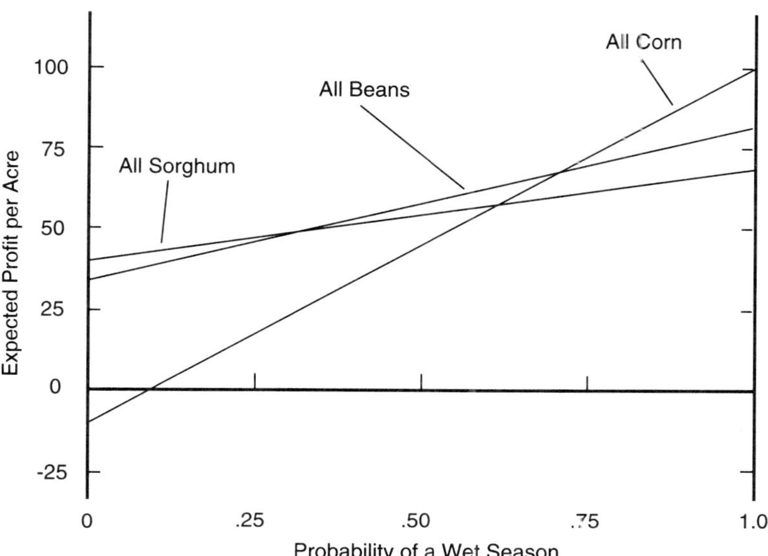

beans is $(3/8)80 + (5/8)35 = \$51.875$ per acre. The expected profit from behaving optimally is almost 20% greater than just behaving "reasonably." The qualitative conclusion to draw from this small example is:

> *The best decision for today, when faced with a number of different outcomes for the future, is in general not equal to the "average" of the decisions that would be best for each specific future outcome.*

For a problem this simple, one does not need LP; however, let us demonstrate the LP for this problem in preparation for more complex problems. There are three first-stage decision variables:

$C =$ acreage planted to corn,
$S =$ acreage planted to sorghum,
$B =$ acreage planted to beans.

Presuming that the probability of a wet season is 3/8, the objective is to

Maximize $(3/8)(100C + 70S + 80B) = (5/8)(-10C + 40S + 35B)$
subject to $C + S + B \le 1$.

The solitary constraint specifies that we are interested only in how to plant one acre. When the expressions in the objective are calculated and simplified, we get:

Maximize $31.25C + 51.25S + 51.875B$
subject to $C + S + B \le 1$.

The solution is clearly to set $B = 1$; i.e., plant all beans.

The coefficients of corn and sorghum in the objective are simply the expected profits of planting one acre of the respective crop. This illustrates a second important point about planning under uncertainty:

> Certainty Equivalence Theorem: *If the randomness or unpredictability in problem data exists solely in the objective function coefficients, it is correct to solve the LP in regular form after simply using the expected values for the random coefficients in the objective.*

If the randomness exists in a right-hand side or a constraint coefficient, it is not correct to simply replace the random element by its average or expected value.

10.4 A More Complicated Two-Period Planning Problem

The previous example had a trivial second-stage decision. There were no decisions left to be made after nature made its decision. The following example requires some nontrivial second-stage decisions.

It is late summer in a northern city, and the director of streets is making decisions regarding the purchase of fuel and salt to be used in snow removal in the approaching winter. If insufficient supplies are purchased before a severe winter, substantially higher prices must be paid to purchase these supplies quickly during the winter. There are two methods of snow removal: plowing or salting. Salting is generally cheaper, especially during a warm winter; however, excess salt after a warm winter must be carried until next winter. Excess fuel, on the other hand, is readily usable by other city departments, so there is less penalty for stocking too much fuel.

The director of streets classifies a winter as either warm or cold and attaches probabilities 0.4 and 0.6, respectively, to these two possible states of nature. The costs and salvage values of salt and fuel are described in the table below. Decisions made before winter are period 1 decisions, whereas decisions made during or after winter are period 2 decisions. For the convenience of the reader, all figures will be presented in "truck-days," that is, the amount consumed by one truck in one day.

Cost or Value of Supplies vs. Date of Purchase

	Salt	Fuel	Cost Per Truck-Day
Bought in Period 1	$20	$70	
Bought in Period 2 { Warm	$30	$73	$110
Bought in Period 2 { Cold	$32	$73	$120
Salvage Value at End of Period 2	$15	$65	

Notice that the second-period price of salt is a random variable depending upon the weather. If the winter is cold, we expect the price of salt to be higher.

The cost of operating a truck per day, exclusive of fuel and salt, is $110 in a warm winter but $120 in a cold winter. The truck fleet has a capacity of 5,000 truck-days during the winter season. If only plowing but no salting is used, a warm winter will require 3,500 truck-days of snow removal, whereas a cold winter will require 5,100. Salting is a more effective use of trucks than plowing. In a warm winter, one truck salting is equivalent to 1.2 trucks plowing, whereas in a cold winter, the equivalency drops to 1.1. Thus, in a cold winter, the limited truck capacity implies that some salting will be necessary.

At this point it is useful to define variables for the amounts of fuel and salt bought or sold at various times:

$$
\begin{aligned}
\text{BF1} &= \text{truck-days of fuel bought in period 1} \\
\text{BS1} &= \text{truck-days of salt bought in period 1} \\
\text{BFW} &= \text{fuel bought in period 2, warm winter} \\
\text{BSW} &= \text{salt bought in period 2, warm winter} \\
\text{XFW} &= \text{excess fuel at end of warm winter} \\
\text{XSW} &= \text{excess salt at end of warm winter} \\
\text{PW} &= \text{truck-days plowing, warm winter} \\
\text{SW} &= \text{truck-days spreading salt, warm winter} \\
\text{KW} &= \text{costs incurred during a warm winter in dollars} \\
\text{BFC} &= \text{fuel bought in period 2, cold winter} \\
\text{BSC} &= \text{salt bought in period 2, cold winter} \\
\text{XFC} &= \text{excess fuel at end of a cold winter} \\
\text{XSC} &= \text{excess salt at end of a cold winter} \\
\text{PC} &= \text{truck-days plowing, cold winter} \\
\text{SC} &= \text{truck-days spreading salt, cold winter} \\
\text{KC} &= \text{costs incurred during a cold winter in dollars}
\end{aligned}
$$

An important thing to notice is that we have defined unique second-stage decision variables for each of the possible states of nature; e.g., salt bought in period 2 is distinguished as to whether bought in a warm rather than cold winter. This is the key to constructing a correct formulation.

10.4.1 The Warm Winter Solution

If the winter is known to be warm, the relevant LP is:

```
MIN      70 BF1 + 20 BS1 + KW
SUBJECT TO
 2)  -BF1 - BFW + XFW + PW + SW = 0                    !(Fuel Usage)
 3)  -BS1 - BSW + XSW + SW = 0                         !(Salt Usage)
 4)   PW + SW <= 5,000                                 !(Truck Usage)
 5)   PW + 1.2SW >= 3,500                              !(Snow Removal)
 6)   KW - 73 BFW - 30 BSW + 65 XFW - 110 PW - 110 SW = 0 !(Cost)
```

When solved, the solution is:

```
OBJECTIVE FUNCTION VALUE

   1)        583333.300000

VARIABLE          VALUE           REDUCED COST
   BF1         2916.666660          0.000000
   BS1         2916.666660          0.000000
   KW        320833.332000          0.000000
```

```
BFW                  0.000000                3.000000
XFW                  0.000000                5.000000
PW                   0.000000               13.333334
SW                2916.666660                0.000000
BSW                  0.000000               10.000000
XSW                  0.000000                5.000000

ROW                  SLACK              DUAL PRICES
 2)                  0.000000               70.000000
 3)                  0.000000               20.000000
 4)               2083.333340                0.000000
 5)                  0.000000             -166.666666
 6)                  0.000000               -1.000000
```

The solution is, as you would expect if you knew beforehand that the winter is to buy sufficient fuel and salt in the first period to follow a "pure salt spreading" policy in the second period. No supplies are bought, nor is there any excess in period 2.

10.4.2 The Cold Winter Solution

The corresponding LP, if we knew that the winter would be cold, is:

```
MIN          70 BF1 + 20 BS1 + KC
 SUBJECT TO
 2)  -BF1 - BFC + XFC + PC + SC = 0
 3)  -BS1 + SC - BSC + XSC = 0
 4)   PC + SC <= 5,000
 5)   PC + 1.1 SC >= 5,100
 6)   KC - 73 BFC + 65 XFC - 120 PC - 120 SC - 32 BSC + 15 XSC = 0
```

The solution is slightly more complicated. In a cold winter, the assumptions are such as to make plowing slightly more cost effective than salting. A pure plowing policy cannot be used, however, because of scarce truck capacity. Thus, just sufficient salt is used to make the truck capacity sufficient. This is illustrated below:

```
                 OBJECTIVE FUNCTION VALUE

         1)          970000.0

    VARIABLE           VALUE          REDUCED COST
        BF1         5000.0000             0.0000
        BS1         1000.0000             0.0000
         KC       600000.0000             0.0000
        BFC            0.0000             3.0000
        XFC            0.0000             5.0000
         PC         3999.9999             0.0000
         SC         1000.0000             0.0000
        BSC            0.0000            12.0000
        XSC            0.0000             5.0000

        ROW           SLACK            DUAL PRICES
         2)           0.00000             70.000000
         3)           0.00000             20.000000
         4)           0.00000              0.000000
```

```
      5)            0.00000        -200.000000
      6)            0.00000          -1.000000
```

10.4.3 The Unconditional Solution

Neither of these two models or solutions, however, is immediately useful by itself, because it is not known beforehand whether it will be a cold or warm winter. Part of the problem is that the two solutions recommend different first-period purchasing decisions depending upon whether the winter is to be warm or cold. In reality, the first-period decision must be unique, regardless of whether the winter is cold or warm. This is easy to remedy, however; we simply combine the two models into one. Because the same first-stage variables, BF1 and BS1, appear in both sets of constraints, this forces the same first-stage decision to appear regardless of the severity of the winter.

It remains to specify the appropriate objective function for the combined problem. It is obvious that the cost coefficients of the first-stage variables are appropriate as they are; however, the second-stage costs, KW and KC, are really random variables. With probability 0.4, we want KW to apply and KC to be treated as zero, whereas with probability 0.6, we want KC to be in the objective and KW to be treated as zero. The correct resolution is to apply weights 0.4 and 0.6 to KW and KC, respectively, in the objective. Thus, the complete formulation is:

```
MIN    70 BF1 + 20 BS1 + 0.4 KW + 0.6 KC;
SUBJECT TO
 2)  -BF1 - BFW + XFW + PW + SW = 0;
 3)  -BS1 + SW - BSW + XSW = 0;
 4)   PW + SW < 5000;
 5)   PW + 1.2 SW > 3500;
 6)   KW - 73 BFW + 65 XFW - 110 SW - 110 PW - 30 BSW + 15 XSW = 0;
 7)  -BF1 - BFC + XFC + PC + SC = 0;
 8)  -BS1 + SC - BSC + XSC = 0;
 9)   PC + SC < 5000;
10)   PC + 1.1 SC > 5100;
11)   KC - 73 BFC + 65 XFC - 120 PC - 120 SC - 32 BSC + 15 XSC = 0;
END
```

In order to understand this model, it is worth looking at the following PICTURE of its coefficients:

```
        B  B     B  X        B  X     B  X        B  X
        F  S  K  F  F  P  S  S  S  K  F  F  P  S  S  S
        1  1  W  W  W  W  W  W  W  C  C  C  C  C  C  C
   1:   B  B  T                    T                    MIN
   2:  -1        -1  1  1  1                              =
   3:     -1                 1 -1  1                      =
   4:                     1  1                           < D
   5:                     1  A                           > D
   6:            1 -B  B -C -C -B  B                      =
   7:  -1                             -1  1  1  1         =
   8:     -1                              1 -1  1  =
   9:                                     1  1        < D
  10:                                     1  A        > D
  11:                           1 -B  B -C -C -B  B  = 0
```

The model really consists of two submodels, one for a cold winter in the lower right and one for a warm winter above and to the left. These two models would be separate except for the linkage via the common first-stage variables BF1 and BS1 on the extreme left. Another way of stating the problem in words is:

Minimize   first-stage cost + 0.4 (second-stage costs for a warm winter)
            + 0.6 (second-stage costs for a cold winter)

subject to the same first decisions applying regardless of whether the winter is warm or cold.

The solution to the complete problem is:

```
              OBJECTIVE FUNCTION VALUE

        1)            819888.3

     VARIABLE          VALUE            REDUCED COST
        BF1         2916.666660            0.0000
        BS1         2916.666660            0.0000
         KW       320833.332000            0.0000
        BFW            0.000000            3.0000
        XFW            0.000000            0.2000
         PW            0.000000            4.6833
         SW         2916.666660            0.0000
        BSW            0.000000            3.5799
        XSW            0.000000            2.4200
         KC       715091.672000            0.0000
        BFC         1891.666690            0.0000
        XFC            0.000000            4.8000
         PC         1891.666690            0.0000
         SC         2916.666660            0.0000
        BSC            0.000000            7.6200
        XSC            0.000000            2.5799

        ROW            SLACK            DUAL PRICES
         2)            0.000000           26.20000
         3)            0.000000            8.42000
         4)         2083.333340            0.00000
         5)            0.000000          -65.51666
         6)            0.000000           -0.40000
         7)            0.000000           43.80000
         8)            0.000000           11.57999
         9)          191.666645            0.00000
        10)            0.000000         -115.80000
        11)            0.000000           -0.60000
```

The solution is interesting. It recommends buying sufficient salt and fuel in the first period to follow a pure salt spreading policy if the winter is warm. If the winter is cold, extra fuel is bought in the second period to be used for plowing only to gain the needed snow removal capacity. There will be no excess fuel or salt for either outcome.

We are now in position to state the general procedure for developing an LP model of a two-period planning problem under uncertainty:

1. For each possible state of nature, formulate the appropriate LP model.
2. Combine these submodels into one supermodel, making sure that:
   (a) the first-stage variables are common to all submodels but
   (b) the second-stage variables in a submodel appear only in that submodel.
3. The second-stage cost for each submodel appears in the overall objective function weighted by the probability that nature will choose the state corresponding to that submodel.

In a typical application, there will be a debate about the proper values for the probabilities, and therefore you may wish to examine the sensitivity of the results to changes in the probabilities. The following range report indicates some of these sensitivities.

```
RANGES IN WHICH THE BASIS IS UNCHANGED
                         COST COEFFICIENT RANGES
    VARIABLE          CURRENT         ALLOWABLE         ALLOWABLE
                       COEF           INCREASE          DECREASE
      BF1           70.000000         3.000000           0.20000
      BS1           20.000000         3.579999           2.42000
      KW             0.400000         0.003077           0.04109
      BFW            0.000000         INFINITY           3.00000
      XFW            0.000000         INFINITY           0.20000
      PW             0.000000         INFINITY           4.68333
      SW             0.000000         5.619999          78.62000
      BSW            0.000000         INFINITY           3.57999
      XSW            0.000000         INFINITY           2.42000
      KC             0.600000         0.002740           0.04109
      BFC            0.000000         0.200000           3.00000
      XFC            0.000000         INFINITY           4.80000
      PC             0.000000         2.200001           2.34545
      SC             0.000000         2.579999           2.42000
      BSC            0.000000         INFINITY           7.62000
      XSC            0.000000         INFINITY           2.57999

                         RIGHTHAND SIDE RANGES
     ROW              CURRENT          ALLOWABLE         ALLOWABLE
                       RHS             INCREASE          DECREASE
      2              0.000000        2916.666660       1891.666690
      3              0.000000        1916.666550       1719.696990
      4           5000.000000         INFINITY         2083.333340
      5           3500.000000        2063.636380       2299.999760
      6              0.000000         INFINITY       320833.332000
      7              0.000000        1891.666690         INFINITY
      8              0.000000        1719.696990       1916.666550
      9           5000.000000         INFINITY          191.666645
     10           5100.000000         191.666645       1891.666690
     11              0.000000         INFINITY       715091.672000
```

Notice that the objective coefficient ranges for KW and KC are quite small. Thus, it would appear that modest changes in the probabilities, 0.4 and 0.6, might produce very noticeable changes in the solution.

10.5 Expected Value of Perfect Information (EVPI)

Uncertainty has its costs. Therefore, it may be worthwhile to invest in research to reduce the uncertainty. This investment might be in better weather forecasts for problems like the one just considered or it might be in test markets or market surveys for problems relating to new product investment. A bound on the value of better forecasts is obtainable by considering the possibility of getting perfect forecasts, so-called perfect information.

We have sufficient information on the snow removal problem to calculate the value of perfect information. For example, if we knew beforehand that the winter would be warm, we saw from the solution of the warm winter model that the total cost would be 583,333.3. On the other hand, if we knew beforehand that the winter would be cold, we saw that the total cost would be 970,000. Having perfect forecasts will not change the frequency of warm and cold winters. They will presumably still occur with respective probabilities 0.4 and 0.6. Thus, if we had perfect forecasts, the expected cost per season would be:

$$0.4 \times 583{,}333.3 + 0.6 \times 970{,}000 = 815{,}333.3.$$

From the solution of the complete model, we see that the expected cost per season without any additional information is 819,888.3. Thus, the expected value of perfect information is 819,888.3 − 815,333.3 = 4,555.0. Therefore, if a well-dressed weather forecaster claims prior knowledge of the severity of the coming winter, an offer of at most 4,555 should be made to learn his forecast. In reality, his forecast is probably worth considerably less than that, because it is probably not a perfect forecast.

10.6 Expected Value of Modeling Uncertainty (EVMU)

Suppose the EVPI is high. Does this mean that it is important to use stochastic programming, or the scenario approach? Definitely not. Even though the EVPI may be high, it may be that a very simple deterministic model does just as well, e.g., recommends the same decision as a sophisticated stochastic model. The Expected Value of Modeling Uncertainty (EVMU) measures the additional profit possible by using a "correct" stochastic model.

10.6.1 Certainty Equivalence

Constructing a mathematical model of a decision problem under uncertainty takes a lot of work. So, a reasonable question is: "Under what conditions can we replace a random variable in a model by its expected value without changing the action recommended by the model?" If we can justify such a replacement, we have a priori determined that the EVPI is zero for that random variable.

Define:

X = the set of decision variables,
Y_i = some random variable in the model,
$\overline{Y}_i$ = all other random variables in the model, except Y_i,
$\tilde{Y}_i$ = all other random variables that are independent of Y_i.

We are justified in replacing Y_i by its expected value, $E(Y_i)$, if

(a) Y_i appears only in the objective function, and each term containing Y_i either
(b) is not a function of X, or
(c) is linear in Y_i and contains no random variables dependent upon Y_i.

Equivalently, we must be able to write the objective as:

$$\text{Min } F_1\!\left(X,\overline{Y}_i\right) + F_2\!\left(X,\tilde{Y}_i\right) \times Y_i + F_3\!\left(\overline{Y}_i,Y_i\right).$$

If we take expected values :

$$E\!\left[F_1\!\left(X,Y_i\right) + F_2\!\left(X,\tilde{Y}_i\right) \times Y_i + F_3\!\left(\overline{Y}_i,Y_i\right)\right]$$
$$= E\!\left[F_1\!\left(X,\overline{Y}_i\right)\right] + E\!\left[F_2\!\left(X,\tilde{Y}_i\right)\right] \times E\!\left(Y_i\right) + E\!\left[F_3\!\left(\overline{Y}_i,Y_i\right)\right].$$

The third term is a constant with respect to the decision variables, so it can be dropped. Thus, any X that minimizes $E\!\left[F_1\!\left(X,\overline{Y}_i\right) + F_2\!\left(X,\tilde{Y}_i\right) \times Y_i\right]$ also minimizes:

$$E\!\left[F_1\!\left(X,\overline{Y}_i\right) + F_2\!\left(X,\tilde{Y}_i\right) \times E\!\left(Y_i\right)\right].$$

As an example, consider a farmer who must decide how much corn, beans, and milo to plant in the face of random yields and random prices for the crops. Further, suppose the farmer receives a government subsidy that is a complicated function of current crop prices and the farmer's total land holdings but not a function of current yield or planting decisions. Suppose that the price for corn at harvest time is independent of the yield. The farmer's income can be written

(income from beans and milo) + (acreage devoted to corn) × (corn yield)
× (price of corn) + (subsidy based on prices).

The third term is independent of this year's decision, so it can be disregarded. In the middle term, the random variable, "price of corn," can be replaced by its expected value, because it is independent of the two other components of the middle term.

10.7 Risk Aversion

Thus far we have assumed that the decision maker is strictly an expected profits maximizer and is neither risk averse nor risk preferring. Casino gamblers who play games such as roulette must be risk preferring if the roulette wheel is not defective, because their expected profits are negative. A person is risk averse if he or she attaches more weight to a large loss than expected profits maximization would dictate.

In the context of the snow removal problem, the Streets Manager might be embarrassed by a high cost of snow removal in a cold winter even though long-run expected cost minimization would imply an occasional big loss. From the optimal policy for the snow removal problem, we can see that the sum of first-period plus second-period costs, if the winter is cold, is

```
70 BF1 + 20 BS1 + KC = 977,591.
```

On the other hand, if it is known beforehand that the winter will be cold, we have seen that this cost can be reduced to 970,000.

For fear of attracting the attention of a political opponent, the Streets Manager might wish to prevent the possibility of a cost more than $5,000 greater than the minimum possible for the cold winter outcome.

The Manager can incorporate his risk aversion into the LP by adding the constraint:

```
70 BF1 + 20 BS1 + KC <= 975,000.
```

When this is done, the solution is:

```
                OBJECTIVE FUNCTION VALUE

        1)              820061.1

        VARIABLE              VALUE           REDUCED COST
          BF1            3780.557800            0.000000
          BS1            2916.666630            0.000000
          KW           264680.406000            0.000000
          BFW                0.000000            3.199999
          XFW              863.891151            0.000001
          PW                 0.000000            4.611111
          SW             2916.666660            0.000000
          BSW                0.000000            3.533333
          XSW                0.000000            2.466667
          KC           652027.609000            0.000000
          BFC             1027.775540            0.000001
          XFC                0.000000            5.333332
          PC              1891.666690            0.000001
          SC              2916.666630            0.000000
          BSC                0.000000            8.466666
          XSC                0.000000            2.866666
```

The expected cost has increased by about $820,061 - 819,888 = 173$ dollars. A politician might consider this a price worth paying to reduce his worst case (cold winter) cost almost $2,600. Notice, however, that performance in the event of a warm winter does not look as good. The value of XFW indicates that there will be almost 864 units of fuel to be disposed of at the end of a warm winter.

10.7.1 Downside Risk

There are a variety of ways of measuring risk. Variance is probably the most common measure of risk. The variance measure gives equal weight to deviations above the mean as well as below. For a symmetric distribution, this is fine, but for non-symmetric distributions, this is not attractive. Most people worry a lot more about returns that are below average than about ones that are above average.

Downside risk is a reasonably intuitive way of quantifying risk that looks only at returns that are lower than some threshold. In words, downside risk is the expected amount by which return falls short of a specified target. To explain it more carefully, define:

P_s = probability that scenario s occurs,
T = a target return threshold that we specify,
R_s = the return achieved if scenario s occurs,
D_s = the down side if scenario s occurs = max $\{0, T - R_s\}$,
ER = expected downside risk = $P_1 D_1 + P_2 D_2 + \ldots$

10.7.2 Example

Suppose that the farmer of our earlier acquaintance has made two changes in his assessment of things: (a) he assesses the probability of a wet season as 0.7, and (b) he has eliminated beans as a possible crop, so that he has only two choices, corn and sorghum. A reformulation of his model is:

```
MAX       0.7 RW + 0.3 RD
SUBJECT TO
   2)    RW - 100 C - 70 S =      0
   3)    RD + 10 C - 40 S =      0
   4)    C + S =     1
END
FREE          RW
FREE          RD
```

The variables RW and RD are the return (i.e., profit) if the season is wet or dry, respectively. Notice that both RW and RD were declared as FREE because RD in particular could be negative.

When solved, the recommendation is to plant 100% corn, with a resulting expected profit of 67.

```
           OBJECTIVE FUNCTION VALUE

      1)         67.0000000

 VARIABLE          VALUE         REDUCED COST
       RW        100.000000           .000000
       RD        -10.000000           .000000
        C          1.000000           .000000
        S           .000000          6.000000

      ROW     SLACK OR SURPLUS     DUAL PRICES
       2)           .000000           .700000
       3)           .000000           .300000
       4)           .000000         67.000000
```

The solution makes it explicit that, if the season is dry, our profits, RD, will be negative. Let us compute the expected downside risk for a solution to this problem. We must choose a target threshold. A plausible value for this target is one such that the most conservative decision available to us just barely has an expected downside risk of zero. For our farmer, the most conservative decision is sorghum. A target value of 40 would give sorghum a downside risk of zero. To compute the expected downside risk for our problem, we want to add the constraints:

```
DW >= 40 - RW
DD >= 40 - RD
```

and

```
ER = .7DW + .3DD.
```

The constraint `DW >= 40 - RW` effectively sets `DW = max (0, 40 - RW)`. When converted to standard form and appended to our model, we get:

```
MAX      0.7 RW + 0.3 RD
SUBJECT TO
      2)    RW - 100 C - 70 S =     0
      3)    RD + 10 C - 40 S =      0
      4)    C + S =      1
      5)    RW + DW >=     40
      6)    RD + DD >=     40
      7) - 0.7 DW - 0.3 DD + ER =     0
END
FREE        RW
FREE        RD
FREE        ER
```

The solution is:

```
OBJECTIVE FUNCTION VALUE

        1)      67.00000

    VARIABLE          VALUE          REDUCED COST
          RW      100.000000             .000000
          RD      -10.000000             .000000
           C        1.000000             .000000
           S         .000000            6.000000
          DW         .000000             .000000
          DD       50.000000             .000000
          ER       15.000000             .000000
```

Because we put no constraint on expected downside risk, we get the same solution as before, but with the additional information that the expected downside risk is 15.

What happens as we become more risk averse? Suppose we add the constraint `ER <= 10`. We then get the solution:

```
OBJECTIVE FUNCTION VALUE

        1)      65.0000000

    VARIABLE          VALUE          REDUCED COST
          RW       90.000000             .000000
          RD        6.666668             .000000
           C         .666667             .000000
```

```
        S            .333333              .000000
       DW            .000000              .280000
       DD          33.333330              .000000
       ER          10.000000              .000000
```

Notice that the recommendation is now to put 1/3 of the land into sorghum. The profit drops modestly to 65 from 67. If the season is dry, the profit is now 6.67 rather than −10 as before. Finally, let's constrain the expected downside risk to zero with ER ≤ 0. Then the solution is:

```
OBJECTIVE FUNCTION VALUE

       1)      61.000000

    VARIABLE           VALUE          REDUCED COST
       RW           70.000000              .000000
       RD           40.000000              .000000
        C            .000000               .000000
        S           1.000000               .000000
       DW            .000000               .280000
       DD            .000000               .000000
       ER            .000000               .000000
```

Now all the land is planted with sorghum, and expected profit drops to 61.

10.8 Decisions Under Uncertainty with More than Two Periods

The ideas that were discussed for the two-period problem can be extended to an arbitrary number of periods. The sequence of events in the general case is:

1. We make a decision,
2. Nature makes a random decision,
3. We make a decision,
4. Nature makes a random decision,
5. Etc.

The extension can be made by working backwards through time. For example, if we wished to analyze a three-period problem, we would start with the last two periods and formulate the associated two-period stochastic LP model. When the first period is taken into account, the model just developed for the last two periods is treated as the second period of a two-period problem for which now the true first period is really the first period. This process cannot continue for too many periods because the problem size gets too large rapidly. If the number of periods is n and the number of possible states of nature each period is s, the problem size is proportional to s^n. Thus, it is unusual to have manageable stochastic LPs with more than two or three periods.

10.9 Choosing Scenarios

Even when outcomes are naturally discrete, the number of scenarios may be huge from a computational point of view. Consider an electrical utility company that has

20 major transformers scattered over its demand area. In planning its major capital expenditures for the coming year, the only significant source of randomness for the coming year is whether or not each transformer fails. Thus, a configuration of transformer failures constitutes a scenario and therefore there are $2^{20} = 1,048,576$ scenarios. This is too many scenarios for current computational technology. Which scenarios should be included?

Intuitively, a particular scenario should be included in our analysis if the expected cost of not including it is high. The expected cost is directly related to two things: (a) the probability the scenario occurs, and (b) the difference in cost between an optimal stage 1 decision and a nonoptimal one if this scenario occurs in reality. Infanger (1994) presents a sophisticated methodology based on importance sampling for doing the above kind of sampling of scenarios "on-the-fly." A simplified analysis is as follows.

For our transformer example, suppose that transformers fail independently, each with probability 0.01. We can start to list the possible scenarios:

Failure Scenario	Probability	Cumulative
No failures	.818	.818
Transformer 1 fails	.00826	.826
Transformer 2 fails	.00826	.834
$\vdots$	$\vdots$	$\vdots$
Transformer 20 fails	.00826	.983
Transformers 1 & 2 fail	.0000826	.9830826
Transformers 1 & 3 fail	.0000826	.9831652
$\vdots$	$\vdots$	$\vdots$
Transformers 1 through 20 fail	10^{-40}	1.0000

Thus, the first 21 scenarios, consisting of no transformer failures and exactly one failure, account for over 98% of the probability.

To push the analysis a little more, suppose the cost of behaving non-optimally in the face of a transformer failure is at most $10,000, and this cost is additive among transformers. Thus, an upper bound on the expected cost of not including one of the scenarios with exactly one failure is $0.00826 \times 10,000 = \$82.6$. An upper bound on the expected cost of not including one of the scenarios with exactly two failures is $0.0000826 \times (10,000 + 10,000) = \$1.65$.

A very conservative estimate of the expected cost of disregarding all scenarios with more than 1 failure is $(1 - 0.983) \times 20 \times 10,000 = \$3400$.

If we use these 21 scenarios, what probabilities should be used? One choice would be to assign probability 0.818 to the non-failure scenario and $(1 - 0.818)/20 = 0.0091$ to each of the non-failure scenarios. The expected number of failures in the real system is $0.01 \times 20 = 0.2$. If we wished to match this statistic, we would assign a probability of 0.01 to each of the one-failure scenarios and a probability of 0.8 to the non-failure scenario.

10.10 Matching Scenarios Statistics to Targets

Suppose that scenarios represent things such as demand, on the return on investment, or the failure of equipment. Then we might be interested in knowing whether (using our scenarios and associated probabilities) the scenario-based expected demand equals the forecast demand, or the scenario-based expected return on a particular stock matches the forecast return for that stock, or the scenario-based expected number of machine failures matches the forecast number of machine failures.

If scenarios have already been selected, we may wish to choose scenario probabilities so as to match given forecasts. Alternatively, if scenarios have not yet been selected, we may wish to choose both scenarios and probabilities to match forecasts.

10.11 Generating a Set of Scenarios with a Specified Covariance Structure

Carino et al. (1994), in their description of the application of stochastic programming at the Yasuda-Kasai Company, mention that they chose scenarios so as to match forecasted means and variances for forecasted quantities such as interest rates. This "matching" can also be done for covariances.

Suppose we wish to generate m observations or scenarios, on n variables, e.g., returns on investment instruments, such that the *sample* covariance matrix exactly equals a specified covariance matrix V, and the sample means exactly equal a specified vector M. We somewhat arbitrarily decide that each scenario will be equally likely.

We can use a variation of a method described in Bratley, Fox, and Schrage (1987). Do a Cholesky factorization of V to give an upper triangular matrix C so that $C'C = V$. Effectively, C is the square root of V.

Next generate m observations on n (pseudo) random variables so that the *sample* means are all zero and the *sample* covariance matrix is the identity matrix. Note that $m \geq n + 1$ may be required; $m = n + 1$ is always sufficient, so we will assume $m = n + 1$. For example, if $m = 4$ and $n = 3$, a suitable matrix of pseudo random values is:

$$\begin{pmatrix} -1 & 1 & -1 \\ 1 & 1 & 1 \\ -1 & -1 & 1 \\ 1 & -1 & -1 \end{pmatrix}$$

Call this matrix Z.

Next, generate the desired random observations by the transformation:

$$X = M + ZC$$

where

M = vector of desired means.

X = desired set of observations or scenarios.

Note that:

$$(X - M)'\,(X-M) = (ZC)'\,(ZC) = C'\,Z'\,ZC$$

By construction $Z'Z$ is a diagonal matrix with m's on the diagonal. Thus, the sample covariance matrix is $(X-M)'(X-M)/m = m\,C'C/m = C'C = V$.

10.11.1 Generating a Suitable Z Matrix

We provided an example Z matrix for which it was obvious that it satisfied the required features:

$$(1)\quad \sum_{i=1}^{m} z_{ij} = 0 \qquad \text{for } j = 1, 2, \cdots, n,$$

$$(2)\quad \sum_{i=1}^{m} z_{ij}^2 = m \qquad \text{for } j = 1, 2, \cdots, n,$$

$$(3)\quad \sum_{i=1}^{m} z_{ij} z_{ik} = 0 \qquad \text{for all } j,\ k \text{ with } j \neq k.$$

We can subsume condition (1) into condition (3) if we temporarily place a column of 1s in front of Z, i.e., as its first column. Thus, the condition

$$\sum_{i=1}^{m} z_{ij} \times z_{i1} = 0$$

will imply condition (1).

With this convenient device, we can also write conditions (2) and (3) in matrix notation as simply:

(4) $Z'\,Z = m\,I$, where I is the identity matrix with 1s down the diagonal.

There is a procedure called Gram-Schmidt Orthogonalization that can be used for finding a matrix Z that satisfies conditions (2) and (3), or equivalently satisfies condition (4) in matrix notation. The Gram-Schmidt procedure will take as input an $m \times m$ matrix U of linearly independent columns, and output an $m \times m$ matrix V that satisfies condition (3). It is a simple matter to scale each column of V so that condition (2) is also satisfied.

The steps of the Gram-Schmidt procedure are:

For $j = 1, 2, 3, \ldots, m$:

For $t = 1, 2, \ldots, j - 1$

$$\alpha_{tj} = \left(\sum_{i=1}^{m} v_{it} u_{ij} \right) \bigg/ \sum_{i=1}^{m} v_{it} v_{it}$$

For $i = 1, 2, \ldots, m$

$$v_{ij} = u_{ij} - \sum_{t=1}^{j-1} \alpha_{tj} v_{it}$$

The v_{ij}s now satisfy, for $j \neq t$:

$$\sum_{i=1}^{m} v_{ij} v_{it} = 0$$

We finally obtain the matrix Z satisfying condition (2) by discarding the first column of the $\{v_{ii}\}$ and scaling each column as follows:

For $j = 1, 2, \ldots, m - 1$:

$$\sigma_j = \sqrt{\left(\sum_{i=1}^{m} v_{ij+1} v_{ij+1} \right) \Big/ m}$$

For $i = 1, 2, \ldots, m$:

$$z_{ij} = v_{ij+1} \Big/ \sigma_j$$

10.11.2 Example

For the case $m = 4$, a suitable U matrix is:

1	1	0	0
1	0	1	0
1	0	0	1
1	0	0	0

The Gram-Schmidt orthogonalization of it is:

1	.75	0	0
1	−.25	.66667	0
1	−.25	−.33333	.5
1	−.25	−.33333	−.5

After we normalize or scale each column to satisfy condition (2) and drop the first column, we get the Z matrix:

1.73205	0	0
−0.57735	1.63299	0
−0.57735	−0.81650	1.41421
−0.57735	−0.81650	−1.41421

The U matrix that we chose to illustrate the procedure was somewhat arbitrary. The only requirements are that the initial column be a vector of 1's and that the columns be independent. If, for example, we feel that the random variables being simulated are Normal-distributed, we could have chosen the remaining columns of U by making independent draws from a Normal distribution. The values in each column, 2, 3, . . . , m, of the matrix V would then also be independent, identically Normal-distributed. The values in each column of Z would be approximately Normal-distributed as m increases.

Now suppose we wish to match the following covariance matrix:

$V =$	.01080753	.01240721	.01307512
	.01240721	.05839169	.05542639
	.01307512	.05542639	.09422681

and the vector of means:

$$M = \quad 1.089083 \qquad 1.213667 \qquad 1.234583$$

The Cholesky factorization of V is:

$$C = \quad .10395930 \qquad .11934681 \qquad .1257716$$
$$.21011433 \qquad .19235219$$
$$.20349188$$

Using the Z generated above, a set of scenarios that exactly match V and M are:

$$X = \quad 1.269245 \qquad 1.420381 \qquad 1.452425$$
$$1.029062 \qquad 1.487877 \qquad 1.476078$$
$$1.029062 \qquad 0.973204 \qquad 1.292694$$
$$1.029062 \qquad 0.973204 \qquad 0.717132$$

10.11.3 Converting Multistage Problems to Two-Stage Problems

In many systems, the effect of randomness (e.g., demand) does not carry over from one period to the next. Eppen, Martin, and Schrage (1989), for example, assumed this in their analysis of long-range capacity planning for an automobile manufacturer. Effectively, the entire plan for the next five years was decided upon in the first year. If demands are independent from year to year and there is no carryover inventory, when deciding what to do in period $t + 1$, one need not know what random demands occurred in periods 1 through t.

10.12 Decisions Under Uncertainty with an Infinite Number of Periods

We can consider the case of an infinite number of periods if we have a system where:

(a) we can represent the state of the system as one of a finite number of possible states,
(b) we can represent our possible actions as a finite set,
(c) given that we find the system in state s and take action x in a period, nature moves the system to state j the next period with probability $p(s, x, j)$,
(d) a cost $h(s)$ is incurred when we find the system in state s,
(e) a cost $c(s, x)$ is incurred when we take action x from state s.

Such a system is called a Markov Decision Process and is in fact quite general. Our goal is to find the best action to take for each state so as to minimize the average cost per period. Manne (1960) showed how to formulate the problem of determining the best action for each state as a linear program.

He defined:

$$w(s, x) = \text{probability that in the steady state the state is } s \text{ and we take action } x.$$

Manne's LP is then:

$$\text{Min } \Sigma(s, x: (h(s) + c(s, x)) \times (w(s, x))$$

subject to:

$$\Sigma(x, s: w(s, x)) = 1$$

For each state s:

$$\Sigma(x: w(s, x)) = \Sigma(r, x: w(r, x) \times (p(r, x, s))$$

Wang and Zaniewski (1996) describe a system based on a Markov decision process model for scheduling maintenance on Arizona highways. It has been in use since 1982. A state in this application corresponds to a particular condition of a section of roadway. Transition probabilities describe the statistical manner in which a road deteriorates. Actions correspond to possible road repairs, such as patch, resurface, or completely replace.

10.12.1 Example: Cash Balance Management

Suppose we are managing a cash account for which each day there is a random input or output of cash. If the cash level gets too high, we want to transfer some of the cash to a longer term investment account that pays a higher interest rate, whereas if the cash account gets too low, we want to transfer funds from a longer term account into the cash account, so that we always have sufficient cash on hand. Because we require discrete scenarios, let us represent the cash on hand status as multiples of $1000. In order to avoid negative subscripts, let us make the following correspondence between cash on hand and state:

Cash on hand:	−2000	−1000	0	1000	2000	3000	4000	5000
State:	1	2	3	4	6	7	8	9
Cost:	14	7	0	2	4	6	8	10

Only three transitions are possible: go down one state, stay put, or go up one state. Their probabilities are:

$$PDN = .4; PUT = .1; PUP = .5.$$

However, for state one, the probability of going down one state is zero. Likewise, for state eight, the probability of going up one state is zero. So, their probabilities are:

For one	$PDN = 0; PUT = .5; PUP = .5;$
For eight	$PDN = .4; PUT = .6; PUP = 0.$

We can make any state change we want, but there is a fixed cost of making any change:

$$FCOST = 3$$

and a variable cost proportional to the amount of change:

$$VCOST = 5.$$

The model is:

```
MIN     10 W88 + 18 W87 + 23 W86 + 28 W85 + 33 W84 + 38 W83
      + 43 W82 + 48 W81 + 16 W78 +  8 W77 + 16 W76 + 21 W75
      + 26 W74 + 31 W73 + 36 W72 + 41 W71 + 19 W68 + 14 W67
      +  6 W66 + 14 W65 + 19 W64 + 24 W63 + 29 W62 + 34 W61
      + 22 W58 + 17 W57 + 12 W56 +  4 W55 + 12 W54 + 17 W53
      + 22 W52 + 27 W51 + 25 W48 + 20 W47 + 15 W46 + 10 W45
      +  2 W44 + 10 W43 + 15 W42 + 20 W41 + 28 W38 + 23 W37
      + 18 W36 + 13 W35 +  8 W34 +  8 W32 + 13 W31 + 40 W28
      + 35 W27 + 30 W26 + 25 W25 + 20 W24 + 15 W23 +  7 W22
      + 15 W21 + 52 W18 + 47 W17 + 42 W16 + 37 W15 + 32 W14
      + 27 W13 + 22 W12 + 14 W11
SUBJECT TO
INTO1)  - 4 W82  - .5 W81 - .4 W72 - .5 W71 - .4 W62 - .5 W61
      - .4 W52 - .5 W51 - .4 W42 - .5 W41 - .4 W32 - .5 W31
      - .4 W22 - .5 W21 + W18 + W17 + W16 + W15 + W14
      + W13 + .6 W12 + .5 W11 =       0
INTO2)  - .4 W83 - .1 W82  - .5 W81 - .4 W73 - .1 W72 - .5 W71
      -  .4 W63 - .1 W62 - .5 W61 - .4 W53 - .1 W52 - .5 W51
      -  .4 W43 - .1 W42 - .5 W41 - .4 W33 - .1 W32 - .5 W31
      + W28 + W27 + W26 + W25 + W24 + .6 W23 + .9 W22
      + .5 W21 - .4 W13 - .1 W12 - .5 W11 =       0
INTO3)  - .4 W84 - .1 W83 - .5 W82 - .4 W74 - .1 W73 - .5 W72
      -  .4 W64 - .1 W63 - .5 W62 - .4 W54 - .1 W53 - .5 W52
      -  .4 W44 - .1 W43 - .5 W42 + W38 + W37 + W36 + W35
      + .6 W34 + .9 W33 + .5 W32 + W31 - .4 W24 - .1 W23
      -  .5 W22 - .4 W14 - .1 W13 - .5 W12 =       0
INTO4)  - .4 W85 - .1 W84 - .5 W83 - .4 W75 - .1 W74 - .5 W73
      -  .4 W65 - .1 W64 - .5 W63 - .4 W55 - .1 W54 - .5 W53
      + W48 + W47 + W46 + .6 W45 + .9 W44 + .5 W43 + W42
      + W41 - .4 W35 - .1 W34 - .5 W33 - .4 W25 - .1 W24
      -  .5 W23 - .4 W15 - .1 W14 - .5 W13 =       0
INTO5)  - .4 W86 - .1 W85 - .5 W84 - .4 W76 - .1 W75 - .5 W74
      -  .4 W66 - .1 W65 - .5 W64 + W58 + W57 + .6 W56
      + .9 W55 + .5 W54 + W53 + W52 + W51 - .4 W46
      -  .1 W45 - .5 W44 - .4 W36 - .1 W35 - .5 W34 - .4 W26
      -  .1 W25 - .5 W24 - .4 W16 - .1 W15 - .5 W14 =       0
INTO6)  - .4 W87 - .1 W86 - .5 W85 - .4 W77 - .1 W76 - .5 W75
      + W68 + .6 W67 + .9 W66 + .5 W65 + W64 + W63 + W62
      + W61 - .4 W57 - .1 W56 - .5 W55 - .4 W47 - .1 W46
      -  .5 W45 - .4 W37 - .1 W36 - .5 W35 - .4 W27 - .1 W26
      -  .5 W25 - .4 W17 - .1 W16 - .5 W15 =       0
INTO7)  - .64 W88 - .1 W87 - .5 W86 + .6 W78 + .9 W77 + .5 W76
      + W75 + W74 + W73 + W72 + W71 - .4 W68 - .1 W67
      -  .5 W66 - .4 W58 - .1 W57 - .5 W56 - .4 W48 - .1 W47
      -  .5 W46 - .4 W38 - .1 W37 - .5 W36 - .4 W28 - .1 W27
      -  .5 W26 - .4 W18 - .1 W17 - .5 W16 =       0
INTO8)   .4 W88 + .5 W87 + W86 + W85 + W84 + W83 + W82
      + W81 - .6 W78 - .5 W77 - .6 W68 - .5 W67 - .6 W58
      -  .5 W57 - .6 W48 - .5 W47 - .6 W38 - .5 W37 - .6 W28
      -  .5 W27 - .6 W18 - .5 W17 =       0
TOTAL)  W88 + W87 + W86 + W85 + W84 + W83 + W82 + W81
      + W78 + W77 + W76 + W75 + W74 + W73 + W72 + W71
```

```
        + W68 + W67 + W66 + W65 + W64 + W63 + W62 + W61
        + W58 + W57 + W56 + W55 + W54 + W53 + W52 + W51
        + W48 + W47 + W46 + W45 + W44 + W43 + W42 + W41
        + W38 + W37 + W36 + W35 + W34 + W33 + W32 + W31
        + W28 + W27 + W26 + W25 + W24 + W23 + W22 + W21
        + W18 + W17 + W16 + W15 + W14 + W13 + W12 + W11 = 1
   END
```

Part of the solution report is reproduced below:

```
    VARIABLE              VALUE
    W13              0.5245902E-01
    W22              0.1311475
    W33              0.2426229
    W44              0.2663934
    W55              0.2049180
    W64              0.1024590
```

Conclusion:

If the state is 1 or less, we should raise it to state 3;

If the state is 6 or more, we should drop it to state 4;

If the state is 2, 3, 4, or 5, we should stay put.

The above model minimizes the average cost per period in the long run. If discounted present value, rather than average cost per period, is of concern, see d'Epenoux (1963) for a linear programming model, similar to the above, that does discounting.

10.13 Chance Constrained Programs

A drawback of the methods just discussed is that problem size can grow very large if the number of possible states of nature is large. Chance constrained programs do not apply to exactly the same problem and, as a result, do not become large as the number of possible states of nature gets large. The stochastic programs discussed thus far had the feature that every constraint had to be satisfied by some combination of first- and second-period decisions. Chance constrained programs, however, allow each constraint to be violated with a certain specified probability. An advantage to this approach for tolerating uncertainty is that the chance constrained model has essentially the same size as the LP for a corresponding problem with no random elements.

We will illustrate the idea with the snow removal problem. Under the chance constrained approach, there are no second-stage decision variables, and we would have to specify a probability allowance for each constraint. For example, we might specify that, with probability at least 0.75, we must be able to provide the snow removal capacity required by the severity of the winter. For our problem, it is very easy to see that this means that we must provide 5,100 truck-days of snow removal capacity. For example, if only 4,400 truck-days of capacity were provided, the probability of sufficient capacity would only be 0.4. Let us assume that one truck-day of operation costs \$116, and one truck-day of salting equals 1.14 truck-days of plowing; then, the appropriate chance constrained LP is the simple model:

```
Minimize    70 BF1 + 20 BS1 + 116 P + 116 S
subject to   - BF1 + P + S = 0
- BS1 + S        = 0
P + S            <= 5,000
P + 1.14 S    >= 5,100.
```

10.14 PROBLEMS

Problem 1

What is the expected value of perfect information in the corn/soybean/sorghum planting problem?

Problem 2

The farmer in the corn/soybean/sorghum problem is reluctant to plant all soybeans because, if the season is wet, he will make \$20 less per acre than he would if he had planted all corn. Can you react to his risk aversion and recommend a planting *mix* that has the feature that the profit per acre is never more than \$15 from the planting mix that in retrospect would have been best for the particular outcome?

Problem 3

Analyze the snow removal problem of this chapter for the situation where the cost of fuel in a cold winter is \$80 per truck-day rather than \$73 and the cost of salt in a cold winter is \$35 rather than \$32. Include in your analysis the derivation of the expected value of perfect information.

Problem 4

A farmer has 1000 acres available for planting to either corn, sorghum or soybeans. The yields of the three crops, in bushels/acre, as a function of the two possible kinds of season are:

	Corn	Sorghum	Beans
Wet	100	43	45
Dry	45	35	33

The probability of a wet season is 0.6. The probability of a dry season is 0.4. Corn sells for \$2/bushel, whereas sorghum and beans each sell for \$4/bushel. The total production cost for any crop is \$100/acre, regardless of type of season. The farmer can also raise livestock. One unit of livestock uses one hundred bushels of corn. The profit contribution of one unit of livestock, exclusive of its corn consumption, is \$215. Corn can be purchased at any time on the market for \$2.20/bushel. The decisions of how much to raise of livestock and of each crop must be made before the type of season is known.

(a) What should the farmer do?
(b) Formulate and solve the problem by the scenario-based stochastic programming approach.

Problem 5

A firm serves essentially two markets, East and West, and is contemplating the location of one or more distribution centers (DC) to serve these markets. A complicating issue is the uncertainty in demand in each market. The firm has enumerated three representative scenarios to characterize the uncertainty. The table below gives (1) the fixed cost per year of having a DC at each of three candidate locations and (2) the profit per year in each market as a function of the scenario and which DC is supplying the market. Each market will be assigned to that one open DC which results in the most profit. This assignment can be done after we realize the scenario that holds. The DC location decision must be made before the scenario is known.

Profit by Scenario/Region and Supplier DC

DC Location	Fixed Cost	Scenario One		Scenario Two		Scenario Three	
		East	West	East	West	East	West
A	51	120	21	21	40	110	11
B	49	110	28	32	92	70	70
C	52	60	39	20	109	20	88

For example, if Scenario Three holds and we locate DCs at A and C, East would get served from A, West from C, and total profits would be $110 + 88 - 51 - 52 = 95$.

(a) If Scenario One holds, what is the best combination of DCs to have open?
(b) If Scenario Two holds, what is the best combination of DCs to have open?
(c) If Scenario Three holds, what is the best combination of DCs to have open?
(d) If all three scenarios are equally likely, what is the best combination of DCs to have open?

Economic Equilibria as LPs

11.1 What is an Equilibrium?

If one is modeling an economy composed of two or more individuals, each acting in his or her own self-interest, there is no obvious overall objective function that should be maximized. In a market, a solution or equilibrium point is a set of prices such that supply equals demand for each commodity. More generally, an equilibrium for a system is a state in which no individual in the system is motivated to change the state. Thus, at equilibrium there are no arbitrage possibilities, e.g., buy a commodity in one market and sell it in another market at a higher price at no risk.

11.2 Representing Supply and Demand Curves in LPs

The methodology about to be described is the equilibration method used in the PIES (Project Independence Evaluation System) model developed by the Department of Energy. This model and its later versions were extensively used from 1974 onward to evaluate the effect of various U.S. energy policies.

Consider the following example. There is a producer A and a consumer X who have the following supply and demand schedules for a single commodity (e.g., energy):

Producer A		Consumer X	
Market Price/Unit	Amount Willing to Sell	Market Price/Unit	Amount Willing to Buy
$1	2	$9	2
2	4	4.5	4
3	6	3	6
4	8	2.25	8

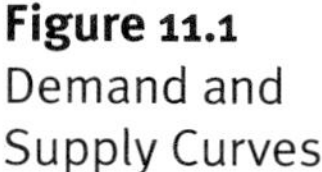

Figure 11.1
Demand and
Supply Curves

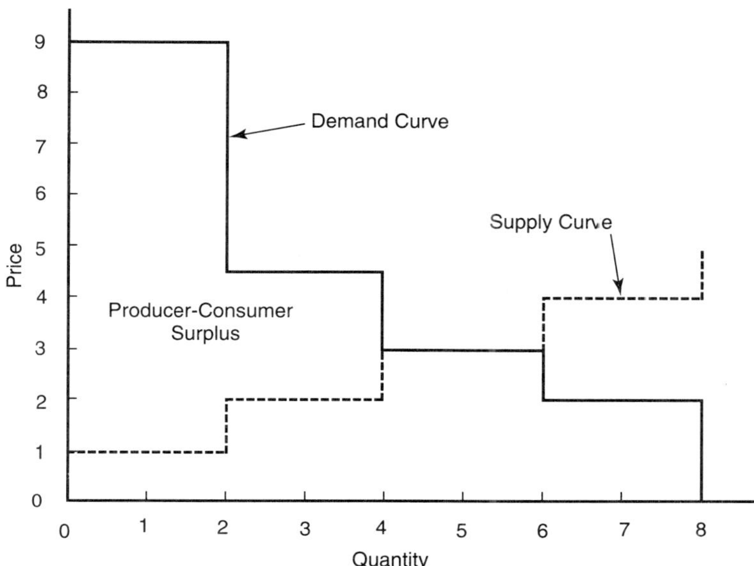

For example, if the price is less than $2 but greater than $1, the producer will produce 2 units; however, the consumer would like to buy at least 8 units at this price. By inspection, note that the equilibrium price is $3 and any quantity from 4 to 6 satisfies equilibrium.

It is easy to find an equilibrium in this market by inspection; nevertheless, it is useful to examine the LP formulation that could be used to find it. Although there is a single market clearing price, it is useful to interpret the supply schedule as if the supplier is willing to sell the first 2 units at $1, the next 2 units at $2 each, etc. Similarly, the consumer is willing to pay $9 each for the first 2 units, $4.5 for the next 2 units, etc. To find the market clearing price such that the amount produced equals the amount consumed, we act as if there is a broker who actually buys and sells at these marginal prices, and all transactions must go through the broker. The broker maximizes his profits. The broker will continue to increase the quantity of goods transferred as long as he can sell them at a price higher than his purchase price. At the broker's optimum, the quantity bought equals the quantity sold, and the price offered by the buyers equals the price demanded by the sellers. This satisfies the conditions for a market equilibrium. Graphically, the situation is shown in Figure 11.1. The area marked "producer-consumer surplus" is the profit obtained by the hypothetical broker. In reality, this profit is allocated between the producer and the consumer according to the equilibrium price. In the case where the equilibrium price is $3, the consumer's profit or surplus is the portion of the producer-consumer surplus area above the $3 horizontal line, whereas the producer's profit or surplus is the portion of the producer-consumer surplus area below $3.

Readers with a mathematical bent may note that the general approach we are using is based on the fact that, for many problems of finding an equilibrium, one can formulate an objective function, which, when optimized, produces a solution satisfying the equilibrium conditions. For purposes of the LP formulation, define:

$A1$ = units sold by producer for \$1 per unit
$A2$ = units sold by producer for \$2 per unit
$A3$ = units sold by producer for \$3 per unit
$A4$ = units sold by producer for \$4 per unit
$X1$ = units bought by consumer for \$9 per unit
$X2$ = units bought by consumer for \$4.5 per unit
$X3$ = units bought by consumer for \$3 per unit
$X4$ = units bought by consumer for \$2.25 per unit

The formulation is:

```
MAX 9X1 + 4.5X2 + 3X3 + 2.25X4          ! Maximize broker's revenue
  -  A1 - 2A    - 3A3 - 4A4             ! minus cost
SUBJECT TO
  A1 + A2 + A3 + A4 - X1 - X2 - X3 - X4 = 0 ! Supply = demand
  A1 <= 2    A2 <= 2    A3 <= 2    A4 <= 2  ! Steps in supply
  X1 <= 2    X2 <= 2    X3 <= 2    X4 <= 2  ! and demand functions
END
```

The solution is:

```
A1 = A2 = X1 = X2 = 2
A3 = A4 = X3 = X4 = 0
```

The dual price on the first constraint is \$3. In general, the dual price on the constraint that sets supply equal to demand is the market clearing price.

Let us complicate the problem by introducing another supplier, B, and another consumer, Y. Their supply and demand curves are, respectively:

Producer B		Consumer Y	
Market Price/Unit	Amount Willing to Sell	Market Price/Unit	Amount Willing to Buy
\$2	2	\$15	2
4	4	8	4
6	6	5	6
8	8	3	8

An additional complication is that shipping costs \$1.5 per unit shipped from A to Y, and \$2 per unit shipped from B to X. What will be the clearing price at the shipping door of A, B, X, and Y? How much will each participant sell or buy?

The corresponding LP can be developed if we define $B1$, $B2$, $B3$, $B4$, $Y1$, $Y2$, $Y3$, and $Y4$ analogous to $A1$, $X1$, etc. Also, we define AX, AY, BX, and BY as the number of units shipped from A to X, A to Y, B to X, and B to Y, respectively. The formulation is:

```
MAX        9X1 + 4.5X2 + 3X3 + 2.25X4 + 15Y1 + 8Y2 + 5Y3 + 3Y4
         - 2BX - 1.5AY - A1 - 2A2 - 3A3 - 4A4 - 2B1 - 4B2 - 6B3
         - 8B4      ! Maximize revenue - cost for broker;
SUBJECT TO
  2)     - AY + A1 + A2 + A3 + A4 - AX = 0   ! amount shipped from A
  3)     - BX + B1 + B2 + B3 + B4 - BY = 0   ! amount shipped from B
  4)     - X1 - X2 - X3 - X4 + BX + AX = 0   ! amount shipped to X
  5)     - Y1 - Y2 - Y3 - Y4 + AY + BY = 0   ! amount shipped to Y
  6)       A1 <= 2
  7)       A2 <= 2
  8)       A3 <= 2
  9)       A4 <= 2
 10)       B1 <= 2
 11)       B2 <= 2
 12)       B3 <= 2
 13)       B4 <= 2
 14)       X1 <= 2
 15)       X2 <= 2
 16)       X3 <= 2
 17)       X4 <= 2
 18)       Y1 <= 2
 19)       Y2 <= 2
 20)       Y3 <= 2
 21)       Y4 <= 2
END
```

Notice from the objective function that the broker is charged $2/unit shipped from *B* to *X*, and $1.5/unit shipped from *A* to *Y*. Most of the constraints are simple upper bound (SUB) constraints. In realistic-size problems, several thousand SUB-type constraints can be tolerated without adversely affecting computational difficulty.

The solution is:

```
OBJECTIVE FUNCTION VALUE
     1)              56.0000000
    VARIABLE            VALUE          REDUCED COST
      X1              2.000000           0.000000
      X2              2.000000           0.000000
      X3              0.000000           0.500000
      X4              0.000000           1.250000
      Y1              2.000000           0.000000
      Y2              2.000000           0.000000
      Y3              2.000000           0.000000
      Y4              0.000000           2.000000
      BX              0.000000           3.500000
      AY              2.000000           0.000000
      A1              2.000000           0.000000
      A2              2.000000           0.000000
      A3              2.000000           0.000000
      A4              0.000000           0.500000
      B1              2.000000           0.000000
      B2              2.000000           0.000000
      B3              0.000000           1.000000
      B4              0.000000           3.000000
      AX              4.000000           0.000000
      BY              4.000000           0.000000
```

```
         ROW                    SLACK              DUAL PRICES
          2)                  0.000000              -3.500000
          3)                  0.000000              -5.000000
          4)                  0.000000              -3.500000
          5)                  0.000000              -5.000000
          6)                  0.000000               2.500000
          7)                  0.000000               1.500000
          8)                  0.000000               0.500000
          9)                  2.000000               3.000000
         10)                  0.000000               1.000000
         11)                  0.000000               0.000000
         12)                  2.000000               0.000000
         13)                  2.000000               0.000000
         14)                  0.000000               5.500000
         15)                  0.000000               1.000000
         16)                  2.000000               0.000000
         17)                  2.000000               0.000000
         18)                  0.000000              10.000000
         19)                  0.000000               3.000000
         20)                  0.000000               0.000000
         21)                  2.000000               0.000000
```

From the dual prices on rows 2 through 5, we note that the prices at the shipping door of A, B, X, and Y are \$3.5, \$5, \$3.5, and \$5, respectively. At these prices, A and B are willing to produce 6 and 4 units, respectively, whereas X and Y are willing to buy 4 and 6 units, respectively. A ships 2 units to Y, where the \$1.5 shipping charge causes them to sell for \$5. A ships 4 units to X, where they sell for \$3.5. B ships 4 units to Y, where they sell for \$5.

11.3 Auctions as Economic Equilibria

The concept of a broker who maximizes producer-consumer surplus can also be applied to auctions. LP is useful if the auction is complicated by features that might be interpreted as bidders with demand curves. The example presented here is based on a design by R. L. Graves for a course registration system used since 1981 at the University of Chicago, in which students bid on courses.

Suppose there are N types of objects to be sold (e.g., courses), and there are M bidders (students). Bidder i is willing to pay up to b_{ij}, $b_{ij} \geq 0$ for one unit of object type j. Further, a bidder is interested in at most one unit of each object type. Let S_j be the number of units of object type j available for sale.

There are a variety of ways of holding the auction. Let us suppose that it is a sealed-bid auction and we want to find a single, market-clearing price, p_j, for each object type j, such that:

(a) at most, S_j units of object j are sold;
(b) any bid for j less than p_j does not buy a unit;
(c) $p_j = 0$ if less than S_j units of j are sold;
(d) any bid for j greater than p_j does buy a unit.

It is easy to determine the equilibrium p_js by simply sorting the bids and allocating each unit to the higher bidder first. Nevertheless, in order to prepare for more complicated auctions, let us consider how to solve this problem as an optimization problem. Again, we take the view of a broker who sells at as high (buys at as low) a price as possible and maximizes profits.

Define:

$x_{ij} = 1$ if bidder i buys a unit of object j, else 0.

The LP is:

$$\text{Maximize} \quad \sum_{i=1}^{M} \sum_{j=1}^{N} x_{ij}\, b_{ij}$$

$$\text{subject to} \quad \sum_{i=1}^{M} b_{ij} \le S_j \quad \text{for } j = 1 \text{ to } N$$

$$x_{ij} \le 1 \quad \text{for all } i \text{ and } j.$$

The dual prices on the first N constraints can be used, with minor modification, as the clearing prices p_j. The possible modifications have to do with the fact that, with step function demand and/or supply curves, there is usually a small range of acceptable clearing prices. The LP solution will choose one price in this range, usually at one end of the range. One may wish to choose a price within the interior of the range to break ties.

Now we complicate this auction slightly by adding the condition that no bidder wants to buy more than 3 units total. Consider the following specific situation:

Maximum Price Willing to Pay

		Objects				
		1	2	3	4	5
Bidders	1	9	2	8	5	3
	2	6	7	9	1	5
	3	7	8	6	3	4
	4	5	4	3	2	1
Capacity		1	2	3	3	4

For example, bidder 3 is willing to pay up to 4 for one unit of object 5. There are only 3 units of object 4 available for sale.

We want to find a "market clearing" price for each object and an allocation of units to bidders so that each bidder is willing to accept the units awarded to him at the market clearing price. We must generalize the previous condition d to d': a bidder is satisfied with a particular unit if he cannot find another unit with a bigger difference between his maximum offer price and the market clearing price. This is equivalent to saying that each bidder maximizes his consumer surplus.

The associated LP is:

```
MAX 9 X11 + 2 X12 + 8 X13 + 6 X14 + 3 X15 + 6 X21 + 7 X22 + 9 X23
    +   X24 + 5 X25 + 7 X31 + 8 X32 + 6 X33 + 3 X34 + 4 X35 + 5 X41
    + 4 X42 + 3 X43 + 2 X44 +   X45        !(Maximize broker revenues)
SUBJECT TO
   2)   X11 + X21 + X31 + X41 <=  1        !(Units of object 1 available)
   3)   X12 + X22 + X32 + X42 <=  2
```

```
 4)   X13 + X23 + X33 + X43 <=   3                    .
 5)   X14 + X24 + X34 + X44 <=   3                    .
 6)   X15 + X25 + X35 + X45 <=   4       !(Units of object 5 available)
 7)   X11 + X12 + X13 + X14 + X15 <= 3 !(Upper limit on buyer 1 demand)
 8)   X21 + X22 + X23 + X24 + X25 <= 3                  .
 9)   X31 + X32 + X33 + X34 + X35 <= 3                  .
10)   X41 + X42 + X43 + X44 + X45 <= 3 !(Upper limit on buyer 2 demand)
11)     X11 <=    1
12)     X21 <=    1
13)     X31 <=    1
14)     X41 <=    1
15)     X12 <=    1
16)     X22 <=    1
17)     X32 <=    1
18)     X42 <=    1
19)     X13 <=    1
20)     X23 <=    1
21)     X33 <=    1
22)     X43 <=    1
23)     X14 <=    1
24)     X24 <=    1
25)     X34 <=    1
27)     X15 <=    1
28)     X25 <=    1
29)     X35 <=    1
30)     X45 <=    1
END
```

The solution is:

```
OBJECTIVE FUNCTION VALUE
 1)            65.0000000
VARIABLE           VALUE          REDUCED COST
X11             1.000000           0.000000
X12             0.000000           7.000000
X13             1.000000           0.000000
X14             1.000000           0.000000
X15             0.000000           1.000000
X21             0.000000           1.000000
Y22             1.000000           0.000000
X23             1.000000           0.000000
X24             0.000000           1.000000
X25             1.000000           0.000000
X31             0.000000           1.000000
X32             1.000000           0.000000
X33             1.000000           0.000000
X34             0.000000           0.000000
X35             1.000000           0.000000
X41             0.000000           0.000000
X42             0.000000           1.000000
X43             0.000000           0.000000
X44             1.000000           0.000000
X45             1.000000           0.000000
ROW               SLACK          DUAL PRICES
 2)             0.000000           5.000000
 3)             0.000000           5.000000
```

4)	0.000000	3.000000
5)	1.000000	0.000000
6)	1.000000	0.000000
7)	0.000000	4.000000
8)	0.000000	2.000000
9)	0.000000	3.000000
10)	1.000000	0.000000
11)	0.000000	0.000000
12)	1.000000	0.000000
13)	1.000000	0.000000
14)	1.000000	0.000000
15)	1.000000	0.000000
16)	0.000000	0.000000
17)	0.000000	0.000000
18)	1.000000	0.000000
19)	0.000000	1.000000
20)	0.000000	4.000000
21)	0.000000	0.000000
22)	1.000000	0.000000
23)	0.000000	2.000000
24)	1.000000	0.000000
25)	1.000000	0.000000
26)	0.000000	2.000000
27)	1.000000	0.000000
28)	0.000000	3.000000
29)	0.000000	1.000000
30)	0.000000	1.000000

The dual prices on the first five constraints essentially provide us with the needed market clearing prices. To avoid ties, we may wish to add or subtract a small number to each of these prices. We claim that acceptable market clearing prices for objects 1, 2, 3, 4, and 5 are 5, 5, 3, 0, and 0, respectively.

Now note that at these prices the market clears. Bidder 1 is awarded the sole unit of object 1 at a price of \$5.00. If the price were lower, bidder 4 could claim the unit. If the price were more than 6, bidder 1's surplus on object 1 would be less than $9 - 6 = 3$, and, therefore, he would prefer object 5 instead, where his surplus is $3 - 0 = 3$. If object 2's price were less than 4, bidder 4 could claim the unit. If the price were greater than 5, bidder 3 would prefer to give up his type-2 unit (with surplus $8 - 5 = 3$) and take a type-4 unit, which has a surplus of $3 - 0 = 3$. Similar arguments apply to objects 3, 4, and 5.

11.4 Transportation Equilibria

When designing a highway or street system, traffic engineers usually use models of some sophistication to predict the volume of traffic and the expected travel time on each link in the system. For each link, the engineers specify estimated average travel time as a (nondecreasing) function of traffic volume on the link.

The determination of the volume on each link is usually based upon a rule called Wardrup's Principle: If a set of commuters wish to travel from A to B, then the

Figure 11.2
A Transportation
Network

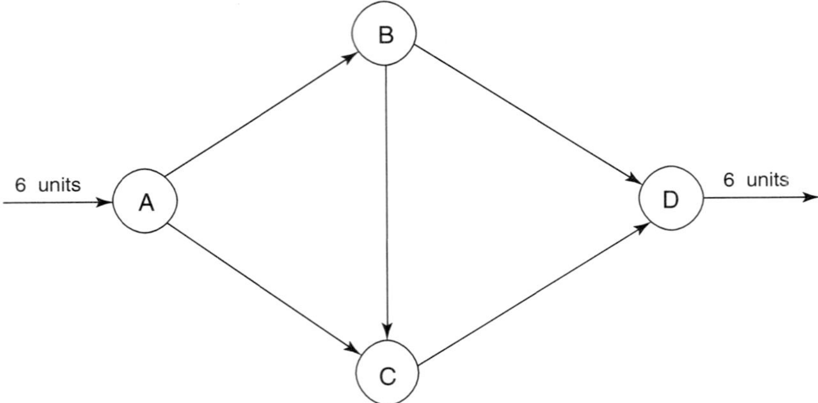

commuters will take the shortest route in the travel time sense. The effect of this is that, if there are alternative routes from A to B, commuters will distribute themselves over these two routes so that either travel times are equal over the two alternates or none of the A to B commuters use the longer alternate.

As an example, consider the network in Figure 11.2. Six units of traffic (e.g., in thousands of cars) want to get from A to B.

The travel time on any link as a function of the traffic volume is given in the table below:

For All Volumes Less Than or Equal To:	Link Travel Time in Minutes				
	AB	AC	BC	BD	CD
2	20	52	12	52	20
3	30	53	13	53	30
4	40	54	14	54	40

The dramatically different functions for the various links might be due to such features as number of lanes, or whether a link has traffic lights rather than stop signs.

We are interested in how traffic will distribute itself over the three possible routes *ABD, ACD,* and *ABCD* if each unit behaves individually optimally. That is, we want to find the flows for which a user is indifferent between the three routes.

This can be formulated as an LP analogous to the previous equilibrium problems if the travel time schedules are interpreted as supply curves.

Define variables as follows. Two letter variable names, e.g., AB or CD, denote the total flow along a given arc, e.g., the arc AB or the arc CD. Variables with a numeric suffix denote the incremental flow along a link; e.g., AB2 measures flow up to 2 units on link $A \rightarrow B$, and AB3 measures the incremental flow above 2 but less than 3.

The formulation is then:

```
MIN 20 AB2 + 30 AB3 + 40 AB4 + 52 AC2 + 53 AC3 + 54 AC4 + 12 BC2
   + 13 BC3 + 14 BC4 + 52 BD2 + 53 BD3 + 54 BD4 + 20 CD2 + 30 CD3
   + 40 CD4 !Minimize congestion costs of each incremental unit;
SUBJECT TO
   2)    - AB2 -   AB3 -   AB4 +   AB =   0   !Definition of AB
   3)    - AC2 -   AC3 -   AC4 +   AC =   0
   4)    - BC2 -   BC3 -   BC4 +   BC =   0   !     etc.
   5)    - BD2 -   BD3 -   BD4 +   BD =   0
   6)    - CD2 -   CD3 -   CD4 +   CD =   0
   7)      AB +   AC  =   6                   !Flow out of A
   8)      AB -   BC -   BD  =   0            !Flow through B
   9)      AC +   BC -   CD  =   0            !Flow through C
  10)      BD +   CD =   6                    !Flow into D
  11)      AB2 <=   2                         !Definition of the steps in
  12)      AB3 <=   1                         !supply cost schedule
  13)      AB4 <=   1
  14)      AC2 <=   2
  15)      AC3 <=   1
  16)      AC4 <=   1
  17)      BC2 <=   2
  18)      BC3 <=   1
  19)      BC4 <=   1
  20)      BD2 <=   2
  21)      BD3 <=   1
  22)      BD4 <=   1
  23)      CD2 <=   2
  24)      CD3 <=   1
  25)      CD4 <=   1
END
```

The objective requires a little bit of explanation. It minimizes the incremental
congestion seen by each incremental individual unit as it "selects" its route. It does
not take into account the additional congestion that the incremental unit imposes on
units already taking the route. Because additional traffic typically hurts rather than
helps, this suggests that this objective will understate true total congestion costs. Let
us see if this is the case.

The solution is:

```
                              OBJECTIVE FUNCTION VALUE

        1)            452.0000000
VARIABLE              VALUE            REDUCED COST
  AB2                2.000000            0.000000
  AB3                1.000000            0.000000
  AB4                1.000000            0.000000
  AC2                2.000000            0.000000
  AC3                0.000000            1.000000
  AC4                0.000000            2.000000
  BC2                2.000000            0.000000
  BC3                0.000000            1.000000
  BC4                0.000000            2.000000
  BD2                2.000000            0.000000
  BD3                0.000000            1.000000
```

```
           BD4                   0.000000                   2.000000
           CD2                   2.000000                   0.000000
           CD3                   1.000000                   0.000000
           CD4                   1.000000                   0.000000
           AB                    4.000000                   0.000000
           AC                    2.000000                   0.000000
           BC                    2.000000                   0.000000
           BD                    2.000000                   0.000000
           CD                    4.000000                   0.000000

           ROW                    SLACK                 DUAL PRICES
            2)                   0.000000                  40.000000
            3)                   0.000000                  52.000000
            4)                   0.000000                  12.000000
            5)                   0.000000                  52.000000
            6)                   0.000000                  40.000000
            7)                   0.000000                 -92.000000
            8)                   0.000000                  52.000000
            9)                   0.000000                  40.000000
           10)                   0.000000                   0.000000
           11)                   0.000000                  20.000000
           12)                   0.000000                  10.000000
           13)                   0.000000                   0.000000
           14)                   0.000000                   0.000000
           15)                   1.000000                   0.000000
           16)                   1.000000                   0.000000
           17)                   0.000000                   0.000000
           18)                   1.000000                   0.000000
           19)                   1.000000                   0.000000
           20)                   0.000000                   0.000000
           21)                   1.000000                   0.000000
           22)                   1.000000                   0.000000
           23)                   0.000000                  20.000000
           24)                   0.000000                  10.000000
           25)                   0.000000                   0.000000
```

Notice that 2 units of traffic take each of the three possible routes: *ABD*, *ABCD*, and *ACD*. The travel time on each route is 92 minutes. This agrees with our understanding of an equilibrium; i.e., no user is motivated to take a different route.

The total congestion is 6 * 92 = 552, greater than the 452 value of the objective of the LP. This is as we suspected because the objective measures the congestion incurred by the incremental unit. The objective function value has no immediate practical interpretation for this formulation. In this case, the objective function is simply a device to cause Wardrup's Principle to hold when the objective is optimized.

The solution approach based on formulating the traffic equilibrium problem as a standard LP was presented mainly for pedagogical reasons. For larger, real-world problems, there are highly specialized procedures; cf. Florian (1977).

We shall see that for this problem the solution just displayed does not minimize total travel time. In order to minimize total travel time, it is useful to prepare a table of total travel time incurred by users of a link as a function of link volume. This is done in Table 11.1, where "Total" is the product of link volume times travel time at that volume.

Table 11.1   Total and Incremental Travel Time Incurred on a Link

Traffic Volume	AB		AC		BC		BD		CD	
	Total	**Rate/ Unit**	**Total**	**Rate/ Unit**	**Total**	**Rate/ Unit**	**Total**	**Rate/ Unit**	**Total**	**Rate/ Unit**
2	40	20	104	52	24	12	104	52	40	20
3	90	50	159	55	39	15	159	55	90	50
4	160	70	216	57	56	17	216	57	160	70

The appropriate formulation is:

```
MIN 20 AB2 + 50 AB3 + 70 AB4 + 52 AC2 + 55 AC3 + 57 AC4 + 12 BC2
   + 15 BC3 + 17 BC4 + 52 BD2 + 55 BD3 + 57 BD4 + 20 CD2 + 50 CD3
   + 70 CD4    ! Minimize total congestion
SUBJECT TO
    2)   -  AB2 - AB3 - AB4 +    AB =    0    !Definition of AB
    3)   -  AC2 - AC3 - AC4 +    AC =    0    ! and AC,
    4)   -  BC2 - BC3 - BC4 +    BC =    0    ! BC
    5)   -  BD2 - BD3 - BD4 +    BD =    0    ! BD
    6)   -  CD2 - CD3 - CD4 +    CD =    0    ! and CD
    7)      AB  +  AC  =    6                 ! Flow out of A
    8)      AB  -  BC  -  BD  =    0          ! Flow through B
    9)      AC  +  BC  -  CD  =    0          ! Flow through C
   10)      BD  +  CD  =    6                 ! Flow into D
   11)      AB2 <=    2                       ! Steps in supply schedule
   12)      AB3 <=    1
   13)      AB4 <=    1
   14)      AC2 <=    2
   15)      AC3 <=    1
   16)      AC4 <=    1
   17)      BC2 <=    2
   18)      BC3 <=    1
   19)      BC4 <=    1
   20)      BD2 <=    2
   21)      BD3 <=    1
   22)      BD4 <=    1
   23)      CD2 <=    2
   24)      CD3 <=    1
   25)      CD4 <=    1
END
```

The solution is:

```
              OBJECTIVE FUNCTION VALUE

   1)          498.000000
   VARIABLE         VALUE           REDUCED COST
      AB2          2.000000           0.000000
      AB3          1.000000           0.000000
      AB4          0.000000          20.000000
```

AC2	2.000000	0.000000
AC3	1.000000	0.000000
AC4	0.000000	2.000000
BC2	0.000000	0.000000
BC3	0.000000	3.000000
BC4	0.000000	5.000000
BD2	2.000000	0.000000
BD3	1.000000	0.000000
BD4	0.000000	2.000000
CD2	2.000000	0.000000
CD3	1.000000	0.000000
CD4	0.000000	20.000000
AB	3.000000	0.000000
AC	3.000000	0.000000
BC	0.000000	7.000000
BD	3.000000	0.000000
CD	3.000000	0.000000

ROW	SLACK	DUAL PRICES
2)	0.000000	50.000000
3)	0.000000	55.000000
4)	0.000000	12.000000
5)	0.000000	55.000000
6)	0.000000	50.000000
7)	0.000000	-105.000000
8)	0.000000	55.000000
9)	0.000000	50.000000
10)	0.000000	0.000000
11)	0.000000	30.000000
12)	0.000000	0.000000
13)	1.000000	0.000000
14)	0.000000	3.000000
15)	0.000000	0.000000
16)	1.000000	0.000000
17)	2.000000	0.000000
18)	1.000000	0.000000
19)	1.000000	0.000000
20)	0.000000	3.000000
21)	0.000000	0.000000
22)	1.000000	0.000000
23)	0.000000	30.000000
24)	0.000000	0.000000
25)	1.000000	0.000000

An interesting feature is that no traffic uses link *BC*. Three units each take routes *ABD* and *ACD*. Even more interesting is the fact that the travel time on both routes is 83 minutes. This is noticeably less than the 92 minutes for the previous solution. With this formulation, the objective function measures the total travel time incurred. Note $498/6 = 83$.

If link *BC* were removed, this latest solution would also be a user equilibrium, because no user would be motivated to switch routes. The interesting paradox is that by adding additional capacity, in this case link *BC*, to a transportation network, the total delay may actually increase. This is known as Braess's Paradox; cf. Braess

(1968) or Murchland (1970). Braess claims to have observed this paradox in a German city when a new link was added to its road network. When traffic got worse rather than better with the new link, the new link was removed.

To see why the paradox occurs, consider what happens when link BC is added. One of the 3 units taking route ABD notices that travel time on link BC is 12 and time on link CD is 30. This total of 42 minutes is better than the 53 minutes the unit is suffering in link BD, so the unit replaces link BD in its route by the sequence BCD. At this point one of the units taking link AC observes that it can reduce its delay in getting to C by replacing link AC (delay 53 minutes) with the two links AB and BC (delay of $30 + 12 = 42$). Unfortunately (and this is the cause of Braess's Paradox), neither of these units that switched took into account the effect of their actions on the rest of the population. The switches increased the load on links AB and CD, two links for which increased volume dramatically increases the travel time of everyone. The general result is that *when individuals each maximize their own objective function, the obvious overall objective function is not necessarily maximized.*

11.5 PROBLEMS

Problem 1

Producer B in the 2-producer–2-consumer market at the beginning of the chapter is actually a foreign producer. The government of the importing country is contemplating putting a \$0.60 per unit tax on units from Producer B.

(a) How is the formulation changed?
(b) How is the equilibrium solution changed?

Problem 2

An organization is interested in selling 5 parcels of land, denoted A, B, C, D, and E, which it owns. It is willing to accept offers for subsets of the 5 parcels. Three buyers, x, y, and z, are interested in making offers. In the privacy of their respective offices, each buyer has identified the maximum price he would be willing to pay for various combinations. This information is summarized as follows:

Buyer	Parcel Combination	Maximum Price
x	A, B, D	95
x	C, D, E	80
y	B, E	60
y	A, D	82
z	B, D, E	90
z	C, E	71

Figure 11.3
A Travel
Network

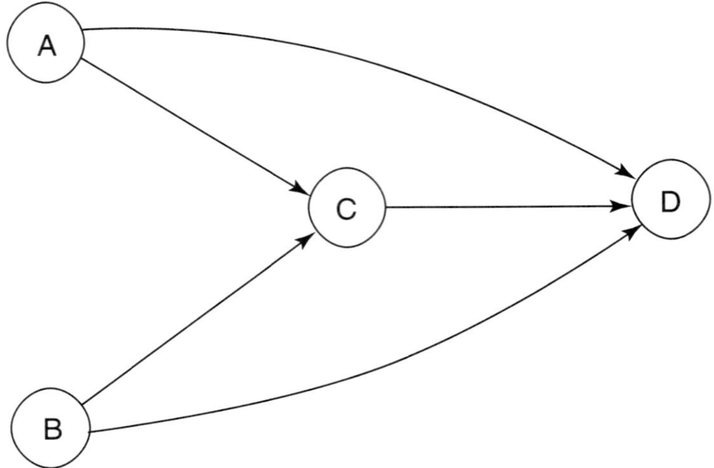

Each buyer wants to buy at most one parcel combination. Suppose the organization is a government and would like to maximize social welfare. What is a possible formulation based on an LP for holding this auction?

Problem 3

Commuters wish to travel from points A, B, and C to point D in the network shown in Figure 11.3. Three units wish to travel from A to D, two units from B to D, and one from C to D. The travel time on the five links as a function of volume are:

For All Volumes	Link Travel Time in Minutes				
Less Than or Equal To:	AD	AC	BC	BD	CD
2	21	50	17	40	12
3	31	51	27	41	13
4	41	52	37	42	14

(a) Display the LP formulation corresponding to a Wardrup's Principle user equilibrium.
(b) Display the LP formulation useful for the total travel time minimizing solution.
(c) What are the solutions to (a) and (b)?

Problem 4

In the sale of real estate and in the sale of rights to portions of the radio frequency spectrum, the value of one item to a buyer may depend upon which other items the buyer is able to buy. A method called a combinatorial auction is sometimes used in such cases. In such an auction, a bidder is allowed to submit a bid on a combination of items. The seller is then faced with the decision of which combination of these "combination" bids to select. Consider the following situation. The Duxbury Ranch is being sold for potential urban development. The ranch has been divided into four parcels, A, B, C, and D, for sale. Parcels A and B both face major roads. Parcel C is a corner parcel at the intersection of the two roads. D is an interior parcel with a narrow access to one of the roads. The following bids have been received for various combinations of parcels:

Bid No.	Amount	Parcels Desired
1	$380,000	A, C
2	$350,000	A, D
3	$800,000	A, B, C, D
4	$140,000	B
5	$120,000	B, C
6	$105,000	B, D
7	$210,000	C
8	$390,000	A, B
9	$205,000	D
10	$160,000	A

Which combination of bids should be selected, so as to maximize revenues, subject to not selling any parcel more than once?

Game Theory

12.1 Introduction

In most decision-making situations, our profits (and losses) are determined not only by our decisions but by the decisions taken by outside forces, e.g., our competitors, the weather, etc. A useful classification is whether the outside force is indifferent or mischievous. We will, for example, classify the weather as indifferent because its decision is indifferent to our actions, despite how we might feel during a rainstorm after washing the car and forgetting the umbrella. A competitor, however, generally takes into account the likelihood of our taking various decisions and, as a result, tends to make decisions that are mischievous relative to our welfare. In this chapter, we analyze situations involving a mischievous outside force. The standard terminology applied to the problem to be considered is game theory. Situations in which these problems might arise are in the choice of a marketing or price strategy, in international affairs, in military combat, and in many negotiation situations. For example, the probability that a competitor executes an oil embargo against us probably depends upon whether we have elected a strategy of building up a strategic petroleum reserve.

12.2 Two-Person Games

In so-called two-person game theory, the key feature is that *each of the two players must make a crucial decision ignorant of the other player's decision.* Only after both players have committed to their respective decisions does each player learn of the other player's decision, and each player receives a payoff that depends solely on the two decisions. Two-person game theory is further classified according to whether the payoffs are constant sum vs. variable sum. In a constant sum game, the total payoff summed over both players is constant. Usually this constant is assumed to be zero so that one player's gain is exactly the other player's loss. The following example illustrates a constant sum game.

A game is to be played between two players called Blue and Gold. It is a single simultaneous move game. Each player must make her single move in ignorance of the other player's move. Both moves are then revealed, and then one player pays the other an amount specified by the payoff table that follows:

Payoff from Blue to Gold

		Blue's Move	
		a	b
Gold's Move	a	4	−6
	b	−5	8
	c	3	−4

Blue must choose one of two moves (a) or (b), whereas Gold has a choice among three moves, (a), (b), or (c). For example, if Gold chooses move (b) and Blue chooses move (a), Gold pays Blue 5 million dollars If Gold chooses (c) and Blue chooses (a), Blue pays Gold 3 million dollars.

12.2.1 The Minimax Strategy

This game does not have an obvious strategy for either player. If Gold is tempted to make move (b) in the hopes of winning the 8 million dollar prize, Blue will be equally tempted to make move (a) so as to win 5 million from Gold. For this example, it is clear that each player will want to consider a random strategy. Any player who follows a pure strategy of always making the same move is easily beaten. Therefore, define:

BM_i = probability Blue makes move i, $i = a$ or b,
GM_i = probability Gold makes move i, $i = a$, b, or c.

How should Blue choose the probabilities BM_i? Blue might observe that:

If Gold chooses move (a), my expected loss is:
```
    4 BMA  -  6 BMB
```
If Gold chooses move (b), my expected loss is:
```
   -5 BMA  +  8 BMB
```
If Gold chooses move (c), my expected loss is:
```
    3 BMA  -  4 BMB
```

So, there are three possible expected losses depending upon which decision is made by Gold. If Blue is conservative, a reasonable criterion is to choose the BM_i so as to minimize the maximum expected loss. This philosophy is called the *minimax* strategy. Stated another way, Blue wants to choose the probabilities BM_i such that no matter what Gold does, Blue's maximum expected loss is minimized. If LB is the maximum expected loss to Blue, then her problem can be stated as the LP:

```
MIN      LB
SUBJECT TO
   2)   BMA + BMB = 1              ! Probabilities must sum to 1
```

```
  3)  -LB + 4 BMA -  6 BMB < 0    ! Expected loss if Gold chooses (a)
  4)  -LB - 5 BMA +  8 BMB < 0    ! Expected loss if Gold chooses (b)
  5)  -LB + 3 BMA -  4 BMB < 0    ! Expected loss if Gold chooses (c)
      END
```

The solution is:

```
            OBJECTIVE FUNCTION VALUE

    1)        0.2000000

    VARIABLE        VALUE          REDUCED COST
      LB          0.2000000         0.000000
      BMA         0.6000000         0.000000
      BMB         0.4000000         0.000000

    ROW           SLACK           DUAL PRICES
     2)         0.000000          -0.20000
     3)         0.200000           0.00000
     4)         0.000000           0.35000
     5)         0.000000           0.65000
```

The interpretation is that if Blue chooses move (a) with probability 0.6 and move (b) with probability 0.4, Blue's expected loss is never greater than 0.2, regardless of Gold's move.

If Gold follows a similar argument but phrases the argument in terms of maximizing the minimum expected profit, PG, instead of minimizing maximum loss, Gold's problem is:

```
MAX   PG
SUBJECT TO
  2)           GMA   + GMB   + GMC = 1 ! Probabilities sum to 1
  3)  -PG + 4 GMA - 5 GMB + 3 GMC > 0 ! Expected profit if Blue chooses (a)
  4)  -PG - 6 GMA + 8 GMB - 4 GMC > 0 ! Expected profit if Blue chooses (b)
      END
```

The solution to Gold's problem is:

```
            OBJECTIVE FUNCTION VALUE

    1)              0.20000000

    VARIABLE        VALUE          REDUCED COST
      PG          0.2000000         0.000000
      GMA         0.0000000         0.000000
      GMB         0.3500000         0.000000
      GMC         0.6500000         0.000000

    ROW           SLACK           DUAL PRICES
     2)         0.000000           0.200000
     3)         0.000000          -0.600000
     4)         0.000000          -0.400000
```

The interpretation is that if Gold chooses move (b) with probability 0.35, move (c) with probability 0.65, and never move (a), Gold's expected profit is never less than 0.2. Notice that Gold's lowest expected profit equals Blue's highest expected loss. From Blue's point of view, the expected transfer to Gold is at least 0.2. The only possible expected transfer is then 0.2. This means that, if both players follow the random strategies just derived, every play of the game there is an expected transfer of 0.2 units from Blue to Gold. The game is biased in Gold's favor at the rate of 0.2 million dollars per play.

If you look closely at the solutions to Blue's LP and to Gold's LP, you will note a surprising similarity. The dual prices of Blue's LP equal the probabilities in Gold's LP, and the negatives of Gold's dual prices equal the probabilities of Blue's LP. Looking more closely, you can note that each LP is really the dual of the other one. This is always true for a two-person game of the type just considered, and mathematicians have long been excited by this fact.

12.3 Nonconstant-Sum Games Involving Two or More Players

The most unrealistic assumption underlying classical two-person constant-sum game theory is that the sum of the payoffs to all players must sum to zero (actually a constant, without loss of generality). In reality, the total benefits are almost never constant; usually, total benefits increase if the players cooperate. In these nonconstant-sum games, the difficulty then becomes one of deciding how these additional benefits due to cooperation should be distributed among the players.

There are two styles for analyzing nonconstant-sum games. If we restrict ourselves to two persons, so-called *bi-matrix game theory* extends the methods for two-person constant-sum games to nonconstant-sum games. If there are three or more players, *n-person game theory* can be used in selecting a decision strategy. Bi-matrix games are considered further in Chapter 15. The following example illustrates the essential concepts of n-person game theory.

Three property owners, *A*, *B*, and *C*, own adjacent lakefront property on a large lake. A piece of property on a large lake has higher value if it is protected from wave action by a seawall. *A*, *B*, and *C* are each considering building a seawall on their properties. A seawall is cheaper to build on a given piece of property if either or both of the neighbors have seawalls. For our example, *A* and *C* already have expensive buildings on their properties. *B* does not have buildings and separates *A* from *C*; i.e., *B* is between *A* and *C*. The net benefits of a seawall for the three owners are summarized below.

Owners Who Cooperate, i.e., Build While Others Do Not	Net Benefit to Cooperating Owners
A alone	1.2
B alone	0
C alone	1
A and *B*	4
A and *C*	3
B and *C*	4
A, *B*, and *C*	7

Obviously, all three owners should cooperate and build a unified seawall, because then their total benefits will be maximized. It appears that B should be compensated in some manner, because he has no motivation to build a seawall by himself. Linear programming can provide some help in selecting an acceptable allocation of benefits.

Denote by v_A, v_B, and v_C the net benefits that are to be allocated to owners A, B, and C. No owner or set of owners will accept an allocation that is less than that which they would enjoy if they acted alone. Thus, we can conclude:

$$v_A \geq 1.2$$
$$v_B \geq 0$$
$$v_C \geq 1$$
$$v_A + v_B \geq 4$$
$$v_A + v_C \geq 3$$
$$v_B + v_C \geq 4$$
$$v_A + v_B + v_C \leq 7$$

That is, any allocation satisfying the above constraints should be self-enforcing. No owner would be motivated not to cooperate. He cannot do better by himself. The above constraints describe what is called the "core" of the game. Any solution satisfying these constraints (e.g., $v_A = 3$, $v_B = 1$, $v_C = 3$) is said to be in the core.

Various objective functions might be appended to this set of constraints to give an LP. The objective could take into account secondary considerations. For example, we might choose to maximize the minimum benefit. The LP in this case is:

Maximize z

subject to $z \leq v_A;\ z \leq v_B;\ z \leq v_C$
$$v_A \geq 1.2$$
$$v_C \geq 1$$
$$v_A + v_B \geq 4$$
$$v_A + v_C \geq 3$$
$$v_A + v_B + v_C \leq 7$$

A solution is $v_A = v_B = v_C = 2.3333$.

Note that the core can be empty. That is, there is no feasible solution. This would be true, for example, if the value of the coalition A, B, C was 5.4 rather than 7. This situation is rather interesting. Total benefits are maximized by everyone cooperating; however, total cooperation is inherently unstable when benefits are 5.4. There will always be a pair of players who find it advantageous to form a subcoalition and improve their benefits (at the considerable expense of the player left out). As an example, suppose the allocations to A, B, and C under full cooperation are 1.2, 2.1, and 2.1, respectively. At this point, A would suggest to B that the two of them exclude C and cooperate between the two of them. A would suggest to B the allocation of 1.8, 2.2, and 1. This is consistent with the fact that A and B can achieve a total of 4 when cooperating. At this point, C might suggest to A that the two of them cooperate and thereby select an allocation of 1.9, 0, 1.1. This is inconsistent with the fact that A and C can achieve a total of 3 when cooperating. At this point B suggests to C, etc. Thus, when the core is empty, it may be that everyone agrees that full cooperation can be better for everyone; there must nevertheless be an enforcement mechanism to prevent "greedy" members from pulling out of the coalition.

12.4 PROBLEMS

Problem 1

Both Big Blue, Inc., and Golden Apple, Inc., are "market oriented" companies and feel that market share is everything. The two of them have 100% of the market for a certain industrial product. Blue and Gold are now planning the marketing campaigns for the upcoming selling season. Each company has three alternative marketing strategies available for the season. Gold's market shares as a function of both the Blue and Gold decisions are tabulated below:

Payment to Blue by Gold as a Function of Both Decisions

		Blue Decision		
		A	B	C
Gold Decision	X	.4	.8	.6
	Y	.3	.7	.4
	Z	.5	.9	.5

Both Blue and Gold know that the above matrix applies. Each must make their decision before learning the decision of the other. There are no other considerations.

(a) What decision do you recommend for Gold?
(b) What decision do you recommend for Blue?

Problem 2

Formulate an LP for finding the optimal policies for Blue and Gold when confronted with the following game.

Payment to Blue by Gold as a Function of Both Decisions

		Blue Decision			
		A	B	C	D
Gold Decision	X	2	-2	1	6
	Y	-1	4	5	-1

Problem 3

Two competing manufacturing firms are contemplating their advertising options for the upcoming season. The profits for each firm as a function of the actions of both firms are shown below. This table is known by both firms.

Fulcher Fasteners

	Option A	Option B	Option C
Option Y	4	8	6
	10	4	6
Option X	8	12	10
	8	2	4

Repicky Rivets

(a) Which pair of actions is most profitable for the pair?

(b) Which pairs of actions are stable?

(c) Presuming that side payments were legal, how much would which firm have to pay the other firm in order to convince them to stick with the most profitable pair of actions?

Problem 4

The three neighboring communities of Parched, Cactus, and Tombstone are located in the desert and are analyzing their options for improving their water supplies. An aqueduct to the mountains would satisfy all their needs and cost in total \$730,000. Alternatively, Parched and Cactus could dig and share an artesian well of sufficient capacity, which would cost \$580,000. A similar option for Cactus and Tombstone would cost \$500,000. Parched, Cactus, and Tombstone could each individually distribute shallow wells over their respective surface areas to satisfy their needs for respective costs of \$300,000, \$350,000, and \$250,000.

Formulate and solve a simple LP for finding a plausible way of allocating the \$730,000 cost of an aqueduct among the three communities.

Problem 5

Sportcasters say Team i is out of the running if the number of games already won by i plus the number of remaining games for Team i is less than the games already won by the league leader. It is frequently the case that a team is mathematically out of the running even before that point is reached. By Team i being mathematically out of the running, we mean that there is no combination of wins and losses for the remaining games in the season such that Team i could end the season having won more games than any other team. A third-place team might find itself mathematically, though not obviously, out of the running if the first- and second-place teams have all their remaining games against each other.

Formulate a linear program which will not have a feasible solution if Team i is no longer in the running.

The following variables may be of interest:

x_{jk} = number of times Team j may beat Team k in the season's remaining games and Team i still win more games than anyone else.

The following constants should be used:

R_{jk} = number of remaining games between Team j and Team k. Note the number of times that j beats k plus the number of times that k beats j must equal R_{jk}.

T_k = total number of games won by Team k to date. Thus, the number of games won at season's end by Team k is T_k plus the number of times it beat other teams.

Problem 6

In the 1983 NBA basketball draft, two teams were tied for having the first draft pick, the reason being that they had equally dismal records the previous year. The tie was resolved by two flips of a coin. Houston was given the opportunity to call the first flip. Houston called it correctly and therefore was eligible to call the second flip. Houston also called the second flip correctly and thereby won the right to negotiate with the top-ranked college star, Ralph Sampson. Suppose that you are in a similar two-flip situation. You suspect that the special coin used may be biased, but you have no idea which way. If you are given the opportunity to call the first flip, should you definitely accept, be indifferent to, or definitely reject the opportunity (and let the other team call the first flip)? State your assumptions explicitly.

Quadratic Programming

13.1 Introduction

Quadratic programming is the name applied to the class of models in which the objective function is a quadratic function and the constraints are linear. Thus, the objective function is allowed to have terms that are products of two variables such as x^2 and $x \times y$. The principal applications of quadratic programming appear mainly in the following areas:

1. Financial portfolio models,
2. Production/demand curve models,
3. Constrained least squares regression,
4. Two-person, nonconstant-sum games.

Strictly speaking, (4) is not a quadratic program; however, essentially the same solution algorithm applies to (4) as to (1), (2), and (3), so we cavalierly include it.

Quadratic programming is computationally appealing because the algorithms for linear programs can be applied to quadratic programming with only modest modifications. Loosely speaking, the reason that only modest modification is required is that the first derivative of a quadratic function is a linear function.

The following sections illustrate the application of quadratic programming to the above problem areas.

13.2 The Markowitz Mean/Variance Portfolio Model

The portfolio model introduced by Markowitz (1959) assumes that an investor has but two considerations when constructing an investment portfolio: expected return and variance in return. The investor wants the former to be high and the latter to be low. Variance measures the variability in realized return around the expected return, giving equal weight to realizations below the expected and above the expected return. The Markowitz model might be mildly criticized in this regard because the typical investor is probably concerned only with variability below the expected return, so-called downside risk. If the distribution of return from the portfolio is symmetric and the investor is risk averse, the Markowitz model is reasonable. Part of the appeal of the Markowitz model is that it can be solved by efficient quadratic programming methods.

The model requires two major kinds of information: (1) the estimated expected return for each candidate investment and (2) the covariance matrix of returns. The covariance matrix characterizes not only the individual variability of the return on each investment but also how each investment's return tends to move with other investments. We assume the reader is familiar with the concepts of variance and covariance as are described in most intermediate statistics texts.

13.2.1 Example

We will use some publicly available data from Markowitz (1959). Eppen, Gould, and Schmidt (1991) use the same data. The increase in price, including dividends, for three stocks over a twelve-year period is shown below.

Year	Growth in			
	S&P 500	**ATT**	**GMC**	**USX**
43	1.258997	1.3	1.225	1.149
44	1.197526	1.103	1.29	1.26
45	1.364361	1.216	1.216	1.419
46	0.919287	0.954	0.728	0.922
47	1.05708	1.929	1.144	1.169
48	1.055012	1.056	1.107	0.965
49	1.187925	1.038	1.321	1.133
50	1.31713	1.089	1.305	1.732
51	1.240164	1.09	1.195	1.021
52	1.183675	1.083	1.39	1.131
53	0.990108	1.035	0.928	1.006
54	1.526236	1.176	1.715	1.908

For reference later, we have also included the change each year in the S&P 500 stock index. To illustrate, in the first year, ATT appreciated in value by 30%. In the second year, GMC appreciated in value by 29%. Based on the twelve years of data, we can use any standard statistical package, such as Minitab, or even spreadsheet programs such as Excel, to calculate a covariance matrix for three stocks: ATT, GMC, and USX. The matrix is:

	ATT	**GMC**	**USX**
ATT	.01080754	.01240721	.01307513
GMC	.01240721	.05839170	.05542639
USX	.01307513	.05542639	.09422631

From the same data, we estimate the expected return per year, including dividends, for ATT, GMC, and USX as 0.0890833, 0.213667, and 0.234583, respectively.

Let the symbols ATT, GMC, USX represent the fraction of the portfolio devoted to each of the three stocks. Suppose we desire a 15% yearly return. The entire model in general algebraic form can be written as:

Min   .01080754 × ATT × ATT + .01240721 × ATT × GMC + .01307513 × ATT × USX + .01240721 × GMC × ATT + .05839170 × GMC × GMC + .05542639 × GMC × USX + .01307513 × USX × ATT + .05542639 × USX × GMC + .09422681 × USX × USX

Subject to:

ATT + GMC + USX = 1   ! Use exactly 100% of the starting budget;
1.089083 ATT + 1.213667 GMC + 1.234583 USX ≥ 1.15   ! Required wealth at end of period.

Note that the two constraints are effectively in the same units. The first constraint is effectively a "beginning inventory" constraint, whereas the second constraint is an "ending inventory" constraint. Note that we could have just as easily stated the expected return constraint as:

.0890833 ATT + .213667 GMC + .234583 USX ≥ .15.

Although perfectly correct, this latter style does not measure end-of-period state in quite the same way as start-of-period state.

The objective function is *not* entered into LINDO in quite the above form. LINDO requires all rows to be linear. For example, .01080754 × ATT × ATT is not linear. The derivative of a quadratic expression is linear, however. To prepare a quadratic model for LINDO, we must do the following:

1. Write the objective function in minimization form, e.g., multiplying through by −1 if you naturally think of the objective function in the maximization form. The objective function in this form is actually *not* input to LINDO.
2. The first-order condition for variable X is composed of:
   (a) the derivative of the objective function with respect to X,
   (b) plus the sum over all "<" and "=" rows of Xs coefficient in the row times the dual variable of the row,
   (c) minus the sum over all ">" rows of Xs coefficient in the row times the dual variable of the row.

The input procedure for LINDO is LP-based and requires an objective function, even though there is no explicit objective listed in the first-order conditions. The first row input serves an important purpose, however, in that it is used to identify the order of variables, which, in turn, determines the correspondence between variables and rows.

LINDO requires that the true constraints (e.g., ATT + GMC + USX = 1, etc.) appear last. Finally, the command QCP must be used to specify which constraint is the first of the real constraints. The complete input is:

```
! PBUD and PRET are the dual prices or LaGrange multipliers
! on the BUDGET and RETURN constraints;
! The MIN row simply gives the order of the variables;
 MIN ATT + GMC + USX + PBUD + PRET
   Subject to
! The first order conditions, essentially,
!      2 × Cov × X + PBUD - Return × PRET >= 0;
FATT) .02161508 ATT + .02481442 GMC + .02615026 USX
        + PBUD - 1.089083 PRET >= 0
FGMC) .02481442 ATT + .11678340 GMC + .11085278 USX
        + PBUD - 1.213667 PRET >= 0
FUSX) .02615026 ATT + .11085278 GMC + .18845362 USX
        + PBUD - 1.234583 PRET >= 0
!
! The Budget constraint;
BUD) ATT + GMC + USX = 1
! The target Return constraint;
RET) 1.089083 ATT + 1.213667 GMC + 1.234583 USX >= 1.15
END
! Tell LINDO that this is a quadratic problem with
!  first real constraint being row 5;
QCP 5
```

The order of the variables in the very first row (MIN ATT + GMC, etc.) is important. The so-called complementary slackness conditions require that, if ATT is greater than zero, the first constraint:

```
.02161508 ATT + .02481442 GMC + .02615026 USX
     + PBUD - 1.089083 PRET >= 0,
```

must be binding, i.e., hold as an equality. Similar comments apply to GMC and USX. Thus, LINDO must know this correspondence between variables and constraints to enforce these conditions.

We solve the problem as follows:

```
: go

          OBJECTIVE FUNCTION VALUE

        1)        0.2241381E-01

   VARIABLE          VALUE          REDUCED COST
        ATT          0.530091         0.000000
        GMC          0.356412         0.000000
        USX          0.113497         0.000000
       PBUD          0.362138         0.000000
       PRET         -0.353883         0.000000

        ROW     SLACK OR SURPLUS      DUAL PRICES
       FATT)         0.000000        -0.530091
       FGMC)         0.000000        -0.356412
       FUSX)         0.000000        -0.113497
        BUD)         0.000000         0.362138
        RET)         0.000000        -0.353883
```

The solution recommends that about 53% of the portfolio be put in ATT, about 36% in GMC, and just over 11% in USX. The expected return is 15%, with a variance of 0.02241381, or equivalently, a standard deviation of about 0.1497123.

We based the model simply on straightforward statistical data based on yearly returns. In practice, it may be more typical to use monthly rather than yearly data as a basis for calculating a covariance. Also, rather than use historical data for estimating the expected return of an asset, a decision maker might base the expected return estimate on more current, proprietary information about expected future performance of the asset. In practice, one may wish to use considerable care in estimating the covariances and the expected returns.

13.3 Efficient Frontier and Parametric Analysis

There is no precise way for an investor to determine the "correct" tradeoff between risk and return. Thus, one is frequently interested in looking at the tradeoff between the two. If an investor wants a higher expected return, she generally has to "pay for it" with higher risk. In finance terminology, we would like to trace out the efficient frontier of return and risk. LINDO has a command, PARA(metric) for doing this analysis. To illustrate, consider the original Markowitz model, but with the highest possible expected return we can hope to achieve (without borrowing) 23.45%, by investing entirely in USX.

```
MIN       ATT + GMC + USX + PBUD + PRET
SUBJECT TO
 FATT)    0.021615 ATT + 0.0248144 GMC + 0.0261502 USX
            + PBUD - 1.089083 PRET >= 0
 FGMC)    0.0248144 ATT + 0.1167834 GMC + 0.1108528 USX
            + PBUD - 1.213667 PRET >= 0
 FUSX)    0.0261502 ATT + 0.1108528 GMC + 0.1884536 USX
            + PBUD - 1.234583 PRET >= 0
  BUD)    ATT + GMC + USX = 1
  RET)    1.089083 ATT + 1.213667 GMC + 1.234583 USX >= 1.2345
END
QCP=      5
```

When we solve it, we find:

```
OBJECTIVE VALUE =   0.939197540E-01

            OBJECTIVE FUNCTION VALUE

        1)      0.9391975E-01

    VARIABLE          VALUE           REDUCED COST
         ATT        0.000000            0.375517
         GMC        0.003967            0.000000
         USX        0.996033            0.000000
        PBUD        4.372746            0.000000
        PRET        3.694277            0.000000
```

We can ask LINDO to list the "pivot points" as we parametrically decrease our desired expected return to 0% from 23%. Simply type:

```
: para                  ! Execute the PARA command;
  ROW: 6                 ! The row whose RHS we wish to vary;
  NEW RHS VAL= 0.0       ! The ending value:
```

VAR OUT	VAR IN	PIVOT ROW	RHS VAL	DUAL PRICE BEFORE PIVOT	OBJ VAL
			1.23450	-3.69428	0.939198E-01
SLK 2	ATT	6	1.21894	-0.723501	0.595519E-01
USX	SLK 4	3	1.09357	-0.513495E-01	0.109804E-01
PRET	SLK 3	2	1.08908	-0.256807E-01	0.317673E-01
GMC	SLK 6	5	1.08908	0.000000	0.108075E-01
			0.000000	0.000000	0.108075E-01

Recall that row 6 is the target return constraint. The PARA command has requested that the changes in the portfolio be traced out as the required return is decreased to 0.0 from 23.45%. One line of output is printed each time one of the following occurs:

(a) a new asset enters the optimal portfolio,
(b) an asset is removed from the optimal portfolio,
(c) a binding constraint becomes nonbinding,
(d) a nonbinding constraint becomes binding.

As we drop the required return, the first thing that happens is that ATT enters the portfolio and the slack (SLK 2) in its first-order condition (necessarily) goes to zero. When the required return drops to 9.357%, USX is dropped from the portfolio. When the required return is dropped to 8.908%, GMC is dropped from the portfolio, leaving only ATT in the portfolio. Note that cash has not been listed as a possible "investment," so when the required return is dropped to zero, the variance of the portfolio does not go to zero, but remains at 0.0108075, the variance of ATT.

LINDO prints the objective function value only at the "pivot points." For linear programs, the objective function changes linearly between pivot points. For quadratic programs, the objective function changes quadratically between pivot points. Suppose we wish to interpolate between two adjacent pivot points, labelled 1 and 2. Define:

$V(i)$ = objective value at point i, for $i = 1$ or 2,
$R(i)$ = RHS value at point i, for $i = 1$ or 2,
$D(2)$ = dual price of the constraint being parameterized, just before point 2,
r = some RHS value between $R(1)$ and $R(2)$,
d = $(R(2) - r)/(R(2) - R(1))$.

The objective value with a RHS of r is then:

$$V(2) + d \times D(2) \times [R(2) - R(1)] + d \times d \times (V(1) - V(2) - D(2) \times [R(2) - R(1)]).$$

When plotted, we get the efficient frontier graph in Figure 13.1

Notice the "knee" in the curve as the required expected return increases past 1.21894. This is the point where ATT drops out of the portfolio.

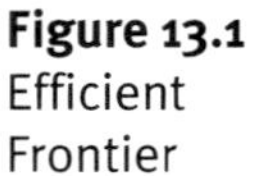

Figure 13.1
Efficient
Frontier

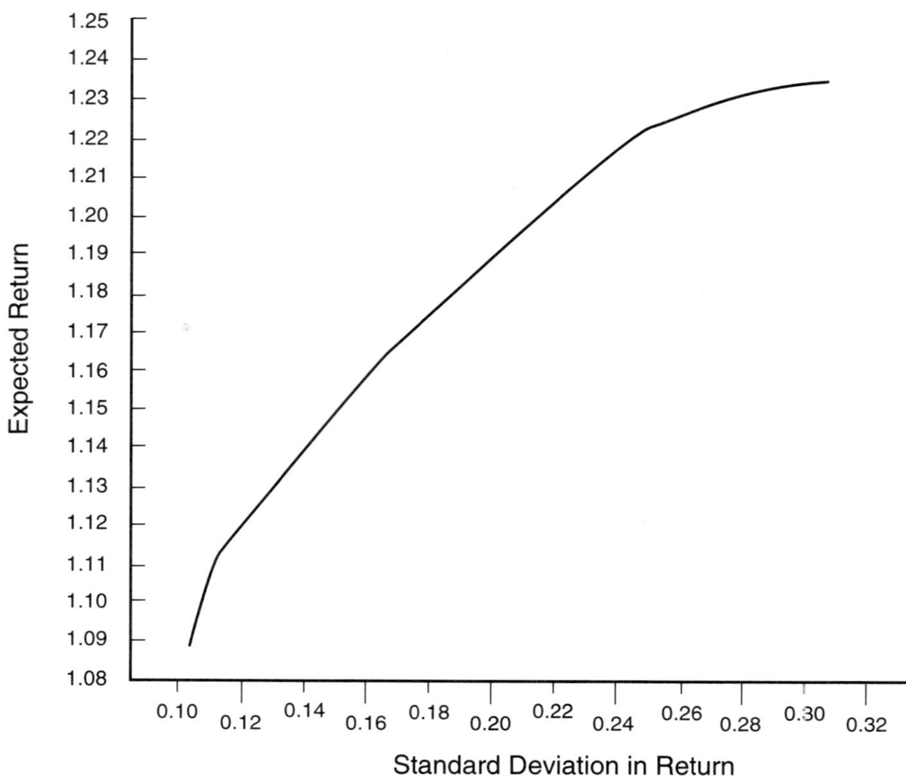

13.3.1 Portfolios with a Risk-Free Asset

When one of the investments available is risk free, the optimal portfolio composition has a particularly simple form. Suppose the opportunity to invest money risk free (e.g., in government treasury bills) at 5% per year has just become available. Working with our previous example, we now have a fourth investment instrument that has zero variance and zero covariance. There is no limit on how much can be invested at 5%. We ask the question: How does the portfolio composition change as the desired rate of return changes from 15% to 5%?

We will use the following slight generalization of the original Markowitz example model. Notice that a fourth instrument, treasury bills (TBILL), has been added.

```
! The Markowitz model with a risk free asset
! The original Markowitz portfolio problem formulated for
  LINDO
! PBUD and PRET are the dual prices or LaGrange multipliers
! on the BUDGET and RETURN constraints;
! The MIN row simply gives the order of the variables;
  MIN ATT + GMC + USX + TBILL + PBUD + PRET
ST
```

```
! The first order conditions, essentially,
!     2 * COV * X + PBUD + Return * X;
 FATT) .0216150 ATT + .0248144 GMC + .0261502 USX
        + PBUD - 1.089083 PRET >= 0
 FGMC) .0248144 ATT + .1167834 GMC + .1108528 USX
        + PBUD - 1.213667 PRET >= 0
 FUSX) .0261502 ATT + .1108528 GMC + .1884536 USX
        + PBUD - 1.234583 PRET >= 0
 FTBILL)    PBUD - 1.05 PRET >= 0
! The actual constraints;
! The Budget constraint;
  BUD) ATT + GMC + USX + RFREE = 1
! The target Return constraint;
  RET) 1.089083 ATT + 1.213667 GMC + 1.234583 USX
        + 1.05 TBILL >= 1.15
END
! Tell LINDO that this is a quadratic problem with
!  first real constraint being row 6;
QCP 6
```

When solved, we find:

```
          OBJECTIVE FUNCTION VALUE

     1)       0.2080344E-01

       VARIABLE         VALUE          REDUCED COST
          ATT         0.086867          0.000000
          GMC         0.428528          0.000000
          USX         0.143399          0.000000
        TBILL         0.341206          0.000000
         PBUD         0.436872          0.000000
         PRET         0.416069          0.000000

         ROW     SLACK OR SURPLUS       DUAL PRICES
        FATT)         0.000000         -0.086867
        FGMC)         0.000000         -0.428528
        FUSX)         0.000000         -0.143399
      FTBILL)         0.000000         -0.341206
         BUD)         0.000000          0.436872
         RET)         0.000000         -0.416069
```

Notice that more than 34% of the portfolio was invested in the risk-free investment, even though its return rate, 5%, is less than the target of 15%.

What happens as we decrease the target return toward 5%? Clearly, at 5%, we would put zero in ATT, GMC, and USX. A simple form of solution would be to keep the same proportions in ATT, GMC, and USX, but just change the allocation between the risk-free asset and the risky ones. Let us check an intermediate point. When we decrease the required return to 10%, we get the following solution:

```
          OBJECTIVE FUNCTION VALUE

     1)       0.5200865E-02

       VARIABLE         VALUE          REDUCED COST
          ATT         0.043433          0.000000
          GMC         0.214264          0.000000
```

```
        USX          0.071700          0.000000
       TBILL         0.670603          0.000000
        PBUD         0.218436          0.000000
        PRET         0.208035          0.000000

        ROW     SLACK OR SURPLUS     DUAL PRICES
       FATT)         0.000000         -0.043433
       FGMC)         0.000000         -0.214264
       FUSX)         0.000000         -0.071700
      FTBILL)        0.000000         -0.670603
        BUD)         0.000000          0.218436
        RET)         0.000000         -0.208035
```

This solution supports our conjecture: As we change our required return, the relative proportions devoted to risky investments do not change; only the allocation between the risk-free asset and the risky assets changes. From the above solution, we observe that, except for roundoff error, the amount invested in ATT, GMC, and USX is allocated in the same way in both solutions. Thus, two investors with different risk preferences would nevertheless both carry the same mix of risky stocks in their portfolio. Their portfolios would differ only in the proportion devoted to the risk-free asset. Our observation from the above example in fact holds in general. Thus, the decision of how to allocate funds among stocks, given the amount to be invested in stocks, can be separated from the question of risk preference. Tobin received the Nobel Prize in 1981, largely for noticing the above feature, the so-called Separation Theorem. So if you noticed it, you must be Nobel Prize caliber.

13.4 Important Variations of the Portfolio Model

There are several issues that may concern you when you think about applying the Markowitz model in its simple form.

1. As we increase the number of assets to consider, the size of the covariance matrix becomes overwhelming. For example, 1000 assets implies 1,000,000 covariance terms, or at least 500,000 if symmetry is exploited.
2. If the model is applied every time that new data becomes available (e.g., weekly), we would "rebalance" the portfolio frequently, making small, possibly unimportant adjustments in the portfolio.
3. There are no upper bounds on how much can be held of each asset. In practice, there might be legal or regulatory reasons for restricting the amount of any one asset to more than, say, 5% of the total portfolio. Some portfolio managers may set the upper limit on a stock to, say, one day's trading volume for the stock, the reasoning being that, if the manager wants to "unload" the stock quickly, the market price would be affected significantly by selling so much.

Two approaches for simplifying the covariance structure have been proposed: the scenario approach and the factor approach. For the issue of portfolio "nervousness," the incorporation of transactions costs is useful.

13.4.1 Portfolios with Transaction Costs

The models above do not tell us much about how frequently to adjust our portfolio as new information becomes available, i.e., new estimates of expected return and new estimates of variance. If we applied the above models every time new information became available, we would be constantly adjusting our portfolio. This might make our broker happy, but that should be at best a secondary objective.

The method we will describe assumes transaction costs are paid at the beginning of the period. It is a straightforward exercise to modify the model to handle the case of transaction costs paid at the end of the period. The major modifications to the basic portfolio model are:

(a) we must introduce two additional variables for each asset, an "amount bought" variable and an "amount sold" variable;
(b) the budget constraint must be modified to include money spent on commissions;
(c) an additional constraint must be included for each asset to enforce the requirement: amount invested in asset I

= (initial holding of I)

+ (amount bought of I)

− (amount sold of I).

13.4.2 Example

Suppose that we have to pay a 1% transaction fee on the amount bought or sold of any stock, and our current portfolio is 50% ATT, 35% GMC, and 15% USX. This is pretty close to the optimal mix. Should we incur the cost of adjusting? The following is the relevant model.

```
MIN    ATT + GMC + USX + BA + SA + BG + SG + BU + SU
       + PBUD + PRET + PTA + PTG + PTU
SUBJECT TO
! First order conditions on the amount invested in each asset;
    FATT)  0.021615 ATT + 0.0248144 GMC + 0.0261502 USX
              + PBUD - 1.089083 PRET + PTA >= 0
    FGMC)  0.0248144 ATT + 0.1167834 GMC + 0.1108528 USX
              + PBUD - 1.213667 PRET + PTG >= 0
    FUSX)  0.0261502 ATT + 0.1108528 GMC + 0.1884536 USX
              + PBUD - 1.234583 PRET + PTU >= 0
! First order condition on amount bought of ATT;
     FBA)    0.01 PBUD - PTA >=  0
! First order condition on amount sold of ATT;
     FSA)    0.01 PBUD + PTA >=  0
! First order condition on amount bought of GMC, etc.
     FBG)    0.01 PBUD - PTG >=  0
     FSG)    0.01 PBUD + PTG >=  0
     FBU)    0.01 PBUD - PTU >=  0
     FSU)    0.01 PBUD + PTU >=  0
! Budget constraint at beginning of period;
      BUD) ATT + GMC + USX + 0.01 BA + 0.01 SA
         + 0.01 BG + 0.01 SG + 0.01 BU + 0.01 SU = 1
```

```
! Constraint on required return;
     RET)  1.089083 ATT + 1.213667 GMC + 1.234583 USX >= 1.15
! Invested in ATT - bought + sold = initial holding;
      TA)    ATT - BA + SA =  0.5
!  Ditto for GMC, and USX;
      TG)    GMC - BG + SG =  0.35
      TU)    USX - BU + SU =  0.15
  END
  QCP=    11
```

The resulting solution is:

```
          OBJECTIVE FUNCTION VALUE

      1)        0.2261144E-01

  VARIABLE           VALUE          REDUCED COST
       ATT         0.526475            0.000000
       GMC         0.350000            0.000000
       USX         0.122990            0.000000
        BA         0.026475            0.000000
        SA         0.000000            0.006371
        BG         0.000000            0.004825
        SG         0.000000            0.001546
        BU         0.000000            0.006371
        SU         0.027010            0.000000
      PBUD         0.318538            0.000000
      PRET         0.316784            0.000000
       PTA         0.003185            0.000000
       PTG        -0.001640            0.000000
       PTU        -0.003185            0.000000
```

The solution recommends buying a little bit more ATT, neither buy nor sell any GMC, and sell a little USX.

13.4.3 Factors Model for Simplifying the Covariance Structure

Sharpe (1963) introduced a substantial simplification to the modeling of the random behavior of stock market prices. He proposed that there is a "market factor" that has a significant effect on the movement of a stock. The market factor might be the Dow-Jones Industrial average, the S&P 500 average, or the Nikkei index. If we define:

$$M = \text{the market factor,}$$
$$m_0 = E(M),$$
$$s_0^2 = \text{var}(M),$$
$$e_i = \text{random movement specific to stock } i.$$

Sharpe's approximation assumes that (where $E(\ )$ denotes expected value):

$$E(e_i) = 0,$$
$$E(e_i e_j) = 0 \quad \text{for } i \neq j,$$
$$E(e_i M) = 0,$$
$$s_i^2 = \text{var}(e_i).$$

Then, according to the Sharpe single factor model, the return of one dollar invested in stock or asset i is:

$$u_i + b_i M + e_i.$$

The parameters u_i and b_i are obtained by regression, e.g., least squares, of the return of asset i on the market factor. The parameter b_i is known as the "beta" of the asset. Let

$$X_i = \text{amount invested in asset } i.$$

The variance in return of the portfolio is:

$$\begin{aligned}
&\text{var}[\Sigma X_i(u_i + b_i M + e_i)] \\
&= \text{var}(\Sigma X_i b_i M) + \text{var}(\Sigma X_i e_i) \\
&= \Sigma (X_i b_i)^2 s_o^2 + \Sigma X_i^2 s_i^2.
\end{aligned}$$

Thus, our problem can be written:

$$\begin{aligned}
\text{Min} \quad & Z^2 s_o^2 + \Sigma X_i^2 s_i^2 \\
\text{s.t.} \quad & \\
& Z - \Sigma X_i b_i = 0 \\
& \Sigma X_i = 1 \\
& \Sigma X_i (u_i + b_i m_o) \geq r.
\end{aligned}$$

So, at the expense of adding one constraint and one variable, we have reduced a dense covariance matrix to a diagonal covariance matrix.

In practice, perhaps a half dozen factors might be used to represent the "systematic risk." That is, the return of an asset is assumed to be correlated with a number of indices or factors. Typical factors might be a market index such as the S&P 500, interest rates, inflation, defense spending, energy prices, gross national product, correlation with the business cycle, and various industry indices. For example, bond prices are very much affected by interest rate movements.

13.4.4 Example of the Factor Model

To illustrate the factor model, we used multiple regression to regress the returns of ATT, GMC, and USX on the market index, the Standard and Poors 500, for the same 12 periods. The regression formula was:

$$\text{Return}(i) = \text{Alpha}(i) + \text{Beta}(i) * \text{SP500} + \text{residual error}.$$

The results of the regression gave the following estimates for the Alphas, Betas, and the standard deviation in the residual error.

	ATT	GMC	USX
ALPHA =	.004702	−.023700	−.057160
BETA =	.440726	1.2398	1.52380
SIGMA =	.075817	.125070	.173930

The mean and standard deviation of SP500 were:

$$RETSP = .191460;$$
$$SIGSP = .162302;$$

The resulting model is:

```
MIN   Z + ATT + GMC + USX + PDEF + PBUD + PRET
 SUBJECT TO
  FZ)  0.0526839 Z + PDEF >= 0
FATT)  0.0114964 ATT - 0.440726 PDEF + PBUD - 1.089083 PRET >= 0
FGMC)  0.031285 GMC - 1.2398 PDEF + PBUD - 1.21367 PRET >= 0
FUSX)  0.0605033 USX - 1.5238 PDEF + PBUD - 1.234588 PRET >= 0
DEF)  Z - 0.440726 ATT - 1.2398 GMC - 1.5238 USX = 0
BUD)  ATT + GMC + USX =  1
RET)  1.089083 ATT + 1.21367 GMC + 1.234588 USX >= 1.15
END
 QCP=  6
```

When solved, we get the following solution:

```
         OBJECTIVE FUNCTION VALUE

      1)        0.2294247E-01

VARIABLE          VALUE            REDUCED COST
       Z        0.846199            0.000000
     ATT        0.527593            0.000000
     GMC        0.373867            0.000000
     USX        0.098540            0.000000
    PDEF       -0.044581            0.000000
    PBUD        0.334915            0.000000
    PRET        0.331131            0.000000
```

Notice that the portfolio makeup is slightly different; however, the estimated variance of the portfolio is very close to that of our original portfolio.

13.4.5 Scenario Model for Representing Uncertainty

The scenario approach to modeling uncertainty assumes that the possible future situations can be represented by a small number of "scenarios." The smallest number used is typically three, e.g., "optimistic," "most likely," and "pessimistic." Some of the original ideas underlying the scenario approach come from the approach known as stochastic programming; see Madansky (1962), for example. For a discussion of the scenario approach for large portfolios, see Markowitz and Perold (1981) and Perold (1984). For a thorough discussion of the general approach of stochastic programming, see Infanger (1992). Eppen, Martin, and Schrage (1988) use the scenario approach for capacity planning in the automobile industry.

Let:

P_s = Probability that scenario s occurs,

u_{is} = return of asset i if the scenario is s,

X_s = investment in asset i,

Y_s = deviation of actual return from the mean if the scenario is s,
$$= \Sigma_i X_i(u_{i\,s} - \Sigma_q Pu).$$

Our problem in algebraic form is

Minimize $\Sigma_s P_s Y_s^2$
subject to
$Y_s - \Sigma_i X_i(u_{is} - \Sigma \Sigma_q P_q u_{i\,q}) = 0$ (deviation from mean of each scenario, s)
$\Sigma_i X_i = 1$ (budget constraint)
$\Sigma_i X_i \Sigma_s P_s u_{is} \geq r$ (desired return).

If asset i has an inherent variability v_i^2, the objective generalizes to:

Min $\Sigma_i X_i^2 v_i^2 + \Sigma_s P_s Y_s^2$

The key feature is that even though this formulation has a few more constraints, the covariance matrix is diagonal, and thus very sparse.

You will generally also want to put upper limits on what fraction of the portfolio is invested in each asset. Otherwise, if there are no upper bounds or inherent variabilities specified, the optimization will tend to invest in only as many assets as there are scenarios.

13.4.6 Example: Scenario Model for Representing Uncertainty

We will use the original data from Markowitz once again. We simply treat each of the 12 years as being a separate scenario, independent of the other 11 years.

```
! The MIN row simply gives the order of the
! primal variables . . . ;
 MIN Y1 + Y2 + Y3 + Y4  + Y5  + Y6 + Y7 + Y8 - Y9 + Y10 + Y11 + Y12
    + ATT + GMC + USX + MEAN
! and the dual/price variables;
    + PS1 + PS2 + PS3 + PS4  + PS5  + PS6 + PS7 + PS8 + PS9 + PS10
    + PS11 + PS12 + PBUD + PDEF + PRET
 Subject to
! The first order conditions on the Y's
 FY1)  .1666666 Y1 + PS1 = 0
 FY2)  .1666666 Y2 + PS2 = 0
 FY3)  .1666666 Y3 + PS3 = 0
 FY4)  .1666666 Y4 + PS4 = 0
 FY5)  .1666666 Y5 + PS5 = 0
 FY6)  .1666666 Y6 + PS6 = 0
 FY7)  .1666666 Y7 + PS7 = 0
 FY8)  .1666666 Y8 + PS3 = 0
 FY9)  .1666666 Y9 + PS9 = 0
FY10)  .1666666 Y10 + PS10 = 0
FY11)  .1666666 Y11 + PS11 = 0
FY12)  .1666666 Y12 + PS12 = 0
! First order conditions on the investments;
 FATT)  + 1.3 PS1 + 1.103 PS2 + 1.216 PS3 + 0.954 PS4 + 0.929 PS5
        + 1.056 PS6 + 1.038 PS7 + 1.089 PS8 + 1.09 PS9 + 1.083 PS10
        + 1.035 PS11 + 1.176 PS12 + PBUD + 1.089083 PDEF >= 0
```

```
FGMC)  + 1.225 PS1 + 1.29 PS2 + 1.216 PS3 + 0.728 PS4 + 1.144 PS5
       + 1.107 PS6 + 1.321 PS7 + 1.305 PS8 + 1.195 PS9 + 1.39 PS10
       + 0.928 PS11 + 1.715 PS12 + PBUD + 1.213667 PDEF >= 0
FUSX)  + 1.149 PS1 + 1.26 PS2  + 1.419 PS3 + 0.922 PS4 + 1.169 PS5
       + 0.965 PS6 + 1.133 PS7 + 1.732 PS8 + 1.021 PS9 + 1.131 PS10
       + 1.006 PS11 + 1.908 PS12 + PBUD + 1.234583 PDEF >= 0
! First order conditions on the mean;
 FMEAN) - PS1 - PS2 - PS3 - PS4 - PS5 - PS6 - PS7 - PS8
 - PS9 - PS10 - PS11 - PS12 - PDEF - PRET >= 0
! Here are the real constraints, compute Y for each scenario;
 S1)   Y1 + 1.3   ATT + 1.225 GMC + 1.149 USX - MEAN = 0
 S2)   Y2 + 1.103 ATT + 1.29  GMC + 1.26  USX - MEAN = 0
 S3)   Y3 + 1.216 ATT + 1.216 GMC + 1.419 USX - MEAN = 0
 S4)   Y4 + 0.954 ATT + 0.728 GMC + 0.922 USX - MEAN = 0
 S5)   Y5 + 0.929 ATT + 1.144 GMC + 1.169 USX - MEAN = 0
 S6)   Y6 + 1.056 ATT + 1.107 GMC + 0.965 USX - MEAN = 0
 S7)   Y7 + 1.038 ATT + 1.321 GMC + 1.133 USX - MEAN = 0
 S8)   Y8 + 1.089 ATT + 1.305 GMC + 1.732 USX - MEAN = 0
 S9)   Y9 + 1.09  ATT + 1.195 GMC + 1.021 USX - MEAN = 0
 S10) Y10 + 1.083 ATT + 1.39  GMC + 1.131 USX - MEAN = 0
 S11) Y11 + 1.035 ATT + 0.928 GMC + 1.006 USX - MEAN = 0
 S12) Y12 + 1.176 ATT + 1.715 GMC + 1.908 USX - MEAN = 0
! The Budget constraint;
BUD) ATT + GMC + USX = 1
! compute the mean;
 DEF) 1.089083 ATT + 1.213667 GMC + 1.234583 USX - MEAN = 0
! The target Return constraint;
RET) MEAN >= 1.15
END
! Tell LINDO that this is a quadratic problem with
!  first real constraint being row 18
QCP 18
```

When we solve it, we get the following familiar solution:

```
OBJECTIVE FUNCTION VALUE

        1)      0.2054597E-01

    VARIABLE         VALUE          REDUCED COST
         Y1        -0.106131          0.000000
         Y2        -0.037468          0.000000
         Y3        -0.089040          0.000000
         Y4         0.280181          0.000000
         Y5         0.117132          0.000000
         Y6         0.086151          0.000000
         Y7         0.000353          0.000000
         Y8        -0.088963          0.000000
         Y9         0.030408          0.000000
        Y10        -0.301186          0.000000
        Y11         0.156427          0.000000
        Y12         0.301186          0.000000
        ATT         0.530091          0.000000
        GMC         0.356412          0.000000
        USX         0.113497          0.000000
       MEAN         1.150000          0.000000
        PS1         0.017689          0.000000
```

PS2	0.006245	0.000000
PS3	0.014840	0.000000
PS4	-0.046697	0.000000
PS5	-0.019522	0.000000
PS6	-0.014359	0.000000
PS7	-0.000059	0.000000
PS8	0.014827	0.000000
PS9	-0.005068	0.000000
PS10	0.007978	0.000000
PS11	-0.026071	0.000000
PS12	0.050198	0.000000
PBUD	0.331960	0.000000
PDEF	-0.324393	0.000000
PRET	0.324393	0.000000

ROW	SLACK OR SURPLUS	DUAL PRICES
FY1)	0.000000	-0.106131
FY2)	0.000000	-0.037468
FY3)	0.000000	-0.089040
FY4)	0.000000	0.280181
FY5)	0.000000	0.117132
FY6)	0.000000	0.086151
FY7)	0.000000	0.000353
FY8)	0.000000	-0.088963
FY9)	0.000000	0.030408
FY10)	0.000000	-0.047366
FY11)	0.000000	0.156427
FY12)	0.000000	-0.301186
FATT)	0.000000	-0.530091
FGMC)	0.000000	-0.356412
FUSX)	0.000000	-0.113497
FMEAN)	0.000000	-1.150000
S1)	0.000000	0.017689
S2)	0.000000	0.006245
S3)	0.000000	0.014840
S4)	0.000000	-0.046697
S5)	0.000000	-0.019522
S6)	0.000000	-0.014359
S7)	0.000000	-0.000059
S8)	0.000000	0.014827
S9)	0.000000	-0.005068
S10)	0.000000	0.007978
S11)	0.000000	-0.026071
S12)	0.000000	0.050198
BUD)	0.000000	0.331960
DEF)	0.000000	-0.324393
RET)	0.000000	-0.324393

NO. ITERATIONS=   32

The perceptive reader will have noticed that the solution suggests *exactly the same portfolio* as our original model based on the covariance matrix (based on the same 12 years of data as in the above scenario model). This, in fact, is a general result: if the covariance matrix and expected returns are calculated directly from the original data by the traditional statistical formulae, the covariance model and the scenario model based on the same data will recommend exactly the same portfolio.

The careful reader will have noticed that the objective function from the scenario model (0.02054597) is slightly less than that of the covariance model (0.02241381). The exceptionally perceptive reader may have noticed that $12 \times 0.02054597/11 = 0.02241381$. The difference in objective value is a result simply of the fact that standard statistics packages tend to divide by $N - 1$ rather than N when computing variances and covariances, where N is the number of observations. Thus, a slightly more general statement is that if the covariance matrix is computed using a divisor of N rather than $N - 1$, the covariance model and the scenario model will give the same solution, including objective value.

13.5 Measures of Risk Other Than Variance

The most common measure of risk is variance (or its square root, the standard deviation). This is a reasonable measure for assets that have a symmetric distribution and are traded in a so-called "efficient" market. If these two features do not hold, however, variance has some drawbacks. Consider the four possible growth distributions in Figure 13.2.

Investments A, B, and C are equivalent according to the variance measure, because each has an expected growth of 1.10 (an expected return of 10%) and a variance of 0.04 (standard deviation around the mean of 0.20). Risk-averse investors would, however, probably not be indifferent among the three. Under distribution (A), you would never lose any of your original investment, and there is a 0.2 probability of the investment growing by a factor of 1.5, i.e., a 50% return. Distribution (C), on the other hand, has a 0.2 probability of an investment decreasing to 0.7 of its original value, i.e., a negative 30% return. Risk-averse investors would tend to prefer (A) most and prefer (C) least. This illustrates that variance need not be a good measure of risk if the distribution of returns is not symmetric.

Investment (D) is an inefficient investment. It is dominated by (A). Suppose the only investments available are (A) and (D) and our goal is to have an expected return of at least 5%, i.e., a growth factor of 1.05, and the lowest possible variance. The solution is to put 50% of our investment in each of (A) and (D). The resulting variance is 0.01 (standard deviation = 0.1) If we invested 100% in (A), the standard deviation would be 0.20. Nevertheless, we would prefer to invest 100% in (A). It is true that the return is more random; however, our profits are always at least as high under every outcome. (If the randomness in profits is an issue, we can always give profits to a worthy educational institution when our profits are high so as to reduce the variance.) Thus, the variance objective may cause us to choose inefficient investments.

In active and efficient markets, such as major stock markets, you will tend not to find investments such as (D), because investors will realize that (A) dominates (D), and thus the market price of (D) will drop until its return approaches that of competing investments. In investment decisions regarding new physical facilities, however, there are no strong market forces making all investment candidates "efficient," so the variance risk measure may be less appropriate in such situations.

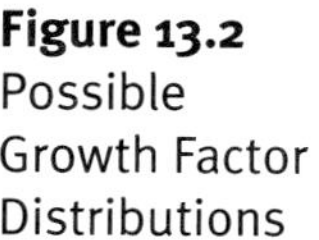

Figure 13.2
Possible
Growth Factor
Distributions

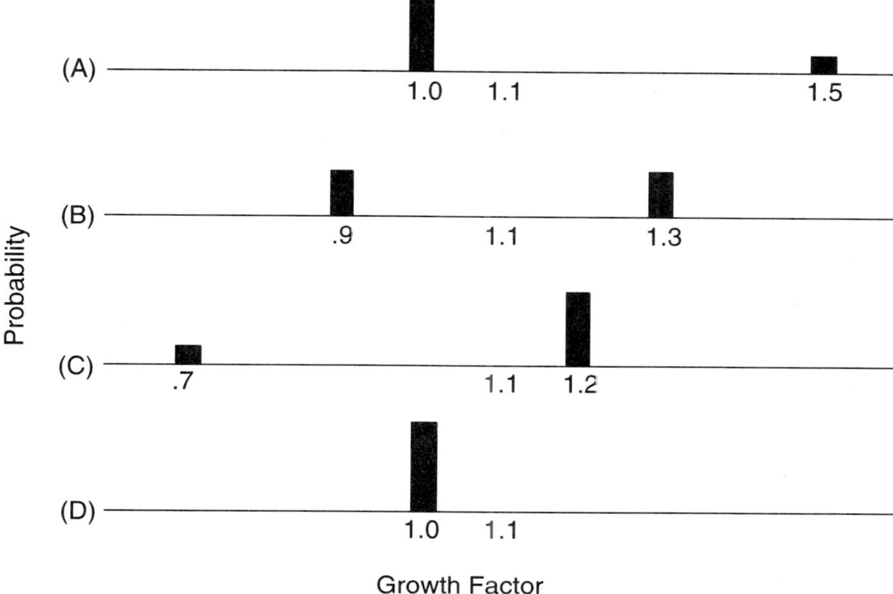

13.6 Maximizing the Minimum Return

A very conservative investor might react to risk by maximizing the minimum return over scenarios. There are some curious implications from this. Suppose the only investments available are A and C above and the two scenarios are:

Scenario	Probability	Payoff from A	Payoff from C
1	0.8	1.0	1.2
2	0.2	1.5	0.7

If we wish to maximize the minimum possible wealth, the probability of a scenario does not matter, as long as the probability is positive. Thus, the following LP is appropriate:

```
MAX       WMIN
   SUBJECT TO
 !  Initial budget constraint;
        2)    A + C =    1
 !  Wealth under scenario 1;
        3)  - WMIN + A + 1.2 C >=   0
 !  Wealth under scenario 2;
        4)  - WMIN + 1.5 A + 0.7 C >=   0
   END
```

The solution is:

```
OBJECTIVE FUNCTION VALUE
        1)              1.100000

    VARIABLE          VALUE          REDUCED COST
        WMIN          1.100000         0.000000
           A          0.500000         0.000000
           C          0.500000         0.000000

     ROW    SLACK OR SURPLUS         DUAL PRICES
        2)          0.000000           1.100000
        3)          0.000000          -0.800000
        4)          0.000000          -0.200000
```

Given that both investments have an expected return of 10%, it is not surprising that the expected growth factor is 1.10, that is, a return of 10%. The possibly surprising thing is that there is no risk. Regardless of which scenario occurs, the $1 initial investment will grow to $1.10 if 50 cents is placed in each of A and C.

Now suppose an extremely reliable friend provides us with the interesting news that "if scenario 1 occurs, investment C will payoff 1.3 rather than 1.2." This is certainly good news. The expected return for C has just gone up, and its downside risk has certainly not gotten worse. How should we react to it? We make the obvious modification in our model:

```
    MAX    WMIN
    SUBJECT TO
!  Initial budget constraint;
        2)    A + C =      1
!  Wealth under scenario 1;
        3) - WMIN + A + 1.3 C >=    0
!  Wealth under scenario 2;
        4) - WMIN + 1.5 A + 0.7 C >=    0
    END
```

and re-solve it to find:

```
OBJECTIVE FUNCTION VALUE
        1)              1.136364

    VARIABLE          VALUE          REDUCED COST
        WMIN          1.136364         0.000000
           A          0.545455         0.000000
           C          0.454545         0.000000

     ROW    SLACK OR SURPLUS         DUAL PRICES
        2)          0.000000           1.136364
        3)          0.000000          -0.727273
        4)          0.000000          -0.272727
```

This is a bit curious. We have decreased our investment in C. This is as if our friend had continued on: "I have this very favorable news regarding stock C; let's sell it before the market has a chance to react." Why the anomaly? The problem is that we are basing our measure of goodness on a single point among the possible payoffs, in this case, the worst possible. For a further discussion of these issues, see Clyman (1995).

13.7 Scenario Model and Minimizing Downside Risk

Minimizing the variance in return is appropriate if either: (1) the actual return is Normal distributed, or (2) the portfolio owner has a quadratic utility function. In practice, it is difficult to show that either condition holds. Thus, it may be of interest to use a more intuitive measure of risk. One such measure is the downside risk, which intuitively is the expected amount by which the return is less than a specified target return. The approach can be described if we define:

T = user specified target threshold. Typically, less than the maximum expected return when risk is disregarded, and greater than the return under the worst scenario, when risk is disregarded.

Y_s = max $\{0, T - \Sigma X_i u_{is}\}$

= amount by which the return under scenario s falls short of target.

The model in algebraic form is then:

Min $\Sigma P_s Y_s$ Minimize expected downside risk

s.t.

(compute deviation below target of each scenario, s):

$Y_s - T + \Sigma X_i u_{is} \geq 0$

$\Sigma X_i = 1$ (budget constraint)

$\Sigma X_i \Sigma P_s u_{is} \geq r$ (desired return).

Notice that this is just a linear program.

13.7.1 Semivariance and Downside Risk

Another common alternative suggested to variance as a measure of risk is semivariance. It is essentially variance, except that only deviations below the mean are counted as risk. The scenario model is well suited to such measures. The previous scenario model needs only a slight modification to convert it to a semivariance model. The Y variables are redefined to measure the deviation below the mean only, zero otherwise.

The resulting model is:

```
! Minimize the semivariance
! The MIN row simply gives the order of the
! primal variables . . . ;
  MIN Y1 + Y2 + Y3 + Y4  + Y5  + Y6
    + Y7 + Y8 + Y9 + Y10 + Y11 + Y12
    + ATT + GMC + USX + MEAN
! and the dual/price variables;
    + PS1 + PS2 + PS3 + PS4  + PS5  + PS6
    + PS7 + PS8 + PS9 + PS10 + PS11 + PS12
```

```
    + PBUD + PDEF + PRET
  Subject to
! The first order conditions on the Y's
 FY1)  .1666666 Y1 - PS1 >= 0
 FY2)  .1666666 Y2 - PS2 >= 0
 FY3)  .1666666 Y3 - PS3 >= 0
 FY4)  .1666666 Y4 - PS4 >= 0
 FY5)  .1666666 Y5 - PS5 >= 0
 FY6)  .1666666 Y6 - PS6 >= 0
 FY7)  .1666666 Y7 - PS7 >= 0
 FY8)  .1666666 Y8 - PS8 >= 0
 FY9)  .1666666 Y9 - PS9 >= 0
 FY10) .1666666 Y10 - PS10 >= 0
 FY11) .1666666 Y11 - PS11 >= 0
 FY12) .1666666 Y12 - PS12 >= 0
! First order conditions on the investments;
 FATT) - 1.3 PS1 - 1.103 PS2 - 1.216 PS3 - 0.954 PS4
         - 0.929 PS5 - 1.056 PS6 - 1.038 PS7 - 1.089 PS8
         - 1.09 PS9 - 1.083 PS10 - 1.035 PS11 - 1.176 PS12
         + PBUD + 1.089083 PDEF >= 0
 FGMC) - 1.225 PS1 - 1.29 PS2 - 1.216 PS3 - 0.728 PS4
         - 1.144 PS5 - 1.107 PS6 - 1.321 PS7 - 1.305 PS8
         - 1.195 PS9 - 1.39 PS10 - 0.928 PS11 - 1.715 PS12
         + PBUD  + 1.213667 PDEF >= 0
 FUSX - 1.149 PS1 - 1.26 PS2 - 1.419 PS - 0.922 PS4
         - 1.169 PS5 - 0.965 PS6 - 1.133 PS7 - 1.732 PS8
         - 1.021 PS9 - 1.131 PS10 - 1.006 PS11 - 1.908 PS12
         + PBUD + 1.234583 PDEF >= 0
! First order conditions on the mean;
 FMEAN) + PS1  + PS2  + PS3  + PS4 + PS5 + PS6 + PS7 + PS8
         + PS9  + PS10 + PS11 + PS12 - PDEF - PRET >= 0
! Here are the real constraints, compute Y, the deviation
  below target, for each scenario;
 S1)   Y1 + 1.3   ATT + 1.225 GMC + 1.149 USX - MEAN >= 0
 S2)   Y2 + 1.103 ATT + 1.29  GMC + 1.26  USX - MEAN >= 0
 S3)   Y3 + 1.216 ATT + 1.216 GMC + 1.419 USX - MEAN >= 0
 S4)   Y4 + 0.954 ATT + 0.728 GMC + 0.922 USX - MEAN >= 0
 S5)   Y5 + 0.929 ATT + 1.144 GMC + 1.169 USX - MEAN >= 0
 S6)   Y6 + 1.056 ATT + 1.107 GMC + 0.965 USX - MEAN >= 0
 S7)   Y7 + 1.038 ATT + 1.321 GMC + 1.133 USX - MEAN >= 0
 S8)   Y8 + 1.089 ATT + 1.305 GMC + 1.732 USX - MEAN >= 0
 S9)   Y9 + 1.09  ATT + 1.195 GMC + 1.021 USX - MEAN >= 0
 S10) Y10 + 1.083 ATT + 1.39  GMC + 1.131 USX - MEAN >= 0
 S11) Y11 + 1.035 ATT + 0.928 GMC + 1.006 USX - MEAN >= 0
 S12) Y12 + 1.176 ATT + 1.715 GMC + 1.908 USX - MEAN >= 0
! The Budget constraint;
BUD) ATT + GMC + USX = 1
! compute the mean;
 DEF) 1.089083 ATT + 1.213667 GMC + 1.234583 USX - MEAN = 0
! The target Return constraint;
RET) MEAN >= 1.15
END
! Tell LINDO that this is a quadratic problem with
!  first real constraint being row 18;
QCP 18
```

The resulting solution is:

```
          OBJECTIVE FUNCTION VALUE

     1)        0.8917106E-02

    VARIABLE           VALUE        REDUCED COST
        Y1          0.000000          0.000000
        Y2          0.000000          0.000000
        Y3          0.000000          0.000000
        Y4          0.217060          0.000000
        Y5          0.120152          0.000000
        Y6          0.127125          0.000000
        Y7          0.064445          0.000000
        Y8          0.000000          0.000000
        Y9          0.082557          0.000000
       Y10          0.036644          0.000000
       Y11          0.130312          0.000000
       Y12          0.000000          0.000000
       ATT          0.575780          0.000000
       GMC          0.038585          0.000000
       USX          0.385635          0.000000
      MEAN          1.150000          0.000000
       PS1          0.000000          0.088875
       PS2          0.000000          0.020760
       PS3          0.000000          0.144284
       PS4          0.036177          0.000000
       PS5          0.020025          0.000000
       PS6          0.021187          0.000000
       PS7          0.010741          0.000000
       PS8          0.000000          0.195298
       PS9          0.013760          0.000000
      PS10          0.006107          0.000000
      PS11          0.021719          0.000000
      PS12          0.000000          0.329082
      PBUD          0.119842          0.000000
      PDEF          0.009997          0.000000
      PRET          0.119718          0.000000
```

Notice that the objective value is less than half that of the variance model. We would expect it to be at most half, because it considers only the down, not the up deviations. The most noticeable change in the portfolio is that substantial funds have been moved to USX from GMC. This is not surprising if you look at the original data. In the years in which ATT performs poorly, USX tends to perform better than GMC.

13.7.2 Scenarios Based Directly Upon a Covariance Matrix

If only a covariance matrix is available, rather than original data, it is nevertheless possible to construct scenarios that match the covariance matrix. The following example uses just four scenarios to represent the possible returns that might be obtained from the three assets: ATT, GMC, and USX. These scenarios have been constructed so that they mimic behavior consistent with the original covariance matrix.

```
MIN   Y1 + Y2 + Y3 + Y4 + ATT + GMC + USX + MEAN
    + PS1 + PS2 + PS3 + PS4 + PBUD + PDEF + PRET
SUBJECT TO
! The first order conditions on the Y's
  FY1)   0.5 Y1 + PS1 = 0
  FY2)   0.5 Y2 + PS2 = 0
  FY3)   0.5 Y3 + PS3 = 0
  FY4)   0.5 Y4 + PS4 = 0
! First order conditions on the investments
  FATT) - 0.9851237 PS1 - 1.193042 PS2 - 0.9851237 PS3
        - 1.193042 PS4 + PBUD + 1.089083 PDEF >= 0
  FGMC) - 1.304437 PS1 - 1.543131 PS2 - 0.8842088 PS3
        - 1.122902 PS4 + PBUD + 1.213667 PDEF >= 0
  FUSX) - 1.097669 PS1 - 1.756196 PS2 - 1.119948 PS3
        - 0.9645076 PS4 + PBUD + 1.234583 PDEF >= 0
! First order conditions on the mean;
  FMEAN) PS1 + PS2 + PS3 + PS4 - PDEF - PRET >=   0
! Here are the real constraints;
!  Compute the return under each of 4 scenarios;
    S1) Y1 - 0.9851237 ATT - 1.304437 GMC - 1.097669 USX
        + MEAN = 0
    S2) Y2 - 1.193042 ATT - 1.543131 GMC - 1.756196 USX
        + MEAN = 0
    S3) Y3 - 0.9851237 ATT - 0.8842088 GMC - 1.119948 USX
        + MEAN = 0
    S4) Y4 - 1.193042 ATT - 1.122902 GMC - 0.9645076 USX
        + MEAN = 0

! The Budget constraint;
    BUD)   ATT + GMC + USX = 1
! Define or compute the mean;
    DEF) 1.089083 ATT + 1.213667 GMC + 1.234583 USX
        - MEAN = 0
! Target return;
      RET)   MEAN >=   1.15
  END
! The first real constraint starts with row 10;
  QCP=   10
```

When solved, we get the familiar solution:

```
      OBJECTIVE FUNCTION VALUE

      1)      0.2241380E-01

  VARIABLE          VALUE         REDUCED COST
       Y1        -0.038296           0.000000
       Y2         0.231734           0.000000
       Y3        -0.185541           0.000000
       Y4        -0.007894           0.000000
      ATT         0.530091           0.000000
      GMC         0.356412           0.000000
      USX         0.113497           0.000000
     MEAN         1.150000           0.000000
      PS1         0.019148           0.000000
      PS2        -0.115867           0.000000
      PS3         0.092771           0.000000
```

```
         PS4          0.003947          0.000000
        PBUD          0.362138          0.000000
        PDEF         -0.353885          0.000000
        PRET          0.353883          0.000000

         ROW    SLACK OR SURPLUS      DUAL PRICES
        FCY1)          0.000000         -0.038296
        FCY2)          0.000000          0.231734
        FCY3)          0.000000         -0.185541
        FCY4)          0.000000         -0.007894
        FATT)          0.000000         -0.530091
        FGMC)          0.000000         -0.356412
        FUSX)          0.000000         -0.113497
       FMEAN)          0.000000         -1.150000
          S1)          0.000000          0.019148
          S2)          0.000000         -0.115867
          S3)          0.000000          0.092771
          S4)          0.000000          0.003947
         BUD)          0.000000          0.362138
         DEF)          0.000000         -0.353885
         RET)          0.000000         -0.353883

   NO. ITERATIONS=         16
```

Notice that the objective function value and the allocation of funds over ATT, GMC, and USX are essentially identical to those of our original portfolio example. For a discussion of how to generate scenarios that exactly match a given set of covariances, see Chapter 10.

13.8 Hedging, Matching, and Program Trading

13.8.1 Portfolio Hedging

Given a "benchmark" portfolio B, we say that we hedge B if we construct another portfolio C such that taken together B and C have essentially the same return as B but lower risk than B. Typically, our portfolio B contains certain components that cannot be removed; thus, we want to buy some components that are negatively correlated with the existing ones. Examples are: (a) An airline knows that it will have to purchase a lot of fuel in the next three months; it would like to be insulated from unexpected fuel price increases. (b) A farmer is confident that his fields will yield $200,000 worth of corn in the next two months. He is happy with the current price for corn and thus would like to "lock in" the current price.

13.8.2 Portfolio Matching, Tracking, and Program Trading

Given a benchmark portfolio B, we say we construct a matching or tracking portfolio if we construct a new portfolio C that has stochastic behavior very similar to B but excluding certain instruments that are in B. Example situations are: (a) A portfolio manager does not wish to look bad relative to some well-known index of performance such as the S&P 500 but for various reasons cannot purchase certain of the instruments in the index. (b) An arbitrager with the ability to make fast, low-cost trades wants to exploit market inefficiencies, i.e., instruments mispriced by the market. If he can construct a portfolio that perfectly matches the future behavior of the well-defined portfolio, but costs less today, he has an arbitrage profit opportunity if he can act before this "mispricing" disappears. (c) A retired person is concerned mainly about inflation risk; thus, a portfolio that tracks inflation is desired. As an example of (a), a certain so-called "green" mutual fund will not include in its portfolio companies which derive more than 2% of their gross revenues from the sale of military weapons, or own directly or operate nuclear power plants, or participate in business related to the nuclear fuel cycle.

The following table, for example, compares the performance of six Vanguard portfolios with the indices the portfolios were designed to track; see Vanguard (1995).

Total Return
Six Months Ended June 30, 1995

Vanguard Portfolio Name	Portfolio Growth	Comparative Growth Index	Index Name
500 Portfolio	+20.1%	+20.2%	S&P 500
Growth Portfolio	+21.1	+21.2	S&P 500/BARRA Growth
Value Portfolio	+19.1	+19.2	S&P 500/BARRA Value
Extended Market Portfolio	+17.1%	+16.8%	Wilshire 4500 Index
SmallCap Portfolio	+14.5	+14.4	Russell 2000 Index
Total Stock Market Portfolio	+19.2%	+19.2%	Wilshire 5000 Index

Notice that even though there is substantial difference in the performance of the portfolios, each matches its benchmark index quite well.

13.9 Methods for Constructing Benchmark Portfolios

A variety of approaches have been used for constructing hedging and matching portfolios. For matching portfolios, an intuitive approach has been to generalize the Markowitz model so that the objective is to minimize the variance in the difference in return between the target portfolio and the tracking portfolio. The approach below, in contrast, is based on the idea of scenarios.

13.9.1 A Downside Risk Version of the Portfolio Matching/Hedging Problem

Key objects are: (a) scenarios or possible outcomes, and (b) instruments, such as stocks, bonds, options, and futures contracts, that we can purchase.

Scenarios may correspond to interest changes, election outcomes, inflation, weather, etc.

13.9.2 Parameters

P_s = Prob {scenario s occurs},
v_j = initial cost per unit of instrument j,
u_{js} = end-of-period value per unit of instrument j if the scenario is s,
T_s = target value for the portfolio if scenario s occurs,
U_o = initial budget,
U_e = desired expected value of portfolio at end of period.

13.9.3 Variables

x_j = units of instrument j to purchase; because of transaction costs it may be worthwhile to distinguish between buying and short selling,
R_s = value of portfolio if scenario s occurs,
D_s = deviation below target if scenario s occurs.

The standard downside risk linear model is:

Minimize risk

$$(1) \quad \text{Min} \ \sum_s p_s D_s$$

subject to:

Initial budget:

$$(2) \quad \sum_j v_j x_j = U_o$$

Compute value under scenario s:

$$(3) \quad R_s = \sum_j v_{js} x_j$$

Desired expected ending value:

$$(4) \quad \sum_s p_s R_s \geq U_e$$

Measure downside risk:

$$(5) \quad D_s \geq T_s - R_s$$

The objective (1) ensures that the constructed portfolio C does not differ any more than necessary from portfolio B with regard to return. Other attributes of the constructed portfolio might be constrained similarly. For example, the duration or convexity of the target portfolio might be constrained to be similar to the duration and convexity of the benchmark portfolio B.

For simplicity, we have used a linear objective. If we wish to penalize large unfavorable deviations from target, we could use the quadratic objective:

$$\text{Min} \ \sum_s p_s D_s^2$$

This is substantially more difficult to solve than the linear case.

13.9.4 Hedging, Matching, and Program Trading: Setting Scenario Targets

Given an existing portfolio B, we (a) *hedge B* if we find another portfolio that is highly negatively correlated with B; (b) *match B* if we find another portfolio that is highly positively correlated with B.

More specifically:

Let N_s = value of our existing portfolio B if scenario s holds. Then, loosely speaking:

To construct a hedging portfolio, we set

$$T_s = -N_s.$$

To construct a matching portfolio, we set

$$T_s = N_s.$$

13.9.5 Efficient Benchmark Portfolios

We say a portfolio is on the efficient frontier if there is no other portfolio that has both higher expected return and lower risk.

Let:

r_i = expected return on asset i,
t = an arbitrary target return for the portfolio.

A portfolio, with weight m_i on asset i, is efficient if there exists some target t for which the portfolio is a solution to the problem:

Minimize risk
subject to

$$\sum_{i=0}^{n} m_i = 1 \qquad \text{(budget constraint)}$$

$$\sum_{i=0}^{n} r_i m_i \geq t \qquad \text{(return target constraint)}.$$

Portfolio managers are frequently evaluated on their performance relative to some benchmark portfolio. Let b_i = the weight on asset i in the benchmark portfolio. If the benchmark portfolio is not on the efficient frontier, an interesting question is: What are the weights of the portfolio on the efficient frontier that is closest to the benchmark portfolio, in the sense that the risk of the efficient portfolio relative to the benchmark is minimized?

There is a particularly simple answer when the measure of risk is portfolio variance, there is a risk-free asset, borrowing is allowed at the risk-free rate, and short sales are permitted. Let m_o = the weight on the risk-free asset. An elegant result in this case is that there is a so-called "market" portfolio with weights m_i on asset i, such that effectively only m_o varies as the return target varies. Specifically, there are constants m_i, for $i = 1, 2, \ldots, n$, such that the weight on asset i is simply $(1 - m_o) \times m_i$.

Define:

$q = 1 - m_o$ = weight to put on the market portfolio,
R_i = random return on asset i.

Then the variance of any efficient portfolio relative to the benchmark portfolio can be written as:

$$\mathrm{var}\left(\sum_{i=1}^{n} R_i \left[qm_i - b_i \right] \right)$$

$$= \sum_{i=1}^{n} \left(qm_i - b_i \right)^2 \mathrm{var}\left(R_i \right) + 2 \sum_{j>i} \left(qm_i - b_i \right)\left(qm_j - b_j \right) \mathrm{Cov}\left(R_i, R_j \right)$$

Setting the derivative of this expression with respect to q equal to zero gives the result:

$$q = \frac{\displaystyle\sum_{i=1}^{n} m_i b_i \, \mathrm{var}\left(R_i \right) + \sum_{j>i} \left(m_i b_j + m_j b_i \right) \mathrm{Cov}\left(R_i, R_j \right)}{\displaystyle\sum_{i=1}^{n} m_i^2 \, \mathrm{var}\left(R_i \right) + 2 \sum_{j>i} m_i m_j \, \mathrm{Cov}\left(R_i, R_j \right)}$$

For example, if the benchmark portfolio is on the efficient frontier with weight b_o on the risk-free asset, $b_i = (1 - b_o)m_i$ and, therefore, $q = 1 - b_o$.

Thus, a manager who is told to outperform the benchmark portfolio $\{b_o, b_1, \ldots b_n\}$ should perhaps in fact be compensated according to his performance relative to the efficient portfolio given by q above.

13.10 Quadratic Programming Applied to Simultaneous Price/Production Decisions

A firm that has the choice of setting either price or quantity for its products may wish to set them simultaneously. If the production process can be modeled as a linear program and the demand curves are linear, the problem of simultaneously setting price and production is a quadratic program. The following example illustrates.

A firm produces and sells two products A and B at price P_A and P_B and in quantities X_A and X_B. Profit-maximizing values for P_A, P_B, X_A, and X_B are to be determined. The quantities (sold) are related to the prices by the demand curves:

$$X_A = 60 - 21\, P_A + 0.1\, P_B$$
$$X_B = 50 - 25\, P_B + 0.1\, P_A$$

Notice that the two products are mild substitutes. As the price of one is raised, it causes a modest increase in the demand for the other item.

The production side has the following features:

	A	B
Variable Cost per Unit	$0.20	$0.30
Production Capacity	25	30

Further, the total production is limited by the constraint:

$$X_A + 2X_B \leq 50.$$

The problem can be written as:

$$\begin{aligned}
\text{Minimize} \quad &-(P_A - 0.20)X_A - (P_B - 0.30)X_B \\
\text{subject to} \quad &X_A + 21P_A - 0.1P_B = 60 \qquad \text{(Demand curve definition)} \\
&X_B + 25P_B - 0.1P_A = 50 \\
&\qquad\qquad\quad X_A \leq 25 \qquad \text{(Supply restrictions)} \\
&\qquad\qquad\quad X_B \leq 30 \\
&\qquad X_A + 2X_B \leq 50
\end{aligned}$$

Notice that the objective function is quadratic, rather than linear, because it contains product terms such as $P_A \times X_A$. Also note that we have written it in minimization form.

The problem must be converted to linear form by writing the first-order conditions for all the variables. To do this, we must introduce dual variables for each of the constraints. We shall associate the dual variables D_A, D_B, C_A, C_B, and C_{AB} with the five original constraints of the model. When we write the first-order conditions for the four decision variables, we have a total of nine constraints.

The complete formulation in LINDO style is:

```
MIN        XA + XB + PA + PB + DA + DB + CA + CB + CAB
SUBJECT TO
    2)    -PA + DA + CA +   CAB >= -0.2
    3)    -PB + DB + CB + 2CAB >= -0.3
    4)    -XA + 21 DA -  0.1 DB >= 0
    5)    -XB + 25 DB -  0.1 DA >= 0
    6)     XA + 21 PA -  0.1 PB = 60
    7)     XB -  0.1 PA + 25 PB = 50
    8)     XA <= 25
    9)     XB <= 30
   10)     XA + 2 XB <= 50
END
QCP 6
```

The solution is:

```
              OBJECTIVE FUNCTION VALUE
      1)         -51.9510580

   VARIABLE          VALUE          REDUCED COST
      XA          24.390556           0.000000
      XB          12.804722           0.000000
      PA           1.702805           0.000000
      PB           1.494622           0.000000
      DA           1.163916           0.000000
      DB           0.516845           0.000000
      CA           0.000000           0.609444
      CB           0.000000           7.195278
      CAB          0.338889           0.000000
```

Note that it is the joint capacity constraint $X_A + 2X_B \leq 50$ that is binding. The total profit contribution is \$51.951058.

13.11 Least Squares Regression

Suppose we are given the following observations:

Observation	X_{i0}	X_{i1}	X_{i2}	Y_i
1	1	2	6	8
2	1	3	9	14
3	1	5	7	12
4	1	7	8	17
5	1	8	10	18

We wish to explain or predict Y_i in terms of X_{i0}, X_{i1} and X_{i2}. Notice that the column 0 is a constant column of 1's. A common way of doing this is via least squares regression.

The form of the explanatory equation is:

$$Y_i = B_0 X_{i0} + B_1 X_{i1} + B_2 X_{i2} + e_i$$

where e_i is the error in explaining observation Y_i. Because $X_{i0} = 1$ for every observation i, this equation is equivalent to $Y_i = B_0 X_{i0} + B_1 X_{i_} + B_2 X_{i2} + e_i$. Least squares regression chooses B_0, B_1, and B_2 so as to minimize the sum of the squared errors, i.e., $\Sigma^5_{i=1} e_i^2$.

We can rewrite this as

$$\text{Min} \; \sum_{i=1}^{5} \left(Y_i - B_0 X_{i0} - B_1 X_{i1} - B_2 X_{i2} \right)^2$$

It is convenient to divide by 2 times the number of observations and rewrite as:

$$\text{Min} \; \sum_{i=1}^{5} \left[\left(Y_i - B_0 X_{i0} - B_1 X_{i1} - B_2 X_{i2} \right) \right]^2 / 10$$

$$= \sum_{i=1}^{5} \left[Y_i^2 - 2Y_i \left(B_0 X_{i0} + B_1 X_{i1} + B_2 X_{i2} \right) + \left(B_0 X_{i0} + B_1 X_{i1} + B_2 X_{i2} \right)^2 \right] /$$

The term $\sum_{i=1}^{5} Y_i^2$ is a constant and can be disregarded.

Taking derivatives with respect to B_0, B_1, and B_2 gives the first-order conditions:

$$\sum_{i=1}^{5} \left[\left(B_0 X_{i0} + B_1 X_{i1} + B_2 X_{i2} \right) X_{i0} \right] / 5 = \sum_{i=1}^{5} Y_i X_{i0} / 5$$

$$\sum_{i=1}^{5} \left[\left(B_0 X_{i0} + B_1 X_{i1} + B_2 X_{i2} \right) X_{i1} \right] / 5 = \sum_{i=1}^{5} Y_i X_{i1} / 5$$

$$\sum_{i=1}^{5} \left[\left(B_0 X_{i0} + B_1 X_{i1} + B_2 X_{i2} \right) X_{i2} \right] / 5 = \sum_{i=1}^{5} Y_i X_{i2} / 5$$

Thus we are interested in means of cross products of the form $\sum_i X_{ij} X_{ik}/5$ and $\sum_i X_{ij} Y_i/5$. These are tabulated below for our example:

	$\bar{X}_0$	$\bar{X}_1$	$\bar{X}_2$	$\bar{Y}$
$\bar{X}_0$	1	5	8	13.8
$\bar{X}_1$	5	30.2	42	76.2
$\bar{X}_2$	8	42	66	114.8
$\bar{Y}$	13.8	76.2	114.8	203.4

The problem can now be written in LINDO format as:

```
MIN      B0 + B1 + B2
  SUBJECT TO
     B0 +  5 B1 +  8 B2 = 13.8
   5 B0 + 30.2 B1 + 42 B2 = 7612
   8 B0 + 42 B1 + 66 B2 = 114.8
  END
  QCP
  ROW OF FIRST CONSTRAINT =
  5
```

Note that row 1, MIN B0 + B1 + B2, simply provides the ordering of the variables. Rows 2, 3, and 4 describe the first-order conditions. Because there are no real constraints, the QCP command specifies a row number one more than the total number of rows. When the problem is solved, we get the following:

```
            QP OPTIMUM FOUND AT STEP     4

            OBJECTIVE FUNCTION VALUE

  1)              -101.285000

          VARIABLE           VALUE           REDUCED COST
             B0            -1.175000             0.000000
             B1             0.875000             0.000000
             B2             1.325000             0.000000

          ROW         SLACK OR SURPLUS        DUAL PRICES
             2)            0.000000             -1.175000
             3)            0.000000              0.875000
             4)            0.000000              1.325000
```

The proposed form of the regression equation is:

$$Y_i = -1.175 + 0.875 X_{i1} + 1.325 X_{i2}.$$

Recall that, on the way to developing the formulation, we divided the objective by two times the number of observations and subtracted the term

$$\sum_{i=1}^{5} Y_i^2.$$

Undoing these actions, we find the sum of squares as

$$(-101.285 \times 10) + 203.4 \times 5 = 4.15.$$

Thus far, all we have done is conventional least squares regression, and quadratic programming was unneeded.

13.11.1 Constrained Least Squares

When using regression, one frequently encounters results where some of the coefficients in the regression equation seem obviously wrong; e.g., the formula might predict that lowering the price of a product lowers the demand for the product. So one might want to do a constrained regression in which this coefficient is constrained to be nonnegative, say. Forecasters in the retail food industry have commented that using quadratic programming to do constrained least squares leads to about a 2% improvement in forecasting accuracy. We will illustrate constrained regression using the previous example.

Now suppose we have some additional information that causes us to require

$$B_0 + B_1 + B_2 > 1.5.$$

A dual variable, SIDEC, associated with this constraint must be added to the formulation. The new formulation is:

```
MIN      B0 + B1 + B2 + SIDEC
SUBJECT TO
     2)   B0 + 5 B1 + 8 B2 - SIDEC = 13.8
     3)   5 B0 + 30.2 B1 + 42 B2 - SIDEC = 13.8
     4)   8 B0 + 42 B1 + 66 B2 - SIDEC = 114.8
     5)   B0 + B1 + B2 >= 1.5
END
QCP 5
```

The solution is:

```
           OBJECTIVE FUNCTION VALUE

       1)             -101.281015

   VARIABLE           VALUE            REDUCED COST
      B0              -0.641280           0.000000
      B1               0.890728           0.000000
      B2               1.250552           0.000000
      SIDEC            0.016777           0.000000

    ROW          SLACK OR SURPLUS      DUAL PRICES
       2)             0.000000           -0.641280
       3)             0.000000            0.890728
       4)             0.000000            1.250552
       5)             0.000000           -0.016777

   NO. ITERATIONS = 5
```

The sum of squares has increased to

$$101.28105 \times 10 + 203.4 \times 5 = 4.18985.$$

13.12 Two-Person Nonconstant-Sum Games

There are many situations where the welfare, utility, or profit of one person depends not only on his decisions but on the decisions of others. A two-person game is a special case of the above in which (1) there are exactly two players/decision makers, (2) each must make one decision, (3) in ignorance of the other's decision, and (4) the loss incurred by each is a function of both decisions. A two-person constant-sum game (frequently more narrowly called a zero sum game) is the special case of the above where (4a) the losses to both are in the same commodity, e.g., dollars, and (4b) the total loss is a constant independent of players' decisions. Thus, in a constant-sum game, the sole effect of the decisions is to determine how a "constant-sized pie" is allocated. Ordinary linear programming can be used to solve two-person constant-sum games. When (1), (2), and (3) apply but (4b) does not, we have a two-person nonconstant-sum game. Ordinary linear programming cannot be used to solve these games; however, the algorithm commonly applied to quadratic programs does apply. Sometimes a two-person nonconstant-sum game is also called a bimatrix game.

As an example, consider two firms, each of which is about to introduce an improved version of an already popular consumer product. The versions are very similar, so one firm's profit is very much affected by its own advertising decision as well as the decision of its competitor. The major decision for each firm is presumed to be simply the level of advertising. Suppose that the losses (in millions of dollars) as a function of decision are given by Figure 13.3. The example illustrates that each player need not have exactly the same kinds of alternatives.

Negative losses correspond to profits.

13.12.1 Prisoner's Dilemma

This cost matrix has the so-called prisoner's dilemma cost structure. This name arises from a setting in which there are two criminal accomplices in jail. If neither prisoner cooperates with the authorities (thus the two cooperate), both will receive a medium punishment. If one of them provides evidence against the other, the other will get severe punishment, whereas the one who provides evidence will get light punishment, *if the other does not provide evidence against the first*. If each provides evidence against the other, they both receive severe punishment. Clearly the best thing for the two as a group is for the two to cooperate with each other. However, individually there is a strong temptation to defect.

The same situation exists with our two firms. For example, if A does not advertise but B does, A makes 1 million and B makes 5 million of profit. Total profit would be maximized if neither advertised; however, if either knew that the other would not advertise, the one who thought he had such clairvoyance would have a temptation to advertise.

Later, it will be useful to have a loss table with all entries strictly positive. The relative attractiveness of an alternative is not affected if the same constant is added to all entries. Figure 13.4 was obtained by adding $+6$ to every entry in Figure 13.3.

We will henceforth work with the data in Figure 13.4.

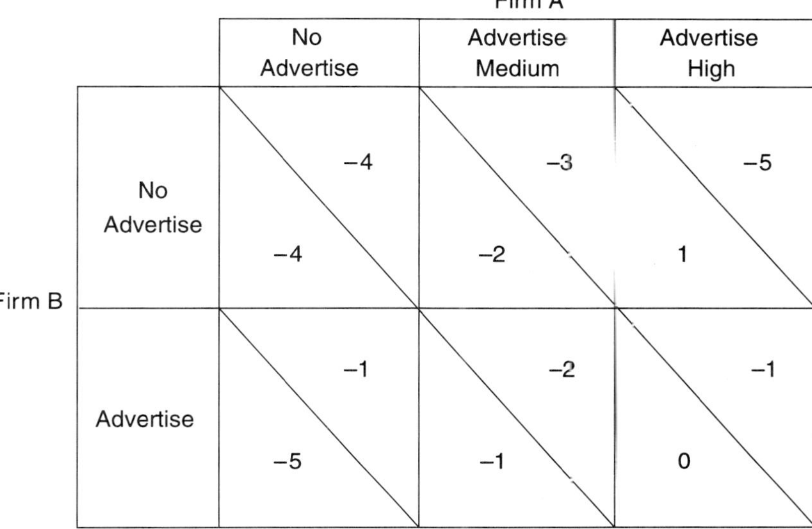

Figure 13.3
Two-Person
Nonconstant-
Sum Game

Figure 13.4
Two-Person
Nonconstant-
Sum Game

13.12.2 Choosing a Strategy

Our example problem illustrates that we might wish our own choice to be (i) somewhat unpredictable by our competitor and (ii) robust in the sense that, regardless of how unpredictable our competitor is, our expected profit is high. Thus, we are lead to the idea of a random strategy. By making our decision random, e.g., by flipping a coin, we tend to satisfy (i). By biasing the coin appropriately we tend to satisfy (ii).

For our example, define a_1, a_2, a_3 as the probability that A chooses the alternative "No advertise," "Advertise Medium," and "Advertise High," respectively. Similarly, b_1 and b_2 are the probabilities that B applies to alternatives "No Advertise" and "Advertise," respectively. How should firm A choose a_1, a_2, and a_3? How should firm B choose b_1 and b_2?

For a bimatrix game, it is difficult to define a solution that is simultaneously optimum for both. We can, however, define an equilibrium stable set of strategies. A stable solution has the feature that given B's choice for b_1 and b_2, A is not motivated to change his probabilities a_1, a_2, and a_3. Likewise, given a_1, a_2, and a_3, B is not motivated to change b_1 and b_2. There may be bimatrix games with several stable solutions.

What can we say beforehand about a strategy of A's that is stable? Some of the a_i's may be zero, whereas for others we may have $a_i > 0$. An important observation not immediately obvious is the following: The expected loss to A of choosing alternative i is the same over all i for which $a_i > 0$. If this were not true, A could reduce his overall expected loss by increasing the probability associated with the lower loss alternative. Denote the expected loss to A by v_A. Also, the fact that $a_i = 0$ must imply that the expected loss from choosing i is $> v_A$. These observations imply that, with regard to A's behavior, we must have:

$$2b_1 + 5b_2 \geq v_A \text{ (with equality if } a_1 > 0),$$
$$3b_1 + 4b_2 \geq v_A \text{ (with equality if } a_2 > 0),$$
$$b_1 + 5b_2 \geq v_A \text{ (with equality if } a_3 > 0).$$

Symmetric arguments for B imply:

$$2a_1 + 4a_2 + 7a_3 \geq v_B \text{ (with equality if } b_1 > 0),$$
$$a_1 + 5a_2 + 6a_3 \geq v_B \text{ (with equality if } b_2 > 0).$$

We also have the nonnegativity constraints

$$a_i \geq 0 \text{ and } b_1 \geq 0, \text{ for all alternatives } i.$$

Because the a_i and b_i are probabilities, we wish to add the constraints $a_1 + a_2 + a_3 = 1$ and $b_1 + b_2 = 1$. The above is what is known as a linear complementarity problem.

Formulated for the LINDO computer program, we have:

```
MIN       A1 + A2 + A3 + B1 + B2 + VA + VB
SUBJECT TO
    2)    2 B1 + 5 B2 - VA >= 0
    3)    3 B1 + 4 B2 - VA >= 0
    4)      B1 + 5 B2 - VA >= 0
    5)    2 A1 + 4 A2 + 7 A3 - VB >= 0
    6)      A1 + 5 A2 + 6 A3 - VB >= 0
    7)      A1 + A2 + A3 = 1
    8)      B1 + B2 = 1
END
QCP  9
```

As before, the objective row serves only to specify an order for the decision variables consistent with the constraint order. There are and can be no real constraints, only first-order conditions in a bimatrix game, so the QC? 9 indicates that the problem is a "quadratic/complementary pivoting" problem and that the first six rows specify the first-order condition.

When the problem is solved, we get the following:

```
VARIABLE         VALUE           REDUCED COST
   A1           0.000000          0.333333
   A2           0.500000          0.000000
   A3           0.500000          0.000000
   B1           0.333333          0.000000
   B2           0.666667          0.000000
   VA           3.666667          0.000000
   VB           5.500000          0.000000
```

The solution indicates that firm A should not use option 1 and should randomly choose with equal probability between options 2 and 3. Firm B should choose its option 2 twice as frequently as it chooses its option 1.

The objective function value, reduced costs, and dual prices can be disregarded. Using our original loss table, we can calculate the following:

Situation			Weighted Contribution to Total Loss of	
A	B	Probability	A	B
No Ads	No Ads	$0 \times 1/3$	0	0
No Ads	Ads	$0 \times 2/3$	0	0
Advertise Medium	No Ads	$1/2 \times 1/3$	$(1/6) \times (-3)$	$(1/6) \times (-2)$
Advertise Medium	Ads	$1/2 \times 2/3$	$(1/3) \times (-2)$	$(1/3) \times (-1)$
Advertise High	No Ads	$1/2 \times 1/3$	$(1/6) \times (-5)$	$(1/6) \times (1)$
Advertise	Ads	$1/2 \times 2/3$	$(1/3) \times (-1)$	$(1/3) \times (0)$
			-2.3333	-0.5

Thus, following the randomized strategy suggested, A would have an expected profit of 2.33 million, whereas B would have an expected profit of 0.5 million. Contrast this with the fact that if A and B cooperated, they could each have an expected profit of 4 million.

13.12.3 Bimatrix Games with Several Solutions

When a nonconstant sum game has several stable solutions, life gets more complicated. The essential observation is that we must look outside our narrow definition of "stable solution" to decide which of the stable solutions, if any, would be selected in reality.

Consider the following two-person nonconstant-sum game:

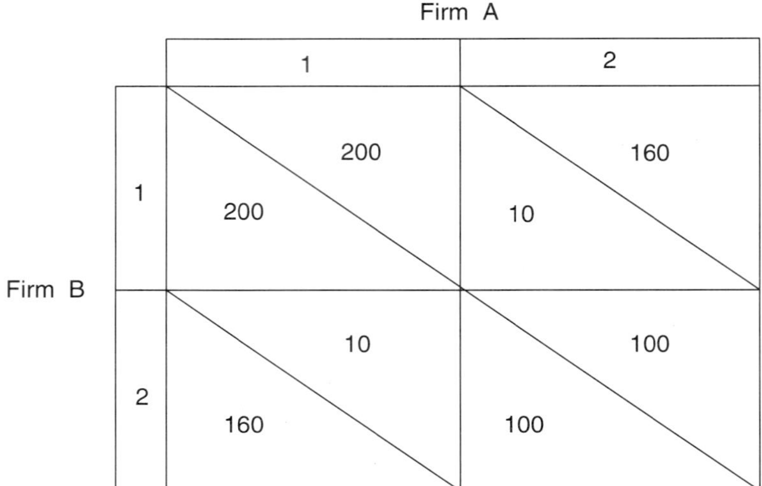

As before, the numbers represent losses.

First, observe that one solution is stable according to our definition: (I) Firm *A* always chooses option 1, and Firm *B* always chooses option 2. Firm *A* is not motivated to switch to 2, because his losses would increase to 100 from 10. Similarly, *B* would not switch to 1 from 2, because his losses would increase to 200 from 160. The game is symmetric in the players, so similar arguments apply to the solution (II): *B* always chooses 1, and *A* always chooses 2.

Which solution would result in reality? It probably depends upon such things as the relative wealths of the two firms. Suppose (i) *A* is the wealthier firm, (ii) the game is repeated week after week, and (iii) currently the firms are using solution II. After some very elementary analysis, *A* concludes that it much prefers solution I. To move things in this direction, *A* switches to option 1. Now it becomes what applied mathematicians call a game of "chicken." Both players are taking punishment at the rate of 200 per week. Either player could improve his lot by $200 - 160 = 40$ by unilaterally switching to his option 2; however, his lot would be improved a lot more, i.e., $200 - 10 = 190$, if his opponent unilaterally switched. At this point, a rational *B* would probably take a glance at *A*'s balance sheet and decide that *B* switching to option 2 is not such a bad decision.

If it is not clear which firm is wealthier, the two firms may decide that a cooperative solution is best, e.g., alternate between solutions I and II on alternate weeks. At this point, however, federal antitrust authorities might express a keen interest in this bimatrix game.

We conclude that a "stable" solution is stable only in a local sense. When there are multiple stable solutions, we should really look at all of them and take into account other considerations in addition to the loss matrix.

13.13 PROBLEMS

Problem 1

You are considering three stocks, IBM, GM, and Georgia-Pacific (GP), for your stock portfolio. The covariance matrix of the yearly percentage returns on these stocks is estimated to be:

	IBM	*GM*	*GP*
IBM	10	2.5	1
GM	2.5	4	1.5
GP	1	1.5	9

Thus, if equal amounts were invested in each, the variance would be proportional to $10 + 4 + 9 + 2(2.5 + 1 + 1.5)$. The predicted yearly percentage returns for IBM, GM, and GP are 9, 6, and 5, respectively. Find a minimum variance portfolio of these three stocks for which the yearly return is at least 7, at most 80% of the portfolio is invested in IBM, and at least 10% is invested in GP.

Problem 2

Modify your formulation of problem 1 to incorporate the fact that your current portfolio is 50% IBM and 50% GP. Further, transactions costs on a buy or sell transaction are 1% of the amount traded.

Problem 3

The manager of an investment fund hypothesizes that three different scenarios might characterize the economy one year hence. These scenarios are denoted Green, Yellow, and Red, and subjective probabilities 0.7, 0.1, and 0.2 are associated with them. The manager wishes to decide how a model portfolio should be allocated among stocks, bonds, real estate, and gold in the face of these possible scenarios. His estimated returns in percent per year as a function of asset and scenario are given in the table below:

	Stocks	Bonds	Real Estate	Gold
Green	9	7	8	−2
Yellow	−1	5	10	12
Red	10	4	−1	15

Formulate and solve the asset allocation problem of minimizing the variance in return subject to having an expected return of at least 6.5.

Problem 4

Conglomerate Motors (CM) manufactures and sells three sizes of automobiles: Rambler, Mercury, and Cadillac. CM's operations research department has just completed an extensive market analysis. One of the results of that study is a set of demand curves for the three products. If sales are measured in thousands of cars and price/car is measured in thousands of dollars, the demand curves can be written as

$$Q_R = 1600 - 100P_R + 4P_M,$$
$$Q_M = 495 - 13P_M + 3P_R + P_C,$$
$$Q_C = 180 - 4P_C + 2P_M,$$

where Q_R = number of Ramblers sold in 1000s, P_R = the price of the Rambler in 1000s, etc.

Federal regulations regarding "fleet mileage" place a restriction on the mix of cars that CM may manufacture. Specifically, the average miles per gallon (mpg) taken over all cars manufactured must be greater than or equal to 24. The Rambler, Mercury, and Cadillac have mpg ratings of 29, 23, and 19, respectively. The average is based on the presumption that all cars are driven equal distance. CM has five plants. Plant D can manufacture only Ramblers. The variable cost/unit is $7000, and the plant has a capacity of 500,000 cars/year. Plant E can manufacture either Ramblers or Mercurys in any mix totaling no more than 100,000 cars/year. The variable cost of a car in this plant is $800 for a Rambler and $12,000 for a Mercury. Plant F can produce only Mercurys. It has a capacity of 200,000 cars per year, and the variable cost per car is $10,500. Plant G can produce either Mercurys or Cadillacs in any mix totaling no more than 50,000 cars/year. The variable costs of Mercurys and Cadillacs in this plant are $12,500 and $17,000 per car, respectively. Plant H can produce only Cadillacs. The variable cost per unit is $15,600. The yearly capacity is 50,000. How many cars of each type should CM produce? At what price should CM plan to sell each type?

Problem 5

Two not necessarily friendly nations, Blue and Gold, are contemplating their military options for the next few years. Each has three general options: Aggressive, Defensive, and Minimal. The losses to each as a function of option chosen are summarized in the following table.

Gold

Blue \ Gold		A	D	M
	A	11 / 10	8 / 4	−5 / 11
	D	5 / 3	6 / 4	5 / 1
	M	12 / −6	1 / 2	1 / 1

Find a strategy for each country which is stable in the game theory sense.

Problem 6

From time to time a department store will reallocate some space among its various departments. One simple approach is to approximate the average profit per square meter per year for a department as a linear function of the space allocated to the department. One then tries to find an allocation that maximizes the total profit. Suppose that we have a modest little store with but two departments: Odds and Ends. The managers of these departments were asked to each give two point estimates of the yearly profit per square meter as a function of the number of square meters allocated. These are shown below:

	Odds		Ends	
	Square Meters of Space	Profits Per Square Meter Per Year	Square Meters of Space	Profits Per Square Meter Per Year
min space	9	$12,000	12	$15,000
max space	50	$5,000	45	$4,000

There are a total of 65 square meters of space to be allocated. Further, each department will be allocated neither less than the minimum space shown for it in the above table nor more than the maximum space. It is assumed that between the minimum and maximum allocations the average profit/(square meter per year) is a linear function of space allocated.

(a) Formulate this allocation problem as a quadratic program.
(b) Solve it.
(c) Suppose that any space not allocated to Odds and Ends can be rented out for a constant $800/(square meter per year) of profit. Now what should be the allocation?
(d) How would you motivate managers to give accurate estimates of the numbers needed in the table above?

Problem 7

In each round of the game of Even/Odd, player A writes one of the numbers 2, 4, or 6, while player B writes one of the numbers 1, 3, or 5. Both players then reveal their selection. If the difference is greater than 1, the player with the lower number pays the other player the difference. If the difference is exactly 1, the player with the higher number pays the other player the sum of the two numbers.

(a) Write the loss matrix.
(b) Write the conditions for a stable solution.
(c) Is the implied solution likely to be good in the sense that globally optimizing players would in fact settle upon a solution satisfying the conditions in (b)?
(d) Which player seems to have the advantage?

Problem 8

Consider the ATT/GMC/USX portfolio problem discussed earlier. The desired or target rate of return in the solved model was 15%.

(a) Suppose we desire 16% rate of return. Using just the solution report, what can you predict about the standard deviation in portfolio return of the new portfolio?

(b) We illustrated the situation where the opportunity to invest money risk free at 5% per year became available. That is, this 4th option has zero variance and zero covariance. Now suppose the risk-free rate is 4% per year rather than 5%. As before, there is no limit on how much can be invested at 4%. Based on only the solution report available for the original version of the problem (where the desired rate of return is 15% per year), discuss whether this new option is attractive when the desired return for the portfolio is 15%.

(c) You have $100,000 to invest. What modifications would need to be made to the original ATT/GMC/USX model so that the answers in the solution report would come in the appropriate units, e.g., no multiplying of the numbers in the solution by 100,000, etc.

(d) What is the estimated standard deviation in the value of your end-of-period portfolio in (c) if invested as the solution recommends?

CHAPTER 14

Formulating and Solving Integer Programs

14.1 Introduction

In most applications of LP, one would really like the decision variables to be restricted to integer values. One is likely to tolerate a solution recommending that GM produce 1,524,328.37 Chevrolets. No one will mind if this recommendation is rounded up or down. If, however, a different study recommends that the optimum number of aircraft carriers to build is 1.37, a lot of people around the world will be very interested in how this number is rounded. It is clear that the validity and value of many LP models could be improved markedly if one could restrict selected decision variables to integer values.

All good commercial LP modeling systems are augmented with a capability that allows the user to restrict certain decision variables to integer values. The manner in which the user informs the program of this requirement varies from program to program. For example, in LINDO one way of indicating that variable X is to be restricted to integer values 0 or 1 is to type the command INTEGER X. The important point is that it is straightforward to specify this restriction. We shall see later that, even though easy to specify, sometimes it may be difficult to solve problems with this restriction. The methods for formulating and solving problems with integrality are called Integer Programming.

The integrality enforcing capability is perhaps more powerful than the reader at first realizes. A frequent use of an integer variable in a model is as a zero/one variable to represent a go/no-go decision. It is probably true that the majority of real-world integer programs are of the zero/one variety.

14.2 Computational Difficulty of Integer Programs

Integer programs can be very difficult to solve. This is in marked contrast to LP problems. The solution time for an LP is fairly predictable. For an LP, the time increases approximately proportionally with the number of variables and with the number of constraints squared. For a given IP problem, the time may in fact decrease as the number of constraints is increased. As the number of integer variables is increased, the solution time may increase dramatically. Some small IPs (e.g., 60 constraints, 60 variables) are extremely difficult to solve.

Just as with LPs, there may be alternate IP formulations of a given problem. With IPs, however, the solution time generally depends critically upon the formulation. Producing a good IP formulation requires skill. For many of the problems in the remainder of this chapter, the difference between a good formulation and a poor formulation may be the difference between whether the problem is solvable or not.

14.2.1 Types of Variables

One general classification is according to types of variables:

(a) *Pure vs. mixed.* In a pure integer program, all variables are restricted to integer values. In a mixed formulation, only certain of the variables are integer, whereas the rest are allowed to be continuous.

(b) *0/1 vs. general.* In many applications the only integer values allowed are 0/1; therefore, some integer programming codes assume that integer variables are restricted to the values 0 or 1.

14.3 Exploiting the IP Capability: Standard Applications

You will frequently encounter problems that are LPs with the exception of just a few combinatorial complications. Many of these complications are fairly standard. The next several sections describe many of the standard complications along with the methods for incorporating them into an IP formulation. Most of these complications only require the 0/1 capability rather than the general integer capability. Binary variables can be used to represent a wide variety of go/no-go, or make-or-buy decisions. In the latter use, they are sometimes referred to as "Hamlet" variables, as in: "To buy or not to buy, that is the question." Binary variables are sometimes also called Boolean variables in honor of the logician George Boole. He developed the rules of the special algebra, now known as Boolean algebra, for manipulating variables that can take on only two values. In Boole's case, the values were "True" and "False"; however, it is a minor conceptual leap to represent "True" by the value 1 and "False" by the value 0. The power of these methods developed by Boole is undoubtedly the genesis of the modern compliment: "Strong, like Boole."

14.3.1 Binary Representation of General Integer Variables

Some algorithms apply only to problems with only 0/1 integer variables. Conceptually, this is no limitation, as any general integer variable with a finite range can be represented by a set of 0/1 variables. For example, suppose X is restricted to the set $[0, 1, 2, \ldots, 15]$. Introduce the four 0/1 variables: y_1, y_2, y_3, and y_4. Replace every occurrence of X by $y_1 + 2 * y_2 + 4 * y_3 + 8 * y_4$. Note that every possible integer in $[0, 1, 2, \ldots, 15]$ can be represented by some setting of the values of y_1, y_2, y_3, and

y_4. Verify that, if the maximum value X can take on is 31, you will need 5 0/1 variables. If the maximum value is 63, you will need 6 0/1 variables. In fact, if you use k 0/1 variables, the maximum value that can be represented is 2^k-1. You can write: VMAX $= 2^k-1$. Taking logs, you can observe that the number of 0/1 variables required in this so-called binary expansion is approximately proportional to the log of the maximum value that X can take on.

Although this substitution is valid, it should be avoided if possible. Most integer programming algorithms are not very efficient when applied to models containing this substitution.

14.3.2 Minimum Batch Size Constraints

When there are substantial economies of scale in undertaking an activity regardless of its level, many decision makers will specify a minimum "batch" size for the activity. For example, a large brokerage firm may require that, if you buy any bonds from the firm, you must buy at least 100. A zero/one variable can enforce this restriction as follows. Let:

x = activity level to be determined, e.g., no. of bonds purchased,
y = a zero/one variable = 1, if and only if $x > 0$,
B = minimum batch size for x, e.g., 100, and
U = known upper limit on the value of x.

The following two constraints enforce the minimum batch size condition:

$$x \le Uy$$
$$By \le x$$

If $y = 0$, the first constraint forces $x = 0$, whereas if $y = 1$, the second constraint forces x to be at least B. Thus, y acts as a switch that forces x to be either 0 or greater than B. The constant U should be chosen with care. For reasons of computational efficiency, it should be as small as validly possible.

Some IP packages allow the user to directly represent minimum batch size requirements by way of so-called semi-continuous variables. A variable x is semi-continuous if it is either 0 or in the range $B \le x \le \infty$. No binary variable need be explicitly introduced.

14.3.3 Fixed Charge Problems

A situation closely related to the minimum batch size situation is one where the cost function for an activity is of the fixed plus linear type indicated in Figure 14.1.

Define x, y, and U as before, and let K be the fixed cost incurred if $x > 0$. Then the following components should appear in the formulation:

Minimize $Ky + cx + \ldots$
subject to
$$x \le Uy$$
$$\vdots$$

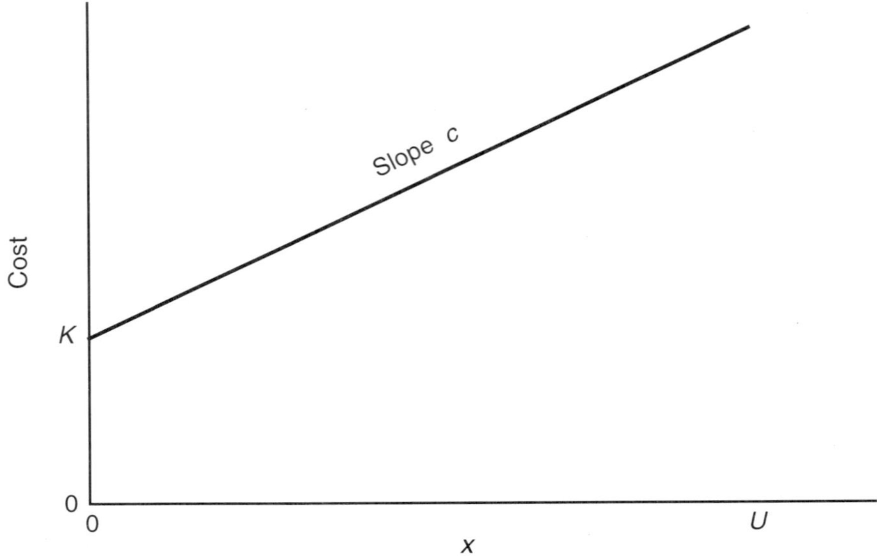

Figure 14.1
A Fixed Plus
Linear Cost
Curve

The constraint and the term Ky in the objective imply that x cannot be greater than 0 unless a cost K is incurred. Again, for computational efficiency, U should be as small as validly possible.

14.3.4 The Simple Plant Location Problem

The Simple Plant Location Problem (SPL) is a commonly encountered form of fixed charge problem. It is specified as follows:

n = the number of sites at which a plant may be located or opened,
m = the number of customer or demand points, each of which must be assigned to a plant,
k = the number of plants that may be opened,
f_i = the fixed cost (e.g., per year) of having a plant at site i, for $i = 1, 2, \ldots, n$,
c_{ij} = cost (e.g., per year) of assigning customer j to a plant at site i, for $i = 1, 2, \ldots, n$ and $j = 1, 2, \ldots, m$.

The goal is to determine the set of sites at which plants should be located and which site should service each customer.

A situation giving rise to the SPL problem is the lockbox location problem encountered by a firm with customers scattered over a wide area. The plant sites, in this case, correspond to sites at which the firm might locate a postal lockbox that is managed by a bank at the site. The customer points would correspond to, say, the 100 largest metropolitan areas in the firm's market. A customer would mail his or her monthly payments to the closest lockbox. The reason for resorting to multiple lockboxes rather than having all payments mailed to a single site is that several days of mail time may be saved. Suppose that a firm receives $60 million per year through the mail, the yearly cost of capital to the firm is 10% per year and it could reduce the mail time by two days. This reduction has a yearly value of about $30,000.

The f_i for a particular site would equal the yearly cost of having a lockbox at site i regardless of the volume processed through the site. The cost term c_{ij} would approximately equal the product: (daily cost of capital) × (mail time in days between i and j) × (yearly dollar volume mailed from area j).

Define the decision variables:

$y_i = 1$ if a plant is located at site i, else 0,
$x_{ij} = 1$ if the customer j is assigned to a plant site i, else 0.

A compact formulation of this problem as an IP is:

$$\text{Minimize} \quad \sum_{i=1}^{n} f_i y_i + \sum_{i=1}^{n} \sum_{j=1}^{m} c_{ij} x_{ij} \tag{1}$$

$$\text{Subject to} \quad \sum_{i=1}^{n} x_{ij} = 1 \qquad \text{for } j = 1 \text{ to } m, \tag{2}$$

$$\sum_{j=1}^{m} x_{ij} \leq m y_i \qquad \text{for } i = 1 \text{ to } n, \tag{3}$$

$$\sum_{i=1}^{n} y_i = k, \tag{4}$$

$$y_i = 0 \text{ or } 1 \qquad \text{for } i = 1 \text{ to } n, \tag{5}$$

$$x_{ij} = 0 \text{ or } 1 \qquad \text{for } i = 1 \text{ to } n, \tag{6}$$

$$j = 1 \text{ to } m.$$

Constraints (2) force each customer j to be assigned to exactly one site. Constraints (3) force a plant to be located at site i if any customer is assigned to site i.

The reader should be cautioned against trying to solve a problem formulated in this fashion, because the solution process may require embarrassingly much computer time for all but the smallest problem. The difficulty arises because, when the problem is solved as an LP; i.e., with conditions (5) and (6) deleted, the solution tends to be highly fractional and with little similarity to the optimal IP solution.

A "tighter" formulation, which frequently produces an integer solution naturally when solved as an LP, is obtained by replacing constraints (3) by the constraints:

$$x_{ij} \leq y_i \quad \text{for } i = 1 \text{ to } n, j = 1 \text{ to } m. \quad (3')$$

At first glance, replacing (3) by (3') may seem counterproductive. If there are 20 possible plant sites and 60 customers, set (3) would contain 20 constraints whereas set (3') would contain $20 \times 60 = 1{,}200$ constraints. Empirically, however, it appears to be the rule rather than the exception that, when the problem is solved as an LP with (3') rather than (3), the solution is naturally integer.

14.3.5 The Capacitated Plant Location Problem (CPL)

The CPL problem arises from the SPL problem if the volume of demand processed through a particular plant is an important consideration. In particular, the CPL problem assumes that each customer has a known volume and each plant site has a known volume limit on total volume assigned to it. The additional parameters to be defined are:

D_j = volume or demand associated with customer j,
K_i = capacity of a plant located at i.

The IP formulation is:

$$\text{Min} \quad \sum_{i=1} f_i y_i + \sum_{i=1} \sum_{j-1} c_{ij} y_{ij} \tag{7}$$

$$\text{s.t.} \quad \sum_{i=1}^{n} x_{ij} = 1 \quad \text{for } j = 1 \text{ to } m, \tag{8}$$

$$\sum_{j=1}^{m} D_j x_{ij} \leq K_i y_i \quad \text{for } i = 1 \text{ to } n, \tag{9}$$

$$x_{ij} \leq y_i \quad \text{for } i = 1 \text{ to } n, \ j = 1 \text{ to } m, \tag{10}$$

$$y_i = 0 \text{ or } 1 \quad \text{for } i = 1 \text{ to } n, \tag{11}$$

$$x_{ij} = 0 \text{ or } 1 \quad \text{for } i = 1 \text{ to } n, \ j = 1 \text{ to } m. \tag{12}$$

This is the "single-sourcing" version of the problem. Because the x_{ij} are restricted to 0 or 1, each customer must have all of its volume assigned to a single plant. If "split-sourcing" is allowed, the x_{ij} are allowed to be fractional with the interpretation that x_{ij} is the fraction of customer j's volume assigned to plant site i. In this case condition (12) is dropped.

14.3.6 Example: Capacitated Plant Location

Some of the points just mentioned will be illustrated with the following example.

The Zzyzx Company of Zzyzx, California, currently has a warehouse in each of the following cities: (A) Baltimore, (B) Cheyenne, (C) Salt Lake City, (D) Memphis, and (E) Wichita. These warehouses supply customer regions throughout the U.S. It is convenient to aggregate customer areas and consider the customers to be located in the following cities: (1) Atlanta, (2) Boston, (3) Chicago, (4) Denver, (5) Omaha, and (6) Portland. There is some feeling that Zzyzx is "overwarehoused"; that is, it may be able to save substantial fixed costs by closing some warehouses without unduly increasing transportation and service costs. Relevant data have been collected and assembled on a "per month" basis and are displayed below.

| | | Demand City | | | | | | Monthly Supply Capacity in Tons | Monthly Fixed Cost |
		1	2	3	4	5	6		
	A	1675	400	685	1630	1160	2800	18	7,650
	B	1460	1940	970	100	495	1200	24	3,500
Supply	C	1925	2400	1425	500	950	800	27	5,000
	D	380	1355	543	1045	665	2321	22	4,100
	E	922	1646	700	508	311	1797	31	2,200
Monthly Demand In Tons		10	8	12	6	7	11		

For example, closing the warehouse at A (Baltimore) would result in a monthly fixed cost saving of $7,650. If 5 (Omaha) gets all of its monthly demand from E

(Wichita), the associated transportation cost for supplying Omaha is $7 \times 311 = \$2,177$ per month. A customer need not get all of its supply from a single source. Such "multiple sourcing" may result from the limited capacity of each warehouse; e.g., Cheyenne can only process 24 tons per month. Should Zzyzx close any warehouses and, if so, which ones?

We will compare the performance of four different methods for solving this problem:

1. Loose formulation of the IP,
2. Tight formulation of the IP,
3. Greedy open heuristic: start with no plants open and sequentially open the plant giving the greatest reduction in cost until it is worthless to open further plants.
4. Greedy close heuristic: start with all plants open and sequentially close the plant saving the most money until it is worthless to close further plants.

The advantage of heuristics 3 and 4 is that they are easy to apply. The performance of the four methods is as follows.

Method	Value of Best Solution	Computing Time in Seconds	Plants Open	Value of LP Solution
Loose IP	46,031	3.38	A, B, D	35,662
Tight IP	46,031	1.67	A, B, D	46,031
Greedy Open Heuristic	46,943	nil	A, B, D, E	—
Greedy Close Heuristic	46,443	nil	A, C, D, E	—

Notice that even though the loose IP finds the same optimum as the tight formulation (as it must), it takes about twice as much computing time. For large problems, the difference becomes much more dramatic. Notice that for the tight formulation, however, the objective function value is the same as for the IP solution. When the tight formulation was *solved as an LP*, the solution was naturally integer.

The single product dynamic lotsizing problem is described by the following parameters:

n = number of periods for which production is to be planned for a product
D_j = predicted demand in period j, for $j = 1, 2, \ldots, n$
f_i = fixed cost of making a production run in period i
h_i = cost per unit of product carried from period i to $i + 1$

This problem can be cast as a simple plant location problem if we define:

$$c_{ij} = D_j \sum_{t=1}^{j-1} h_t$$

that is, c_{ij} is the cost of supplying period j's demand from period i production. Each period can be thought of as both a potential plant site (period for a production run) and a customer.

If, further, there is a finite production capacity, K_t, in period i, this capacitated dynamic lotsizing problem is a special case of the capacitated plant location problem.

Figure 14.2
Concave
Piecewise Linear
Cost Curve

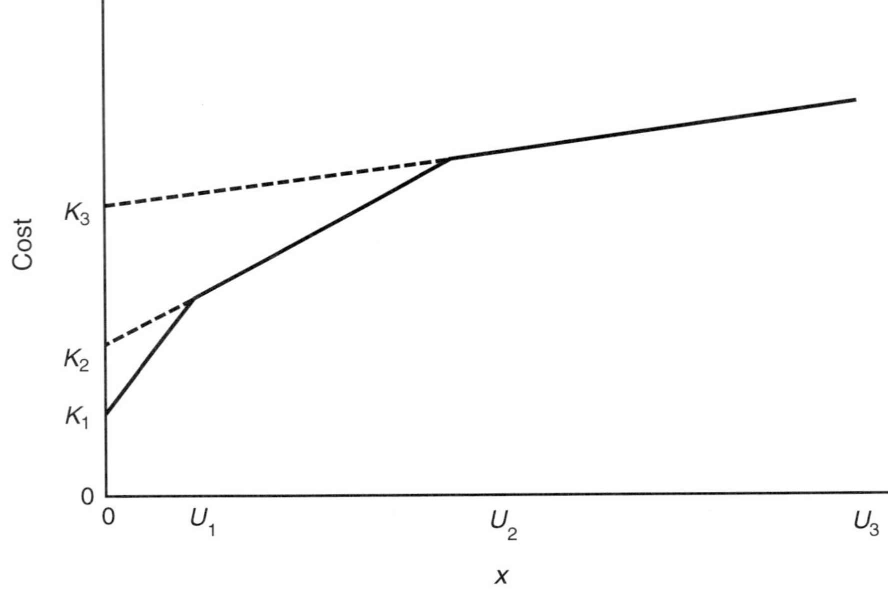

14.3.7 Representing General Cost Curves with Economies of Scale

The fixed-plus linear cost curve seen in plant location models is a special case of the more general cost curve such as that shown in Figure 14.2.

The slopes of the three segments are c_1, c_2, and c_3. The intercepts K_2 and K_3 are determined from the formula $K_{i+1} = K_i + c_i U_i - c_{i+1} U_i$. If $c_{i+1} \le c_i$, the cost curve represents an activity with economies of scale. We are faced with a similar cost curve if we are buying from a vendor that gives quantity discounts.

There are several methods for representing such cost curves. The first method we describe is an extension of the approach used to represent the simple fixed plus linear curve. This method is satisfactory if there are only a few such curves in the overall models or if each such curve has only one or two breakpoints.

Define:

$$y_i = 1 \quad \text{if } U_{i-1} < x \le U_i$$
$$0 \text{ otherwise.}$$

$$x_i = x \quad \text{if } U_{i-1} < x \le U_i$$
$$0 \text{ otherwise.}$$

The formulation should include the terms:

Min $\qquad K_1 y_1 + K_2 y_2 + K_3 y_3 + c_1 x_1 + c_2 x_2 + c_3 x_3 + \ \cdots$
s.t.
(a) $\ x_1 \le U_1 y_1$
$\qquad x_2 \le U_2 y_2$
$\qquad x_3 \le U_3 y_3$

(b) $y_1 + y_2 + y_3 \leq 1$
   $x_2 \geq U_1 y_2$
   $x_3 \geq U_2 y_3$

Anywhere that x appears in the remainder of the formulation, it should be replaced by $x_1 + x_2 + x_3$. If the y_i are required to be 0 or 1, the above will cause the cost function to be correctly represented. Constraint set (b) is not needed if the cost curve is concave (has economies of scales everywhere) and the upper limit on x is not binding.

14.3.8 Example

One part of a larger problem involves the determination of the order quantity for a supplier that gives a quantity discount. The relevant facts are: There is a fixed cost of $150 for placing an order; the first 1,000 gallons of the product can be purchased for $2 per gallon; the price drops to $1.90 per gallon for anything in excess of 1,000 gallons; at most 5,000 gallons will be purchased. The parameters can be now computed as

$K_1 = 150$
$U_1 = 1,000$
$K_2 = 150 + 1,000 \times 2 - 1.90 = 250$
$U_2 = 5,000$

Define the variables:

$y_1 = 1$ if more than 0 but no more than 1,000 gallons are purchased, else 0;
$y_2 = 1$ if more than 1,000 gallons are purchased, else 0;
$x_1 = $ gallons purchased if no more than 1,000 gallons are purchased;
$x_2 = $ gallons purchased if more than 1,000 gallons are purchased.

The formulation would include:

Min $150y_1 + 250y_2 + 2x_1 + 1.9x_2 + \ldots$
s.t.

$x_1 \leq 1,000\, y_1$
$x_2 \leq 5,000\, y_2$
$y_1 + y_2 \leq 1$
y_1 and y_2 are required to be integer.

14.3.9 Alternative Representation of Nonlinear Cost Curves

An alternative method for representing nonlinear cost curves is illustrated with the cost curve in Figure 14.3.

The function is assumed to be linear between the breakpoints $x = U_1$, $x = U_2$, etc. The value of the function at the ith breakpoint is denoted by v_i, i.e., $v_i = f(U_i)$.

Such a function with breakpoints can be represented in a linear integer program if we:

1. Append the constraint $w_1 + w_2 + \ldots + w_n = 1$.
2. Replace each occurrence of x by the expression $w_1 U_1 + w_2 U_2 + \ldots + w_n U_n$.

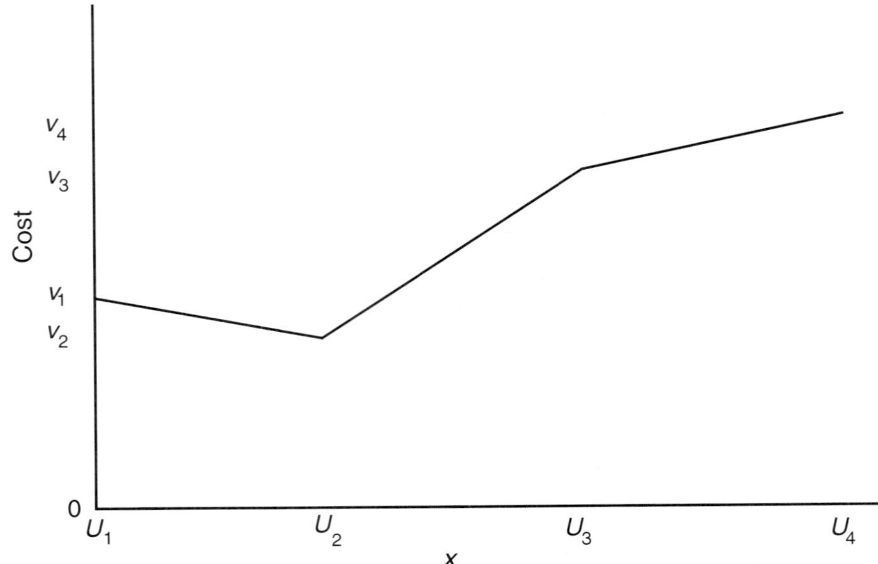

Figure 14.3
Arbitrary
Piecewise Linear
Cost Curve

3. Replace each occurrence of $f(x)$ by the expression $w_1v_1 + w_2v_2 + \ldots + w_nv_n$.
4. Allow at most two w_is to be nonzero and then only if adjacent.

The new variable w_i specifies the weight to be applied to point U_i. If the function $f(x)$ is linear between the two adjacent points $x = U_i$ and $x = U_{i+1}$ and $x = w_iU_i + w_{i+1}U_{i+1}$ with $w_i + w_{i+1} = 1$, $f(x) = w_if(U_i) + w_{i+1}f(U_{i+1}) = w_iv_i + w_{i+1}v_{i+1}$.

Restriction (4) can be enforced in several ways. A number of IP codes allow constraints such as (1) to be identified as so-called "Special Ordered Sets of Type 2" or simply "SOS2." The IP code will guarantee that restriction (4) is satisfied for each constraint identified as SOS2.

If we have a standard IP code but without the SOS2 feature, restriction (4) can be enforced by adding the following constraints:

$$w_1 \le z_1$$
$$w_2 \le z_1 + z_2$$
$$w_3 \le z_2 + z_3$$
$$\vdots$$
$$w_{n-1} \le z_{n-2} + z_{n-1}$$
$$w_n \le z_{n-1}$$
$$z_1 + z_2 + \ldots + z_{n-1} = 1$$
$$z_i = 0 \text{ or } 1.$$

Summarizing, each nonlinear term results in the addition of at least one constraint and n variables. If the SOS2 feature is not available, to this one must further add n constraints and $n - 1$ variables.

The general approach just described is sometimes called the lambda method.

14.3.10 Converting to Separable Functions

The previous method is applicable only to nonlinear functions of one variable. There are some tricks available for transforming a function of several variables so that a function is obtained that is additively separable in the transformed variables. The most common such transformation is for converting a product of two variables into separable form.

Given the function:

$$x_1 x_2$$

Add the linear constraints:

$$y_1 = \left(x_1 + x_2\right)/2$$

$$y_2 = \left(x_1 - x_2\right)/2$$

Then replace every instance of $x_1 x_2$ by the term $y_1^2 - x_2^2$, that is, the claim is:

$$x_1 x_2 = y_1^2 - y_2^2$$

The justification is observed by noting:

$$y_1^2 - y_2^2 = \left(x_1^2 + 2x_1 x_2 + x_2^2\right)/4$$
$$- \left(x_1^2 - 2x_1 x_2 + x_2^2\right)/4$$
$$= 4x_1 x_2 /4 = x_1 x_2$$

This example suggests that, any time you have a product of two variables, you can add two new variables to the model and replace the product term by a sum of two squared variables. If you have n original variables, you could have up to $n(n-1)/2$ cross product terms. This suggests that you might need up to $n(n-1)$ new variables to get rid of all cross product terms. In fact, the above ideas can be generalized (using the technique of Cholesky factorization) so that only n new variables are needed.

14.4 Outline of Integer Programming Methods

The time that a computer requires to solve an IP may depend dramatically on how you formulated it. It is therefore worthwhile to know a little about how IPs are solved. There are two general approaches for solving IPs: "cutting plane" methods and the "branch-and-bound" (B & B) method. The B & B method has thus far proven to be the more reliable. Most commercial IP codes use the B & B method, but aided by some cutting plane features. Fortunately for the reader, the B & B method is the easier to describe. In most general terms, B & B is a form of intelligent enumeration.

More specifically, B & B first solves the problem as an LP. If the LP solution is integer valued in the integer variables, no more work is required. Otherwise, B & B resorts to an intelligent search of all possible ways of rounding the fractional variables.

We shall illustrate the application of the branch-and-bound method to the following problem.

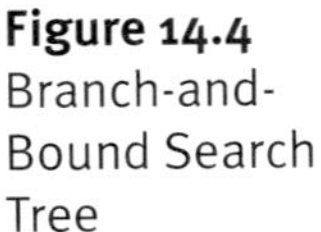

Figure 14.4
Branch-and-
Bound Search
Tree

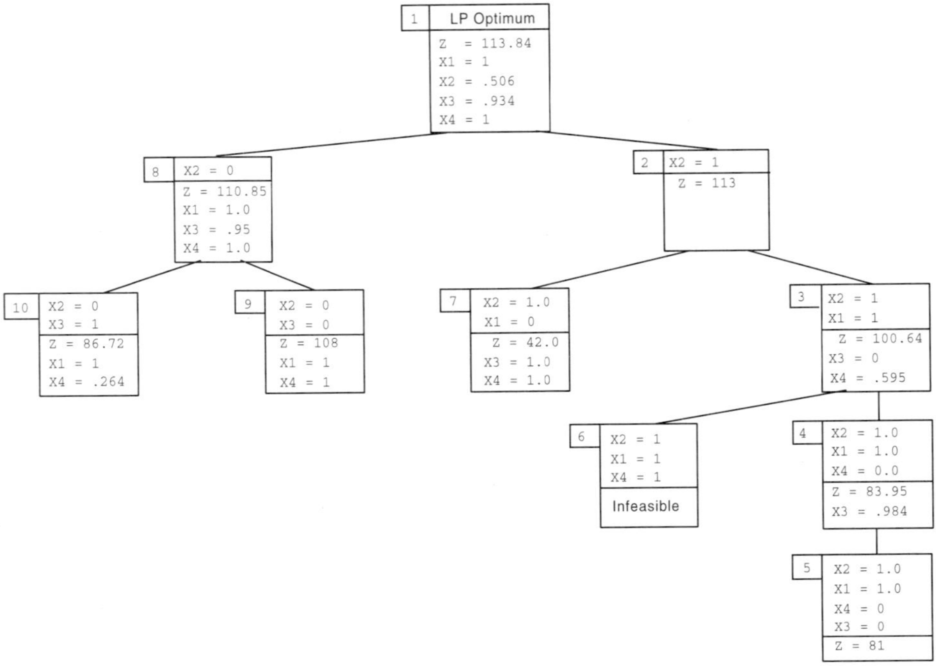


```
MAX  75 X1 +  6 X2 +  3 X3 + 33 X4
SUBJECT  TO
   2)     774 X1 + 76 X2 + 22 X3 + 42 X4 <= 875
   3)      67 X1 + 27 X2 + 794 X3 + 53 X4 <= 875
END
INT  4    !X1, X2, X3, X4  restricted to 0, 1.
```

The search process that a computer might follow in finding an integer optimum is illustrated in Figure 14.4. First the problem is solved as an LP with the constraints X1, X2, X3, X4 <= 1. This solution is summarized in the box labeled 1. The solution has fractional values for X2 and X3 and is therefore unacceptable. At this point, X2 is arbitrarily selected and the following reasoning is applied. At the integer optimum, X2 must equal either 0 or 1.

Therefore, replace the original problem by two new subproblems, one with X2 constrained to equal 1 (box or node 2) and the other with X2 constrained to equal 0 (node 8). If we solve both of these new IPs, the better solution must be the best solution to the original problem. This reasoning is the motivation for using the term "branch." Each subproblem created corresponds to a branch in an enumeration tree.

The numbers to the upper left of each node indicate the order in which the nodes (or equivalently, subproblems) are examined. The variable Z is the objective function value. When the subproblem with X2 constrained to 1 (node 2) is solved as an LP, we find that X1 and X3 take fractional values. Arguing as before, but now with variable X1, we create two new subproblems: one with X1 constrained to 0 (node 7) and one with X1 constrained to 1 (node 3). This process is repeated with X4 and X3 until node 5. At this point an integer solution with $z = 81$ is found. We do not know that this is the optimum integer solution, however, because we must still look at subproblems 6 through 10. Subproblem 6 need not be pursued further because there are no feasible solutions having all of X2, X1, and X4 equal to 1. Subproblem 7 need not be pursued further because it has a z of 42 which is worse than an integer solution already in hand.

At node 9, a new and better integer solution with $z = 108$ is found when X3 is set to 0. Node 10 illustrates the source for the "bound" part of "branch-and-bound." The solution is fractional; however, it is not examined further because the z-value of 86.72 is less than the 108 associated with an integer solution already in hand. The z-value at any node is a bound on the z-value at any offspring node. This is true because an offspring node or subproblem is obtained by appending a constraint to the parent problem. Appending a constraint can only hurt. Interpreted in another light, this means that the z-values cannot improve as one moves down the tree. The tree presented in the preceding figure was only one illustration of how the tree might be searched. Other trees could be developed for the same problem by playing with the following two degrees of freedom:

1. Node selection: Choice of next node to examine, and
2. Branch selection: Choice of how the chosen node is split into two or more subnodes.

For example, if nodes 8 and then 9 were examined immediately after node 1, the solution with $z = 108$ would have been found quickly. Further, nodes 4, 5, and 6 could then have been skipped because the z-value at node 3 (100.64) is worse than a known integer solution (108); therefore, no offspring of node 3 would need examination.

In the example tree, the first node is by branching on the possible values for X2. One could just as well have chosen X3 or even X1 as the first branching variable.

The efficiency of the search is closely related to how wisely the choices are made in (a) and (b) above. Typically, in (b) the split is made by branching on a single variable. For example, if in the continuous solution, $x = 1.5$, the obvious split is to create two subproblems, one with the constraint $x \leq 1$, and the other with the constraint $x \geq 2$. The split need not be made on a single variable; it could be based on an arbitrary constraint. For example, the first subproblem might be based on the constraint $x_1 + x_2 + x_3 \leq 0$, whereas the second is obtained by appending the constraint $x_1 + x_2 + x_3 \geq 1$. Also, the split need not be binary. For example, if the model contains the constraint $y_1 + y_2 + y_3 = 1$, one could create three subproblems corresponding to either $y_1 = 1$, or $y_2 = 1$, or $y_3 = 1$.

If the split is based on a single variable, one wants to choose variables that are "decisive." In general, the computer will make intelligent choices, and the user need not be aware of the details of the search process. The user should, however, keep the general B & B process in mind when formulating a model. If the user has a priori knowledge that an integer variable x is decisive, for the LINDO program it is useful to place x early in the formulation to indicate its importance. This general understanding should drive home the importance of a "tight" LP formulation. A tight LP formulation is one which, when solved, has an objective function value close to the IP optimum. The LP solutions at the subproblems are used as bounds to curtail the search. If the bounds are poor, many early nodes in the tree may be explicitly examined because their bounds look good even though in fact these nodes have no good offspring.

14.5 Problems with Naturally Integer Solutions and the Prayer Algorithm

The solution algorithms for IP are generally based on first solving the IP as an LP by disregarding the integrality requirements and praying that the solution is naturally integer. For example, if x is required to be 0 or 1, the problem is first solved by replacing this requirement by the requirement that simply $0 \leq x \leq 1$. When initiating the analysis of a problem in which integer answers are important, it is useful to know beforehand whether the resulting IP will be easy to solve. After the fact, one generally observes that the IP was easy to solve if the objective function values for the LP optimum and the IP optimum were close. About the only way we can predict beforehand that the objective function values of the LP and IP will be close is if we know beforehand that the LP solution will be almost completely integer valued. Thus, we are interested in knowing what kind of LPs have naturally integer solutions.

The classes of LP problems for which we know beforehand that there is a naturally integer optimum have integer right-hand sides and are in one of the classes:

(a) Network LPs,
(b) MRP or Integral Leontief LPs,
(c) Problems that can be transformed to (a) or (b) by either row operations, or taking the dual.

We first review the distinguishing features of network and MRP LPs.

14.5.1 Network LPs Revisited

An LP is said to be a network LP if, disregarding simple upper and lower bound constraints such as $x \leq 3$, each variable appears in at most two constraints and, if it is two, its coefficients in the two are +1 and −1. If the variable appears in one constraint, its coefficient is either +1 or −1.

Result: *If the right-hand side is integer, there is an integer optimum. If the objective coefficients are all integer, there is an optimum with integral dual prices.*

14.5.2 Integral Leontief Constraints

A constraint set is said to be *integral Leontief* or *MRP* (for Material Requirements Planning) if all of the following are true (see Jeroslow, Martin, et al., 1992):

(a) Each constraint is an equality;
(b) Every column has exactly one positive coefficient and it is a +1;
(c) Each column has 0 or more negative coefficients, every one of which is integer;
(d) Each RHS coefficient is a nonnegative integer.

Result: An LP whose complete constraint set is an MRP set has an optimal solution that is integer. Further, if the objective coefficients are all integer, there is an optimal solution with integral dual prices.

14.5.3 Example: A One-Period MRP Problem

The Schwindle Cycle Company makes three products: unicycles (U), regular bicycles (R), and twinbikes (T). Each product is assembled from a variety of components, including seats (S), wheels (W), hubs (H), spokes (P), chains (C), and links (L). The full bills of materials for each product are shown below. The numbers in parentheses specify how many units of the child are required per parent.

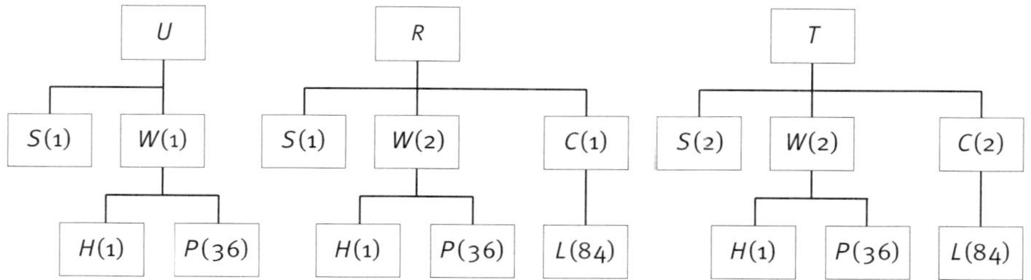

Current inventories are zero. Schwindle needs to supply 100 unicycles, 500 regular bicycles, and 200 twinbikes. Finished products and complete subassemblies can be either manufactured or bought at the following prices:

Item	U	R	T	S	W	C	H	P	L
Bought Price	2.60	5.2	3.10	.25	1.40	.96	.19	.07	.05
Assembly cost	1.04	1.16	1.90	.20	.22	.26	.16	.04	.03

Note that the assembly cost is the immediate cost at the level of assembly; it does not include the cost of the components going into the assembly. How many units of each item should be made or bought so as to satisfy demand at minimum price?

An LP formulation is:

```
MIN      1.04 UM + 2.6 UB + 1.16 RM + 5.2 RB + 1.9 TM + 3.1 TB
       + 0.2 SM + 0.25 SB + 0.22 WM + 1.4 WB + 0.26 CM + 0.96 CB
       + 0.16 HM + 0.19 HB + 0.04 PM + 0.07 PB + 0.03 LM
       + 0.05 LB
SUBJECT TO
UNICYCLE)    UM + UB =       100
 REGULAR)    RM + RB =       500
TWINBIKE)    TM + TB =       200
   SEATS)  - UM - RM - 2 TM + SM + SB =        0
  WHEELS)  - UM - 2 TM + 2 TM + WM + WB =         0
  CHAINS)  - RM - 2 TM + CM + CB =      0
    HUBS)  - WM + HM + HB =       0
  SPOKES)  - 36 WM + PM + PB =       0
   LINKS)  - 84 CM + LM + LB =       0
END
```

In the PICTURE of the formulation in the figure below, notice that it has the MRP structure.

```
                 U U R R T T S S W W C C H H P P L L
                 M B M B M B M B M B M B M B M B M B

           1: A A A A A A T T A T T T T U U U U MIN
  UNICYCLE: 1 1     '       '       '       '         = B
   REGULAR: '   '1 1   '   '   '   '   '   '   '   '   = C
  TWINBIKE:       ' 1 1 '       '                     = C
     SEATS:-1   -1 '-2   1 1     '       '       '     =
    WHEELS:-1   -2 '-2'     '1 1 '   '   '   '   '     =
    CHAINS:     -1 '-2     '     ' 1 1 '       '       =
      HUBS:         '       '  -1 '     1 1     '       =
    SPOKES: '   '   '   '   '  -B '   '   ' '1 1   '   =
     LINKS:         '       '     '-B '       ' 1 1   =
```

The solution is:

```
              OBJECTIVE FUNCTION VALUE

        1)        3440.0000

   VARIABLE           VALUE          REDUCED COST
        UB         100.000000           0.000000
        RM         500.000000           0.000000
        TB         200.000000           0.000000
        SM         500.000000           0.000000
        WB        1000.000000           0.000000
        CB         500.000000           0.000000
```

Notice that it is naturally integer. Thus we should buy all the unicycles and twin-bikes (and paste our own brand name on them). We assemble our own regular bicycles. They are assembled from manufactured seats and bought wheels and chains.

If we put an upper limit of 300 on the number of links manufactured by adding the constraint LM <= 300, we will get a fractional solution, because this constraint violates the MRP structure.

14.5.4 Transformations to Naturally Integer Formulations

A *row operation* consists of either of the following:

(a) multiplication through an equation by some non-zero constant,
(b) adding a finite multiple of one equation to another.

A row operation changes neither the feasible region nor the set of optimal solutions to a problem. Thus, if we can show that a model can be transformed to either a network LP or an MRP LP by row operations, we know there is an integer optimum. We do not actually need to do the transformation to get the solution.

Similarly, if we have a model with an integer right-hand side and we can show that it is the dual of either a network LP or an MRP LP, we know the model has an integer optimum.

14.5.5 Example

Consider the following LP that arose in planning how much to produce in each of four periods:

```
          P P P P P P P P P P
          1 1 1 1 2 2 2 3 3 4
          4 3 2 1 4 3 2 4 3 4
    1:   9 6 4 3 6 4 3 4 3 3 MIN
    2:   1 1 1 1                 = 1
    3:   1 1 1   1 1 1           = 1
    4:   1 1     1 1     1 1     = 1
    5:   1       1       1   1 = 1
```

When the problem is solved as an LP, we obtained the following naturally integer solution:

    P12 = P34 = 1; all others 0.

Could we have predicted a naturally integer solution beforehand? If we perform the row operations: $(5') = (5) - (4)$; $(4') = (4) - (3)$; $(3') = (3) - (2)$, we obtain the equivalent LP:

```
          P P P P P P P P P P
          1 1 1 1 2 2 2 3 3 4
          4 3 2 1 4 3 2 4 3 4
    1:   9 6 4 3 6 4 3 4 3 3 MIN
    2:   1 1 1 1                 = 1
    3:       -1 1 1 1            = 0
    4:     -1        -1 1 1      = 0
    5:   -1       -1     -1 1 = 0
```

This is a network LP, so it has a naturally integer solution.

14.5.6 Example

In trying to find the minimum elapsed time for a certain project composed of seven activities, the following LP was constructed (in PICTURE form):

```
        A B C D E F
   1:-1          '     1 MIN
  AB:-1 1        '       > 3
  AC:-1    '1 '     '    > 2
  BD:    -1    1         > 5
  BE:    -1    ' 1       > 6
  CF: '    -1 '    '1 > 4
  DF:         -1    1 > 7
  EF:            '-1 1 > 6
```

This is neither a network LP (e.g., consider columns A, B, or F) nor an MRP LP (e.g., consider columns A or F). Nevertheless, when solved we get the naturally integer solution:

```
             OBJECTIVE FUNCTION VALUE

       1)      15.0000000

   VARIABLE            VALUE           REDUCED COST
       A              .000000            .000000
       B             3.000000            .000000
       C             2.000000            .000000
       D             8.000000            .000000
       E             9.000000            .000000
       F            15.000000            .000000

      ROW     SLACK OR SURPLUS        DUAL PRICES
      AB)            .000000          -1.000000
      AC)            .000000            .000000
      BD)            .000000          -1.000000
      BE)            .000000            .000000
      CF)           9.000000            .000000
      DF)            .000000          -1.000000
      EF)            .000000            .000000
```

Could we have predicted a naturally integer solution beforehand? If we look at the PICTURE of the model, we see that each constraint has exactly one +1 and one −1; thus, its dual model is a network LP, and expectation of integer answers is justified.

14.6 The Assignment Problem and Related Sequencing and Routing Problems

The assignment problem is a simple LP problem that is frequently encountered as a major component in more complicated practical problems.

The assignment problem is:

Given a matrix of costs:

c_{ij} = cost of assigning object i to object j,

and variables:

$x_{ij} = 1$ if object i is assigned to object j.

Then we want to

Minimize $\sum_i \sum_j c_{ij} x_{ij}$

Subject to $\sum_i x_{ij} = 1$ for each object j

$\sum_j x_{ij} = 1$ for each object i,

$x_{ij} \geq 0.$

This problem is easy to solve as an LP, and the x_{ij} will be naturally integer.

There are a number of problems in routing and sequencing that are closely related to the assignment problem.

14.6.1 Example: The Assignment Problem

Large airlines tend to base their route structure around the hub concept. An airline will try to have a large number of flights arrive at the hub airport during a certain short interval of time, e.g., 9 A.M. to 10 A.M., and then have a large number of flights depart the hub shortly thereafter, e.g., 10 A.M. to 11 A.M. This allows customers of that airline to travel between a large combination of origin/destination cities with one stop and at most one change of planes. For example, United Airlines uses Chicago as a hub, Delta Airlines uses Atlanta, TWA uses St. Louis, and American uses Dallas/Fort Worth.

A desirable goal in using a hub structure is to minimize the amount of changing of planes (and the resulting moving of baggage) at the hub. The following little example illustrates how the assignment model applies to this problem.

A certain airline has six flights arriving at O'Hare airport between 9 and 9:30 A.M. The same six airplanes depart on different flights between 9:40 and 10:20 A.M. The average numbers of people transferring between incoming and leaving flights appear in the table below:

	L01	L02	L03	L04	L05	L06
I01	20	15	16	5	4	7
I02	17	15	33	12	8	6
I03	9	12	18	16	30	13
I04	12	8	11	27	19	14
I05	0	7	10	21	10	32
I06	0	0	0	6	11	13

Flight I05 arrives too late to connect with L01. Similarly, I06 is too late for flights L01, L02, and L03.

All the planes are identical. A decision problem is which incoming flight should be assigned to which outgoing flight. For example, if incoming flight I02 is assigned to leaving flight L03, 33 people (and their baggage) will be able to remain on their plane at the stop at O'Hare. How should incoming flights be assigned to leaving flights so that a minimum number of people need to change planes at the O'Hare stop?

This problem can be formulated as an assignment problem if we define:

$x_{ij} = 1$ if incoming flight i is assigned to outgoing flight j,
    0 otherwise.

The objective is to maximize the number of people not having to change planes. A formulation is:

```
MAX       20 X11 +  15 X12 +  16 X13 +  5 X14 +  4 X15 +  7 X16
        + 17 X21 +  15 X22 +  33 X23 + 12 X24 +  8 X25 +  6 X26
        +  9 X31 +  12 X32 +  18 X33 + 16 X34 + 30 X35 + 13 X36
        + 12 X41 +   8 X42 +  11 X43 + 27 X44 + 19 X45 + 14 X46
        +  7 X52 +  10 X53 +  21 X54 + 10 X55 + 32 X56 +  6 X64
        + 11 X65 +  13 X66
SUBJECT TO
    2)        X11 + X21 + X31 + X41 =       1
    3)        X12 + X22 + X32 + X42 + X52 =       1
    4)        X13 + X23 + X33 + X43 + X53 =       1
    5)        X14 + X24 + X34 + X44 + X54 + X64 =       1
    6)        X15 + X25 + X35 + X45 + X55 + X65 =       1
```

```
 7)      X16 + X26 + X36 + X46 + X56 + X66 =    1
 8)      X11 + X12 + X13 + X14 + X15 + X16 =    1
 9)      X21 + X22 + X23 + X24 + X25 + X26 =    1
10)      X31 + X32 + X33 + X34 + X35 + X36 =    1
11)      X41 + X42 + X43 + X44 + X45 + X46 =    1
12)      X52 + X53 + X54 + X55 + X56 =    1
13)      X64 + X65 + X66 =    1
END
```

A solution is:

```
 OBJECTIVE FUNCTION VALUE

 1)       135.00000

 VARIABLE          VALUE            REDUCED COST
      X11        1.000000               .000000
      X23        1.000000               .000000
      X32        1.000000               .000000
      X44        1.000000               .000000
      X56        1.000000               .000000
      X65        1.000000               .000000
```

Notice that each incoming flight except I03 is able to be assigned to its most attractive outgoing flight.

14.6.2 The Traveling Salesman Problem

One of the more famous optimization problems is the traveling salesman problem (TSP). It is an assignment problem with the additional condition that the assignments chosen must constitute a tour. Lawler et al. (1985) present a tour-de-force on this fascinating problem.

The constraint sets are:

(1)   Each city j must be entered exactly once:

$$\sum_{\substack{i \neq j}}^{n} x_{ij} = 1 \quad \text{for } j = 1 \text{ to } n,$$

(2)   Each city i must be exited exactly once:

$$\sum_{\substack{j \neq i}}^{n} x_{ij} = 1 \quad \text{for } i = 1 \text{ to } n,$$

(3)   No subtours are allowed for any subset of cities S not including city 1:

$$\sum_{i,j \in S} x_{ij} \leq |S| - 1 \quad \text{for every subset } S \text{ where } |S| \text{ is the size of } S,$$

(4)   Alternatively (3) may be replaced by

$$u_j \geq u_i + 1 - \left(1 - x_{ij}\right)n \quad \text{for } j = 2, 3, 4, \ldots \,; \, j \neq i.$$

Effectively, u_j is the sequence number of city j on the trip. Note that (3) is much tighter than (4). Large problems may be computationally intractable if (3) is not used. On the other hand, there are of the order of 2^n constraints of type (3) but only $n - 1$ constraints of type (4). Even though there are a huge number of constraints in

(3), only a few of them (e.g., $\leq n$) will be binding at the optimum. Thus, an iterative approach that adds violated constraints of type (3) as needed works surprisingly well. Padberg and Rinaldi (1987) used essentially this iterative approach and were able to solve to optimality problems with over 2000 cities. The solution time was several hours on a large computer.

For practical problems, it may be important to get good but not necessarily optimal answers in just a few seconds or minutes rather than hours. The most commonly used heuristic for the traveling salesman problem is due to Lin and Kernighan (1973). This heuristic tries to improve a given solution by clever reorderings of cities in the tour. For practical problems (e.g., in operation sequencing on computer controlled machines), the heuristic seems to always find solutions no more than 2% more costly than the optimum. Problems with up to 14,464 "cities" arising from the sequencing of operations on a computer controlled machine are described by Bland and Shallcross (1989). In no case was the Lin-Kernighan heuristic more than 1.7% from the optimal for these problems.

14.6.3 Example of a Traveling Salesman Problem

P. Rose, currently unemployed, has hit upon the following scheme for making some money. He will guide a group of 18 people on a tour of all the National League baseball parks in which he once played. He is betting his life savings on this scheme, so he wants to keep the cost of the tour as low as possible. The tour will start and end in Cincinnati. The following distance matrix has been constructed:

	Atl	Chi	Cin	Hou	LA	Mon	NY	Phi	Pit	StL	SD	SF
Atlanta	0	702	454	842	2396	1196	864	772	714	554	2363	2679
Chicago	702	0	324	1093	2136	764	845	764	459	294	2184	2187
Cincinnati	454	324	0	1137	2180	798	664	572	284	338	2228	2463
Houston	842	1093	1137	0	1616	1857	1706	1614	1421	799	1521	2021
Los Angeles	2396	2136	2180	1616	0	2900	2844	2752	2464	1842	95	405
Montreal	1196	764	798	1857	2900	0	396	424	514	1058	2948	2951
New York	864	845	664	1706	2844	396	0	92	386	1002	2892	3032
Philadelphia	772	764	572	1614	2752	424	92	0	305	910	2800	2951
Pittsburgh	714	459	284	1421	2464	514	386	305	0	622	2512	2646
St. Louis	554	294	338	799	1842	1058	1002	910	622	0	1890	2125
San Diego	2363	2184	2228	1521	95	2948	2892	2800	2512	1890	0	500
San Francisco	2679	2187	2463	2021	405	2951	3032	2951	2646	2125	500	0

14.6.4 Solution

We can exploit the fact that the distance matrix is symmetric. Define the decision variables:

$Y_{ij} = 1$ if the link between cities i and j is used, regardless of the direction of travel;
    $= 0$ otherwise.

Thus, YATLCHI = 1 if the link between ATL and CHI is used. Each city or node must be connected to two links. In words the formulation is:

Minimize   the cost of links selected
subject to   For each city, number of links connected to it that are selected = 2
    Each link can be selected at most once.

A fragment of the LINDO formulation is shown below.

```
MIN       702 YATLCHI + 454 YATLCIN + 842 YATLHOU + 2396 YATLLAX
        + 1196 YATLMON + 864 YATLNYK + 772 YATLPHI + 714 YATLPIT
        + 554 YATLSTL + 2363 YATLSND + 2679 YATLSNF + 324 YCHICIN
        + 1093 YCHIHOU + 2136 YCHILAX + 764 CHIMON + 845 YCHINYK
        + 764 YCHIPHI + 459 YCHIPIT + 294 YCHISTL + 2184 YCHISND
        + 2187 YCHISNF
                                    .
                                    .
                                    .
        + 2512 YPITSND + 2646 YPITSNF + 1890 YSTLSND
        + 2125 YSTLSNF + 500 YSNDSNF
SUBJECT TO
  ATL)   YATLCHI + YATLCIN + YATLHOU + YATLLAX + YATLMON
       + YATLNYK + YATLPHI + YATLPIT + YATLSTL + YATLSND
       + YATLSNF =     2
  CHI)   YATLCHI + YCHICIN + YCHIHOU + YCHILAX + YCHIMON
       + YCHINYK + YCHIPHI + YCHIPIT + YCHISTL + YCHISND
       + YCHISNF =     2
                                    .
                                    .
                                    .
  SNF)   YATLSNF + YCHISNF + YCINSNF + YHOUSNF + YLAXSNF
       + YMONSNF + YNYKSNF + YPHISNF + YPITSNF + YSTLSNF
       + YSNDSNF =   2
END
SUB YATLCHI   1.00
SUB YATLCIN   1.00
SUB YATLHOU   1.00
SUB YATLLAX   1.00
SUB YATLMON   1.00
              .
              .
              .
SUB YSNDSNF   1.00
```

When this model is solved *as an LP*, we get the solution:

```
VARIABLE        VALUE
YATLCIN         1.000000
YATLHOU         1.000000
YCHICIN         1.000000
YCHISTL         1.000000
YHOUSTL         1.000000
YLAXSND         1.000000
YLAXSNF         1.000000
```

Figure 14.5

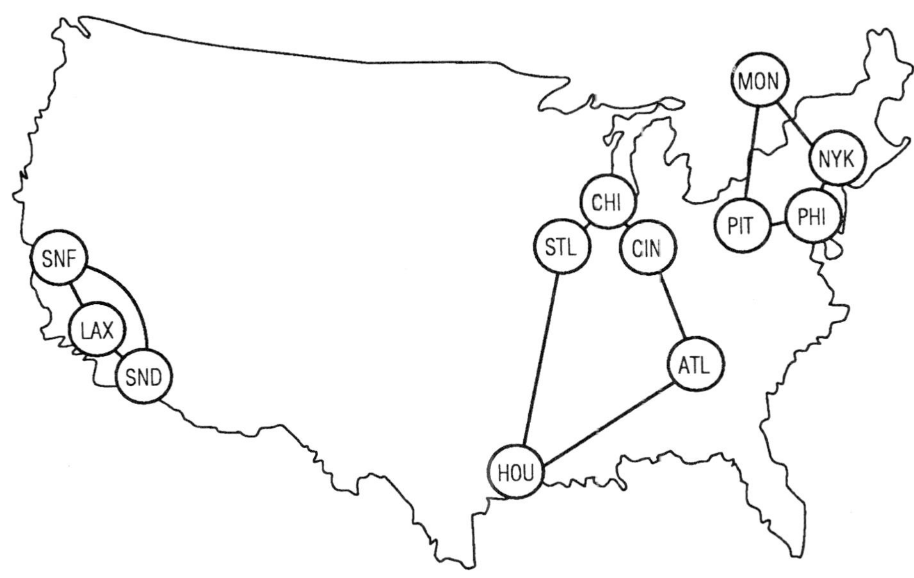


```
YMONNYK           1.000000
YMONPIT           1.000000
YMONPHI           1.000000
YPHIPIT           1.000000
YSNDSNF           1.000000
```

This has a cost of 5020 miles. Graphically it corresponds to Figure 14.5.

Unfortunately, the solution has three subtours. We decide to cut off the smallest subtour by adding the constraint:

```
YLAXSND + YLAXSNF + YSNDSNF <= 2
```

Now, when we solve it *as an LP,* we get a solution with cost 6975, corresponding to Figure 14.6. We cut off the subtour in the southwest by adding the constraint:

```
YLAXSND + YLAXSNF + YSNDSNF + YHOULAX + YHOUSND + YHOUSNF <= 3
```

We continue in this fashion adding subtour elimination cuts:

```
YMONNYK + YMONPHI + YMONPIT + YNYKPHI + YNYKPIT + YPHIPIT <= 3
```

and

```
YMONNYK + YMONPHI + YNYKPHI <= 2
```

Figure 14.6

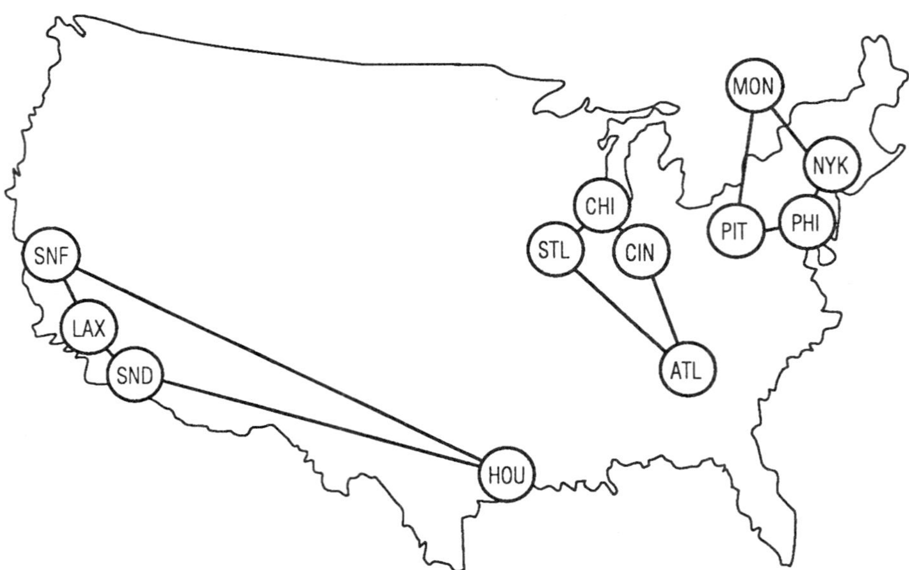

Figure 14.7

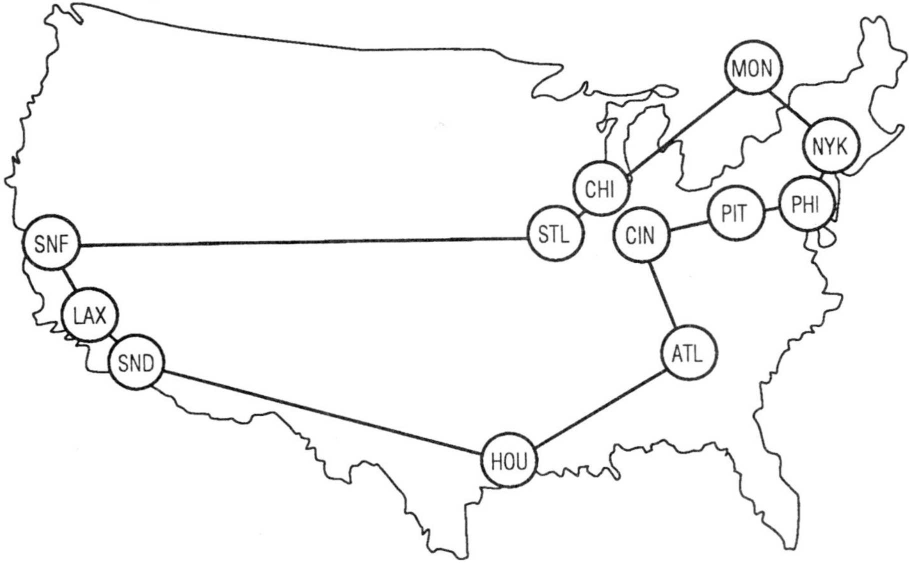

After the above are all added, we get the solution shown in Figure 14.7. It is a complete tour with cost 7577. Note that only LPs were solved. No branch and bound was required.

Could P. Rose have done as well by trial and error? The most obvious heuristic is the "closest unvisited city" heuristic. If one starts in Cincinnati and next goes to the closest unvisited city at each step and finally returns to Cincinnati, the total distance is 8015 miles—about 6% worse than the optimum.

14.6.5 The Optional Stop TSP

If we drop the requirement that every stop must be visited, we then get the optional stop TSP. This might correspond to a job sequencing problem where v_j is the profit from job j if we do it and c_{ij} is the cost of switching from job i to job j. Let:

y_j = 1 if city j is visited, 0 otherwise.

If v_j is the value of visiting city j, the objective is:

$$\text{Min} \sum_i \sum_j c_{ij} x_{ij} - \sum v_j y_j.$$

The constraint sets are:

(1) Each city j can be visited at most once:
$$\sum_{i \neq j} x_{ij} = y_j.$$

(2) If we enter city j, we must exit it:
$$\sum_{k \neq j} x_{jk} = y_j.$$

(3) No subtours allowed for each subset, S, of cities not including the home base 1:
$$\sum_{i,j \in S} x_{ij} \leq |S| - 1, \text{ where } |S| \text{ is the size of } S.$$

For example, if there are n cities, including the home base, there are $(n-1)(n-2)/(3*2)$ subsets of size 3.

(4) Alternatively, (3) may be replaced by
$$u_j \geq u_i + 1 - (1 - x_{ij})n \text{ for } j = 2, 3, \ldots, n.$$

Effectively, u_j is the sequence number of city j in its tour. Constraint set (3) is much tighter than (4).

14.6.6 Capacitated Multiple TSP/ Vehicle Routing Problems

An important practical problem is the routing of vehicles from a central depot. An example is the routing of delivery trucks for a metropolitan newspaper. You can think of this as a multiple traveling salesman problem with finite capacity for each salesperson. A formulation is:

Given
V = capacity of a vehicle
d_j = demand of city or stop j

(1) Each city, j, must be visited once for $j > 1$.

$$\sum_j x_{ij} = 1$$

(2) Each city $i > 1$, must be exited once

$$\sum_i x_{ij} = 1$$

(3) No subtours

$$\sum_{i,j \in S} x_{ij} \leq |S| - 1$$

(4) No overloads: For each set of cities T, including 1, which constitute more than a truckload:

$$\sum_{i,j \in T} x_{ij} \leq |T| - k,$$

where k = minimum number of cities which must be dropped from T to reduce it to one load.

This formulation can solve to optimality modest sized problems of, say, 25 cities. For larger or more complicated practical problems, the heuristic method of Clarke and Wright (1964) is a standard starting point for quickly finding good but not necessarily optimal solutions.

14.6.7 Combined DC Location/Vehicle Routing

Frequently, there is a vehicle routing problem associated with opening a new plant or distribution center (DC). Specifically, given the customers to be served from the DC, what trips are made so as to serve the customers at minimum cost? A "complete" solution to the problem would solve the location and routing problems simultaneously.

The following IP formulation illustrates one approach:

Parameters

F_i = fixed cost of having a DC at location i,
C_j = cost of using route j,
a_{ijk} = 1 if route j originates at DC i and serves customer k. There is exactly one DC associated with each route.

Decision variables

y_i = 1 if we use DC i, else 0,
x_j = 1 if we use route j, else 0.

The Model

$$\text{Min} \quad \sum_i F_i y_i + \sum_j c_j x_j$$

Subject to

(Demand constraints) For each customer k:

$$\sum_i \sum_j a_{ijk} x_j = 1$$

(Forcing constraints) For each DC i and customer k:

$$\sum_j a_{ijk} x_j \leq y_i$$

14.6.8 Minimum Spanning Tree

A spanning tree of n nodes is a collection of $n - 1$ arcs so that there is exactly one path between every pair of nodes. A minimum cost spanning tree might be of interest, for example, in designing a communications network.

Assume that node 1 is the root of the tree. Let $x_{ij} = 1$ if the path from 1 to j goes through node i immediately before node j, else $x_{ij} = 0$.

A formulation is

$$\text{Min} \quad \sum_i \sum_j c_{ij} x_{ij}$$

Subject to

$$\sum_i \sum_j x_{ij} = n - 1$$

$$(*) \quad \sum_{i,j \in S} x_{ij} \leq |S| - 1 \quad \text{for every subset } S.$$

$$x_{ij} = 0 \text{ or } 1.$$

An alternative to $(*)$ is

$$u_j \geq u_i + 1 - \left(1 - x_{ij}\right) n \quad \text{for } j = 2, 3, 4, \ldots, n.$$

$$u_j \geq 0.$$

In this case, u_j is the number of arcs between node j and node 1.

If one has a pure spanning tree problem, the "greedy" algorithm of Kruskal (1956) is a fast way of finding optimal solutions.

14.6.9 The Linear Ordering Problem

A variation of the TSP is the linear ordering problem. One wants to find a strict ordering of n objects. Applications are to ranking in sports tournaments, product preference ordering in marketing, job sequencing on one machine, ordering of industries in an input-output matrix, ordering of historical objects in archeology and others. The crucial input data are cost entries c_{ij}. If object i appears *anywhere* before object j in the proposed ordering, c_{ij} is the resulting cost. The decision variables are:

$$x_{ij} = 1 \text{ if object } i \text{ precedes object } j, \text{ either directly or indirectly for all } i \neq j.$$

The problem is

Minimize $\displaystyle\sum_i \sum_j c_{ij} x_{ij}$

Subject to

$(1)\quad x_{ij} + x_{ji} = 1\quad$ for all $i \geq j$

> If i precedes j and j precedes k, we want to imply that i precedes k. This is enforced with the constraints

$(2)\quad x_{ij} + x_{jk} + x_{ki} \leq 2\quad$ for all i, j, k with $i \neq j$, $i \neq k$, $j \neq k$.

The size of the formulation can be cut in two by noting that $x_{ij} = 1 - x_{ji}$. Thus, we substitute out x_{ji} for $j > i$. Constraint set (1) becomes simply $0 < x_{ij} < 1$. Constraint set (2) becomes:

$(2')\quad x_{ij} + x_{jk} - x_{ik} + s_{ijk} = 1\quad$ for all $i < j < k$.

$$0 \leq s_{ijk} \leq 1$$

14.6.10 Quadratic Assignment Problem

The quadratic assignment problem has the same constraint set as the linear assignment problem; however, the objective function contains products of two variables. Notationally, it is:

Min $\displaystyle\sum_i \sum_j \sum_k \sum_l c_{ijkl} x_{ij} x_{kl}$

Subject to

For each j :

$$\sum_i x_{ij} = 1$$

For each i :

$$\sum_j x_{ij} = 1$$

Some examples of this problem are:

1. *Facility layout.* If d_{jl} is the physical distance between room j and room l, s_{ik} is the communication traffic between department i and k, and $x_{ij} = 1$ if department i is assigned to room j, we want to:

   Minimize $\displaystyle\sum_i \sum_j \sum_k \sum_l x_{ij} x_{kl} d_{jl} s_{ik}$

2. *Vehicle to gate assignment at a terminal.* If d_{jl} is the distance between gate j and gate l at an airline terminal or at a truck terminal, s_{ik} is the number of passengers or tons of cargo that need to be transferred between vehicle i and vehicle k, and $x_{ij} = 1$ if vehicle i (incoming or outgoing) is assigned to gate j, we want to:

$$\text{Minimize} \ \sum_i \sum_j \sum_k \sum_l x_{ij} x_{kl} d_{jl} s_{ik}$$

3. *Radio frequency assignment.* If d_{ij} is the physical distance between transmitters i and j, s_{kl} is the distance in frequency k and l, and p_i is the power of transmitter i, we want max $\{p_i, p_j\}\, (1/d_{ij})(1/s_{kl})$ to be small if transmitter i is assigned frequency k and transmitter j is assigned frequency l.
4. *Type wheel design.* Arrange letters and numbers on a type wheel so that (a) the most frequently used ones appear together and (b) characters that tend to get typed together, e.g., qu, appear close together on the wheel.
5. *Disk file allocation.* If w_{ij} is the interference if files i and j are assigned to the same disk, we want to assign files to disk so that total interference is minimized.

The quadratic assignment problem is a notoriously difficult problem. If someone asks you to solve such a problem, you should make every effort to show that the problem is not really a quadratic assignment problem. One indication of its difficulty is that the solution is not naturally integer.

Small quadratic assignment problems can be converted to linear integer programs by the transformation.

(a) Replace the product $x_{ij} x_{kl}$ by z_{ijkl}

(b) If $c_{ijkl} > 0$, add the constraint:

$$z_{ijkl} \geq x_{ij} + x_{jl} - 1$$

(c) If $c_{ijkl} \leq 0$, add the constraints:

$$z_{ijkl} \leq x_{ij}$$

$$z_{ijkl} \leq x_{kl}$$

14.7 Problems of Grouping: Matching, Covering, Partitioning, and Packing

There is a class of problems that have the following essential structure:

(a) There is a set of m objects and
(b) they are to be grouped into subsets so that some criterion is optimized.

Some example situations are:

	Objects	Group	Criteria for a group
(i)	Dormitory inhabitants	Roommates	At most two to a room, no smokers with nonsmokers.
(ii)	Deliveries to customers	Trip	Total weight assigned to trip is less than vehicle capacity, customers in same trip are close together.

(iii)	Sessions at a scientific meeting	Sessions scheduled for same time slot	No two sessions on same general topic; enough rooms of sufficient size.
(iv)	Exams to be scheduled	Exams scheduled for the same time slot	No student has more than one exam in the time slot.
(v)	Sportsmen	Foursome, e.g., in golf or tennis doubles	Members are of comparable ability, appropriate combination of sexes as in tennis mixed doubles.
(vi)	States on map to be colored	All states of a given color	States in same group/color cannot be adjacent.

If each object can belong to at most one group, it is called a *packing* problem. If each object must belong to exactly one group, it is called a *partitioning* problem. If each object must belong to at least one group, it is called a *covering* problem. A packing or partitioning problem with group sizes limited to two or less is called a *matching* problem. Specialized and fast algorithms exist for matching problems. A problem that is closely related to covering problems is the cutting stock problem. It arises in paper, printing, textile, and steel industries. In this problem, we want to determine cutting patterns to be used in cutting up large pieces of raw material into finished good size pieces. This problem was discussed in Chapter 6.

Although grouping problems may be very easy to state, it may be very difficult to find a provably optimal solution.

There are two common approaches to formulating grouping problems: (1) assignment style, or (2) the packing method. The former is convenient for small problems, but it quickly becomes useless as the number of objects gets large.

14.7.1 Formulation as an Assignment Problem

The most obvious formulation for the general grouping problem is based around the following definition of 0/1 decision variables:

$X_{ij} = 1$ if object j is assigned to group i, 0 otherwise.

A drawback of this formulation is that there are many alternate optimal solutions, all of which essentially are identical. For example, assigning golfers A, B, C, and D to group 1 and golfers E, F, G, and H to group 2 is essentially the same as assigning golfers E, F, G, and H to group 1 and golfers A, B, C, and D to group 2. These alternate optima make the typical integer programming algorithm take much longer than necessary.

For packing and partitioning problems, we can eliminate these alternate optima with no loss of optimality if we agree to the following restrictions: (i) object 1 can only be assigned to group 1; (ii) object 2 can only be assigned to groups 1 or 2 and only to 1 if object 1 is not assigned; (iii) object 3 can only be assigned to groups 1, 2, or 3 and only to groups 1 or 2 if object 2 is not assigned to group 2, and only to group 1 if neither object 1 nor object 2 are assigned; (iv) etc.

This restriction can be enforced with the following 2 sets of constraints:

1. For each object $j = 2, 3, \ldots, N$:

$$X_{j,j-1} + X_{j+1,j-1} + \ldots X_{Mj-1} = 0.$$

(You do not actually add this constraint; rather just do not bother to generate the variables in it.)

You may also add the constraints for $i = 2, 3, \ldots, N$, $j = 2, 3, \ldots$, min $\{i, M\}$:

2. $X_{ij} \leq X_{i-1,1} + X_{i-1,2} + X_{i-1,j-1}.$

In words, if object j is assigned to group i, some lower numbered object must be assigned to group $i-1$.

Even with constraints (1) and (2), this formulation tends to be hard to solve if the number of groups is greater than about a half dozen.

14.7.2 Formulation as a Packing Problem

An alternative approach is to first enumerate either all possible or all interesting feasible groups and then solve an optimization problem of the form:

Maximize value of the groups selected,
s.t.
Each object is in at most one of the selected groups.

The advantage of this formulation is that, when it can be used, it typically can be solved more easily than the assignment formulation. The disadvantages are that it may have a huge number of decision variables, especially if the typical group size is more than three. For example, if there are 21 objects, all groups are of size three and all groups of size three are feasible, the problem is to choose the best set of 7 groups out of a set of 1330 groups.

14.7.3 Example: Packing Financial Instruments

A financial services firm has financial objects (e.g., mortgages) that it wants to "package" and sell. One of the features of a package is that it must contain a combination of objects whose values total at least one million dollars. For our purposes, we will assume that this is the only qualification in synthesizing a package. Suppose we have nine objects with the values:

Object:	A	B	C	D	E	F	G	H	I
Value in $1000:	910	870	810	640	550	250	120	95	55

We want to maximize the number of packages that we form.

The packing approach to formulating a model for this problem constructs all possible packages or groups that just satisfy the one million minimum. The general form of the LP/IP is:

Maximize number of packages selected
s.t.
Each object appears in at most one selected package.

In the actual formulation below, we will use variable names like AB, BGH, etc., to represent packages of (A and B), (B, G, and H). The resulting LP/IP model in PICTURE form is:

```
                                                    D E
                                B B B          C    D F F
        A A A A A A A B B B B G G H C C C G D F H G
        B C D E F G H C D E F H I I D E F H E G I H
  1:  1 1 1 1 1 1 1 1 1 1 1 1 1 1 1 1 1 1 1 1 1 1 MAX
  A:  1 1 1 1 1 1 1         '         '         '         '         ' < 1
  B:  1   '   '   '   ' 1'1 1 1'1 1 1'   '   '   '   '   ' < 1
  C:    1   '       ' 1   '         '   1 1 1 1 '       ' < 1
  D:      1 '       '   1 '         '   1 '     1 1 1 ' < 1
  E:  '   '   1 '   '   '   1 '   '   '   1 '   1   ' 1 < 1
  F:        ' 1   '       ' 1   '       ' 1   ' 1 1 1 < 1
  G:          '   1 '       '   1 1       '   1 ' 1   1 < 1
  H:  '   '   '   ' 1   '   ' '1 ' 1'   '   '1 '   '1 1 < 1
  I:          '       '       '   1 1   '       '   1 ' < 1
```

When solved as an LP, it produces the following naturally integer solution:

```
OBJECTIVE FUNCTION VALUE

      1)      4.00000000

VARIABLE            VALUE            REDUCED COST
      AH          1.000000              0.000000
     BGI          1.000000              0.000000
      CF          1.000000              0.000000
      DE          1.000000              0.000000
```

Thus, four packages are constructed, namely: AH, BGI, CF, and DE. It happens that every object appears in some package. There are alternate packings of all the objects into four groups. Thus, one may wish to consider secondary criteria for choosing one alternate optimum over another; e.g., the largest package should be as close as possible to one million in size.

14.8 Linearizing Products of Variables

We have previously seen that products of 0/1 variables, such as y_1, y_2, and y_1^2, can be represented by linear expressions by means of a simple transformation. This transformation generalizes to the case of the product of a 0/1 variable and a continuous variable.

To illustrate, suppose the product xy appears in a model, where y is 0/1 while x is nonnegative continuous. We want to replace this nonlinear component by a (somewhat bigger) linear component. If we have an upper bound, M_x, on the value of x, an upper bound, M_y, on the product xy, and we define $P = xy$, the following linear constraints will cause P to take on the correct value:

$$P \le x$$
$$P \le M_y y$$

$$P \geq x - M_x(1 - y)$$

Hanson and Martin (1990) show how this approach is useful in setting prices for products when we allow bundling of products. Bundle pricing is a form of quantity discounting. Examples of products that might be bundled are (a) airfare, hotel, rental car, tours, and meals or (b) computer, monitor, printer, and hard disk. Stigler (1963) showed how a movie distributor might improve profits by leasing bundles of movies rather than leasing individual movies. Bundling assumes that it is easy for the seller to assemble the bundle and difficult for a buyer to unbundle. Otherwise a reseller could buy the bundle at a discount and then sell the individual components at a markup.

14.8.1 Example: Bundling of Products

Microland Software has recently acquired an excellent word processing product to complement its own recently developed spreadsheet product. Microland is contemplating offering the combination of the two products for a discount. After demonstrating the products at a number of diverse professional meetings, Microland developed the following characterization of the market.

Market Segment	Size in 10,000	Maximum Price Market Segment is Willing to Pay for Various Bundles		
		Spreadsheet Only	Word Processor Only	Both
Business/Scientific	7	450	110	530
Legal/Administrative	5	75	430	480
Educational	6	290	250	410
Home	4.5	220	380	390

We will refer to each market segment as simply a "customer." Economic theory suggests that a customer will buy the product that gives it the greatest consumer surplus, where consumer surplus is defined as the price the customer is willing to pay for the product (the "reservation price") minus the market price for the product. For example, if the prices for the three bundles—spreadsheet only, word processor only, and both together—were set, respectively, at 400, 150, and 500, the Business/Scientific market would buy the spreadsheet alone because the consumer surplus is 50 vs. −40, and 30 for the other two bundles.

To give a general model of this situation, define:

R_{ij} = reservation price of customer i for bundle j,
N_i = "size" of customer i, i.e., number of individual customers in segment i,
s_i = consumer surplus achieved by customer i,
y_{ij} = 1 if customer i buys bundle j, 0 otherwise,
x_j = price of bundle j set by the seller.

We will treat the empty bundle as just another bundle so that we can say that every customer buys exactly one bundle.

The seller, Microland, would like to choose the x_j to:

$$\text{Maximize} \qquad \sum_i \sum_j N_i y_{ij} x_j.$$

The fact that each customer will buy exactly one bundle is enforced with:

For each customer i:

$$\sum_j y_{ij} = 1.$$

For each customer i, its achieved customer surplus is:

$$s_i = \sum_j \left(R_{ij} - x_j\right) y_{ij}.$$

Customer i will buy only that bundle j for which its consumer surplus, s_i, is maximum. This is enforced by the constraints:

For each customer i and bundle j:

$$s_i \geq R_{ij} - x_j.$$

A difficulty with the objective function and the consumer surplus constraints is that they involve the product $y_{ij} x_j$. Let us follow our previous little example and replace the product $y_{ij} x_j$ by P_{ij}. If M_j is an upper bound on x_j, proceeding as before, to enforce the definition that $P_{ij} = y_{ij} x_j$ we need the constraints:

$$P_{ij} \leq x_j$$
$$P_{ij} \leq R_{ij} y_{ij}$$
$$P_{ij} \geq x_j - (1 - y_{ij}) M_j.$$

Making these adjustments to the model, we get:

$$\text{Max} \ \ \sum_i \sum_j N_i P_{ij}$$

Subject to:

For each customer i

$$\sum_j y_{ij} = 1$$

For each customer i, bundle j:

$$s_i \geq R_{ij} - x_j$$

For each customer i:

$$s_i = \sum_j \left(R_{ij} y_{ij} - P_{ij}\right)$$

and to enforce the nonlinear condition $P_{ij} = y_{ij} x_j$, we have for each i and j:

$$P_{ij} \leq x_j$$
$$P_{ij} \leq R_{ij} y_{ij}$$
$$P_{ij} \geq x_j - (1 - y_{ij}) M_j.$$

For all i and j

$y_{ij} = 0$ or 1.

In explicit form, the LINDO model is:

```
MAX      7 PBZZ + 7 PBSZ + 7 PBZW + 7 PBSW -
         5 PLZZ + 5 PLSZ + 5 PLZW + 5 PLSW -
         6 PEZZ + 6 PESZ + 6 PEZW + 6 PESW +
       4.5 PHZZ + 4.5 PHSZ + 4.5 PHZW + 4.5 PHSW
SUBJECT TO
 ! Each customer buys exactly one bundle:
    2)    YBZZ + YBSZ + YBZW + YBSW =     1
    3)    YLZZ + YLSZ + YLZW + YLSW =     1
    4)    YEZZ + YESZ + YEZW + YESW =     1
    5)    YHZZ + YHSZ + YHZW + YHSW =     1
 ! Each customer's achieved surplus, S, must be at least
 !  as good as that possible from every bundle
    6)    XSZ + SB >=    450
    7)    XZW + SB >=    110
    8)    XSW + SB >=    530
    9)    XSZ + SL >=    75
   10)    XZW + SL >=    430
   11)    XSW + SL >=    480
   12)    XSZ + SE >=    290
   13)    XZW + SE >=    250
   14)    XSW + SE >=    410
   15)    XSZ + SH >=    220
   16)    XZW + SH >=    380
   17)    XSW + SH >=    390
 ! Compute the achieved surplus for each customer;
   18) - 450 YBSZ - 110 YBZW - 530 YBSW + PBZZ + PBSZ
       + PBZW + PBSW + SB =    0
   19) - 75 YLSZ - 430 YLZW - 480 YLSW + PLZZ + PLSZ
       + PLZW + PLSW + SL =    0
   20) - 290 YESZ - 250 YEZW - 410 YESW + PEZZ + PESZ
       + PEZW + PESW + SE =    0
   21) - 220 YHSZ - 380 YHZW - 390 YHSW + PHZZ + PHSZ
       + PHZW + PHSW + SH =    0
 ! Each product variable Pij must be..
 !   <= Xj
 !   <= Rij * Yij
 !   >= Xj - M + M * Yij
   22)    PBZZ <=    0    ! Empty bundle must have price = 0;
   23) - 600 YBZZ + PBZZ >= - 600
   24)    PBSZ - XSZ <=    0
   25) - 450 YBSZ + PBSZ <=    0
   26) - 600 YBSZ + PBSZ - XSZ >= - 600
   27)    PBZW - XZW <=    0
   28) - 110 YBZW + PBZW <=    0
   29) - 600 YBZW + PBZW - XZW >= - 600
   30)    PBSW - XSW <=    0
   31) - 530 YBSW + PBSW <=    0
   32) - 600 YBSW + PBSW - XSW >= - 600
```

```
 33)    PLZZ <=    0
 34)  - 600 YLZZ + PLZZ >= - 600
 35)    PLSZ - XSZ <=    0
 36)  - 75 YLSZ + PLSZ <=    0
 37)  - 600 YLSZ + PLSZ - XSZ >= - 600
 38)    PLZW - XZW <=    0
 39)  - 430 YLZW + PLZW <=    0
 40)  - 600 YLZW + PLZW - XZW >= - 600
 41)    PLSW - XSW <=    0
 42)  - 480 YLSW + PLSW <=    0
 43)  - 600 YLSW + PLSW - XSW >= - 600
 44)    PEZZ <=    0
 45)  - 600 YEZZ + PEZZ >= - 600
 46)    PESZ - XSZ <=    0
 47)  - 290 YESZ + PESZ <=    0
 48)  - 600 YESZ + PESZ - XSZ >= - 600
 49)    PEZW - XZW <=    0
 50)  - 250 YEZW + PEZW <=    0
 51)  - 600 YEZW + PEZW - XZW >= - 600
 52)    PESW - XSW <=    0
 53)  - 410 YESW + PESW <=    0
 54)  - 600 YESW + PESW - XSW >= - 600
 55)    PHZZ <=    0
 56)  - 600 YHZZ + PHZZ >= - 600
 57)    PHSZ - XSZ <=    0
 58)  - 220 YHSZ + PHSZ <=    0
 59)  - 600 YHSZ + PHSZ - XSZ >= - 600
 60)    PHZW - XZW <=    0
 61)  - 380 YHZW + PHZW <=    0
 62)  - 600 YHZW + PHZW - XZW >= - 600
 63)    PHSW - XSW <=    0
 64)  - 390 YHSW + PHSW <=    0
 65)  - 600 YHSW + PHSW - XSW >= - 600
! Price of bundle should be <= sum of component prices;
 66)  - XSZ - XZW + XSW <=    0
! Price of bundle should be >= price of any component;
 67)  - XSZ + XSW >=    0
 68)  - XZW + XSW >=    0
END
! Make the "pick a bundle" variables 0/1
INTEGER        YBZZ
INTEGER        YBSZ
INTEGER        YBZW
INTEGER        YBSW
INTEGER        YLZZ
INTEGER        YLSZ
INTEGER        YLZW
INTEGER        YLSW
INTEGER        YEZZ
INTEGER        YESZ
INTEGER        YEZW
INTEGER        YESW
INTEGER        YHZZ
INTEGER        YHSZ
INTEGER        YHZW
INTEGER        YHSW
```

For the Microland problem, the solution is to set the following prices:

	Spreadsheet Only	Word Processing Only	Both
Bundle Price:	410	380	410

Thus, the business, legal, and educational markets will buy the bundle of both products. The home market will buy only the word processor. Total revenues obtained by Microland are 90,900,000. The interested reader may show that, if bundling is not possible, the highest revenue that Microland can achieve is only 67,150,000.

14.9 Representing Logical Conditions

For some applications, it may be convenient, perhaps even logical, to state requirements using logical expressions. A logical variable can take on only the values TRUE or FALSE. Likewise, a logical expression involving logical variables can take on only the values TRUE or FALSE. There are two major logical operators, .AND. and .OR., that are useful in logical expressions.

The logical expression A .AND. B is TRUE if and only if both A and B are TRUE. The logical expression A .OR. B is TRUE if and only if at least one of A and B is TRUE.

It is sometimes useful to also have the logical operator, *implication*, written $\Rightarrow$, with the meaning that $A \Rightarrow B$ means that if A is true, B must be true. Logical variables are trivially representable by binary variables, with TRUE being represented by 1, and FALSE being represented by 0.

If A, B, and C are 0/1 variables, the following constraint combinations can be used to represent the various fundamental logical expressions:

Logical Expression	Mathematical Constraints
$C = A$ .AND. B	$C \leq A$
	$C \leq B$
	$C \geq A + B - 1$
$C = A$ .OR. B	$C \geq A$
	$C \geq B$
	$C \leq A + B$
$A \Rightarrow C$	$A \leq C$

14.9.1 Simplifying Difficult Integer Programs

Modest sized integer programs can nevertheless be very difficult to solve. There are a number of rules that can be kept in mind when facing such problems. Several of the most useful rules for difficult integer programs are:

1. Do Not Distinguish the Indistinguishable,
2. Presolve subproblems.

The following example illustrates.

You are a coal supplier and you have a nonexclusive contract with a consumer owned and managed electric utility, Power to the People (PTTP). You supply PTTP by barge. Your contract with PTTP stipulates that the coal you deliver must have at least 13000 BTUs per ton, no more than 0.63% sulfur, no more than 6.5% ash, and no more than 7% moisture. Historically, PTTP would not accept a barge if it did not meet the above requirements. After apprehensively noticing your rising coal inventories and reading the fine print of your PTTP contract carefully, you recently initiated some discussions with PTTP about how to interpret the above requirements. After some intense discussions, PTTP agreed to reinterpret the wording of the agreement and the above requirements to collections of up to three barges. That is, if the average quality taken over a set of N barges, N less than four, meets the above quality requirements, that set of N barges is acceptable. You may specify how the sets of barges are assembled. Each barge can be in at most one set. All the barges in a set must be in the same shipment.

You currently have the following barge loads available. What is the maximum number of barge loads you can ship to PTTP from this collection and how do you convince PTTP of the acceptability of the shipment?

	BTU/Ton	Sulfur %	Ash %	Moisture %
(1)	13029	0.57	5.56	6.2
(2)	14201	0.88	6.76	5.1
(3)	10630	0.11	4.36	4.6
(4)	13200	0.71	6.66	7.6
(5)	13029	0.57	5.56	6.2
(6)	14201	0.88	6.76	5.1
(7)	13200	0.71	6.66	7.6
(8)	10630	0.11	4.36	4.6
(9)	14201	0.88	6.76	5.1
(10)	13029	0.57	5.56	6.2
(11)	13200	0.71	6.66	7.6
(12)	14201	0.88	6.76	5.1

Looking at the original data, we see that, even though there are twelve barges, there are only four distinct barge types represented by the original first four barges. In reality you would expect this, each barge type corresponding to a specific mine with associated coal type.

Modeling the barge grouping problem as an assignment problem is relatively straightforward. The essential decision variable is defined as $X(I, J)$ = number of barges of type I assigned to group J. Note that we have retained the convention of not distinguishing between barges of the same type. Knowing that there are twelve barges, we can restrict ourselves to at most six groups without looking further at the data. The reasoning is: suppose there were seven nonempty groups. Then at least two of the groups must be singletons. If two singletons are feasible, so is the group obtained by combining them. Thus, we can write the following LINDO model.

```
      ! Maximize no. of barges assigned;
      MAX      XB11 + XB12 + XB13 + XB14 + XB15 + XB16 + XB21
               + XB22 + XB23 + XB24 + XB25 + XB26 + XB31 + XB32
               + XB33 + XB34 + XB35 + XB36 + XB41 + XB42 + XB43
               + XB44 + XB45 + XB46
        SUBJECT TO
      ! At most 3 per group;
          2)     XB11 + XB21 + XB31 + XB41 <=     3
          3)     XB12 + XB22 + XB32 + XB42 <=     3
          4)     XB13 + XB23 + XB33 + XB43 <=     3
          5)     XB14 + XB24 + XB34 + XB44 <=     3
          6)     XB15 + XB25 + XB35 + XB45 <=     3
          7)     XB16 + XB26 + XB36 + XB46 <=     3
      ! Assign no more of a type than are available;
          8)     XB11 + XB12 + XB13 + XB14 + XB15 + XB16 <=     3
          9)     XB21 + XB22 + XB23 + XB24 + XB25 - XB26 <=     4
         10)     XB31 + XB32 + XB33 + XB34 + XB35 - XB36 <=     2
         11)     XB41 + XB42 + XB43 + XB44 + XB45 - XB46 <=     3
      ! The blending constraints for each group;
         12)     29 XB11 + 1201 XB21 - 2370 XB31 + 200 XB41 >= 0
         13)  - 0.06 XB11 + 0.25 XB21 - 0.52 XB31 + 0.08 XB41 <= 0
         14)  - 0.94 XB11 + 0.26 XB21 - 2.14 XB31 + 0.16 XB41 <= 0
         15)  - 0.8 XB11 - 1.9 XB21 - 2.4 XB31 + 0.6 XB41 <= 0
         16)     29 XB12 + 1201 XB22 - 2370 XB32 + 200 XB42 >= 0
         17)  - 0.06 XB12 + 0.25 XB22 - 0.52 XB32 + 0.08 XB42 <= 0
         18)  - 0.94 XB12 + 0.26 XB22 - 2.14 XB32 + 0.16 XB42 <= 0
         19)  - 0.8 XB12 - 1.9 XB22 - 2.4 XB32 + 0.6 XB42 <=     0
         20)     29 XB13 + 1201 XB23 - 2370 XB33 - 200 XB43 >=    0
         21)  - 0.06 XB13 + 0.25 XB23 - 0.52 XB33 + 0.08 XB43 <= 0
         22)  - 0.94 XB13 + 0.26 XB23 - 2.14 XB33 + 0.16 XB43 <= 0
         23)  - 0.8 XB13 - 1.9 XB23 - 2.4 XB33 + 0.6 XB43 <=     0
         24)     29 XB14 + 1201 XB24 - 2370 XB34 - 200 XB44 >=    0
         25)  - 0.06 XB14 + 0.25 XB24 - 0.52 XB34 + 0.08 XB44 <= 0
         26)  - 0.94 XB14 + 0.26 XB24 - 2.14 XB34 + 0.16 XB44 <= 0
         27)  - 0.8 XB14 - 1.9 XB24 - 2.4 XB34 + 0.6 XB44 <=     0
         28)     29 XB15 + 1201 XB25 - 2370 XB35 + 200 XB45 >=    0
         29)  - 0.06 XB15 + 0.25 XB25 - 0.52 XB35 + 0.08 XB45 <= 0
         30)  - 0.94 XB15 + 0.26 XB25 - 2.14 XB35 + 0.16 XB45 <= 0
         31)  - 0.8 XB15 - 1.9 XB25 - 2.4 XB35 + 0.6 XB45 <=     0
         32)     29 XB16 + 1201 XB26 - 2370 XB36 + 200 XB46 >=    0
         33)  - 0.06 XB16 + 0.25 XB26 - 0.52 XB36 + 0.08 XB46 <= 0
         34)  - 0.94 XB16 + 0.26 XB26 - 2.14 XB36 + 0.16 XB46 <= 0
         35)  - 0.8 XB16 - 1.9 XB26 - 2.4 XB36 + 0.6 XB46 <=     0
      END
      GIN       24
```

Although easy to formulate, this model is nontrivial to solve.

This problem can be solved almost "by hand" with the matching or grouping (as opposed to the assignment) approach. Applying the rule "Presolve subproblems," we can enumerate all feasible combinations of three or less barges selected from the four types. Applying the "Don't distinguish" rule again, we do not have to consider combinations like (1,1) and (2,2,2), because such sets are feasible if and only if the singleton sets, e.g., (1) and (2) are also feasible. Thus, disregarding quality, there are four singleton sets, six doubleton sets, four distinct triplets (e.g., (1,2,3)) and twelve paired triplets (e.g., (1,1,2)) for a total of 26 combinations. It is not hard to show, even manually, that the only feasible combinations are: (1), (1,1,4), and (2,2,3). Thus, the matching-like IP we want to solve to maximize the number of barges sold is:

```
Max S001 + 3 S114 + 3 S223
S.T.
      S001 + 2 S114  <= 3  ( No. of type 1 barges)
      2 S223         <= 4  ( No. of type 2 barges)
      S223           <= 2  ( No. of type 3 barges)
      S114           <= 3  ( No. of type 4 barges)
```

This is easily solved to give $S001 = 1$, $S114 = 1$, and $S223 = 2$, with an objective value of 10.

For the given data, we can ship at most ten barges. One such way of matching them so that each set satisfies the quality requirements is as follows:

Barges in Set	Average Quality of the Set			
	BTU %	Sulfur %	Ash %	Moisture %
1	13029	0.57	5.56	6.2
4, 5, 10	13086	0.6167	5.927	6.667
2, 3, 6	13010	0.6233	5.96	4.933
8, 9, 12	13010	0.6233	5.96	4.933

14.9.2 Multiproduct, Constrained Dynamic Lot Size Problems

A common scheduling problem is that of deciding which product to produce in which period on a machine with limited capacity. This situation can be thought of as a single stage Material Requirements Planning (MRP) problem where production capacities, setup costs, and holding costs are explicitly considered and optimum solutions are sought.

Examples might be the scheduling of production runs of different types of home appliances on an appliance assembly line or the scheduling of different types of automotive tires onto a tire production line. In the applications described by Lasdon and Terjung (1971) and King and Love (1981), several dozen tire types compete for scarce capacity on a few expensive tire molding machines.

The general situation can be described formally by the following notation.

Input Data

P = number of products,
T = number of time periods,
d_{it} = demand for product i in period t , for $i = 1, 2, \ldots , P$; $t = 1, 2, \ldots , T$,
h_{it} = holding cost charged for each unit of product i in stock at end of period t,

c_{it} = cost per unit of each product produced in period t,

s_{it} = setup cost charged if there is any production of product i in period t,

a_t = production capacity in period t. We assume that the units (e.g., ounces, pounds, grams, etc.) have been chosen for each product so that producing one unit of any product uses one unit of production capacity.

There have been many mathematical programming formulations of this problem, most of them bad. Lasdon and Terjung (1971) describe a good formulation that has been profitably used for many years at the Kelly-Springfield Tire Company. The following formulation due to Eppen and Martin (1987) appears to be one of the best and enjoys the additional benefit of being moderately easy to describe. The decision variables used in this formulation are:

x_{ist} = fraction of demand in periods s through t of product i that is produced in period s, where $1 < s < t < T$.

   = 0 otherwise.

y_{it} = 1 if any product i is produced in period t.

   = 0 otherwise.

It is useful to compute the variable cost associated with variable x_{ist}. It is:

$$g_{ist} = c_{is}\left(d_{is} + d_{i,s+1} + \cdots + d_{it}\right) + d_{i,s+1} + h_{is} + d_{i,s+2}\left(h_{is} - h_{i,s+1}\right)$$
$$+ \cdots + d_{it}\left(h_{is} + h_{i,s+1} + \cdots + h_{i,t-1}\right)$$

Similarly, it is useful to compute the amount of production, p_{ist}, in period s that is associated with using variable x_{ist},

$$p_{ist} = d_{is} + d_{i,s+1} + \cdots + d_{it}$$

The objective function can now be written

$$\text{Min} \quad \sum_{i=1}^{P}\left(\sum_{t=1}^{T} s_{it}y_{it} + \sum_{s=1}^{T} \sum_{t=s}^{T} g_{ist}x_{ist}\right)$$

There will be three types of constraints, specifically, (a) constraints that cause demand to be met each period for each product, (b) constraints that for each product and period force a setup cost to be incurred if there was any production of that product, and (c) constraints that force total production to be within capacity each period. The constraints can be written as:

(a) $\displaystyle\sum_{t=1}^{T} x_{i1t} = 1$, for $i = 1, 2, \ldots, P$

$\displaystyle\sum_{t=s}^{T} x_{ist} - \sum_{r=1}^{s-1} x_{i,r,s-1} = 0$, for $i = 1, 2, \ldots, P$ and $s = 2, 3, \ldots, T$

(b) $y_{is} - x_{iss} - x_{is,s+1} - \cdots - x_{is,T} \geq 0$, for $i = 1, 2, \ldots, P$ and $s = 1, 2, \ldots, T$

(c) $\displaystyle\sum_{i-1}^{P} \sum_{t=s}^{T} p_{ist}x_{ist} \leq a_s$, for $s = 1, 2, \ldots, T$

All variables are required to be nonnegative. y_{it} is required to be either 0 or 1.

If any of the $d_{it} = 0$, there must be a slight modification in the formulation. In particular, if $p_{ist} = 0$, x_{ist} should not appear in constraint set (b). Also, if $p_{ist} = 0$ and $s < t$, variable x_{ist} may be dropped completely from the formulation.

The following example illustrates the model.

14.9.3 Example

The parameters of a two-product, constrained, dynamic lotsize problem are as follows:

		May	June	July	Aug	Sept	Oct
Demand							
	Product A:	40	60	100	40	100	200
	Product B:	20	30	40	30	25	35
Setup Cost							
	Product A:	100	100	150	150	200	200
	Product B:	30	40	30	55	45	45
Variable Cost/Unit							
	Product A:	5	6	7	8	9	10
	Product B:	2	4	4	5	5	5
Unit Holding Cost/Period							
	Product A:	1	1	2	2	3	2
	Product B:	2	1	1	2	1	2

Production capacity is 200 units per period, regardless of product. Two products can be produced in a period.

The LP/IP formulation for this example appears below.

```
! Two Product Capacitated Lotsizing Problem.
!    Yit = 1 if product i is produced in period t,
!    XAst = 1 if demands in periods s through t are
!      satisfied from production in period s, for product A,
!    XBst = 1 etc. for product B.

  MIN  = 100 YA1 + 100 YA2 + 150 YA3 + 150 YA4 + 200 YA5
         + 200 YA6 + 30 YB1 + 40 YB2 + 30 YB3 + 55 YB4
         + 45 YB5 + 45 YB6 + 200 XA11 + 560 XA12 + 1260 XA13
         + 1620 XA14 + 2720 XA15 + 5520 XA16 + 360 XA22
         + 1060 XA23 + 1420 XA24 + 2520 XA25 + 5320 XA26
         + 700 XA33 + 1060 XA34 + 2160 XA35 + 4960 XA36
         + 320 XA44 + 1320 XA45 + 3920 XA46 + 900 XA55
         + 3300 XA56 + 2000 XA66 + 40 XB11 + 160 XB12
         + 360 XB13 + 540 XB14 + 740 XB15 + 1055 XB16
         + 120 XB22 + 320 XB23 + 500 XB24 + 700 XB25
```

```
             + 1015 XB26 + 160 XB33 + 310 XB34 + 485 XB35
             + 765 XB36 + 150 XB44 + 325 XB45 + 605 XB46
             + 125 XB55 + 335 XB56 + 175 XB66;
!    For product A:
!    If a production lot was depleted in period i-1 (the - terms),
!       then a production run of some sort must be started in
!       period i (the  + terms);
        [A1] + XA11 + XA12 + XA13 + XA14 + XA15 + XA16 =  + 1;
        [A2] - XA11 + XA22 + XA23 + XA24 + XA25 + XA26 =    0;
        [A3] - XA12 - XA22 + XA33 + XA34 + XA35 + XA36 =    0;
        [A4] - XA13 - XA23 - XA33 + XA44 + XA45 + XA46 =    0;
        [A5] - XA14 - XA24 - XA34 - XA44 + XA55 + XA56 =    0;
        [A6] - XA15 - XA25 - XA35 - XA45 - XA55 + XA66 =    0;
!    The setup forcing constraints for A;
    [FA1]   YA1 - XA11 - XA12 - XA13 - XA14 - XA15 - XA16 >= 0;
    [FA2]   YA2 - XA22 - XA23 - XA24 - XA25 - XA26 >=    0;
    [FA3]   YA3 - XA33 - XA34 - XA35 - XA36 >=      0;
    [FA4]   YA4 - XA44 - XA45 - XA46 >=        0;
    [FA5]   YA5 - XA55 - XA56 >=      0;
    [FA6]   YA6 - XA66 >=        0;
!    Same constraints for product B:
        [B1] + XB11 + XB12 + XB13 + XB14 + XB15 + XB16 =  + 1;
        [B2] - XB11 + XB22 + XB23 + XB24 + XB25 + XB26 =    0;
        [B3] - XB12 - XB22 + XB33 + XB34 + XB35 + XB36 =    0;
        [B4] - XB13 - XB23 - XB33 + XB44 + XB45 + XB46 =    0;
        [B5] - XB14 - XB24 - XB34 - XB44 + XB55 + XB56 =    0;
        [B6] - XB15 - XB25 - XB35 - XB45 - XB55 + XB66 =    0;
!    The setup forcing constraints;
    [FB1]   YB1 - XB11 - XB12 - XB13 - XB14 - XB15 - XB16 >= 0;
    [FB2]   YB2 - XB22 - XB23 - XB24 - XB25 - XB26 >=    0;
    [FB3]   YB3 - XB33 - XB34 - XB35 - XB36 >=    0;
    [FB4]   YB4 - XB44 - XB45 - XB46 >=        0;
    [FB5]   YB5 - XB55 - XB56 >=      0;
    [FB6]   YB6 - XB66 >=        0;
!    Here are the capacity constraints for each period;
!     The coefficient of a variable is the associated lotsize;
    [CAP1]   40 XA11 + 100 XA12 + 200 XA13 - 240 XA14
           + 340 XA15 + 540 XA16 + 20 XB11 + 50 XB12
           + 90 XB13 + 120 XB14  + 145 XB15 + 180 XB16
           <=   200;
    [CAP2]   60 XA22 + 160 XA23 + 200 XA24 + 300 XA25
           + 500 XA26 + 30 XB22 + 70 XB23 + 100 XB24
           + 125 XB25 + 160 XB26 <=   200;
    [CAP3]   100 XA33 + 140 XA34 + 240 XA35 + 440 XA36
           + 40 XB33 + 70 XB34 + 95 XB35 + 130 XB36 <=   200;
    [CAP4] 40 XA44 + 140 XA45 + 340 XA46 + 30 XB44
           + 55 XB45 + 90 XB46 <=   200;
    [CAP5]   100 XA55 + 300 XA56 + 25 XB55 + 60 XB56
           <=   200;
    [CAP6]   200 XA66 + 35 XB66 <=   200;
END
```

Variables YA1, YA2, . . . , YB1, . . . YB6 are restricted to the values 0 or 1.

The interpretation of the x_{ijk} variables and the constraint rows 2 through 7 can perhaps be better understood with the picture in the figure below.

Example Solution

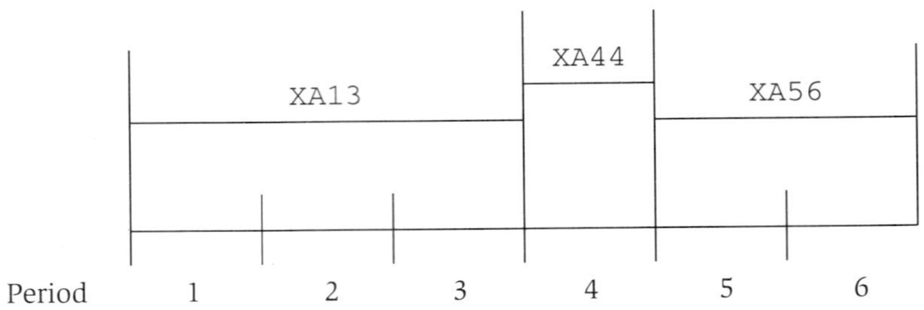

The constraints 2 through 7 force us to choose a set of batch sizes to exactly cover the interval from 1 to 6.

If we solve it as an LP (i.e., with the constraints $Y_{it} = 0$ or 1 relaxed to $0 \le Y_{it} \le 1$) we get a solution with cost 5968.125.

When solved as an IP, we get the following solution:

```
OBJECTIVE FUNCTION VALUE

1)              6030.00000

VARIABLE        VALUE
YA1             1.000000
YA2             1.000000
YA6             1.000000
YB1             1.000000
YB3             1.000000
YB5             1.000000
XA11            0.666667
XA15            0.333333
XA25            0.666667
XA66            1.000000
XB12            1.000000
XB34            1.000000
XB56            1.000000
```

The production amounts can be read off the coefficients of the nonzero X variables in the capacity constraints of the LP. This solution can be summarized as follows:

<table>
<tr><th colspan="3">Product A</th><th colspan="2">Product B</th></tr>
<tr><th>Period</th><th>Production</th><th></th><th>Period</th><th>Production</th></tr>
<tr><td>1</td><td>140</td><td>(.6667*40+.3333*340)</td><td>1</td><td>50</td></tr>
<tr><td>2</td><td>200</td><td>(.6667*300)</td><td>2</td><td>0</td></tr>
<tr><td>3</td><td>0</td><td></td><td>3</td><td>70</td></tr>
<tr><td>4</td><td>0</td><td></td><td>4</td><td>0</td></tr>
<tr><td>5</td><td>0</td><td></td><td>5</td><td>60</td></tr>
<tr><td>6</td><td>200</td><td></td><td>6</td><td>0</td></tr>
</table>

Extensions

There are a variety of extensions to this model that may be of practical interest, e.g:

    (a) *Carry-over setups.* It may be that a setup cost is incurred in period s only if there was production in period s, but no production in period $s - 1$. A straightforward though not necessarily good way of handling this is by introducing a new variable, z_{it} that is related to y_{it} by the relationship $z_{it} \geq y_{it} - y_{i,t-1}$. The setup cost is charged to z_{it} rather than y_{it}.

    (b) *Multiple machines in parallel.* There may be a choice among M machines on which a product can be run. This may be handled by appending an additional subscript m, for $m = 1, 2, \ldots, M$, to the x_{ist} and y_{it} variables. The constraints become:

$$(a') \quad \sum_{t=1}^{T} \sum_{m=1}^{M} x_{i1tm} = 1 \quad \text{for } i = 1, 2, \ldots, P,$$

$$\sum_{t=s}^{T} \sum_{m=1}^{M} x_{istm} - \sum_{r=1}^{s-1} \sum_{m=1}^{M} x_{i,r,s-1,m} = 0 \quad \text{for } i = 2, \ldots, P; \text{ and } s = 2, \ldots, T.$$

$$(b') \quad y_{ism} - x_{issm} - x_{i,s+1,m} - \cdots - x_{i,s,T,m} \leq 0 \quad \text{for } i = 1, 2, \ldots, P;$$

$$s = 1, 2, \ldots, T; m = 1, 2, \ldots, M.$$

$$(c') \quad \sum_{i=1}^{P} \sum_{t=s}^{T} p_{pstm} x_{istm} \leq a_{sm} \quad \text{for } s = 1, 2, \ldots, T; m = 1, 2, \ldots, M.$$

If the machines are nonidentical, the manner in which p_{istm} is calculated will be machine dependent.

14.10 PROBLEMS

Problem 1

The following problem is known as a segregated storage problem. A feed processor has various amounts of four different commodities that must be stored in seven different silos. Each silo can contain at most one commodity. Associated with each commodity and silo combination is a loading cost. Each silo has a finite capacity so some commodities may have to be split over several silos. The following table contains the data for this problem.

		Loading Cost/Ton Silo							Amount of Commodity to be
		1	2	3	4	5	6	7	Stored (in tons)
	A	1	2	2	3	4	5	5	75
	B	2	3	3	3	1	5	5	50
Commodity	C	4	4	3	2	1	5	5	25
	D	1	1	2	2	3	5	5	80
Silo Capacity in Tons		25	25	40	60	80	100	100	

(a) Present a formulation for solving this class of problems.

(b) Find the minimum cost solution for this particular example.

(c) How would your formulation change if additionally there was a fixed cost associated with each silo that is incurred if anything is stored in the silo?

Problem 2

You are the scheduling coordinator for a small growing airline. You must schedule exactly one flight out of Chicago to each of the following cities: Atlanta, Los Angeles, New York, and Peoria. The available departure slots are 8 A.M., 10 A.M., and 12 noon. Your airline has only two departure lounges, so at most two flights can be scheduled per slot. Demand data suggest the following expected profit contribution per flight as a function of departure time:

Expected Profit Contribution in 1000s

	Time		
Destination	8	10	12
Atlanta	10	9	8.5
Los Angeles	11	10.5	9.5
New York	17	16	15
Peoria	6.4	2.5	−1

Formulate a model for solving this problem.

Problem 3

A problem faced by an electrical utility each day is that of deciding which generators to start up. The utility in question has three generators with the following characteristics:

Generator	Fixed Startup Cost	Fixed Cost per Period of Operation	Maximum Cost per Period per Megawatt Used	Capacity in Megawatts Each Period
A	3000	700	5	2100
B	2000	800	4	1800
C	1000	900	7	3000

There are two periods in a day, and the number of megawatts needed in the first period is 2900. The second period requires 3900 megawatts. A generator started in the first period may be used in the second period without incurring an additional startup cost. All major generators (e.g., A, B, and C above) are turned off at the end of each day.

(a) First assume that fixed costs are zero and thus can be disregarded. What are the decision variables?

(b) Give the LP formulation for the case where fixed costs are zero.

(c) Now take into account the fixed costs. What are the additional (zero/one) variables to define?

(d) What additional terms should be added to the objective function? What additional constraints should be added?

Problem 4

Crude Integer Programming. Recently the U.S. Government began to sell crude oil from its Naval Petroleum Reserve in sealed bid auctions. There are typically six commodities or products to be sold in the auction, corresponding to the crude oil at the six major production and shipping points. A "bid package" from a potential buyer consists of (a) a number indicating an upper limit on how many barrels (bbl) the buyer is willing to buy overall in this auction and (b) any number of "product bids." Each product bid consists of a product name and three numbers representing, respectively, the bid price per bbls of this product, the minimum acceptable quantity of this product at this price, and the maximum acceptable quantity of this product at this price. Not all product bids of a buyer need be successful. The government usually places an arbitrary upper limit, e.g., 20%, on the percentage of the total bbls over all six products that one firm is allowed to purchase.

To illustrate the principal ideas, let us simplify slightly and suppose there are only two supply sources/products that are denoted by A and B. There are 17,000 bbls available at A, whereas B has 13,000. Also, there are only two bidders, the Mobon and the Exxil companies. The government arbitrarily decides that either one can purchase at most 65% of the total available crude. The two bid packages are as follows.

Mobon
Maximum desired = 16,000 bbls total.

Product	Bid/Bbl	Min Bbl Accepted	Max Bbl Wanted
A	43	9000	16000
B	51	6000	12000

Exxil
Maximum desired = No limit.

Product	Bid/Bbl	Min Bbl Accepted	Max Bbl Wanted
A	47	5000	10000
B	50	5000	10000

Formulate and solve an appropriate IP for the seller.

Problem 5

A certain state allows a restricted form of branch banking; specifically, a bank can do business in county i if the bank has a "principal place of business" in county i or in a county sharing a nonzero length border with county i. Figure 14.8 is a map of the state in question.

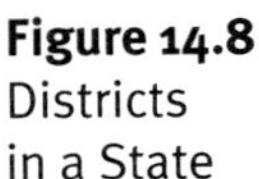

Figure 14.8
Districts
in a State

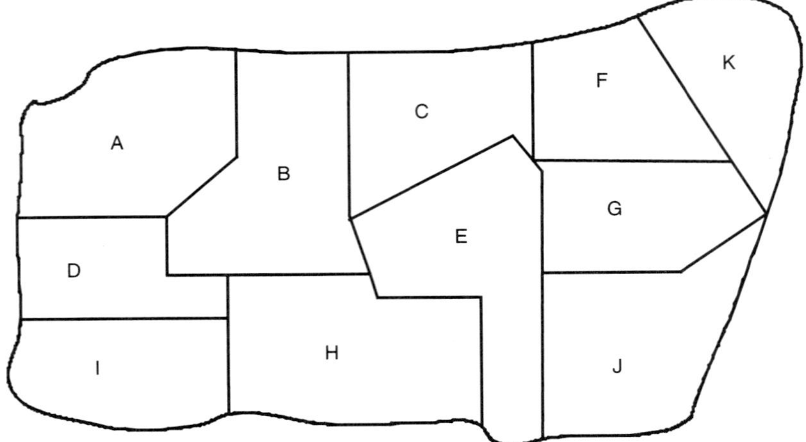

Formulate the problem of locating a minimum number of principal places of business in the state so that a bank can do business in every county in the state. If the problem is formulated as a covering problem, how many rows and columns will it have? What is an optimal solution? Which formulation is tighter, set covering or simple plant location?

Problem 6

Data Set Allocation Problem. There are 10 datasets, each of which is to be allocated to 1 of 3 identical disk storage devices. A disk storage device has 885 cylinders of capacity. Within a storage device a dataset will be assigned to a contiguous set of cylinders. Dataset sizes and interactions between datasets are shown in the table below. Two datasets with high interaction rates should not be assigned to the same device. For example, if datasets C and E are assigned to the same disk, an interaction cost of 46 is incurred. If they are assigned to different disks, there is no interaction cost between C and E.

Dataset for Interaction (Seek Transition) Rates

	A	B	C	D	E	F	G	H	I	J	Dataset Size in Cylinders
A											110
B	43										238
C	120	10									425
D	57	111	188								338
E	96	78	46	88							55

F	83	58	421	60	63					391
G	77	198	207	109	73	74				267
H	31	50	43	47	51	21	88			105
I	38	69	55	21	36	391	47	96		256
J	212	91	84	53	71	40	37	35	221	64
										2250

Find an assignment of datasets to disks so that total interaction cost is minimized and no disk capacity is exceeded.

Problem 7

The game of mastermind pits two players, a "coder" and a "decoder," against each other. The game is played with a pegboard and a large number of colored pegs. The pegboard has an array of 4×12 holes. For our purposes, we assume that there are only six colors: red, blue, clear, purple, gold, and green. Each peg has only one color. The coder starts the game by selecting four pegs and arranging them in a fixed order, all out of sight of the decoder. This ordering remains fixed throughout the game and is called the code. At each play of the game, the decoder tries to match the coder's ordering by placing four pegs in a row on the board. The coder then provides two pieces of information about how close the decoder's latest guess is to the coder's order:

1. The number of pegs in the correct position, i.e., color matching the coder's peg in that position, and
2. The maximum number of pegs that would be in correct position if the decoder were allowed to permute the ordering of the decoder's latest guess.

Call these two numbers m and n. The object of the decoder is to discover the code in a minimum number of plays.

The decoder may find the following IP of interest.

```
MAX        XRED1

SUBJECT TO
    2)    XRED1 + XBLUE1 + XCLEAR1 + XPURP1 + XGOLD1 + XGREEN1 = 1
    3)    XRED2 + XBLUE2 + XCLEAR2 + XPURP2 + XGOLD2 + XGREEN2 = 1
    4)    XRED3 + XBLUE3 + XCLEAR3 + XPURP3 + XGOLD3 + XGREEN3 = 1
    5)    XRED4 + XBLUE4 + XCLEAR4 + XPURP4 + XGOLD4 + XGREEN4 = 1
    6) XRED1 + XRED2   + XRED3 + XRED4 - RED = 0
    7) XBLUE1 + XBLUE2  + XBLUE3 + XBLUE4 - BLUE = 0
    8) XCLEAR1 + XCLEAR2 + XCLEAR3 + XCLEAR4 - CLEAR = 0
    9) XPURP1 + XPURP2 + XPURP3 + XPURP4 - PURP =  0
   10) XGOLD1 + XGOLD2 + XGOLD3 + XGOLD4 - GOLD = 0
   11) XGREEN1 + XGREEN2 + XGREEN3 + XGREEN4 - GREEN = 0
    END
```

All variables are required to be integer. The interpretation of the variables are as follows. XRED1 = 1 if a red peg is in position 1, otherwise 0; XGREEN4 = 1 if a green peg is in position 4, otherwise 0. Rows 2 through 5 enforce the requirement that exactly one peg be placed in each position. Rows 6 through 11 are simply accounting constraints that count the number of pegs of each color. For example, RED = the number of red pegs in any position 1 through 4. The objective is unimportant. All variables are (implicitly) required to be nonnegative.

At each play of the game, the decoder can add new constraints to this IP to record the information gained. Any feasible solution to the current formulation is a reasonable guess for the next play. An interesting question is what constraints can be added at each play.

To illustrate, suppose the decoder guesses the solution XBLUE1 = XBLUE2 = XBLUE3 = XRED4 = 1, and the coder responds with the information that $m = 1$ and $m - n = 1$, that is, one peg is in the correct position, and if permutations were allowed, at most two pegs would be in the correct position. What constraints can be added to the IP to incorporate the new information?

Problem 8

The Mathematical Football League (MFL) is composed of M teams (M is even). In a season of $2(M - 1)$ consecutive Sundays, each team will play $(2M - 1)$ games. Each team must play each other team twice, once at home and once at the other team's home stadium. Each Sunday, k games from the MFL are televised. We are given a matrix $\{v_{ij}\}$ where v_{ij} is the viewing audience on a given Sunday if a game between teams i and j playing at team j's stadium is televised.

   (a) Formulate a model for generating a schedule for the MFL that maximizes the viewing audience over the entire season. Assume that viewing audiences are additive.
   (b) Are some values of k easier to accommodate than others? How?

Problem 9

The typical automobile has close to two dozen electric motors; however, if you examine these motors you will see that only about a half dozen distinct motor types are used. For inventory and maintenance reasons, the automobile manufacturer would like to use as few distinct types as possible. For cost, quality, and weight reasons, one would like to use as many distinct motor types as possible so that the most appropriate motor can be applied to each application. The table at the top of the following page describes the design possibilities for a certain automobile.

For example, two motors are required to operate the head lamps. If type D motors are used for head lamps, the estimated probability of a head lamp motor failure in two years is about 0.01. If no entry appears for a particular combination of motor type and application, it means that the motor type is inappropriate for that application, e.g., because of size.

24-Month Failure Probability

Application	Number Required	Motor Type				
		A	*B*	*C*	*D*	*E*
Head lamps	2	.002	.01		.01	.007
Radiator fan	2		.01	.002		.004
Wipers	2				.007	
Seat	4	.003			.006	.008
Mirrors	2			.004	.001	
Heater fan	1		.006	.001		
Sun roof	1	.002			.003	.009
Windows	4	.004	.008	.005		
Antenna	1	.003		.003	.002	
Weight		2	3	1.5	1	4
Cost per Motor		24	20	36	28	39

Formulate a solvable linear integer program for deciding which motor type to use for each application so that at most M motor types are used, the total weight of the motors used is less than W, total cost of motors used is less than or equal to K, and probability of any failure in two years is approximately minimized.

Problem 10

We have a rectangular three-dimensional container that is 30 * 50 * 50. We want to pack in it rectangular three dimensional boxes of the three different sizes:

(a) 5 * 5 * 10, (b) 5 * 10 * 10, and (c) 5 * 15 * 25.

A particular packing of boxes into the container is undominated if there is no other packing that contains at least as many of each of the three box types and strictly more of one of the box types.

Show that there are no more than 3101 undominated packings.

Problem 11

Given the illustration at the right, if two opposite corners of the checkerboard are made unavailable, prove that there is no way of exactly covering the remaining grid with 17 dominoes.

Checkerboard

Domino

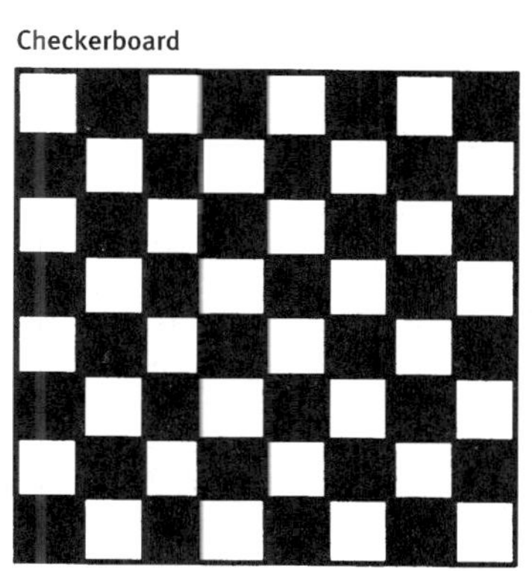

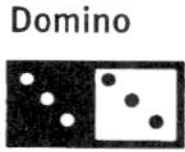

Problem 12

Which of the following requirements could be represented exactly with linear constraints? (You are allowed to use transformations if you wish.)

   (a) $(3 * x + 4 * y)/(2 * x + 3 * y) \leq 12$;
   (b) $\mathrm{MAX}(x, y) < 8$;
   (c) $3 * x + 4 * y * y \geq 11$;
       where y is 0 or 1;
   (d) $\mathrm{ABS}\,(10 - x) \leq 7$; (Note ABS means absolute value).
   (e) $\mathrm{MIN}(x, y) < 12$.

Problem 13

A common way of controlling access in many systems, such as information systems or the military, is with priority levels. Each user i is assigned a clearance level U_i. Each object j is assigned a security level L_j. A user i does not have access to object j if the security level of j is higher than the clearance level of i. Given a set of users and for each user a list of which objects that user is not to have access to, and a list of objects for which it should have access to, can we assign U_i's and L_j's so that these access rights and denials are satisfied? Formulate as an integer program and solve.

Problem 14

One of the big consumption items in the U.S. is automotive fuel. Any petroleum distributor who can deliver this fuel reliably and efficiently to the hundreds of filling stations in a typical distribution region has a competitive advantage. This distribution problem is complicated by the fact that a typical customer (i.e., filling station) requires three major products: premium gasoline, an intermediate octane grade (e.g., "Silver"), and regular gasoline. A typical situation is described below. A delivery tank truck has four compartments with capacities in liters of 13600, 11200, 10800, and 4400. We would like to load the truck according to the following limits:

	Liters of		
	Premium	Intermediate	Regular
At least:	8800	12000	12800
At most:	13200	17200	16400

Only one gasoline type can be stored per compartment in the delivery vehicle. Subject to the previous considerations, we would like to maximize the amount of fuel loaded on the truck.

   (a) Define the decision variables you would use in formulating this problem as an IP.
   (b) Give a formulation of this problem.
   (c) What allocation do you recommend?

Problem 15

Most lotteries are of the form:

> Choose n numbers, e.g., $n = 6$, from the set of numbers $\{1, 2, \ldots, m\}$,
> e.g., $m = 54$.

You win the grand prize if you buy a ticket and choose a set of n numbers that are identical to the n numbers eventually chosen by lottery management. Smaller prizes are awarded to people who match k of the n numbers. For $n = 6$, typical values for k are 4 and 5. Consider a modest little lottery with $m = 7$, $n = 3$, and $k = 2$. How many tickets would you have to buy to guarantee winning a prize? Can you set this up as a grouping/covering problem?

Application to Statistical Estimation

15.1 Introduction

LP can be used for linear regression in much the same way that least squares is used. Classical least squares estimation finds the prediction formula that minimizes the sum of squared differences between the observed and the prediction. LP is applicable if, instead of minimizing the sum of squared errors, one wishes to either:

(a) Minimize the sum of the absolute errors.
(b) Minimize the maximum absolute error.
(c) Minimize the error in predicting the ranking of items, so-called ordinal regression.

A standard notation we shall use is:

$$n = \text{number of observations,}$$
$$k = \text{number of explanatory variables,}$$
$$d_i = \text{value of the dependent variable in observation } i, \text{ for } i = 1, 2, \ldots, n,$$
$$e_{ij} = \text{value of the } j\text{th independent variable in observation } i, \text{ for } i = 1, 2, \ldots,$$
$$n \text{ and } j = 1, 2, \ldots, k.$$

We want to determine:

$$x_j = \text{prediction coefficient applied to the } j\text{th explanatory variable,}$$
$$w_i = \text{error of the forecast formula applied to the } i\text{th observation.}$$

Least squares regression then finds values for the x_j's that:

$$\text{Minimize} \quad w_1^2 + w_1^2 + \ldots w_n^2$$

$$\text{Subject to} \quad w_i = d_i - x_0 - \sum_{j=1}^{k} e_{ij} x_j$$

$$x_j, w_i \text{ unconstrained in sign}$$

15.2 Least Absolute Deviations (LAD) Estimation

An alternative objective might be to minimize the sum of the absolute values of the errors. That is:

$$\text{Minimize } |w_1| + |w_2| + |w_3| + \ldots + |w_n|.$$

A LAD regression is less affected by extreme outliers. Thus, it is appropriate to use if the data contain a few extreme observations that would otherwise affect the predictions more than is deemed proper.

Linear programming can be applied to this problem if we define:

$$u_i - v_i = w_i.$$

The difference, $u_i - v_i$, is introduced because w_i is unconstrained in sign, whereas LP is designed for variables constrained to be nonnegative. The problem of minimizing the sum of absolute errors can now be written:

$$\text{Min } u_1 + v_1 + u_2 + v_2 + \ldots + u_n + v_n$$

subject to

$$u_i - v_i = x_0 - \sum_{j=1}^{k} e_{ij} x_j \quad \text{for } i = 1, 2, \ldots, n.$$

$$x_j \text{ unconstrained in sign.}$$

15.2.1 Example

We have five observations on a single explanatory variable.

d_i	e_{i1}
2	1
3	2
4	4
5	6
8	7

The plot of d_i versus e_{i1} appears in Figure 15.1. With the exception of the last point $(8, 7)$, a straight line would provide a good fit.

The LP specific for this problem is:

```
MIN       U1 + V1 + U2 + V2 + U3 + V3 + U4 + V4 + U5 + V5
SUBJECT TO
   2)     U1 - V1 + X0 + X1  =    2
   3)     U2 - V2 + X0 + 2 X1 =   3
   4)     U3 - V3 + X0 + 4 X1 =   4
   5)     U4 - V4 + X0 + 6 X1 =   5
   6)     U5 - V5 + X0 + 7 X1 =   8
END
```

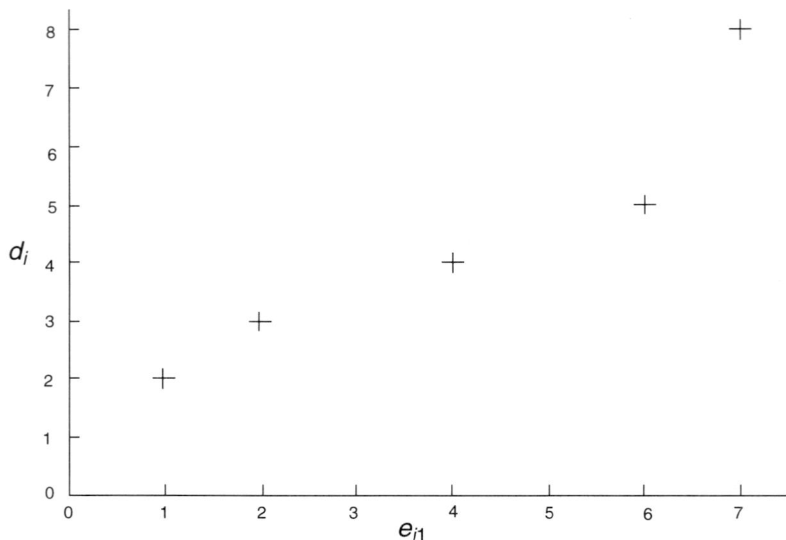

Figure 15.1
Observations on
a Dependent and
an Explanatory
Variable

The PICTURE of the matrix is more revealing of the problem's structure:

```
PICTURE
          U V U V U V U V U V X X
          1 1 2 2 3 3 4 4 5 5 0 1
     1:   1 1 1 1 1 1 1 1 1 1        MIN
     2:   1-1                   1 1 = 2
     3:       1-1               1 2 = 3
     4:           1-1           1 4 = 4
     5:               1-1       1 6 = 5
     6:                   1-1 1 7 = 8
```

The solution is:

```
         LP OPTIMUM FOUND
               OBJECTIVE FUNCTION VALUE
     1)              2.666667
     VARIABLE             VALUE          REDUCED COST
       U1               0.000000           1.333333
       V1               0.000000           0.666667
       U2               0.333333           0.000000
       V2               0.000000           2.000000
       U3               0.000000           1.666667
       V3               0.000000           0.333333
       U4               0.000000           2.000000
       V4               0.333333           0.000000
       U5               2.000000           0.000000
       V5               0.000000           2.000000
       X0               1.333333           0.000000
       X1               0.666667           0.000000
```

```
ROW                     SLACK                DUAL PRICES
 2)                  0.000000                  0.333333
 3)                  1.000000                 -1.000000
 4)                  0.000000                  0.666667
 5)                  0.000000                  1.000000
 6)                  0.000000                 -1.000000

NO.  ITERATIONS=           6
```

The values for X0 and X1 specify the prediction formula:

$$y_i = 1.3333 + .666667\, e_{i1}.$$

15.2.2 Measuring Goodness of Fit for LAD

In classical least-squares, the goodness of fit is measured by a statistic usually called the R^2. This statistic equals the fraction of the variability in the d_is that is explained or eliminated by the prediction model. An analogous statistic can be computed for the LAD regression if we define m to be the median of the d_i. E.g., for our example data, $m = 4$. The analogous R^2 (the so-called "adjusted") is then:

$$1 - \frac{\left(u_1 + v_1 + \cdots + u_n + v_n\right)/\left(n - k - 1\right)}{\left(\left|d_1 - m\right| + \cdots + \left|d_n - m\right|\right)/\left(n - 1\right)}$$

For our example, this statistic is:

$$1 - \frac{\left(2.66667\right)/\left(3\right)}{\left(2 + 1 + 0 + 1 + 4\right)/\left(4\right)} = 0.55556$$

For reference, we will present the least squares solution to this prediction problem. It is:

$$d_i = 1.015 + 0.846\, e_{i2}.$$

The adjusted R^2 for this formula is 0.8374.

15.3 Least Maximum (LMAX) Deviation Regression

LMAX regression is at the opposite end of the spectrum from LAD regression. LMAX minimizes the worst error of forecast that occurs on any observation. A single extreme observation will have a dramatic effect upon the estimates derived. The general form of an LP model for an LMAX regression is:

$$\text{Min } z$$
s.t.
$$x_0 + e_{i1}x_1 + e_{i2}x_2 + \ldots e_{ik}x_k + u_i - v_i = d_i \qquad \text{for } i = 1, 2, \ldots, n.$$
$$z - u_i - v_i \geq 0 \qquad \text{for } i = 1, 2, \ldots, n.$$
$$x_j \text{ unconstrained in sign.}$$

This formulation exploits the fact that, at an optimal solution, at most one of u_i and v_i will be nonzero. Therefore, $z \geq u_i$ and $z \geq v_i$ is equivalent to $z \geq u_i + v_i$.

For our example problem, the formulation is:

```
MIN        Z
SUBJECT TO
  2)      X0  -  Y0  +      X1  +  U1  -  V1  =      2
  3)      X0  -  Y0  +   2 X1  +  U2  -  V2  =      3
  4)      X0  -  Y0  +   4 X1  +  U3  -  V3  =      4
  5)      X0  -  Y0  +   6 X1  +  U4  -  V4  =      5
  6)      X0  -  Y0  +   7 X1  +  U5  -  V4  =      8
  7)      Z-U1  -  V1  >=      0
  8)      Z-U2  -  V2  >=      0
  9)      Z-U3  -  V3  >=      0
 10)      Z-U4  -  V4  >=      0
 11)      Z-U5  -  V5  >=      0
END
```

Notice that the variable X0 has been replaced by the difference X0 - Y0, because the original X0 is unconstrained in sign.

The PICTURE of the matrix reveals more of the structure of this formulation:

```
PICTURE
                        X Y X U V U V U V U V U V
                      Z 0 0 1 1 1 2 2 3 3 4 4 5 5
            1:    1                                          MIN
            2:        1-1 1 1-1                              = 2
            3:        1-1 2       1-1                        = 3
            4:        1-1 4             1-1                  = 4
            5:        1-1 6                   1-1            = 5
            6:        1-1 7                         1-1  = 8
            7:    1        -1-1                             >
            8:    1             -1-1                        >
            9:    1                  -1-1                   >
           10:    1                       -1-1             >
           11:    1                            -1-1  >
```

The solution is:

```
            LP OPTIMUM FOUND
                  OBJECTIVE FUNCTION VALUE
        1)              1.000000
     VARIABLE              VALUE              REDUCED COST
        Z                1.000000              0.000000
        X0               0.000000              0.000000
        Y0               0.000000              0.000000
        X1               1.000000              0.000000
        U1               1.000000              0.000000
        V1               0.000000              0.000000
        U2               1.000000              0.000000
        V2               0.000000              0.200000
        U3               0.000000              0.000000
```

```
        V3                      0.000000                 0.000000
        U4                      0.000000                 1.000000
        V4                      1.000000                 0.000000
        U5                      1.000000                 0.000000
        V5                      0.000000                 0.800000

       ROW                        SLACK                 DUAL  PRICES
        2)                      0.000000                 0.000000
        3)                      0.000000                -0.000000
        4)                      0.000000                 0.000000
        5)                      0.000000                 0.500000
        6)                      0.000000                -0.400000
        7)                      0.000000                 0.000000
        8)                      0.000000                -0.100000
        9)                      0.000000                 0.000000
       10)                      0.000000                -0.500000
       11)                      0.000000                -0.400000

    NO.  ITERATIONS=        9
```

The values of X0 $-$ Y0 and X1 reveal that the prediction formula is:

$$y_i = e_{i1}.$$

15.3.1 Measuring Goodness of Fit, LMAX Case

Define r to be equal to the range of the d_i's, that is, $\max\{d_i\}-\min\{d_i\}$. The analog of the adjusted R^2 is then:

$$1 - \frac{\max\{u_i + v_i\}/(n - k - 1)}{r/(n - 1)}.$$

For our example, this statistic equals:

$$1 - \frac{1/3}{8 - 2/4} = 0.778.$$

The three different prediction curves resulting from the three different methods applied to the example data are displayed in Figure 15.2. Notice that Least Maximum Deviation is most affected by the outlier at (8, 7), whereas Least Absolute Deviation is least affected by the outlier.

15.4 Exploiting the Dual to Obtain a More Compact Formulation

The amount of work required to solve an LP is much more highly correlated with the number of rows than with the number of columns. Because the solution to the dual problem provides the same information as the solution to the primal, one may wish to solve the dual if it has fewer rows.

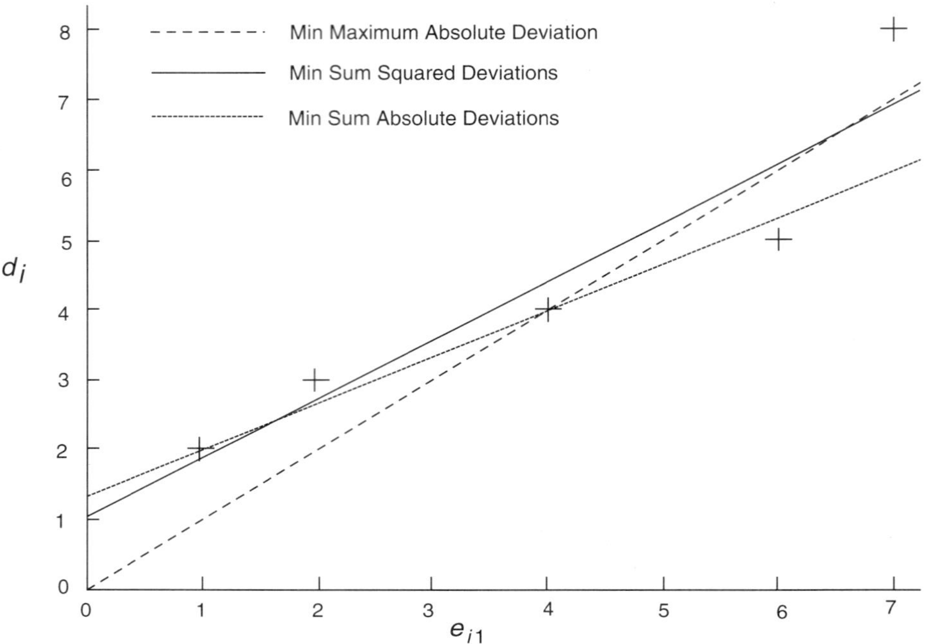

Figure 15.2
Prediction Line
According to
Error Measure

15.4.1 Dual of LAD Formulation

First we will examine the Least Absolute Deviation problem. The dual of the previous formulation is:

$$\text{Max} \quad \lambda_1 d_1 + \lambda_2 d_2 + \ldots + \lambda_n d_n$$

s.t.

$$\lambda_1 e_{1j} + \lambda_2 e_{2j} + \ldots + \lambda_n d_{nj} = 0 \quad \text{for } j = 0, 1, \ldots, k$$
$$\lambda_i \leq 1$$
$$\lambda_i \geq -1$$

This formulation is simplified slightly if we define:

$$L_i = \lambda_i + 1 \text{ so } \lambda_i = L_i - 1.$$

When this substitution is made, the formulation becomes:

$$\text{Max} \quad L_1 d_1 + L_2 d_2 + \ldots + L_n d_n - d_1 - d_2 - \ldots - d_n$$

s.t.

$$L_1 e_{ij} + L_2 e_{2j} + \ldots + L_n e_{nj} = e_{1j} + e_{2j} + \ldots + e_{nj} \quad \text{for } j = 0, 1, \ldots, k.$$
$$L_i \leq 2 \quad \text{for } i = 1, 2, \ldots, n.$$

This formulation has $n + k$ rows as compared to only n in the primal formulation; however, n of the constraints are of the very simple form $L_i \leq 2$.

Most LP codes exploit this simple form. This formulation and its shorthand picture appear below. The constant

$$-d_1 - d_2 - \ldots - d_n$$

in the objective function has no effect, so it is not included.

```
MAX     2 L1 + 3 L2 + 4 L3 + 5 L4 + 8 L5
SUBJECT TO
  2)       L1 +  L2 +  L3 +  L4 +  L5            <=  5
  3)       L1 + 2 L2 +  4 L3 +  6 L4 +  7 L5 <= 20
  4)       L1  <= 2
  5)       L2  <= 2
  6)       L3  <= 2
  7)       L4  <= 2
  8)       L5  <= 2
END

    PICTURE
              L L L L L
              1 2 3 4 5

        1:  2 3 4 5 8 MAX
        2:  1 1 1 1 1 < 5
        3:  1 2 4 6 7 < B
        4:  1           < 2
        5:    1         < 2
        6:      1       < 2
        7:        1     < 2
        8:          1 < 2
```

The solution is:

```
                LP OPTIMUM FOUND

                    OBJECTIVE FUNCTION VALUE
      1)                24.666670
      VARIABLE            VALUE          REDUCED COST
        L1              0.666667           0.000000
        L2              2.000000           0.000000
        L3              0.333333           0.000000
        L4              0.000000           0.333333
        L5              2.000000           0.000000

        ROW              SLACK            DUAL PRICES
       2)              0.000000           1.333333
       3)              0.000000           0.666667
       4)              1.333333           0.000000
       5)              0.000000           0.333333
       6)              1.666667           0.000000
       7)              2.000000           0.000000
       8)              0.000000           2.000000
    NO. ITERATIONS=        5
```

The dual prices on constraints (2) and (3), 1.3333 and 0.6667, correspond to X_0 and X_1. Notice that only five iterations were required to solve it as compared with six iterations for the primal formulation.

15.4.2 The Dual of the LMAX Formulation

The dual of the Least Maximum Deviation Formulation is:

Max $\sum_i \lambda_i d_i$

s.t.

$\sum_i \lambda_i e_{ij} = 0$ for $j = 1, 2, \ldots, k,$

$\lambda_i - \alpha_i \leq 0$ for $i = 1, 2, \ldots, n,$

$-\lambda_i - \alpha_i \leq 0$ for $i = 1, 2, \ldots, n,$

$\sum_i \alpha_i \leq 1$

λ_i unconstrained in sign

This formulation can be rearranged to a more convenient form if we define the variables g_i and h_i such that:

$g_i + h_i = \alpha_i$

$g_i - h_i = \lambda_i,$

with g_i and h_i unconstrained in sign. Substituting for both α_i and λ_i, the formulation becomes:

Max $\sum_i (g_i - h_i) d_i$

s.t.

$\sum_i (g_i - h_i) e_{ij} = 0$ for $j = 1, 2, \ldots, k,$

$g_i - h_i - (g_i + h_i) \leq 0$ or $-2h_i \leq 0$ or $h_i \geq 0$ for $i = 1, 2, \ldots, n,$

$-(g_i - h_i) - (g_i + h_i) \leq 0$ or $-2g_i \leq 0$ or $g_i \geq 0$ for $i = 1, 2, \ldots, n,$

$\sum_i (g_i - h_i) \leq 1$

The nonnegativity constraints $h_i \geq 0$ and $g_i \geq 0$ are assumed by any LP code, so they need not be explicitly stated.

The formulation and PICTURE applied to the example data are given below.

```
MAX 2 G1 - 2 H1 + 3 G2 - 3 H2 + 4 G3 - 4 H3 + 5 G4 - 5   H4
        + 8 G5 - 8 H5

SUBJECT TO
 2)  G1 - H1 + G2 - H2 + G3 - H3 + G4 - H4 + G5 - H5 = 0
 3)  G1 - H1 + 2 G2 - 2 H2 + 4 G3 - 4 H3 + 6 G4 - 6 H4 + 7 G5
        - 7 H5 = 0
 4)  G1 + H1 + G2 + H2 + G3 + H3 + G4 + H4 + G5 + H5 <=   0
END

   PICTURE
            G H G H G H G H G H
            1 1 2 2 3 3 4 4 5 5

        1:  2-2 3-3 4-4 5-5 8-8 MAX
        2:  1-1 1-1 1-1 1-1 1-1 =
        3:  1-1 2-2 4-4 6-6 7-7 =
        4:  1 1 1 1 1 1 1 1 1 1 < 1
```

The solution is:

```
            LP OPTIMUM FOUND
                OBJECTIVE FUNCTION VALUE
        1)              1.000000
     VARIABLE           VALUE           REDUCED COST
        G1              0.083333          0.000000
        H1              0.000000          2.000000
        G2              0.000000          0.000000
        H2              1.000000          2.000000
        G3              1.000000          1.000000
        H3              0.000000          1.000000
        G4              0.000000          2.000000
        H4              0.500000          0.000000
        G5              0.416667          0.000000
        H5              0.000000          2.000000

      ROW               SLACK           DUAL PRICES
       2)              0.000000          0.000000
       3)              0.000000          1.000000
       4)              0.000000          1.000000

   NO. ITERATIONS=          3
```

The dual prices for rows (2) and (3) are the values of $X0$ and $X1$.

Notice that this formulation had only three rows and required three iterations, as compared with ten constraints and nine iterations for the primal formulation.

15.5 Ordinal Regression

The regression methods discussed in the previous section apply when all the data are in numeric form. Sometimes, however, data are found in a more subjective or qualitative form. Consider, for example, a marketing study in which you are trying to predict what determines consumer preferences for various products in a class, e.g., breakfast foods. The data from a consumer survey might consist simply of preference statements of the form "I prefer Wheaties to Cheerios." There is available additional independent quantitative data on each breakfast food describing its characteristics, e.g., sweetness, nutritional value, and price. The desire is to determine how ranking by consumers depends upon the product characteristics.

This problem can be attacked via LP. Consider the following example. Five different cars, denoted by B, C, F, L, and M, have been evaluated by a consumer panel. These evaluations are in the form of eight different pairwise comparisons by different members of the panel. The results are as follows:

Comparison Number	Less Preferred Car	More Preferred Car
1	C	L
2	M	B
3	F	L
4	F	C
5	B	F
6	L	M
7	M	C
8	M	F

For example, the first comparison indicates that some consumers preferred an L to a C, whereas the last comparison indicates that some consumers preferred an F to a B.

Although one could, we have not required that these pairwise rankings be consistent or transitive. Indeed, if these rankings are collected from a number of people, we would expect some inconsistency among them. For example, you can note an inconsistency among rankings (3), (6), (2), and (5). Ranking (3) says F is inferior to L; however, rankings (6), (2), and (5) suggest that L is inferior to F.

We suspect that consumer preferences are affected by the four characteristics: price, weight, length, and mpg. These characteristics for the five cars are listed below:

Car	Price (1,000s)	Weight (1,000s)	Length (feet)	Mpg
B	9	4	15	17
C	6	3	13	21
F	7	2.8	13.5	20
L	10	4.2	15.5	16
M	8	3.9	14	18

Can you develop a scoring formula based on these characteristics such that higher scoring cars will tend to be the more preferred ones? Such a formula would help in identifying the relative importance of various characteristics. The following is an approach for developing such a scoring formula.

Define:

e_{ij} = value of characteristic j for car i,

x_j = scoring weight to be applied to characteristic j;

i.e., the score of car i is $x_1 e_{i1} + x_2 e_{i2} + \ldots + x_4 e_{i4}$,

z_k = the scoring error on the kth observation.

We want to choose the x_js so that the resulting scores agree as much as possible with the eight preference rankings given previously. We will say the scoring agrees with the first of the eight rankings, for example, if car L receives a higher score than car *C*. It agrees with the last ranking if car *F* receives a higher score than car *B*. To see how to compute the scoring error, z_k, suppose that car *F* is preferred to car *L* in the *k*th preference; then the following constraint will cause z_k to take on the proper value:

$$(e_{F1} - e_{L1})x_1 + (e_{F2} - e_{L2})x_2 + \ldots (e_{F4} - e_{L4})x_4 + z_k \geq 0$$

The left-hand side of this constraint is the score of *F* minus the score of $L + z_k$.

A reasonable objective is then to:

$$\text{Minimize } z_1 + z_2 + \ldots + z_8.$$

Using a right-hand side of zero only forces the score of *F* to at least equal the score of *L*. It does not force the score of *F* to exceed the score of *L*. If this is desired, the zero might be replaced by a small positive number, e.g., 0.001. This is illustrated in a later example.

We need a "normalizing" constraint to prohibit the useless solution: $x_1 = x_2 = x_3 = x_4 = 0$. The simplest possible normalizing constraint is $x_1 + x_2 + x_3 + x_4 = 1$.

This, however, ignores the fact that the various characteristics have different units; e.g., mpg may range from 10 to 40, whereas price may have a much higher range of from 2,000 to 20,000. Thus, you probably want to use different weights on the x_js. A reasonable weighted normalizing constraint is:

$$\sum_{j=1}^{4} \sum_{i=1}^{8} \left(e_{rj} - e_{sj}\right)x_j = 1$$

Realize that the x_j are unconstrained in sign; therefore, in the LP formulation, the x_js will be replaced by the difference $x_j - y_j$. The complete formulation and PICTURE for our example follow.

```
 MIN   Z1 +   Z2 +   Z3 +   Z4 +   Z5 +   Z6 +   Z7 +   Z8
 SUBJECT TO
   2)   Z1 + 4 X1 - 4 Y1 + 1.2 X2 - 1.2 Y2 + 2.5 X3 - 2.5 Y3 - 5 X4
        + 5 Y4   >= 0
   3)   Z2 +   X1 -   Y1 + 0.1 X2 - 0.1 Y2 +   X3 -   Y3 - X4
        -   Y4   >=  0
   4)   Z3 + 3 X1 - 3 Y1 + 1.4 X2 - 1.4 Y2 + 2 X3 - 2 Y3 - 4 X4
        + 4 Y4   >=  0
   5)   Z4 -   X1 +   Y1 + 0.2 X2 - 0.2 Y2 - 0.5 X3 + 0.5 X3 +   X4
        -   Y4   >=  0
   6)   Z5 - 2 X1 + 2 Y1 - 1.2 X2 + 1.2 Y2 - 1.5 X3 + 1.5 Y3 + 3 X4
        - 3 Y4   >=  0
   7)   Z6 - 2 X1 + 2 Y1 - 0.3 X2 + 0.3 Y2 - 1.5 X3 + 1.5 Y3 + 2 X4
        - 2 Y4   >=  0
   8)   Z7 - 2 X1 + 2 Y1 - 0.9 X2 + 0.9 Y2 -   X3 +   Y3 + 3 X4
        - 3 Y4   >=  0
   9)   Z8 -   X1 +   Y1 - 1.1 X2 + 1.1 Y2 - 0.5 X3 + 0.5 Y3 + 2 X4
        - 2 Y4   >=  0
  10)   - 0.6 X2 + 0.6 Y2 + 0.5 X3 - 0.5 Y3 + 3 X4 - 3 Y4 =  1
 END
```

```
PICTURE
      Z Z Z Z Z Z Z Z X Y X Y X Y X Y
      1 2 3 4 5 6 7 8 1 1 2 2 3 3 4 4
 1:  1 1 1 1 1 1 1 1                         MIN
 2:  1                 4-4 A-A A-A-5 5 >
 3:    1               1-1 U-U 1-1-1-1 >
 4:      1             3-3 A-A 2-2-4 4 >
 5:        1           -1 1 T-T-T T 1-1 >
 6:          1         -2 2-A A-A A 3-3 >
 7:            1       -2 2-T T-A A 2-2 >
 8:              1     -2 2-T T-1 1 3-3 >
 9:                    1-1 1-A A-T T 2-2 >
10:                    -T T T-T 3-3 = 1
```

The solution report is:

```
                   LP OPTIMUM FOUND

                 OBJECTIVE FUNCTION VALUE

        1)             0.07692308

        VARIABLE          VALUE          REDUCED COST
          Z1           0.000000            0.576923
          Z2           0.000000            0.500000
          Z3           0.000000            1.000000
          Z4           0.000000            1.000000
          Z5           0.000000            1.000000
          Z6           0.076923            0.000000
          Z7           0.000000            1.000000
          Z8           0.000000            0.807692
          X1           0.461538            0.000000
          Y1           0.000000            0.000000
          X2           0.384615            0.000000
          Y2           0.000000            0.000000
          X3           0.000000            0.000000
          Y3           0.076923            0.000000
          X4           0.423077            0.000000
          Y4           0.000000            1.000000

          ROW            SLACK          DUAL PRICES
          2)           0.000000           -0.423077
          3)           0.000000           -0.500000
          4)           0.076923            0.000000
          5)           0.076923            0.000000
          6)           0.000000            0.000000
          7)           0.000000           -1.000000
          8)           0.076923            0.000000
          9)           0.000000           -0.192308
         10)           0.000000           -0.076923

     NO. ITERATIONS=          7
```

The implication of the report is that the scoring formula for a car should be (for the case of a zero right-hand side for constraints 2 to 9):

Score = 0.461538 Price + 0.384615 Weight − 0.076923 Length + 0.423077 MPG, whereas the formula with an RHS of 0.001 for constraints (2) through (9) is:

$$Score = 0.461385\ Price + 0.381154\ Weight - 0.076231\ Length + 0.422269\ MPG.$$

The resulting scores for the five cars are:

	Score	
Car	(RHS = 0.000)	(RHS = 0.001)
B	11.73077	11.71219
C	11.80769	11.78842
F	11.73077	11.71319
L	11.80769	11.78942
M	11.73077	11.71119

Observe that the scores are in the correct order for all eight of the pairwise rankings except for the sixth one, "M is preferred to L."

15.5.1 Goodness of Ordinal Fit

If we let z be the optimal objective function value, n the number of ranking observations, and k the number of parameters estimated for the ordinal regression, a measure of goodness of fit somewhat analogous to the adjusted R^2 of least squares regression is:

$$1/[1 + z/(n - k)].$$

For our example, the goodness of fit is:

$$1/[1 + 0.0769/(8 - 4)] = 0.981.$$

15.5.2 Exploiting the Dual to Reduce the Formulation Size

As with other LP regression formulations, the dual tends to be easier to solve. The primal formulation in general form is below. In all of the following, r is the object preferred to object s in the ith pairwise ranking.

$$\text{Min}\quad z_1 + z_2 + \ldots + z_n$$

s.t.

$$\sum_{j=1}^{k} \left(e_{rj} - e_{sj}\right) x_j + z_i \geq 0$$

where r is preferred to s in the ith observation, $i = 1, 2, \ldots, n$

$$\sum_{j=1}^{k} \sum_{i=1}^{n} \left(e_{rj} - e_{sj}\right) x_j = 1$$

$$x_j \text{ unconstrained in sign.}$$

The dual is

Max u

s.t.

$$\sum_{i=1}^{n}\left(e_{rj} - e_{sj}\right)v_i + \sum_{i=1}^{n}\left(e_{rj} - e_{sj}\right)u = 0 \quad \text{for } j = 1, 2, \ldots, k$$

$$v_i \leq 1 \quad \text{for } i = 1, 2, \ldots, n,$$

u unconstrained in sign.

This formulation has a lot of constraints; however, the majority of them, n out of $n + k$, are of the simple upper bound variety.

The dual formulation for the example problem follows. Note that the unconstrained variable u is replaced by the difference $u_1 - u_2$.

```
MAX    U1 - U2
SUBJECT TO
 2)   4 V1 +   V2 + 3 V3 - V4 - 2 V5 - 2 V6 - 2 V7 - V8 =      0
 3) - 0.6 U1 + 0.6 U2 + 1.2 V1 + 0.1 V2 + 1.4 V3 + 0.2 V4
    - 1.2 V5 - 0.3 V6 - 0.9 V7 - 1.1 V8 =      0
 4)   0.5 U1 - 0.5 U2 + 2.5 V1 +   V2 + 2 V3 - 0.5 V4 - 1.5 V5
    - 1.5 V6 - V7 - 0.5 V8 =      0
 5)   3 U1 - 3 U2 - 5 V1 - V2 - 4 V3 +   V4 + 3 V5 + 2 V6 + 3 V7
    + 2 V8 =      0
 6)     V1 ≤  1
 7)     V2 ≤  1
 8)     V3 ≤  1
 9)     V4 ≤  1
10)     V5 ≤  1
11)     V6 ≤  1
12)     V7 ≤  1
13)     V8 ≤  1
END
```

It is helpful to compare the PICTURE of this formulation with that of the primal.

```
?:PICTURE
                 U U V V V V V V V V
                 1 2 1 2 3 4 5 6 7 8

        1:  1-1                        MAX
        2:        4 1 3-1-2-2-2-1 =
        3:-T T A U A T-A-T-T-A =
        4: T-T A 1 2-T-A-A-1-T =
        5: 3-3-5-1-4 1 3 2 3 2 =
        6:        1                    < 1
        7:          1                  < 1
        8:            1                < 1
        9:              1              < 1
       10:                1            < 1
       11:                  1          < 1
       12:                    1        < 1
       13:                      1 < 1
```

The solution of the dual is:

```
LP OPTIMUM FOUND
                          OBJECTIVE FUNCTION VALUE
             1)                  0.07692308

         VARIABLE            VALUE            REDUCED COST
            U1              0.076923             0.000000
            U2              0.000000             0.000000
            V1              0.423077             0.000000
            V2              0.692308             0.000000
            V3              0.000000             0.076923
            V4              0.000000             0.076923
            V5              0.192308             0.000000
            V6              1.000000             0.000000
            V7              0.000000             0.076923
            V8              0.000000             0.000000

          ROW              SLACK             DUAL PRICES
           2)             0.000000             0.461538
           3)             0.000000             0.384615
           4)             0.000000            -0.076923
           5)             0.000000             0.423077
           6)             0.576923             0.000000
           7)             0.307692             0.000000
           8)             1.000000             0.000000
           9)             1.000000             0.000000
          10)             0.807692             0.000000
          11)             0.000000             0.076923
          12)             1.000000             0.000000
          13)             1.000000             0.000000

   NO.  ITERATIONS=         6
```

Notice that it took only six iterations as compared to seven for the primal. The dual variables on constraints (2) through (5) provide the values for the x_j variables of the primal formulation. The scoring formula is again:

$$\text{Score} = 0.461538 \text{ Price} + 0.384615 \text{ Weight} - 0.076923 \text{ Length} + 0.423077 \text{ MPG}$$

For a further discussion of ordinal linear regression, see Srinivasan (1976).

15.6 PROBLEMS

Problem 1

A table of statistical data contains a small fraction of data transcription errors, e.g., typing mistakes. These errors in the data are very difficult to track down. Which type of regression, LAD, LMAX, or least squares would be least affected by these outlier type errors?

Problem 2

In the simple linear regression model the ith observation is written in the form:

$$r_i = a + bs_i + e_i$$

where r_i, s_i, and e_i are, respectively, the dependent variable, the explanatory variable, and t he error term. Which regression model, LAD, LMAX, or least squares, is most appropriate if the e_i are (a) uniformly distributed over a finite but unknown range, (b) Normal distributed, (c) distributed according to a distribution with fatter tails than the Normal?

Problem 3

Consider the following table for a multiple regression problem:

r	s	t
7	3	12
10	4	11
11	7	9
13	8	8

Formulate and solve the relevant LP for regressing the dependent variable r on the two explanatory variables, s and t, using (a) LMAX regression, (b) LAD regression.

Problem 4

The Geneco Steel Company provides structural steel for construction projects. Typical projects are shopping centers, warehouses, and manufacturing plants. The two major operations performed by Geneco are: (1) cut I-beams to length, and (2) punch bolt holes in the ends of the cut beams. The time spent making cuts is related largely to the number of cuts being made and the cross-section of the cuts, measured in square centimeters. The time to punch a hole is relatively constant, independent of the thickness of the material punched. Geneco wants to improve its estimating formulae used in quoting the time to do a proposed job. Below are tabulated some statistics for several recent completed jobs for the total time in minutes to do the cutting and punching.

Job	Total Time	Number of Cuts	Total Cut Cross-Section	Total Holes
1	452	50	11,200	170
2	675	84	21,300	240
3	787	110	19,200	225
4	180	25	7,500	52
5	1578	210	35,220	540
6	835	95	19,590	380

Geneco would like to derive a linear estimating formula based on these three explanatory factors. From industrial engineering studies, Geneco has derived upper and lower bounds on the coefficients. The derived estimating formula should have coefficients that fall within their respective ranges.

	Number of Cuts	Total Cut Cross-Section	Total Holes
Upper bound:	3.7	.016	1.3
Lower bound:	2.9	.011	0.9

Derive a good estimating formula for Geneco.

Design and Implementation of Optimization-Based Decision Support Systems

16.1 General Structure of the Modeling Process

The overall modeling process is one of:

1. Developing the model; and
2. Implementing the model.

If the purpose of the model is to do a one-time analysis (e.g., to decide whether or not to make a certain investment), step (2) will be relatively less laborious.

16.1.1 Developing the Model: Detail and Maintenance

Whether the model is intended for a one-time study or is to be used regularly has some influence on how you develop the model. If the model is to be used regularly, you want to worry especially about the following:

Problem: *The real world changes rapidly, e.g., prices, company structure, and suppliers. We must be able to update the model just as fast.*

Resolution: *There are two relevant philosophies.*

1. Keep worthless detail out of the model, follow the KISS (Keep It Simple, . . .) admonition.
2. Put as much of the model as possible into data tables rather than hard-coded into the model structure.

16.2 Appropriate Level of Detail, Verification and Validation

If unimportant details are kept out of the model, the model should be not only easier to modify but also easier to use.

16.2.1 Example

In developing a long-range ship scheduling model, a question of the appropriate unit of time arose. Tides follow a roughly 13-hour cycle, and this is an important consideration in the scheduling of ships into shallow ports. Deep draft ships can enter a shallow port only at high tide. Thus, in developing a multiperiod model for ship scheduling, it appeared that 13 hours should be the length of a period.

We found, however, that ship travel times were sufficiently random that scheduling to the day was satisfactory. Thus, to model a month of activity, 30 time periods, rather than about 60, were satisfactory. Halving the number of periods greatly simplified the computations. The moral is that when it comes to incorporating detail into the model, a little bit of selective laziness may be a good thing.

Simplifying approximations can be categorized roughly as follows.

Approximations: *If there is an art to modeling, it is in identifying the simplifications or approximations that can be made without sacrificing the useful accuracy of the model.*

1. *Functional approximation*; e.g., use a linear function to approximate a slightly nonlinear one.
2. *Aggregation*
   2.1 *Temporal* aggregation; e.g., all events occurring during a given day (or week, month, etc.) are treated as having occurred at the end of the day.
   2.2 *Cross-sectional* aggregation; e.g., all customers in a given mail code region are lumped together to be treated as one large customer, or in a consumer products firm all detergents are treated as a single product.
3. *Statistical approximation*; e.g., replace a random variable by its expectation. For example, even though future sales are a random variable, most planners use a single number forecast in planning.
4. *Decomposition.* If a system is overwhelming in its complexity, decomposition is an approach that may be useful for simplifying the structure. Under this approach a sequence of models is solved, each nailing down more detail of the complete solution.

Rogers, Plante, Wong, and Evans (1991) give an extensive survey of techniques for aggregation in optimization problems. The steps in using an approximate model can be summarized as follows:

1. Obtain detailed input data.
2. Derive the approximate (hopefully small) model.
3. Solve the approximate model.
4. Convert the solution of the approximate model back to the real world.

The difficult step is 4. The worst thing that can happen is that it is impossible to convert the approximate solution back to a feasible real world solution.

16.2.2 Should We Behave Nonoptimally?

One of the arts of modeling is knowing which details to leave out of the model. Unfortunately, one of the first kinds of details left out of a model are the things that are difficult to quantify. One kind of difficult-to-quantify feature is the value of information. There are a number of situations where, if value of information is left out of the model, one may wish not to implement exactly an optimal solution. Some examples follow.

An optimal inventory model may recommend using a very large order size. If we use a smaller order size, however, we will be giving more timely information to our supplier about retail demand for his product. In between orders, the supplier has no additional information about how his product is selling. In the extreme, if we used an order size of 1, the supplier would have very up-to-date information about retail demand and could do better planning.

A firm that extends credit to customers may occasionally wish to behave nonoptimally in order to gain additional information. If the firm's initial credit optimization model says never give credit to customers with profile X, the firm should occasionally extend credit to X in order to have up-to-date information on customers with that profile.

In addition to occasionally behaving nonoptimally to gain additional information, one may also wish to behave nonoptimally in order not to reveal too much information. Any good poker player knows that one must occasionally bluff by placing a large bet, even though the odds associated with the given hand do not justify a large bet. If other players know you never bluff, they will drop out every time you place a large bet.

There was a rumor at the end of World War II that Great Britain allowed the bombing of Coventry on one occasion because, if the British had sent up a large fleet of fighters in advance to meet the incoming German bombers, the Germans would have known that the British had broken the German communications codes.

16.2.3 Verification and Validation

The term *verification* is usually applied to the process of verifying that the model as implemented is actually doing what we think it should. Effectively, verification is checking that the model has no unintentional "bugs." *Validation* is the process of demonstrating that the approximations to reality that are intentionally incorporated in the model are tolerable and do not sully the quality of the results from the model. Validation should begin with understanding the real world that is to be modeled. A common problem is that the people willing to speak most authoritatively about the process to be modeled are not always the most informed. A good rule of thumb is always to check your "facts" with a second source. Rothstein (1985) mentions that in a conversation with a vice president of a major airline, the vice president assured him that the airline never engaged in overbooking. A short time later, in a discussion with operating personnel, he learned that in fact the airline had a sophisticated overbooking system used everywhere in that airline.

16.2.4 When Your Model and the RW Disagree, Bet on the RW

As part of the validation process, you compare the output of your model with what happened in the real world (RW). When there is a discrepancy, there are two possibilities: (1) People in the RW are not behaving optimally and you have an opportunity to make some money by using your model, or (2) Your model still has some flaws.

Black (1989) described the situation quite well while he was trying to validate an option pricing model:

> *We estimated the volatility of the stock for each of a group of companies. . . . We noticed that several warrants looked like very good buys. The best buy of all seemed to be National General. . . . I and others jumped right in and bought a bunch. . . . Then a company called American Financial announced a tender offer for National General . . . the tender offer had the effect of sharply reducing the value of the warrants. . . . In other words, the market knew something that our formula didn't know . . . and that's why the warrants seemed so low in price.*

16.3 Separation of Data and System Structure

There are two reasons for separating data from model structure:

1. It allows us to adjust the model easily and quickly to changes in the real world;
2. The person responsible for making day-to-day changes in the data need not be familiar with the technical details of the model structure.

A flexible system is table driven. In LINDO, essentially all data are "in the model." In more powerful systems such as LINGO and What'sBest!, parameters such as interest rates can be input at a single place by a clerk, even though they appear numerous places in the model structure.

16.3.1 System Structure

In the typical case, a model will be used regularly, e.g., weekly in an operational environment. In this case, the model system can be thought of as having the structure shown in Figure 16.1. Notice that the arrow between the data files and the formulation generator is double-headed. This is because the generator may obtain parameters such as capacities from the data files. There is an arrow from the data files to the report writer because there are data, such as addresses of customers, that are needed for the output reports but are not needed in the formulation. The success of spreadsheet programs such as Lotus 1-2-3 is due in part to the fact that they incorporate all the above components in a relatively seamless fashion.

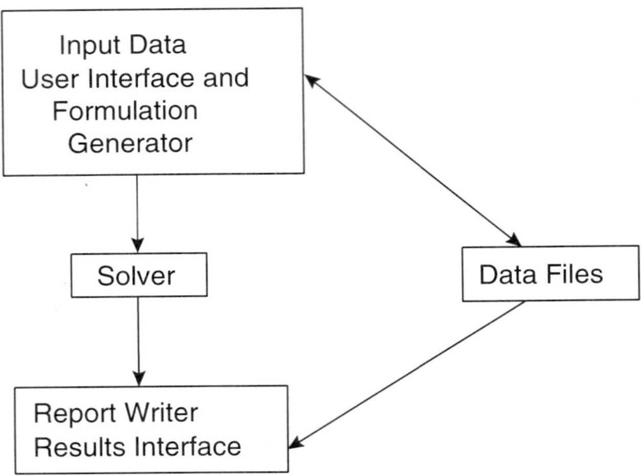

Figure 16.1
System
Structure

16.4 Marketing the Model

It is important to keep in mind: Who will be the users/clients?

Frequently there are two types of clients in a single organization:

1. The Model champion, e.g., a CEO;
2. Actual user, e.g., a foreman working 12 hours/day and whose major concern is getting the work out and meeting deadlines.

Client 1 will commit to model development based on expected profit improvement. Client 2 will actually use the model if it simplifies his/her life. He may get fired if he misses a production deadline. There is a modest probability of a raise if he improves profitability and takes the trouble to document it. Thus, for client 2, the input and output user interfaces are very important.

16.4.1 Reports

A model has an impact largely via the reports it produces. If a standard report already exists in the organization, try to use it. The model simply puts better numbers in it.

> ***Example.*** An LP-based scheduling system was developed for shoe factories. It was a success in the first factory where it was tried. Production improved by about 15%. The system never got off the ground in a second factory. The reason for the difference in success was apparently as follows. The first factory had an existing scheduling report or work order. This report format was retained. The results of the LP scheduling model simply put better

numbers in it. The second factory had been using an ad hoc or informal scheduling and reporting system. The combination of installing both a new reporting system and a new scheduling system was too big a barrier to change.

Designing Reports

The proper attitude in designing reports is to ask: How will the results be used?

In operations settings, there frequently are three types of reports implied by the results of a model run:

1. Raw material acquisition recommendations. For example, in extreme cases the model might generate purchase orders directly.
2. Production orders. For example, how are the raw materials to be processed into finished goods?
3. Finished goods summaries. If the production process is complicated (e.g., several different alternative processes are used to achieve the total production of a specific product), it may not be clear from (1) and (2) how much of a particular finished good was produced.

Example. *Reports in a Blending Facility.* In a facility that blends raw materials into finished goods, reports of the following type might be appropriate.

1.

Raw Material Purchases			
Raw Material	Total Required	Beginning Inventory	Required Purchases

2.

Production			
Batch 1. Product:		**Batch 2.** Product:	
Inputs:		Inputs:	
Raw Material	Amount	Raw Material	Amount

3.

Finished Goods Summary				
Product	Beginning Inventory	Goods Produced	Total Required	Surplus

Dimensional View of Reports

A more mechanical view of report generation is to take a dimensional view of a system; i.e., a problem and its solution have a number of dimensions. Each report is a sort and summary by dimensions.

> *Example.* *Multiperiod Shipping*
>
> *Dimensions:* Origins, Destinations, Time Periods. The major decision variables might be of the form X_{ijt}, where X_{ijt} is the number of tons to be shipped from supplier i to customer j in time period t. The types of reports might be:
>
> *Supplier's Report:* Sorted by Origin, Time, Destination (or summed over destination).
>
> *Shipping Manager:* Sorted by Time, Origin, Destination.
>
> *Customer's Report:* Sorted by Destination, Time, Origin (or perhaps summed over origin).

Most spreadsheets and database systems have multilevel sorting capability.

Report Details/Passing the Snicker Test

Results should be phrased in terms that the user finds easy to use. For example, reporting that a steel bar should be cut to a length of 58.36 inches may cause snickers in some places because "everybody knows" that this commodity (like U.S. stock prices) is measured in multiples of $1/8$ inches, or dollars, as the case may be. So it would be better to round the result to 58.375 inches or, even better, report it as 58 and $3/8$ inches.

Other examples: Dates should be reported not only in day of the month (taking into account leap years), but also day of the week. Different parts of the world use different formats for displaying dates, e.g., 14 March 1991 vs. 3/14/91, etc. Use a format appropriate for the location where used.

Example. *Vehicle Routing/Passing the Snicker Test*

Customers are grouped into trips so that customers on the same trip are served by the same vehicle. The actual model decomposed the problem into two phases:

1. Allocate to trips   ←   Big savings here.
2. Sequence each trip   ←   Users notice this the most.

If your system does an excellent job of allocating customers to trips (where the big savings exist), but does not always get the optimal sequence of customers within a trip, users may notice the latter weakness. Even though there may be no big savings possible by improving the sequence, users may have less faith in the system because of this small weakness.

Models Should Always Have Feasible Solutions

In a large model where the input data are prepared by many people, there may be no assurance that the data are perfectly consistent. For example, production capacity as estimated by the production department may be insufficient to satisfy sales forecasts as estimated by the marketing department. If the model has a constraint that requires production to equal forecasted sales, there may be no feasible solution. The terse message "No feasible solution" is not very helpful.

A better approach is to have in the model a *superworker* or superfacility that can make any product at infinite speed, but at a rather high cost. There will always be feasible solutions although some parts of the solution may look somewhat funny.

Another device is to allow *demand to be backlogged* at a high cost.

In each case, the solution will give sensible indications of where one should install extra capacity or cut back on projected sales, etc.

A model may be fundamentally good but incomplete in certain minor details. As a result, some of its recommendations may be slightly but blatantly incorrect.

For example, in reality almost every activity has a finite upper bound.

Similarly, there may be obvious *bounds on the dual* prices of certain resources. For example, if land is a scarce resource in the real world, its dual price should never be zero. You should *include sellout or buy activities* corresponding to such things as renting out excess land to put lower and upper bounds on dual prices.

"Signing Off" on System Structure

If a prospective model (a) is likely to be complicated and (b) the group that will use the model is distinct from the group that will design the model, it will be worthwhile to have beforehand a written document describing exactly what the model does. Effectively, the "User's Manual" is written before the system is implemented. The prospective users should "sign off" on the design, e.g., by providing a letter that says "Yes, this is what we want *and we will accept* if it provides this."

This document would include descriptions of:

(a) the form in which input will be provided,
(b) the form in which output will be provided,
(c) test data sets that must be successfully processed.

The model will be accepted if and only if these are satisfied.

16.5 Reducing Model Size

Practical LP models tend to be large. Thus, it makes sense to talk about the management of these models. Some of the important issues are:

1. Choosing an appropriate formulation. Frequently there are two conflicting considerations: (a) the model should be large enough to capture all important details of reality, and (b) the model should be solvable in reasonable time.
2. What input data are needed? How is it collected?
3. How do we create an explicit model from the current data? This process has traditionally been called matrix generation.
4. How is the model solved? Is it solvable in reasonable time? In reality, some optimization program must be selected. For our purposes, we assume LINDO has been chosen.

In this section, we discuss issues (1) and (3). The selection of an appropriate formulation also has implications for how easily a model is solved (issue 4).

We begin our discussion with how to choose a formulation that is small and thus more easily solved (usually).

The computational difficulty of an LP is closely related to three features of the LP: the number of rows, the number of columns, and the number of nonzeroes in the constraint matrix. For linear programs, the computation time tends to increase with the square of the number of nonzeroes. Thus, there is some motivation to (re)formulate LP models so that they are small in the above-mentioned three dimensions.

A number of commercial LP solvers have built-in commands with names like REDUCE, which will mechanically do simple kinds of algebraic substitutions and eliminations necessary for reduction. Brearley, Mitra, and Williams (1975) give a thorough description of these reductions.

16.5.1 Reducing the Number of Rows and Columns: Reduction by Substitution

The standard method for reducing the number of rows and columns is to use a row (for simplicity, we assume the last row) to solve for one of the columns (say, the last one) and then use this row to substitute out the last variable in all the other rows. That is, if there are currently m rows and n columns, write the last row as:

$$X_n = \sum_{j=1}^{n-1} a_{mj} X_j + a_{m0}.$$

In rows 1 through $m - 1$, every occurrence of X_n is replaced by the right-hand side in the above equation. Now row m and column n can be dropped if (a) there are no implicit constraints, such as $X_n \geq 0$, which might be violated as a result, and (b) X_n is not an integer variable. One should further note that this substitution, although it reduces the number of rows and columns by one, may increase the number of nonzeroes. Also, some parametric analyses may be invalidated by this substitution.

Frequently, the constraint on which the substitution is based starts out as an inequality constraint. The simplest example is a constraint of the form:

$$ay \leq X$$

where the constant $a > 0$ and the variable $y \geq 0$. In this case, the constraint $X \geq 0$ cannot be binding because the expression ay is always nonnegative. Adding a slack variable we have:

$$ay + s = X$$
$$y \geq 0,\, s \geq 0,\, X \geq 0.$$

Every occurrence of X in the model can be replaced by $ay + s$, and the constraint $ay + s = X$ can be dropped. Thus, the number of constraints is reduced by 1, at the expense of generating $k - 1$ additional nonzeroes, where k is the original number of nonzeroes in the X column.

16.5.2 Example

This reduction can be significant. Certain electrical distribution models (cf. Dutton, Hinman, and Millham, 1974) have essentially the following structure. Parameters (all ≥ 0) are: c_{ij}, d_{ij}, e_j, p_j, S_i, Q_i, a_{ij} and b_{ij}. The decision variables are: X_{ij} is the electrical energy supplied from i to j, and Y_{ij} is the peak power supplied from i to j.

$$\text{Minimize} \quad \sum_{i=1}^{m} \sum_{j=1}^{n} \left(c_{ij} X_{ij} + d_{ij} Y_{ij} \right)$$

subject to   For each demand area $j = 1, 2, \ldots, n$:

Energy requirements:

$$\sum_i X_{ij} = e_j$$

Peak power requirements:

$$\sum_i Y_{ij} = p_j$$

For each supply station i, $i = 1, 2, \ldots, m$:

Energy availability:

$$\sum_i X_{ij} \leq S_i$$

Peak power availability:

$$\sum_i Y_{ij} \leq Q_i$$

For each shipment combination: $i = 1, 2, \ldots, m$ and $j = 1, 2, \ldots, n$. Peak power and energy must be loosely related:

$$a_{ij} Y_{ij} \leq X_{ij}$$
$$X_{ij} \leq b_{ij} Y_{ij}$$
$$X_{ij} \geq 0$$
$$Y_{ij} \geq 0$$

If there are 10 supply points and 100 demand areas, this model has 2120 constraints. This is not prohibitive in size, but it would be nice if it were smaller. What can we do to reduce the size? Introducing a slack variable s_{ij}, all occurrences of X_{ij} can be replaced by $a_{ij} Y_{ij} + s_{ij}$. The explicit constraint $a_{ij} Y_{ij} \leq X_{ij}$ is replaced by $s_{ij} \geq 0$. The constraint $X_{ij} \leq b_{ij} Y_{ij}$ becomes $a_{ij} Y_{ij} + s_{ij} \leq b_{ij} Y_{ij}$ or $s_{ij} \leq (b_{ij} - a_{ij}) Y_{ij}$. Repeating the process by adding the slack variable U_{ij}, we have:

$$s_{ij} + U_{ij} = (b_{ij} - a_{ij}) Y_{ij}$$

Now all occurrences of Y_{ij} can be replaced by:

$$s_{ij} (b_{ij} - a_{ij}) + U_{ij} / (b_{ij} - a_{ij}).$$

When all substitutions are completed, the new model is:

$$\text{Minimize} \quad \sum_{i=1}^{m} \sum_{j=1}^{n} \frac{\left(c_{ij} b_{ij} + d_{ij}\right)}{\left(b_{ij} - a_{ij}\right)} s_{ij} + \frac{\left(c_{ij} a_{ij} + d_{ij}\right)}{\left(b_{ij} - a_{ij}\right)}$$

subject to   For $j = 1, 2, \ldots, n$:

$$\sum_i \left(b_{ij} s_{ij} + a_{ij} u_{ij}\right) / \left(b_{ij} - a_{ij}\right) \leq S_i$$

$$\sum_i \left(s_{ij} + u_{ij}\right) / \left(b_{ij} - a_{ij}\right) = P_j$$

For $i = 1, 2, \ldots, m$:

$$\sum_j \left(b_{ij} s_{ij} + a_{ij} u_{ij}\right) / \left(b_{ij} - a_{ij}\right) \leq S_i$$

$$\sum_j \left(s_{ij} + u_{ij}\right) / \left(b_{ij} - a_{ij}\right) \leq Q_i$$

For $i = 1, 2, \ldots, m$ and $j = 1, 2, \ldots, n$:

$$0 \leq s_{ij}$$

$$0 \leq u_{ij}$$

The nonnegativity constraints are not carried explicitly.

The original formulation has $2n + 2m + 2mn$ explicit constraints, whereas the new formulation has $2n + 2m$ explicit constraints. For example, if $m = 10$ and $n = 20$, the original formulation has 460 constraints, whereas the new formulation has 60 constraints. The latter is small enough to be solved on a small personal computer.

16.5.3 Reduction by Aggregation

We say that we aggregate a set of variables if we replace a set of variables by a single variable. We aggregate a set of constraints if we replace a set of constraints by a single constraint. If we do aggregation we must resolve several issues:

1. After solving the LP, there must be a postprocessing/disaggregation phase to deduce the disaggregate values from the aggregate values.
2. If row aggregation was performed, the solution to the aggregate problem may not be feasible to the true disaggregate problem.
3. If variable aggregation was performed, the solution to the aggregate problem may not be optimal to the true disaggregate problem.

To illustrate (2), consider the LP:

$$\begin{array}{ll} \text{Maximize} & 2x + y \\ \text{subject to} & x \leq 1 \\ & y \leq 1 \\ & x, y \geq 0 \end{array}$$

The optimal solution is $x = y = 1$; with objective value equal to 3. We could aggregate the rows to get:

$$\begin{array}{ll} \text{Maximize} & 2x + y \\ \text{subject to} & x + y \leq 2 \\ & x, y \geq 0 \end{array}$$

The optimal solution to this aggregate problem is $x = 2$, $y = 0$, with objective value equal to 4. This solution, however, is not feasible to the original problem.

To illustrate (3), consider the LP:

$$\begin{array}{ll} \text{Minimize} & x_1 + x_2 \\ \text{subject to} & x_1 \geq 2 \\ & x_2 \geq 1 \\ & x_1, x_2 \geq 0 \end{array}$$

The optimal solution is $x_1 = 2$, $x_2 = 1$, with objective value equal to 3. We could aggregate variables to get the LP:

$$\begin{array}{ll} \text{Minimize} & 2x \\ \text{subject to} & x \geq 2 \\ & x \geq 1 \\ & x \geq 0 \end{array}$$

The optimal solution to the aggregate problem is $x = 2$, with objective value equal to 4. This solution is, however, not optimal for the original, disaggregate LP.

16.5.4 Example: The Room Scheduling Problem

We will illustrate both variable and constraint aggregation with a problem confronted by any large hotel that has extensive conference facilities for business meetings. The hotel has r conference rooms available of various sizes. Over the next t time periods, e.g., days, the hotel must schedule g groups of people into these rooms. Each group has a hard requirement for a room of at least a certain size. Each group may also have a preference of certain time periods over others. Each group requires a room for exactly one time period. The obvious formulation is:

V_{gtr} = value of assigning group g to time period t in room r. This value is provided by group g, presumably as a ranking. The decision variables are:

X_{gtr} = 1 if group g is assigned to room r in time period t. This variable is defined for each group g, each time period t, and each room r that is big enough to accommodate group g.

= 0 otherwise.

The constraints are :

$$\sum_t \sum_r x_{gtr} = 1 \qquad \text{for each group } g$$

$$\sum_g x_{gtr} \leq 1 \qquad \text{for each room } r, \text{ time period } t$$

$$x_{gtr} = 0 \text{ or } 1 \qquad \text{for all } g, t, \text{ and } r$$

The objective is:

$$\text{Maximize } \sum_g \sum_t \sum_r V_{gtr} x_{gtr}$$

The number of constraints in this problem is $g + r \times t$. The number of variables is approximately $g \times t \times r/2$. The $r/2$ is based on the assumption that for a typical group, about half of the rooms will be big enough.

A typical problem instance might have $g = 250$, $t = 10$, and $r = 30$. Such a problem would have 550 constraints and about 37,500 variables. A problem of that size is nontrivial to solve, so we might wish to work with a smaller formulation.

Aggregation of variables can be used validly if a group is indifferent between rooms b and c, as long as both rooms b and c are large enough to accommodate the group. In terms of our notation, $V_{gtb} = V_{gtc}$ for every g and t if both rooms b and c are large enough for g. More generally, two variables can be aggregated if in each row of the LP they have the same coefficients. Two constraints in an LP can be validly aggregated if in each variable they have the same coefficients. We will do constraint aggregation by aggregating together all rooms of the same size. This aggregation process is representative of a fundamental modeling principle: when it comes to solving the model, *do not distinguish things that do not need distinguishing.*

The aggregate formulation can now be defined:

K = number of distinct room sizes
N_k = number of rooms of size k or larger
S_k = the set of groups which require a room of size k or larger
V_{gt} = value of assigning group g to time period t
x_{gt} = 1 if group g is assigned to a room in time period t
  = 0 otherwise

The constraints are:

$$\sum_i x_{gt} = 1 \qquad \text{for each group } g$$

$$\sum_{g \in S_k} x_{gt} \leq N_k \qquad \text{for each room size } k.$$

The objective is:

$$\text{Maximize} \qquad \sum_g \sum_t \sum_r V_{gt} X_{gt}$$

This formulation will have $g + k \times t$ constraints and $g \times t$ decision variables. For the case $g = 250$, $t = 10$, and $r = 30$, we might have $k = 4$. Thus, the aggregate formulation would have 290 constraints and 2500 variables, compared with 550 constraints and 37,500 variables for the disaggregate formulation.

The post processing required to extract a disaggregate solution from an aggregate solution to our room scheduling problem is straightforward. For each time period, the groups assigned to that time period are ranked from largest to smallest. The largest group is assigned to the largest room, the second largest group to the second largest room, etc. Such an assignment will always be feasible as well as optimal to the original problem.

16.5.5 Example 2: Reducing Rows by Adding Additional Variables

If two parties, A and B, to a financial agreement, want the agreement to be treated as a lease for tax purposes, the payment schedule typically must satisfy certain conditions specified by the taxing agency. Suppose that P_i is the payment that A is scheduled to make to B in month i of a seven-year agreement. Parties A and B want to choose at the outset a set of P_js that satisfy a tax regulation that no payment in any given month can be less than $2/3$ of the payment in any earlier month. If there are T periods, the most obvious way of writing these constraints is:

> For $i = 2$, T:
> For $j = 1$, $i - 1$:
> $\quad P_i \geq 0.66666\, P_j$

This would require $T(T - 1)/2$ constraints. A less obvious approach would be to define PM_i as the largest payment occurring any period before i. The requirement could be enforced with:

> $PM_1 = 0$
> For $i = 2$ to T:
> $\quad P_i \geq 0.66666\, PM_i$
> $PM_i \geq PM_{i-1}$
> $PM_i \geq P_{i-1}$

This would require $3T$ constraints rather than $T(T - 1)/2$. For $T = 84$ the difference is between 3486 constraints and 252.

16.5.6 Reducing the Number of Nonzeroes

If a certain linear expression is used more than once in a model, you may be able to reduce the number of nonzeroes by substituting it out. For example, consider the two-sided constraints that are frequently encountered in metal blending models:

$$L_i \leq \frac{\sum_j q_{ij} X_j}{\sum_j X_j} \leq U_i \quad \text{(for each quality characteristic } i\text{)}.$$

In these situations, L_k and U_k are lower and upper limits on the ith quality requirement, and q_{ij} is the quality of ingredient j with respect to the ith quality. The "obvious" way of writing this constraint in linear form is:

$$\sum_j \left(q_{ij} - L_i\right)X_j \geq 0,$$

$$\sum_j \left(q_{ij} - U_k\right)X_j \leq 0.$$

By introducing a batch size variable B and a slack variable s_i, things can be rewritten

$$B - \sum_j X_j = 0$$

$$\sum_j q_{ij}X_j + s_i = U_i \times B$$

$$s_i \leq \left(U_k - L_i\right) \times B$$

If there are m qualities and n ingredients, the original formulation had $2 \times m \times n$ nonzeroes. The modified formulation has $n + 1 + m \times (n + 2) + m \times 2 = n + 1 + m \times (n + 4)$ nonzeroes. For large n, the modified formulation has approximately 50% fewer nonzeroes.

16.5.7 Reducing the Number of Nonzeroes in Covering Problems

A common feature in some covering and some multiperiod financial planning models is that each column will have the same coefficient, e.g., $+1$, in a large number of rows. A simple transformation may substantially reduce the number of nonzeroes in the model. Suppose that row i is written:

$$\sum_{j=1}^{n} a_{ij}X_j = a_{i0}$$

Now suppose we subtract row $i-1$ from row i, so that row i becomes:

$$\sum_{j=1}^{n} \left(a_{ij} - a_{i-1,j}\right)X_j = a_{i0} - a_{i-1,0}$$

If $a_{ij} = a_{i-1,j} \neq 0$ for most j, the number of nonzeroes in row i is substantially reduced.

16.5.8 Example

Suppose that we must staff a facility around the clock with people who work eight-hour shifts. A shift can start at the beginning of any hour of the day. If r_i is the number of people required to be on duty from hour i to hour $i + 1$, X_i is the number of people starting a shift at the beginning of hour i, and s_i is the surplus variable for hour i, the constraints are:

$$X_1 + X_{18} + X_{19} + X_{20} + X_{21} + X_{22} + X_{23} + X_{24} - s_1 = r_1$$
$$X_1 + X_2 + X_{19} + X_{20} + X_{21} + X_{22} + X_{23} + X_{24} - s_2 = r_2$$
$$X_1 + X_2 + X_3 + X_{20} + X_{21} + X_{22} + X_{23} + X_{24} - s_3 = r_3$$
$$\vdots$$

Suppose we subtract row 23 from row 24, row 22 from row 23, etc. The above constraints will be transformed to:

$$X_1 + X_{18} + X_{19} + X_{20} + X_{21} + X_{22} + X_{23} + X_{24} - s_1 \qquad = r_1$$
$$X_2 - X_{18} \qquad\qquad + s_1 - s_2 \qquad = r_2 - r_1$$
$$X_1 \qquad - X_{19} \qquad\qquad + s_2 - s_3 = r_3 - r_2$$
$$\vdots$$

Thus, a typical constraint will have four nonzeroes rather than nine.

The pattern of nonzeroes for the X variables in the original formulation is shown in Figure 16.2. The pattern of the nonzeroes for the X variables in the transformed formulation is shown in Figure 16.3. The total constraint nonzeroes for X and s variables in the original formulation is 216. The analogous count for the transformed formulation is 101, a very attractive reduction.

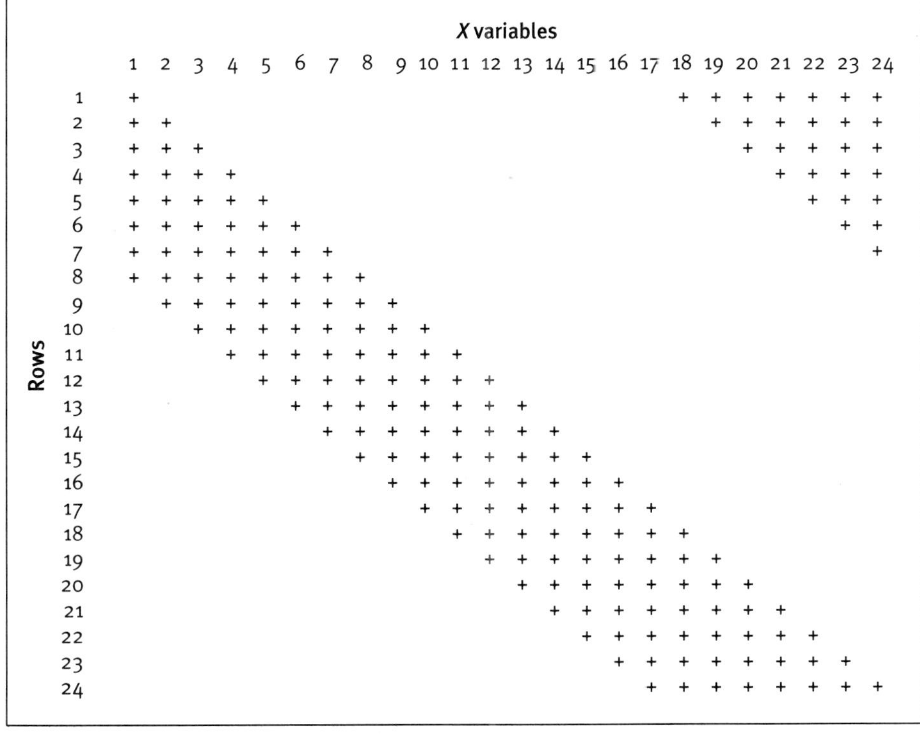

Figure 16.2
Nonzero Pattern for *X* Variables in Original Formulation

X variables

Rows	1	2	3	4	5	6	7	8	9	10	11	12	13	14	15	16	17	18	19	20	21	22	23	24
1	+																	+	+	+	+	+	+	+
2	+	+																	+	+	+	+	+	+
3	+	+	+																	+	+	+	+	+
4	+	+	+	+																	+	+	+	+
5	+	+	+	+	+																	+	+	+
6	+	+	+	+	+	+																	+	+
7	+	+	+	+	+	+	+																	+
8	+	+	+	+	+	+	+	+																
9		+	+	+	+	+	+	+	+															
10			+	+	+	+	+	+	+	+														
11				+	+	+	+	+	+	+	+													
12					+	+	+	+	+	+	+	+												
13						+	+	+	+	+	+	+	+											
14							+	+	+	+	+	+	+	+										
15								+	+	+	+	+	+	+	+									
16									+	+	+	+	+	+	+	+								
17										+	+	+	+	+	+	+	+							
18											+	+	+	+	+	+	+	+						
19												+	+	+	+	+	+	+	+					
20													+	+	+	+	+	+	+	+				
21														+	+	+	+	+	+	+	+			
22															+	+	+	+	+	+	+	+		
23																+	+	+	+	+	+	+	+	
24																	+	+	+	+	+	+	+	+

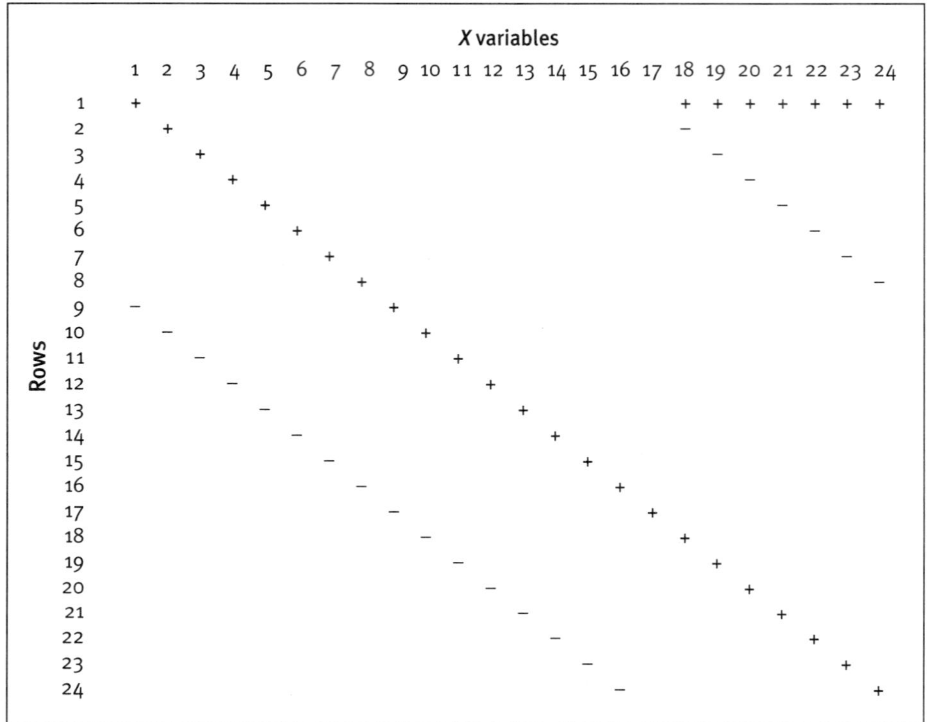

Figure 16.3
Nonzero Pattern for *X* Variables in Transformed Formulation

16.6 Matrix Generators

In large LPs, it is impractical to manually enter all the coefficients of the LP. In these situations, one writes an auxiliary computer program called a matrix generator. This program reads the problem description in an arbitrary format from either a file or the user's terminal and then generates the corresponding LP formulation.

There are two approaches to writing the matrix generator program: (1) use a general purpose programming language such as FORTRAN or C, or (2) use a special purpose language designed expressly for generating LP formulations. These special purpose languages are frequently available from vendors of LP optimization packages.

16.7 On-the-Fly Column Generation

There are a number of generic LP models that have a modest number of rows, e.g., a hundred or so, but a large number of columns, e.g., a million or so. This is frequently the case in cutting stock problems. This could also be the case in staffing problems, where there might be many thousands of different work patterns that people could work. Explicitly generating all these columns is not a task taken lightly. An alternative approach is motivated by the observation that at an optimum there will be no more positive columns than there are rows.

The basic idea is described by the following iterative process.

1. Generate and solve an initial LP that has all the rows of the full model defined, but only a small number (perhaps even zero) of the columns explicitly specified.
2. Given the dual prices of the current solution, generate one or more columns that price out attractively. That is, if a_{0j} is the cost of column j, a_{ij} is its usage of resource i (i.e., its coefficient in rows i for $i = 1, \ldots, m$, and p_i is the dual price of row i) generate or find a new column a such that

$$a_{0j} + p_{1j}a_{ij} + p_2a_{2j} + \ldots + p_ma_{mj} < 0.$$

If no such column exists, stop.

3. Solve the LP with the new column(s) from (2) added.
4. Go to (2).

The crucial step is (2). To use column generation for a specific problem, you must be able to solve the column generation subproblem in (2). In mathematical programming form, the subproblem in (2) is:

Given $\{p_j\}$, solve

Min $a_{0j} + p_1a_{1j} + p_2a_{2j} + K + p_ma_{mj}$
subject to
 The a_{ij} satisfy the conditions defining a valid column.

16.7.1 Example of Column Generation Applied to a Cutting Stock Problem

A common problem encountered in flat goods industries, such as paper, textiles and steel, is the cutting of large pieces of raw material into smaller pieces needed for producing a finished product. Suppose that raw material comes in 72-inch widths and it must be cut up into eight different finished good widths described by the following table.

Product	Width in Inches	Linear Feet Required
1	60	500
2	56	400
3	42	300
4	38	450
5	34	350
6	24	100
7	15	800
8	10	1000

We start the process somewhat arbitrarily by defining the eight pure cutting patterns. A pure pattern produces only one type of finished good width. Let P_i = number of feet of raw material to cut according to the pattern i. We want to minimize the total number of feet cut. The LP with these patterns is:

```
MIN    P001 + P002 + P003 + P004 + P005 + P006 + P007 + P008
SUBJECT TO
  2)     P001 >=   500            (60 inch width)
  3)     P002 >=   400            (56 inch width)
  4)     P003 >=   300            (42 inch width)
  5)     P004 >=   450            (38 inch width)
  6)  2  P005 >=   350            (34 inch width)
  7)  3  P006 >=   100            (24 inch width)
  8)  4  P007 >=   800            (15 inch width)
  9)  7  P008 >=  1000            (10 inch width)
  END
```

The solution is

```
            OBJECTIVE FUNCTION VALUE

        1)              2201.19000

        VARIABLE            VALUE           REDUCED COST
          P001         500.000000             .000000
          P002         400.000000             .000000
          P003         300.000000             .000000
          P004         450.000000             .000000
          P005         175.000000             .000000
          P006          33.333330             .000000
          P007         200.000000             .000000
          P008         142.857100             .000000

          ROW        SLACK OR SURPLUS        DUAL PRICES
          2)              .000000            -1.000000
          3)              .000000            -1.000000
          4)              .000000            -1.000000
          5)              .000000            -1.000000
          6)              .000000             -.500000
          7)              .000000             -.333333
          8)              .000000             -.250000
          9)              .000000             -.142857
```

The dual prices provide information about which finished goods are currently expensive to produce. A new pattern to add to the problem can be found by solving the problem:

$$\text{Minimize} \quad 1 - y_1 - y_2 - y_3 - y_4 - .5y_5 - 0.333333y_6 - 0.25y_7 - 0.142857y_8$$

subject to

$$60y_1 + 56y_2 + 42y_3 + 38y_4 + 34y_5 + 24y_6 + 15y_7 + 10y_8 \leq 72$$

$$y_1 = 0, 1, 2, \ldots \quad \text{for} \quad i = 1, \ldots 8.$$

Note that the objective can be rewritten as

$$\text{Maximize} \quad y_1 + y_2 + y_3 + y_4 + .5y_5 + 0.333333y_6 + 0.25y_7 + 0.142857y_8.$$

This is a knapsack problem. Although knapsack problems are theoretically difficult to solve, there are algorithms that are quite efficient on typical practical knapsack problems. An optimal solution to this knapsack problem is $y_4 = 1$, $y_7 = 2$, i.e., a pattern that cuts one 38-inch width and two 15-inch widths. When this column, P009, is added to the LP we get the formulation (in PICTURE form):

```
         P P P P P P P P P
         0 0 0 0 0 0 0 0 0
         0 0 0 0 0 0 0 0 0
         1 2 3 4 5 6 7 8 9

1:  1 1 1 1 1 1 1 1 1 MIN
2:  1         '         '       > C
3:  ' 1'    '     '    '    '   > C
4:      1 '         '        > C
5:        1        '    1 > C
6:  '   '   ' 2'   '    '    > C
7:          '    3 '         > B
8:          '        4    2 > C
9:  '   '   '   '   ' 7'   > C
```

The solution is

```
OBJECTIVE FUNCTION VALUE

        1)            2201.19000

        VARIABLE          VALUE         REDUCED COST
          P001        500.000000           .000000
          P002        400.000000           .000000
          P003        300.000000           .000000
          P004         50.000000           .000000
          P005        175.000000           .000000
          P006         33.333330           .000000
          P007           .000000          1.000000
          P008        142.857100           .000000
          P009        400.000000           .000000

        ROW       SLACK OR SURPLUS      DUAL PRICES
         2)            .000000            -1.000
         3)            .000000            -1.000000
         4)            .000000            -1.000000
         5)            .000000            -1.000000
         6)            .000000             -.500000
         7)            .000000             -.333333
         8)            .000000             -.000000
         9)            .000000             -.142857
```

The column generation subproblem is

$$\text{Minimize} \quad y_1 + y_2 + y_3 + y_4 + .5y_5 + 0.333333y_6 - 0.142857y_8$$

subject to

$$60y_1 + 56y_2 + 42y_3 + 38y_4 + 34y_5 + 24y_6 + 15y_7 + 10y_8 \leq 72$$

$$y_1 = 0, 1, 2, \ldots \quad \text{for} \quad i = 1, \ldots 8.$$

An optimal solution to this knapsack problem is $y_4 = 1$, $y_5 = 1$, i.e., a pattern that cuts one 38-inch width and one 34-inch width.

We continue generating and adding patterns for a total of eight iterations. At this point the LP formulation is:

```
    P P P P P P P P P P P P P P P
    0 0 0 0 0 0 0 0 0 0 0 0 0 0 0
    0 0 0 0 0 0 0 0 0 1 1 1 1 1 1
    1 2 3 4 5 6 7 8 9 0 1 2 3 4 5

1:  1 1 1 1 1 1 1 1 1 1 1 1 1 1 1 MIN
2:  1         '         '         '         '     1 > C
3:  ' 1'  '   '   '   '   '  '1 '   '     > C
4:      1 '             ' 1   ' 1     > C
5:        1       '   1 1       1       > C
6:  '   '   ' 2'   '   ' 1   '   '   '   > C
7:          '   3 '         '       1       > B
8:          '         4   2 ' 2 1 '       > C
9:  '   '   '   '   ' 7'   '   '   1 3'1 > C
```

The solution is:

```
    OBJECTIVE FUNCTION VALUE

        1)            1664.28600

        VARIABLE           VALUE           REDUCED COST
          P001            .000000             .142857
          P002            .000000             .214285
          P003            .000000             .428571
          P004            .000000             .476191
          P005            .000000             .047619
          P006            .000000             .000000
          P007            .000000             .142857
          P008          14.285710             .000000
          P009            .000000             .047619
          P010         350.000000             .000000
          P011         200.000000             .000000
          P012         400.000000             .000000
          P013         100.000000             .000000
          P014         100.000000             .000000
          P015         500.000000             .000000

        ROW       SLACK OR SURPLUS       DUAL PRICES
        2)            .000000             -.857143
        3)            .000000             -.785714
        4)            .000000             -.571429
        5)            .000000             -.523809
        6)            .000000             -.476191
        7)            .000000             -.333333
        8)            .000000             -.214285
        9)            .000000             -.142857
```

The relevant knapsack problem is:

$$\text{Maximize} \quad 0.857143y_1 + 0.785714y_2 + 0.571429y_3 + 0.523809y_4$$
$$+0.476191y_5 + 0.333333y_6 + 0.214285y_7 + 0.142857y_8$$

subject to

$$60y_1 + 56y_2 + 42y_3 + 38y_4 + 34y_5 + 24y_6 + 15y_7 + 10y_8 \le 72$$
$$y_1 = 0, 1, 2, \ldots \quad \text{for} \quad i = 1, \ldots 8.$$

The optimal solution to the knapsack problem has an objective function value less than or equal to one. Because each column when added to the LP has a "cost" of one in the LP objective, when the proposed column is priced out with the current dual prices it is unattractive to enter. Thus, the previous LP solution specifies the optimal amount to run of all possible patterns. There are in fact 29 different efficient patterns possible, where efficient means the edge waste is less than 10 inches. Thus, the column generation approach allowed us to avoid generating the majority of the patterns.

If an integer solution is required, a simple rounding up heuristic tends to work moderately well. In our example, we know that the optimal integer solution costs at least 1665. By rounding P008 up to 15, we obtain a solution with cost 1665.

16.7.2 Column Generation and Integer Programming

Column generation can be used to easily find an optimum solution to an LP. This is not quite true with IPs. The problem is that with an IP there is no simple equivalent to dual prices. Dual prices may be printed in an IP solution but they have an extremely limited interpretation. For example, it may be that all dual prices are 0 in an IP solution.

Thus, the usual approach when column generation is used to attack IPs is to use column generation only to solve the LP relaxation. A standard IP algorithm is then applied to the problem composed of only the columns generated during the LP. It may be, however, that a true IP optimum includes one or more columns which were not generated during the LP phase. The LP solution, nevertheless, provides a bound on the optimum LP solution. In our previous cutting stock example, this bound was tight.

There is a fine point to be made with regard to the stopping rule. We stop, *not* when the previous column added leads to no improvement in the LP solution, but rather when the latest column generated prices out unattractively.

16.7.3 Row Generation

An analogous approach can be used if the problem intrinsically has many thousands of constraints even though only a few of them will be binding. The basic approach is:

1. Generate some of the constraints.
2. Solve the problem with the existing constraints.
3. Find a constraint that has not been generated but is violated. If none, we are done.
4. Add the violated constraint and go to (2).

16.8 PROBLEMS

Problem 1

Consider the LP:

```
MAX   20 X   + W
s.t.
      X    + Z              <= 70
      Y    + Z              <= 55
      W  - 30 Y - 46 Z   = 0
      X + 2 Y + 3.1     <= 130
END
```

all variables nonnegative. Show how this model can be reduced to a smaller but equivalent LP.

Multiple Criteria and Goal Programming

17.1 Introduction

Until now we have assumed a single objective or criterion. In reality, however, there may be two or more measures of goodness. Our life becomes more difficult, or at least more interesting, if these multiple criteria are incommensurate; i.e., it is difficult to combine them into a single criterion. The overused phrase used in lamenting the difficulty of such situations is that "You can't mix apples and oranges."

Some examples of incommensurate criteria are:

- risk vs. return on investment,
- short-term profits vs. long-term growth of a firm,
- cost vs. service by a government agency,
- the treatment of different individuals under some policy of an administrative agency, e.g., rural vs. urban citizens, residents near an airport vs. travelers using an airport, fishermen vs. water transportation companies vs. farmers using irrigation near a large lake.

Multicriteria situations can be classified into several categories.

1. Criteria are intrinsically different (e.g., risk vs. return, cost vs. service).
   (a) Weights or trade-off rates can be determined.
   (b) Criteria can be strictly ordered by importance. We have so-called preemptive objectives.
2. Criteria are intrinsically similar; i.e., in some sense they should have equal weight.

A rich source of multicriteria problems is the design and operation of public works. A specific example is the huge "Three Gorges" dam on the Yangtze river in China. Interested parties and their criteria include: (a) industrial users of electricity, who would like the average water level in the dam to be high so as to maximize the amount of electricity that can be generated, (b) farmers downstream from the dam, who would like the water level in the dam to be maintained at a low level so that unexpected large rainfalls can be accommodated without overflow and flooding,

(c) river shipping interests, who would like the lake level to be allowed to fluctuate as necessary so as to maintain a steady flow rate out of the dam, thereby allowing year-round river travel by large ships below the dam, (d) lake fishermen and recreational interests, who would like the flow rate out of the dam to be allowed to fluctuate as necessary so as to maintain a steady lake level, and (e) environmental interests, who did not want the dam built in the first place. For the Three Gorges dam in particular, flood control interests have argued for having the water level behind the dam to be held at 459 feet above sea level just before the rainy season, so as to accommodate storm runoff; see, for example, Fillon (1996). Electricity generation interests, however, have argued for a water level of 574 feet above sea level, so as to generate more electricity.

17.1.1 Alternate Optima and Multicriteria

If you have a model with alternate optimal solutions, this is nature's way of telling you that you have multiple criteria. You should probably look at your objective function more closely and add more detail. Users do not like alternate optima. If there are alternate optima, the solution method will usually choose among them essentially randomly. If people's jobs or salaries depend upon the "flip of a coin" in your analysis, they are going to be unhappy. Even if careers are not at stake, alternate optima are at least a nuisance. People find it disconcerting if they get different answers (albeit with the same objective value) when they solve the same problem on different computers.

One resolution of alternate optima that might occur to some readers is to take the average of all distinct alternate optima and use this average solution as the final, unique, well-defined answer. Unfortunately, this is usually not practical because:

(a) it may be difficult to enumerate all alternate optima, and
(b) the average solution may be unattractive or even infeasible because the answer may involve fractional values.

17.2 Approaches to Multicriteria Problems

17.2.1 Pareto Optimal Solutions and Multiple Criteria

A solution to a multicriteria problem is said to be *Pareto optimal* if there is no other solution that is at least as good according to all criteria and strictly better according to at least one criterion. A Pareto optimal solution is not dominated by any other solution. Clearly we want to consider only Pareto optimal solutions. If we do not choose our criteria carefully, we might find ourselves recommending solutions that are not Pareto optimal. There are computer programs for multicriteria linear programming that will generate all the undominated extreme solutions. For a small problem a decision maker could simply choose the most attractive extreme solution

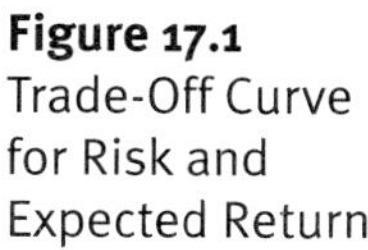

Figure 17.1
Trade-Off Curve
for Risk and
Expected Return

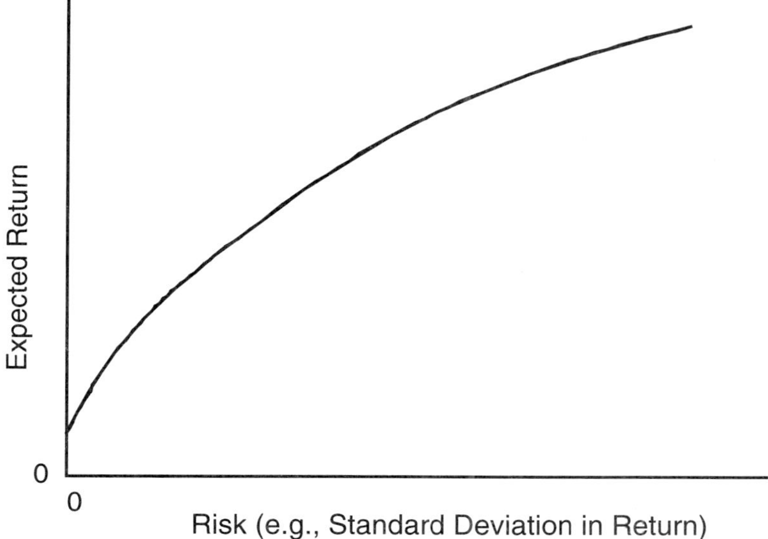

based on subjective criteria. For large problems, the number of undominated extreme solutions may easily exceed 100, and so this approach may be overwhelming.

17.2.2 Utility Function Approach

A solution of the multicriteria problem that is superficially attractive is the definition of a utility function. If the decision variables are $x_1, x_2, \ldots, x_n$, we "simply" construct the utility function $u(x_1, x_2, \ldots, x_n)$ that computes the value or utility of any possible combination of values for the vector $x_1, x_2, \ldots, x_n$. This is a very useful approach for *thinking* about optimization, but it has several practical limitations: (a) it may take a lot of work to construct it, and (b) it will probably be highly nonlinear. Feature (b) means that we probably cannot use LP to solve the problem.

17.2.3 Trade-off Curves

If we have only two or three criteria, the trade-off curve approach has most of the attractive features of the utility function approach but is also fairly practical. We simply construct a curve, the so-called "efficient frontier," that shows how we can trade off one criterion for another. One of the most well known settings in which a trade-off curve is used is to describe the relationship between two criteria in a financial portfolio. The two criteria are expected return on investment and risk. We want return to be high and risk to be low. Figure 17.1 shows the typical relationship between risk and return. Each point on the curve is Pareto optimal. That is, for any point on the curve there is no other point with higher expected return and lower risk.

Even though a decision maker has not gone through the trouble of constructing his utility function, he may be able to look at this trade-off curve and perhaps say: "Gee, I am comfortable with an expected return of 8 percent with standard deviation of 3 percent."

17.2.4 Example: Ad Lib Marketing

Ad Lib is a freewheeling advertising agency that wants to solve a so-called media selection problem for one of its clients. It is considering placing ads in five media: late night TV (TVL), prime time TV (TVP), billboards (BLB), newspapers (NEW), and radio (RAD). These ads are intended to reach seven different demographic groups.

The following table gives the number of exposures obtained in each of the seven markets per dollar of advertising in each of five media. The second last row of the table lists the minimum required number of exposures in each of the seven markets. The feeling is that we must reach this minimum number of readers/viewers, regardless of the cost. The last row of numbers is the saturation level for each market. The feeling is that exposure beyond this level is of no value. Exposures between these two limits will be termed useful exposures.

Exposure Statistics for Ad Lib Marketing

	Exposure in 1000s per $1000 Spent Market Group						
	1	2	3	4	5	6	7
TVL		10	4	50	5		2
TVP		10	30	5	12		
BLB	20					5	3
NEW	8					6	10
RAD		6	5	10	11	4	
Minimum Number of Exposures Needed in 1,000s	25	40	60	120	40	11	15
Saturation Level in 1000s of Exposures	60	70	120	140	80	25	55

How much money should be spent on advertising in each medium? There are really two criteria: (a) cost (that we want to be low), and (b) useful exposures (that we want to be high). At the outset we arbitrarily decided that we will spend no more than $11,000.

A useful model can be formulated if we define:

Decision variables:

TVL, TVP, etc. = dollars spent in 1,000s on advertising in TVL, TVP, etc.;
UX1, UX2, etc. = number of useful excess exposures obtained in market 1, 2, etc., beyond the minimum, i.e., min {saturation level, actual exposures} – minimum required;

```
COST            = total amount spent on advertising,
USEFULX         = total useful exposures.
```

There will be two main sets of constraints, one set that says:

> exposures in a market ≥ minimum required
> + useful excess exposure beyond minimum.

The other says:

> useful excess exposures in a market ≤ saturation level − minimum required.

The explicit formulation is:

```
MAX        USEFULX                  ! Maximize useful exposures;
SUBJECT TO
 LIMCOST)   COST      <= 11 ! With a limit of 11 (in $1,000) on
     cost;
  LIMEXP)    USEFULX <=    0
 DEFCOST)  - COST + TVL + TVP + BLB + NEW + RAD =        0
  DEFEXP)  - USEFULX + UX1 + UX2 + UX3 + UX4 + UX5 + UX6 + UX7 = 0
    MKT1)    20 BLB + 8 NEW - UX1              <=    25
    MKT2)    10 TVL + 10 TVP + 6 RAD - UX2 <=    40
    MKT3)    4 TVL + 30 TVP + 5 RAD - UX3   <=    60
    MKT4)    50 TVL + 5 TVP + 10 RAD - UX4 <=    120
    MKT5)    5 TVL + 12 TVP + 11 RAD - UX5 <=    40
    MKT6)    5 BLB + 6 NEW + 4 RAD - UX6    <=    11
    MKT7)    2 TVL + 3 BLB + 10 NEW - UX7   <=    15
  RANGE1)    UX1 <=    35
  RANGE2)    UX2 <=    30
  RANGE3)    UX3 <=    60
  RANGE4)    UX4 <=    20
  RANGE5)    UX5 <=    40
  RANGE6)    UX6 <=    14
  RANGE7)    UX7 <=    40
END
```

The following is part of the solution to this model.

```
          OBJECTIVE FUNCTION VALUE

     1)      196.762600

  VARIABLE          VALUE           REDUCED COST
  USEFULX        196.762600            .000000
     COST         11.000000            .000000
      TVL          1.997602            .000000
      TVP          3.707434            .000000
      BLB          2.908873            .000000
      NEW           .227818            .000000
      RAD          2.158273            .000000
      UX1         35.000000            .000000
      UX2         30.000000            .000000
      UX3         60.000000            .000000
      UX4         20.000000            .000000
      UX5         38.218220            .000000
      UX6         13.544360            .000000
      UX7          .000000             .007194
```

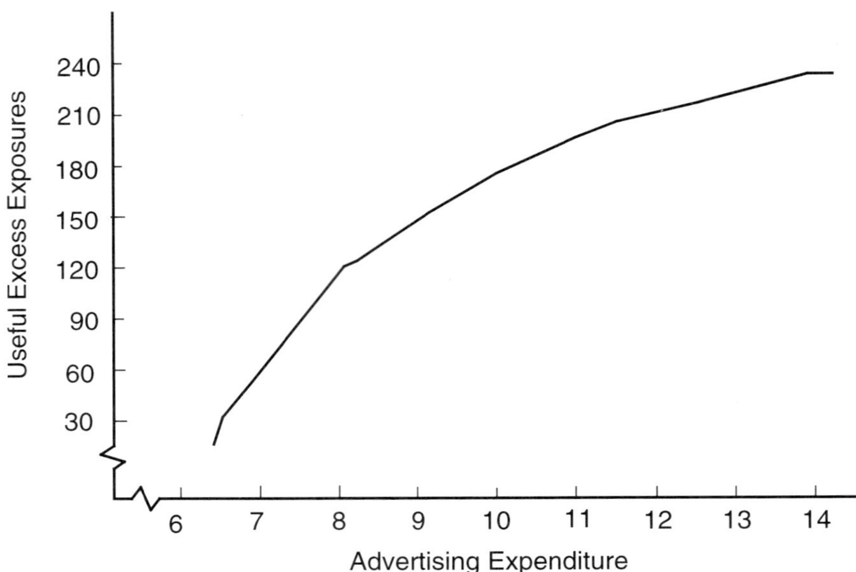

Figure 17.2
Trade-Off Between Exposures and Advertising

ROW	SLACK OR SURPLUS	DUAL PRICES
LIMCOST)	.000000	21.438850
LIMEXP)	196.762600	.000000
DEFCOST)	.000000	21.438850
DEFEXP)	.000000	-1.000000

Notice that we advertise up to the saturation level in markets 1 to 4. In market 7 we advertise just enough to achieve the minimum required.

If you change the cost limit (initially at 11) to various values ranging from 6 to 14, and plot the maximum possible number of useful exposures, you get a trade-off curve, or efficient frontier, like that shown in Figure 17.2.

17.3 Goal Programming and Soft Constraints

Goal Programming is closely related to the concept of multicriteria as well as a simple idea that we dub "soft constraints." Soft constraints and Goal Programming are a response to the following two "laws of the real world":

In the real world,

1. there is always a feasible solution,
2. there are no alternate optima.

In practical terms (1) means that a good manager (or one wishing at least to keep a job) never throws up his or her hands in despair and says "no feasible solution." Law (2) means that a typical decision maker will never be indifferent between two proposed courses of action. There are always sufficient criteria to distinguish some course of action as better than all others.

From a model perspective these two laws mean that a well-formulated model (a) always has a feasible solution and (b) does not have alternate optima.

17.3.1 Example: Secondary Criterion to Choose Among Alternate Optima

Here is a standard, seven-day-per-week staffing problem similar to the one discussed in Chapter 6. The variables M, T, W, R, F, S, N denote the number of people starting their five-day work week on Monday, Tuesday, Wednesday, Thursday, Friday, Saturday, or Sunday, respectively.

```
MIN       9 M + 9 T + 9 W + 9 R + 9 F + 9 S + 9 N

SUBJECT TO
    MON)    M               + R + F + S + N <=    3
    TUE)    M + T               + F + S + N <=    3
    WED)    M + T + W               + S + N <=    8
    THU)    M + T + W + R               + N <=    8
    FRI)    M + T + W + R + F               <=    8
    SAT)        T + W + R + F + S           <=    3
    SUN)            W + R + F + S + N <=    3
END
```

When solved, we get the following solution.

```
        OBJECTIVE FUNCTION VALUE

    1)      72.0000000

  VARIABLE          VALUE          REDUCED CCST
        M          3.000000            0.000000
        T          0.000000            0.000000
        W          5.000000            0.000000
        R          0.000000            9.000000
        F          0.000000            9.000000
        S          0.000000            0.000000
        N          0.000000            0.000000

      ROW    SLACK OR SURPLUS        DUAL PRICES
     MON)          0.000000            0.000000
     TUE)          0.000000            0.000000
     WED)          0.000000           -9.000000
     THU)          0.000000            0.000000
     FRI)          0.000000            0.000000
     SAT)          2.000000            0.000000
     SUN)          2.000000            0.000000
```

Notice that there may be alternate optima; e.g., the slack and dual price in row MON are both zero. This solution puts all the surplus capacity on Saturday and Sunday. The different optima might distribute the surplus capacity in different ways over the days of the week. Saturday and Sunday have a lot of excess capacity, whereas the very similar days, Monday and Tuesday, have no surplus capacity.

In terms of multiple criteria we might say:

(a) our most important criterion is to minimize total staffing cost;
(b) our secondary criterion is to have a little extra capacity, specifically one unit, each day if it will not increase criterion 1.

To encourage more equitable distribution, we add some "excess" variables, XM, XT, etc., that give a tiny credit of –1 for each surplus up to at most 1 on each day. The modified formulation is:

```
MIN      9 M + 9 T + 9 W + 9 R + 9 F + 9 S + 9 N
         - XM - XT - XW - XR - XF - XS - XN
SUBJECT TO
     MON)   M                 +  R   + F    + S    + N   - XM <=   3
     TUE)   M   + T                   + F    + S    + N   - XT <=   3
     WED)   M   + T   + W                    + S    + N   - XW <=   8
     THU)   M   + T   + W   + R                      + N   - XR <=   8
     FRI)   M   + T   + W   + R   + F                      - XF <=   8
     SAT)       T   + W   + R   + F    + S              - XS <=   3
     SUN)             W   + R   + F    + S    + N   - XN <=   3
        9)   XM <=   1
       10)   XT <=   1
       11)   XW <=   1
       12)   XR <=   1
       13)   XF <=   1
       14)   XS <=   1
       15)   XN <=   1
END
```

The solution now is:

```
            OBJECTIVE FUNCTION VALUE

       1)       68.000000

      VARIABLE          VALUE          REDUCED COST
         M            4.000000            0.000000
         T            0.000000            0.000000
         W            4.000000            0.000000
         R            0.000000            4.000000
         F            0.000000            4.000000
         S            0.000000            0.000000
         N            0.000000            0.000000
        XM            1.000000            0.000000
        XT            1.000000            0.000000
        XW            0.000000            4.000000
        XR            0.000000            0.000000
        XF            0.000000            0.000000
        XS            1.000000            0.000000
        XN            1.000000            0.000000
```

Notice that just as before we still hire a total of eight people but now the surplus is evenly distributed over the four days M, T, S, and N. This should be a more attractive solution.

17.3.2 Preemptive/Lexico Goal Programming

The above approach required us to choose the proper relative weights for our two objectives, cost and service. In some situations it may be clear that one objective is orders of magnitude more important than the other. One could choose weights to reflect this (e.g., 99999999 for the first and 0.0000001 for the second), but there are a variety of reasons for not using this approach. First of all, there would probably be numerical problems, especially if there are more than two objectives. A typical computer cannot accurately add numbers that differ by more than 15 orders of magnitude, e.g., 100,000,000 and .0000001.

More importantly, it just seems more straightforward simply to say: "This first objective is far more important than the remaining objectives, the second objective is far more important than the remaining objectives," etc. LINDO has a single command, GLEX, for doing just this. To exploit this command, you must: (1) define a variable for each objective, (2) list these variables in the objective in order of importance, and (3) use the GLEX command, rather than GO, to solve the problem. This approach is sometimes called Preemptive or Lexico goal programming. The following illustrates for our previous staff scheduling example:

```
!Example of Lexico-goal programming

MIN       COST - EXTRA
   SUBJECT TO
         MON)    M + R + F + S + N - XM <=    3
         TUE)    M + F + S + N + T - XT <=    3
         WED)    M + S + N + T + W - XW <=    8
         THU)    M + R + N + T + W - XR <=    8
         FRI)    M + R + F + T + W - XF <=    8
         SAT)    R + F + S + T + W - XS <=    3
         SUN)    R + F + S + N + W - XN <=    3
         XM)    XM <=    1
         XT)    XT <=    1
         XW)    XW <=    1
         XR)    XR <=    1
         XF)    XF <=    1
         XS)    XS <=    1
         XN)    XN <=    1
! Define the two objectives;
        COST)   COST - M - R - F - S - N - T - W =    0
       EXTRA)   EXTRA - XM - XT - XW - XR - XF - XS - XN =  0
   END
   FREE      COST
   FREE     EXTRA

   : terse
   : glex
LP OPTIMUM FOUND AT STEP       4
OBJECTIVE VALUE =    8.00000000
LP OPTIMUM FOUND AT STEP       7
OBJECTIVE VALUE = 4.000000
   : solu
```

```
            OBJECTIVE FUNCTION VALUE

     1)        4.000000

   VARIABLE           VALUE          REDUCED COST
      COST          8.000000           0.000000
     EXTRA          4.000000          -0.750000
         M          4.000000           0.000000
         R          0.000000           0.250000
         F          0.000000           0.250000
         S          0.000000           0.250000
         N          0.000000           0.000000
        XM          1.000000           0.000000
         T          0.000000           0.000000
        XT          1.000000           0.000000
         W          4.000003           0.000000
        XW          0.000003           0.000000
        XR          0.000003           0.000000
        XF          0.000003           0.000000
        XS          1.000000           0.000000
        XN          1.000003           0.000000

       ROW     SLACK OR SURPLUS       DUAL PRICES
      MON)          0.000000           0.000000
      TUE)          0.000000          -0.250000
      WED)          0.000000          -0.250000
      THU)          0.000000          -0.250000
      FRI)          0.000000          -0.250000
      SAT)          0.000003           0.000000
      SUN)          0.000000          -0.250000
       XM)          0.000000           0.250000
       XT)          0.000000           0.000000
       XW)          0.999997           0.000000
       XR)          0.999997           0.000000
       XF)          0.999997           0.000000
       XS)          0.000000           0.250000
       XN)         -0.000003           0.000000
     COST)          0.000000          -1.000000
    EXTRA)          0.000000           0.250000

   NO. ITERATIONS=        3
```

The overall objective value displayed can be disregarded. It is the values of COST and EXTRA that are of interest.

17.4 Minimizing the Maximum Hurt, or Unordered Lexico Minimization

There are some situations in which there are a number of parties that in some sense are equal. There may be certain side conditions, however, that prevent us from treating them exactly equally. An example is representation in a house of representatives. Ideally, we would like each state to have the number of representatives in a state be exactly proportional to the population of the state. The fact that the house of representatives is typically limited to a fixed size and that we cannot have fractional representatives (although some voters may feel they have encountered such an anomaly), we will find that some states have more citizens per representative than others.

In more general settings, an obvious approach for minimizing such inequities is to choose things so that we minimize the maximum inequity or "hurt." Once we have minimized the worst hurt, the obvious next thing is to minimize the second greatest hurt, etc. Such a minimization we will refer to as Unordered Lexico Minimization. For example, if there are four parties and (13, 13, 8, 9) is the vector of taxes to be paid, we would say that the vector (13, 8, 9, 9) is better in the unordered lexicomin sense. The highest tax is the same for both solutions but the second highest tax is lower for the second solution.

17.4.1 Example

This example is based on one in Sankaran (1989). There are six parties, and x_i is the assessment to be paid by party i to satisfy a certain community building project. The x_i must satisfy the set of constraints:

```
A)   X1 + 2 X2 + 4 X3 + 7 X4 >=   16
B) 2.5 X1 + 3.5 X2 + 5.2 X5 >=   17.5
C) 0.4 X2 + 1.3 X4 + 7.2 X6 >=   12
D) 2.5 X2 + 3.5 X3 + 5.2 X5 >=   13.1
E) 3.5 X1 + 3.5 X4 + 5.2 X6 >=   18.2
```

The interested reader may try to improve upon the following set of assessments:

```
X1 = 1.5625
X2 = 1.5625
X3 =  .305357
X4 = 1.463362
X5 = 1.5625
X6 = 1.463362
```

There is no other solution in which

    (a) the highest assessment is less than 1.5625, and
    (b) the second highest assessment is less than 1.5625, and
    (c) the third highest assessment is less than 1.5625, and
    (d) the fourth highest assessment is less than 1.463362, etc.

17.4.2 Finding the Unique Solution Minimizing the Maximum

A quite general approach to finding a unique unordered lexico minimum exists when the feasible region is convex; e.g., there are no integer variables. Let the vector $\{x_1, x_2, \ldots, x_n\}$ denote the cost allocated to each of n parties.

If the feasible region is convex, there is a unique solution, and the following algorithm will find it. Maschler, Peleg, and Shapley (1979) discuss this idea in the game theory setting. If the feasible region is not convex (e.g., the problem has integer variables), the following method is not guaranteed to find the solution. Let S be the original set of constraints on the xs.

(1) Let $J = \{1, 2, \ldots, n\}$, and $k = 0$; (Note: J is the set of parties for whom we do not yet know the final x_i)

(2) Let $k = k + 1$;

(3) Solve the problem:

      Minimize Z

      subject to x feasible to S and,

                $Z \geq x_j$ for j in J;

(Note: this finds the minimum, maximum hurt among parties for which we have not yet fixed the x_js.)

(4) Set $Z_k = Z$ of (3) and add to S the constraints:

      $x_j \leq Z_k$ for all j in J;

(5) Set $L = \{j$ in J for which $x_j = Z_k$ in (3)$\}$;

      For each j in L:

      Solve:

            Minimize x_j

            subject to

                x feasible to S;

      If $x_j = Z_k$, set $J = J - j$, and append to S the constraint $x_j = Z_k$.

(6) If J is not empty, go to (2), else we are done.

To find the minimum maximum assessment for our example problem, we solve the following problem:

```
            MIN       Z
            SUBJECT TO
          ! The physical constraints on the  Xs;
              A)  X1 + 2 X2 + 4 X3 + 7 X4   <=      16
              B)  2.5 X1 + 3.5 X2 + 5.2 X5 <=      17.5
              C)  0.4 X2 + 1.3 X4 + 7.2 X6 <=      12
              D)  2.5 X2 + 3.5 X3 + 5.2 X5 <=      13.1
              E)  3.5 X1 + 3.5 X4 + 5.2 X6 <=      18.2
          ! Constraints to compute the max hurt   Z;
              H1)  Z - X1 <=    0
              H2)  Z - X2 <=    0
              H3)  Z - X3 <=    0
              H4)  Z - X4 <=    0
              H5)  Z - X5 <=    0
              H6)  Z - X6 <=    0
            END
```

Its solution is:

```
              OBJECTIVE FUNCTION VALUE

          1)              1.562500

      VARIABLE          VALUE              REDUCED COST
            Z           1.562500             0.000000
           X1           1.562500             0.000000
           X2           1.562500             0.000000
           X3           1.562500             0.000000
           X4           1.562500             0.000000
           X5           1.562500             0.000000
```

Thus, at least one party will have a "hurt" of 1.5625. Which party or parties will it be?

Because all six X_is equal 1.5625, we solve a series of six problems like the following:

```
MIN    X1
SUBJECT TO
  ! The physical constraints on the  Xs;
    A) X1 + 2 X2 + 4 X3 + 7 X4  <=      16
    B) 2.5 X1 + 3.5 X2 + 5.2 X5 <=      17.5
    C) 0.4 X2 + 1.3 X4 + 7.2 X6 <=      12
    D) 2.5 X2 + 3.5 X3 + 5.2 X5 <=      13.1
    E) 3.5 X1 + 3.5 X4 + 5.2 X6 <=      18.2
  ! Constraints for finding the minmax hurt,  Z;
    H1)       + X1 <=    1.5625
    H2)       + X2 <=    1.5625
    H3)       + X3 <=    1.5625
    H4)       + X4 <=    1.5625
    H5)       + X5 <=    1.5625
    H6)       + X6 <=    1.5625
  END
```

The solution for the case of X1 is:

```
            OBJECTIVE FUNCTION VALUE

    1)              1.562500

VARIABLE            VALUE            REDUCED COST.
    X1            1.562500                .000000
    X2            1.562500                .000000
    X3             .305357                .000000
    X4            1.562500                .000000
    X5            1.562500                .000000
    X6            1.562500                .000000
```

Thus, there is no solution with all the X_is $\le$ 1.5625 but with X1 strictly less than 1.5625. So we can fix X1 at 1.5625. Similar observations turn out to be true for X2 and X5.

So now we wish to solve the following problem:

```
MIN    Z
SUBJECT  TO
  ! The physical constraints on the  Xs;
    A) X1 + 2 X2 + 4 X3 + 7 X4  <=      16
    B) 2.5 X1 + 3.5 X2 + 5.2 X5 <=      17.5
    C) 0.4 X2 + 1.3 X4 + 7.2 X6 <=      12
    D) 2.5 X2 + 3.5 X3 + 5.2 X5 <=      13.1
    E) 3.5 X1 + 3.5 X4 + 5.2 X6 <=      18.2
  ! Constraints for finding the minmax hurt,  Z;
    H1)         X1  = 1.5625
    H2)         X2  = 1.5625
    H3)   - Z + X3 <= 0
    H4)   - Z + X4 <= 0
```

```
    H5)           X5  = 1.5625
    H6)   - Z + X6  <= 0
END
```

Upon solution we see that the second highest "hurt" is 1.463362:

```
        OBJECTIVE FUNCTION VALUE

     1)      1.46336200

   VARIABLE           VALUE          REDUCED COST
       Z            1.463362           .000000
      X1            1.562500           .000000
      X2            1.562500           .000000
      X3            1.463362           .000000
      X4            1.463362           .000000
      X5            1.562500           .000000
      X6            1.463362           .000000
```

Any or all of X3, X4, or X6 could be at this value in the final solution. Which ones? To find out, we solve the following kind of problem for X3, X4, and X6.

```
    MIN     X3
 SUBJECT   TO
   ! The physical constraints on the  Xs;
     A)    X1 + 2 X2 + 4 X3 + 7 X4  <=    16
     B)    2.5 X1 + 3.5 X2 + 5.2 X5 <=    17.5
     C)    0.4 X2 + 1.3 X4 + 7.2 X6 <=    12
     D)    2.5 X2 + 3.5 X3 + 5.2 X5 <=    13.1
     E)    3.5 X1 + 3.5 X4 + 5.2 X6 <=    18.2
   ! Constraints for finding the minmax hurt,  Z;
    H1)    X1  = 1.5625
    H2)    X2  = 1.5625
    H3)    X3 <= 1.463362
    H4)    X4 <= 1.463362
    H5)    X5  = 1.5625
    H6)    X6 <= 1.463362
 END
```

The solution when we minimize X3 is:

```
        OBJECTIVE FUNCTION VALUE

     1)      .305357300

   VARIABLE           VALUE          REDUCED COST
      X3             .305357           .000000
      X1            1.562500           .000000
      X2            1.562500           .000000
      X4            1.463362           .000000
      X5            1.562500           .000000
      X6            1.463362           .000000
```

Thus, X3 need not be as high as 1.463362 in the final solution. We do find, however, that X4 and X6 can be no smaller than 1.463362.

So the final problem we want to solve is:

```
MIN     Z
SUBJECT   TO
  ! The physical constraints on the Xs;
    A)  X1 + 2 X2 + 4 X3 + 7 X4   <=      16
    B)  2.5 X1 + 3.5 X2 + 5.2 X5 <=      17.5
    C)  0.4 X2 + 1.3 X4 + 7.2 X6 <=      12
    D)  2.5 X2 + 3.5 X3 + 5.2 X5 <=      13.1
    E)  3.5 X1 + 3.5 X4 + 5.2 X6 <=      18.2
  ! Constraints for finding the minmax hurt, Z;
  H1)          X1 = 1.5625
  H2)          X2 = 1.5625
  H3)  - Z + X3 = 0
  H4)          X4 = 1.463362
  H5)          X5 = 1.5625
  H6)        + X6 = 1.463362
END
```

We already know that the solution will be:

```
          OBJECTIVE FUNCTION VALUE

     1)      .305357300

VARIABLE          VALUE          REDUCED COST
      Z           .305357           .000000
     X1          1.562500           .000000
     X2          1.562500           .000000
     X3           .305357           .000000
     X4          1.463362           .000000
     X5          1.562500           .000000
     X6          1.463362           .000000
```

The above solution minimizes the maximum X value, as well as the number of Xs at that value. Given that maximum value (of 1.5625), it minimizes the second highest X value, as well as the number at that value, etc.

The approach described requires us to solve a sequence of linear programs. It would be nice if we could formulate a single mathematical program for finding the unordered lexico-min. There are a number of such formulations; unfortunately all of them suffer from numerical problems when implemented on real computers. The formulations assume that arithmetic is done with infinite precision, whereas most computers do arithmetic with at most 15 decimal digits of precision.

17.4.3 Finding Points on the Efficient Frontier

Until now we have considered the problem of how to generate a solution that is on the efficient frontier. Now let us take a slightly different perspective and consider the problem: Given a finite set of points, determine which ones are on the efficient frontier. When there are multiple criteria, it is usually impossible to find a single scoring formula to unambiguously rank all the points or players. The following table comparing on-time performance of two airlines (see Barnett, 1994) illustrates some of the issues.

	Alaska Airlines		America West Airlines	
Destination	% Arrivals on Time	No. of Arrivals	% Arrivals on Time	No. of Arrivals
Los Angeles	88.9	559	85.6	811
Phoenix	94.8	233	92.1	5,255
San Diego	91.4	232	85.5	448
San Francisco	83.1	605	71.3	449
Seattle	85.8	2,146	76.7	262
Weighted 5-Airport Average	86.7%	3,775	89.1%	7,225

The weighted average at the bottom is computed by applying a weight to the performance at airport i proportional to the number of arrivals at that airport. For example, $86.7 = (88.9 \times 559 + \ldots + 85.8 \times 2146)/(559 + \ldots + 2146)$.

According to this scoring, America West has a better on-time performance than Alaska Airlines. A traveler considering flying into San Francisco, however, would almost certainly prefer Alaska Airlines to America West with respect to on-time performance. In fact, the same argument applies to all five airports. Alaska Airlines dominates America West. How could America West have scored higher? The culprit was that a different scoring formula was used for each, and the airport receiving the most weight in America West's formula, sunny Phoenix, had a better on-time performance by America West than Alaska Airline's performance at its busiest airport, rainy Seattle. One should in general be suspicious when different scoring formulae are used for different candidates.

17.4.4 Efficient Points, More-is-Better Case

The previous example was a case of multiple performance dimensions where for each dimension, the higher the performance number, the better the performance. We will now illustrate a method for computing a single score or number, between 0 and 1, for each player. The interpretation of this number or efficiency score will be that a score of 1.0 means the player or organization being measured is on the efficient frontier. In particular, there is no other player better on all dimensions, or even a weighted combination of players so that the weighted averages of their performances surpass the given player on every dimension. On the other hand, a score less than 1.0 means either there is some other player better on all dimensions or there is a weighted combination of players having a weighted average performance better on all dimensions.

Define:

r_{ij} = the performance (or reward) of player i on the jth dimension, e.g., the on-time performance of Alaska Airlines in Seattle,

v_j = the weight or value to be applied to the jth dimension in evaluating overall efficiency.

To evaluate the performance of player k, we will do the following in words:

Choose the v_j so as to maximize score (k)
subject to
    For each player i (including k):
      score $(i) \leq 1$.

More precisely, we want to

Minimize $\sum_j v_j r_{kj}$

subject to

    For every player i, including k:

$$\sum_j v_j r_{ij} \leq 1$$

    For every weight j:

$$v_j \geq e$$

where e is a small positive number.

The reason for requiring every v_j to be slightly positive is as follows. Suppose player k and some other player t are tied for best on one dimension, say j, but player k is worse than t on all other dimensions. Player k would like to place all the weight on dimension j so that it will appear to be just as efficient as player t. Requiring a small positive weight on every dimension will reveal these slightly dominated players.

17.4.5 Example

The performance of five high schools in the "three Rs" of "Reading, Writing and Arithmetic" are tabulated below (see *Chicago Magazine*, February 1995):

School	Reading	Writing	Mathematics
Barrington	296	27	306
Lisle	286	27.1	322
Palatine	290	28.5	303
Hersey	298	27.3	312
Oak Park River Forest (OPRF)	294	28.1	301

Hersey, Palatine, and Lisle are clearly on the efficient frontier because they have the highest scores on Reading, Writing, and Mathematics, respectively. Barrington is clearly not on the efficient frontier because it is dominated by Hersey. What can we say about OPRF?

We formulate OPRF's problem as follows. Notice that we have scaled both the reading and math scores so that all scores are less than 100. This is important if one requires the weight for each attribute to be at least some minimum positive value.

```
MAX        29.4 VR + 28.1 VW + 30.1 VM
SUBJECT TO
  BAR) 29.6 VR + 27   VW + 30.6 VM <= 1
  LIS) 28.6 VR + 27.1 VW + 32.2 VM <= 1
  PAL) 29   VR + 28.5 VW + 30.3 VM <= 1
  HER) 29.8 VR + 27.3 VW + 31.2 VM <= 1
  OPR) 29.4 VR + 28.1 VW + 30.1 VM <= 1
  READ)     VR                        >= 0.0005
  WRIT)             VW                >= 0.0005
  MATH)                        VM >= 0.0005
END
```

When solved:

```
            OBJECTIVE FUNCTION VALUE
        1)        1.000000

    VARIABLE              VALUE         REDUCED COST
         VR            0.022224            0.000000
         VW            0.011799            0.000000
         VM            0.000500            0.000000

         ROW     SLACK OR SURPLUS       DUAL PRICES
        BAR)            0.008285            0.000000
        LIS)            0.028529            0.000000
        PAL)            0.004070            0.000000
        HER)            0.000000            0.000000
        OPR)            0.000000            1.000000
       READ)            0.021724            0.000000
       WRIT)            0.011299            0.000000
       MATH)            0.000000            0.000000
```

The value is 1.0, and thus, OPRF is on the efficient frontier. It should be no surprise that OPRF puts the minimum possible weight on the mathematics score (where it is the lowest of the five).

17.4.6 Efficient Points, Less-is-Better Case

Some measures of performance, such as cost, are of the "less-is-better" nature. Again, we would like to have a measure of performance that gives a score of 1.0 for a player on the efficient frontier, less than 1.0 for one that is not.

Define:

c_{ij} = performance of player i on dimension j
w_j = weight to be applied to the jth dimension.

To evaluate the performance of player k, we want to solve a problem of the following form:

Choose weights w_j so as to maximize the minimum weighted score,
    subject to
        the weighted score of player $k = 1$.

If the objective function value from this problem is less than 1, player k is inefficient, because there is no set of weights such that player k has the best score. More precisely, we want to solve:

Minimize z

subject to

$$\sum_j w_j c_{kj} = 1$$

For each player i, including k :

$$\sum_j w_j c_{ij} \geq z$$

17.4.7 Example

The GBS Construction Materials Company provides steel structural materials to industrial contractors. GBS recently did a survey of price, delivery performance, and quality in order to get an assessment of how it compares with its four major competitors. The results of the survey, with the names of all companies disguised, appears in the following table.

Company	Quality (based on freedom from scale, straightness, etc., based on mean rank, where 1.0 is best)	Delivery Time (days)	Price (in $/cwt)
A	1.8	14	$21
B	4.1	1	$26
C	3.2	3	$25
D	1.2	5	$23
E	2.4	7	$22

Vendors A, B, and D are clearly competitive, based on Price, Delivery Time, and Quality, respectively. For example, a customer for whom quality is paramount will choose D. A customer for whom delivery time is important will choose B. Are C and E competitive? Imagine a customer who uses a linear weighting system to identify the best bid, e.g., score = WQ × Quality + WT × (Delivery time) + WP × Price. Is there a set of weights (all nonnegative) so that Score (C) < Score (i), for $i = A, B, D, E$? Likewise for E?

The model for Company C is:

```
MAX     Z
SUBJECT TO
        A)      - Z + 1.8 WQ + 14 WT + 21 WP <= 0
        B)      - Z + 4.1 WQ + WT + 26 WP    <= 0
        C)      - Z + 3.2 WQ + 3 WT + 25 WP  <= 0
        D)      - Z + 1.2 WQ + 5 WT + 23 WP  <= 0
        E)      - Z + 2.4 WQ + 7 WT + 22 WP  <= 0
   CTARG)       3.2 WQ + 3 WT + 25 WP =      1
    QUAL)       WQ >=       0.0005
    TIME)       WT >=       0.0005
   PRICE)       WP >=       0.0005
END
```

The solution is:

```
          OBJECTIVE FUNCTION VALUE
       1)        0.9814257

  VARIABLE              VALUE           REDUCED COST
        Z            0.981426              0.000000
       WQ            0.000500              0.000000
       WT            0.027811              0.000000
       WP            0.036599              0.000000

      ROW        SLACK OR SURPLUS       DUAL PRICES
       A)            0.177406              0.000000
       B)            0.000000             -0.513761
       C)            0.018574              0.000000
       D)            0.000000             -0.486239
       E)            0.019624              0.000000
   CTARG)            0.000000              0.981651
    QUAL)            0.000000             -0.451376
    TIME)            0.027311              0.000000
   PRICE)            0.036099              0.000000
```

Company C has an efficiency rating of 0.981; thus it is not on the efficient frontier. With a similar model you can show that Company E is on the efficient frontier.

17.4.8 Efficient Points, the Mixed Case

In many situations there may be some dimensions, such as risk, where less is better, whereas there are other dimensions, such as chocolate, where more is better.

In this case, unless we make additional restrictions on the weights, we cannot get a simple score of efficiency between 0 and 1 for a company. We can nevertheless extend the previous approach to determine if a point is on the efficient frontier.

Define:

c_{ij} = level of the jth "less is better" attribute for player i,
r_{ij} = level of the jth "more is better" attribute for player i,
w_j = weight to be applied to the jth "less is better" attribute,
v_j = weight to be applied to the jth "more is better" attribute.

In words, to evaluate the efficiency of player or point k, we want to:

Max score(k)−(best score of any other player)
subject to
sum of the weights = 1

If the objective value is nonnegative, player k is efficient, whereas if the objective is negative, there is no set of weights such that player k scores at least as well as every other player.

If we denote the best score of any other player by z, more specifically, we want to solve:

$$\text{Maximize} \quad \sum_j v_j r_{ij} - \sum_j w_j c_{kj} - z$$

subject to

For each player $i \neq k$

$$z \geq \sum_j v_j r_{ij} - \sum_j w_j c_{kj}$$

and

$$\sum_j v_j + \sum_j w_j = 1$$

$v_j \geq e$, $w_j \geq e$, z unconstrained in sign, where e is a small positive number.

The dual of this problem is to find a set of weights, λ_i, to apply to each of the other players to:

Minimize g

subject to

$$\sum_i \lambda_i = 1$$

For each "more is better" attribute j:

$$g + \sum_{i \neq k} \lambda_i r_{ij} \geq r_{kj}$$

For each "less is better" attribute j:

$$g - \sum_{i \neq k} \lambda_j c_{ij} \geq - c_{kj}$$

g unconstrained in sign.

If g is nonnegative, it means no weighted combination of other points (or players) could be found so that their weighted performance surpasses that of k on every dimension.

17.5 Comparing Performance with Data Envelopment Analysis

Data Envelopment Analysis (DEA) is a method for identifying efficient points in the mixed case, that is, when there are both "less is better" and "more is better" measures. An attractive feature of DEA, relative to the previous method discussed, is that it does produce an efficiency score between 0 and 1. It does this by making slightly stronger assumptions about how efficiency is measured. Specifically, DEA assumes that each performance measure can be classified as either an input or an output. The "score" of a point or a decision-making unit is then the ratio of an output score divided by an input score.

DEA was originated by Charnes, Cooper, and Rhodes (1978) as a means of evaluating the performance of decision-making units. Examples of decision-making units might be hospitals, banks, airports, schools, and managers. For example, Bessent,

Bessent, Kennington, and Reagan (1982) used the approach to evaluate the performance of 167 schools around Houston, Texas. Simple comparisons can be misleading because different units are probably operating in different environments. For example, a school that is operating in a wealthy neighborhood will probably have higher test scores than a school in a poor neighborhood, even though the teachers in the poor school are working harder and require more skill than the teachers in the wealthy school. Also, different decision makers may have different skills. If the teachers in school (A) are well trained in science whereas those in school (B) are well trained in fine arts, a scoring system that applies a lot of weight to science may make the teachers in (B) appear to be inferior, even though they are doing an outstanding job at what they do best.

DEA circumvents both difficulties in clever fashion. If the arts teachers were choosing the performance measures, they would choose one that placed a lot of weight on arts, whereas the science teachers would probably choose a different one. DEA follows the philosophy of a popular fast-food chain, that is, "Have it your way." DEA will derive an "efficiency" score between 0 and 1 for each unit by solving the following problem:

> For each unit k:
> > Choose a scoring function
> so as to:
> > maximize score of unit k
> subject to:
> > For every unit j (including k):
> > > score$_j \leq 1$.

Thus, unit k may choose a scoring function that makes it look as good as possible subject to no other unit getting a score greater than 1 when that same scoring function is applied to the other unit. If a unit k gets a score of 1.0, it means there is no other unit strictly dominating k.

In the version of DEA we consider, the allowed scoring functions are limited to ratios of weighted outputs to weighted inputs, i.e.,

$$\text{score} = \frac{\text{weighted sum of outputs}}{\text{weighted sum of inputs}}$$

We can normalize weights so

> weighted sum of inputs = 1;

then "score ≤ 1" is equivalent to:

> weighted sum of outputs $\leq$ weighted sum of inputs.

Algebraically, the DEA model is:

> Given
> > $n =$ decision-making units,
> > $m =$ no. of inputs,
> > $s =$ no. of outputs,

Observed data:

c_{ij} = level of jth input for unit i,
r_{ij} = level of jth output for unit i,

Variables in the model:

w_j = weight applied to the jth input,
v_j = weight (or value) applied to the jth output.

For unit k, the model to compute the best score is:

$$\text{Maximize} \quad \sum_{j=1}^{s} v_j r_{kj}$$

subject to

$$\sum_{j=1}^{m} w_j c_{kj} = 1$$

For each unit i (including k):

$$\sum_{j=1}^{s} v_j r_{ij} \leq \sum_{j=1}^{m} w_j c_{ij}$$

This model will tend to have more constraints than decision variables; thus if implementation efficiency is a major concern, one may wish to solve the dual of this model rather than the primal.

17.5.1 Example

Below are four performance measures on six high schools: Bloom (BL), Homewood (HW), New Trier (NT), Oak Park (OP), York (YK), and Elgin (EL). Cost/pupil is the number of dollars spent per year per pupil by the school. Percent not-low-income is the fraction of the student body coming from homes not classified as low income. The writing and science scores are the averages over students in a school on a standard writing test and a standard science test. The first two measures are treated as inputs, over which teachers and administrators have no control. The test scores are treated as outputs.

School	Cost/Pupil	Percent Not Low Income	Writing Score	Science Score
BL	8939	64.3	25.2	223
HW	8625	99	28.2	287
NT	10813	99.6	29.4	317
OP	10638	96	26.4	291
YK	6240	96.2	27.2	295
EL	4719	79.9	25.5	222

Which schools would you consider "efficient"? New Trier has the highest score in both writing (29.4) and science (317); however, it also spends the most per pupil,

$10,813, and has the highest fraction not-low-income. A DEA model for maximizing the score of New Trier is:

```
MAX SCORENT
 SUBJECT TO
! Define the numerator for New Trier;
 DEFNUMNT)  SCORENT - 317 WNTSCIN - 29.4 WNTWRIT =      0
! Fix the denominator for New Trier;
 FIXDNMNT)  99.6 WNTRICH + 108.13 WNTCOST =      1
! Numerator/ Denominator < 1 for every school,
!  or equivalently, Numerator < Denominator;
BLNT) 223 WNTSCIN + 25.2 WNTWRIT - 64.3 WNTRICH
      - 89.39 WNTCOST  <= 0
HWNT) 287 WNTSCIN + 28.2 WNTWRIT - 99 WNTRICH
      - 86.25 WNTCOST  <= 0
NTNT) 317 WNTSCIN + 29.4 WNTWRIT - 99.6 WNTRICH
      - 108.13 WNTCOST <= 0
OPNT) 291 WNTSCIN + 26.4 WNTWRIT - 96 WNTRICH
      - 106.38 WNTCOST <= 0
YKNT) 295 WNTSCIN + 27.2 WNTWRIT - 96.2 WNTRICH
      - 62.40 WNTCOST  <= 0
ELNT) 222 WNTSCIN + 25.5 WNTWRIT - 79.9 WNTRICH
      - 47.19 WNTCOST  <= 0
! Each measure must receive a little weight;
 SCINT)   WNTSCIN >=   0.0005
 WRINT)   WNTWRIT >=   0.0005
 RICNT)   WNTRICH >=   0.0005
 COSNT)   WNTCOST >=   0.0005
END
```

The solution is:

```
             OBJECTIVE FUNCTION VALUE

      1)       0.9615804

    VARIABLE          VALUE          REDUCED COST
    SCORENT        0.961580             0.000000
    WNTSCIN        0.002987             0.000000
    WNTWRIT        0.000500             0.000000
    WNTRICH        0.008204             0.000000
    WNTCOST        0.001691             0.000000

        ROW    SLACK OR SURPLUS        DUAL PRICES
   DEFNUMNT)        0.000000             1.000000
   FIXDNMNT)        0.000000             0.963535
      BLNT)         0.000000             0.879526
      HWNT)         0.086703             0.000000
      NTNT)         0.038420             0.000000
      OPNT)         0.085087             0.000000
      YKNT)         0.000000             0.409714
      ELNT)         0.059451             0.000000
     SCINT)         0.002487             0.000000
     WRINT)         0.000000            -3.908283
     RICNT)         0.007704             0.000000
     COSNT)         0.001191             0.000000

  NO.  ITERATIONS=          5
```

The score of New Trier is less than 1.0; thus, according to DEA, New Trier is not efficient. Looking at the solution report, one can deduce that NT is, according to DEA, strictly less efficient than BL and YK . Notice that their "score less than or equal to 1" constraints are binding.

17.6 PROBLEMS

Problem 1

In the example staffing problem of this chapter, the primary criterion was minimizing the number of people hired. The secondary criterion was to spread out any excess capacity as much as possible. The primary criterion received a weight of 9 whereas the secondary criterion received a weight of 1. The minimum number of people required (primary criterion) was 8. How much could the weight on the secondary criterion be increased before the number of people hired increases to more than 8?

Problem 2

Reconsider the advertising media selection problem of this chapter.

(a) Reformulate it so that we achieve at least 197 (in 1000s) useful exposures at minimum cost.
(b) Predict the cost before looking at the solution.

Problem 3

A description of a "project crashing" decision appears in Chapter 7. There were two criteria, project length and project cost. Trace out the efficient frontier describing the trade-off between length and cost.

Problem 4

The various capacities, as reported by a popular consumer rating magazine, of several popular sport utility vehicles, are listed below:

Vehicle	Seats	Cargo Floor Length (in.)	Rear Opening Height (in.)	Cargo Volume (cubic ft)
Blazer	6	75.5	31.5	42.5
Cherokee	5	62.0	33 5	34.5
Land Rover	7	49.5	42 0	42.0
Land Cruiser	8	65.5	38.5	44.5
Explorer	6	78.5	35.0	48.0
Trooper	5	57.0	36.5	42.5

Assuming sport utility vehicle buyers sport a linear utility, which of the above vehicles are on the efficient frontier according to these 4 capacity measures?

Parametric Analysis

18.1 Motivation for Parametric Analysis

The advantage and perhaps the major motivation for using "seat-of-the-pants" decision making is that it obscures the assumptions made in arriving at a decision. If no one knows the assumptions upon which you based your decision, even though they may be uneasy with the decision, they will have a difficult time criticizing your assumptions or decisions.

When a formal model is used in decision making, the assumptions are more apparent to everyone. Therefore, "what if" questions are more likely to be asked. What happens if the assumptions are changed? In an LP model, the most obvious assumptions are the values of each of the coefficients in the model. These coefficients may represent such things as demand for a product, machine capacity, raw material cost, and labor rates. There may be considerable disagreement regarding the exact value of some of these coefficients. The standard LP solution report gives some indication of how the solution is affected by *small* changes in each of the objective function and right-hand-side coefficients.

Parametric analysis or parametric programming is the term applied to tracing out how the solution changes as a specific coefficient (the parameter) changes over a *wide* range. Many LP computer programs have special commands for performing this analysis.

18.2 Types of Parametric Analysis

Parametric procedures found in computer packages typically allow two kinds of parametric changes: (1) cost or objective coefficients parametrics and (2) right-hand-side parametrics. With objective function parametrics one could, for example, trace out how total profit varies as the selling price of a product is varied over a wide range. With right-hand-side parametrics one could similarly trace out profit as the projected sales (a right-hand-side number) of a product is varied over a wide range.

There are three different perspectives from which one might wish to view the effect of a parametric change:

1. How does total profit or cost change as the parameter changes?
2. How does the optimal value and the reduced cost of a specific decision variable change as the parameter changes?
3. How do the dual price and slack of a specific constraint change as the parameter changes?

The following model will be used to illustrate parametric analysis:

```
MAX    20A + 30C
S.T.
   2)   A              <=   60
   3)            C <=   50
   4)   A +  2 C <= 120
   5)  2A +  5 C <= 280
   6)   A -    C <= -40
```

We will examine two changes:

(a) Varying the right-hand side of row (2) from 60 to 0.
(b) Varying the objective function coefficient A from 20 down to whatever level is required to drive A from the solution.

The results of a parametric analysis are usually presented in graphic form. Therefore, let us immediately display the results in this form and then talk about how these results were obtained. Figure 18.1 shows the effect on the total profit and the dual price of row (2) of varying the right-hand side of row 2.

Notice that the total profit is a piecewise linear function of the right-hand side of row (2). The dual price of the constraint is a step function of the right-hand side. In fact, any plot of optimal objective function value and dual price of a constraint as a function of the right-hand side of the constraint will have the following features:

1. The objective function value curve will be piecewise linear and continuous, i.e., without steps or breaks. It will be a straight line between the finite number of points where it bends.
2. The dual price will be a decreasing step function.
3. The objective function value will be concave for Max problems (convex for Min problems); that is, for a Max problem the steepness of the curve diminishes as the right-hand side increases. The slope may in fact go negative. Practically speaking, this is exactly the same as saying that the less you have of something the more valuable is each unit.
4. For a given value of the right-hand side, the slope of the objective function curve equals the level of the dual price curve. As the right-hand side increases from 40 to 60, the objective function curve has slope $(2100 - 2000)/20 = 50$. The dual price over this interval is also 50. Feature (4) with feature (2) implies feature (3).

Each point where the slope changes corresponds to what is called a basis change in the solution. Specifically, as the parameter is increased (or decreased), all vari-

Figure 18.1
Parametric
Analysis of the
Right-Hand Side
of a Constraint

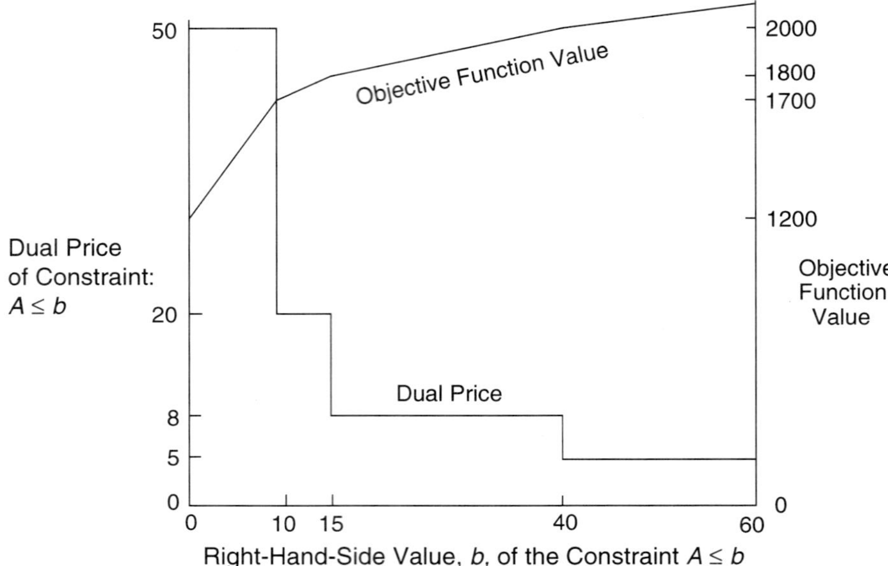

ables that are nonzero change in value smoothly (i.e., linearly) until one of the variables hits zero. At this point a variable that had been zero now starts to increase. When this so-called basis change occurs there is a bend in the objective function curve or a step in the dual price curve.

The Simplex method for solving LPs requires only a minor modification to allow it to trace out the sequence of break points or basis change points in these curves. Even though the method is ostensibly solving as many different LPs as there are break points, the amount of work involved to move from one point to the next is roughly equivalent to doing only one iteration of the Simplex method.

The kind of report produced by a typical computer program for doing parametric analysis on the example problem described earlier might look as follows.

Parametric Analysis on the RHS of Constraint 2

Entering Variable	Departing Variable	RHS Value	New Value of Dual Price	Objective Value
—	—	60	5	2100
Slack(4)	Slack(5)	40	8	2000
Slack(5)	Slack(3)	15	20	1800
Slack(3)	Slack(6)	10	50	1700
Slack(6)	A	0	∞	1200

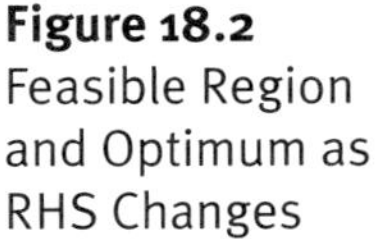

Figure 18.2
Feasible Region
and Optimum as
RHS Changes

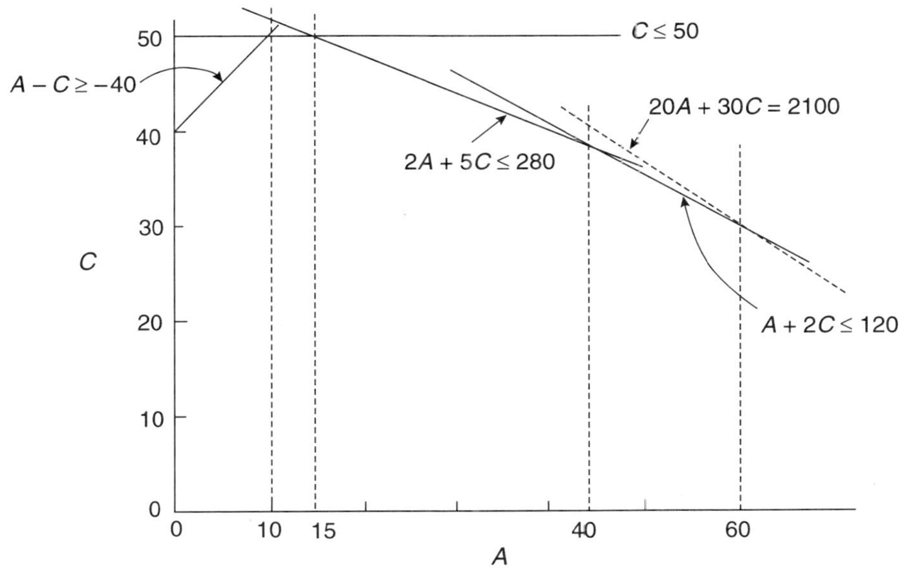

The graph in Figure 18.1 was produced from this table. Right to left in Figure 18.1 corresponds to top to bottom in this table.

18.3 Graphical Derivation of Parametric Profit Curve (RHS)

On a problem with only two variables, a graph of the constraint set can clearly show how the specific shape of the parametric profit curve comes about. Figure 18.2 graphs the constraint set for our example problem. Positions of the constraint $A \leq b$ for the parameter b equal to certain key values are indicated by the vertical dashed lines. The slope of the objective function is indicated by the slanted dashed line. The rightmost vertical line corresponds to the constraint $A \leq 60$. The optimal solution in this case is at the intersection of the two dashed lines. As the constraint $A \leq 60$ is tightened (i.e., as b is decreased from 60), the vertical dashed line moves to the left and the optimal point moves with it to the left along the top of the feasible region. The specific vertical dashed lines in Figure 18.2 correspond to points at which the breaks occur in the curves in Figure 18.1. The breaks occur at the points where the set of binding constraints changes.

One can also observe from Figure 18.2 which variables enter and leave the solution as the constraint $A \leq b$ is tightened. When $b = 60$, the slack in row (5), $2A + 5C \leq 280$, is in the solution at value 10. As b decreases to the breakpoint $b = 40$, the slack in row (4), $A + 2C \leq 120$, begins to increase from zero.

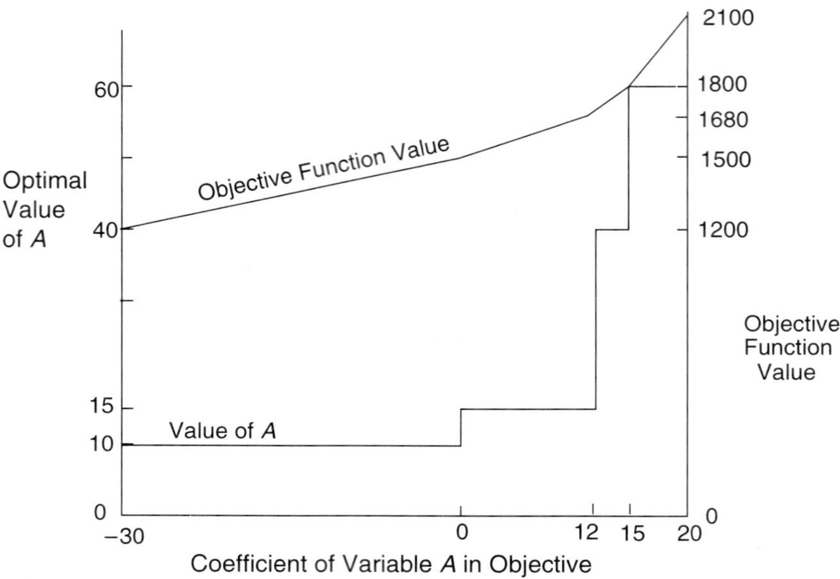

Figure 18.3
Parametric Analysis of an Objective Function Coefficient

At each breakpoint, the solution is degenerate. That is, the number of strictly positive variables (both original and slack) is less than the number of constraints. For example, at $b = 40$ we have $A = 40$, $C = 40$, slack (4) = 0, slack (5) = 0, slack (2) = 0, slack (3) = 10, and slack (6) = 40. There are only 4 nonzero variables even though there are 5 constraints.

Figure 18.3 shows how the optimal objective function value and the value of the variable A change as the profit contribution of A is reduced.

Again, the total profit is a piecewise linear function of the profit contribution of A. In fact, the plot of the optimal objective value and the value of a decision variable as a function of the profit contribution of that decision variable for any LP will have the following features:

1. The objective value will be piecewise linear.
2. The decision variable's value will be an increasing step function as the profit contribution of the variable is increased.
3. The objective value curve will be convex for Max problems (concave for Min). Practically speaking, this is the same as saying that if the profit contribution per unit of a product is very small (e.g., negative), increasing the per unit contribution by a fixed amount will have small effect on total profit. This is because at the optimum we produce very little of the product. If, however, the contribution per unit is large, we tend to produce a lot of the product; therefore, improving the per unit contribution of the product by a fixed amount will tend to produce a large improvement in total profit. Stated another way, reducing the production cost of a Chevrolet by \$1 will have a much more dramatic effect on total profits of GM than reducing the production cost of a Cadillac Seville by \$1 because so many Chevrolets are produced.

4. For a given value of the coefficient in the objective, the slope of the objective function curve equals the level of the decision variable curve (see Figure 18.3). As the profit contribution of A increases from 15 to 20, the objective curve has slope $(2100 - 1800)/5 = 60$. The value of A over this interval is 60. Feature (4) with feature (2) implies feature (3).

As with changes in a right-hand-side coefficient, the set of nonzero variables remains the same between breakpoints. As the parameter is changed past a breakpoint, some variable decreases to zero and is replaced by a variable that had been zero but increases from zero as the breakpoint is passed.

The standard solution method for linear programs, the Simplex method, requires only minor modifications to trace out the effect of changing an objective coefficient. The computational work in moving from one breakpoint to the next is roughly equivalent to one iteration of the Simplex method.

The kind of report produced by a typical program for doing the parametric analysis of an objective coefficient for the previous example might look as follows:

```
PARAMETRIC ANALYSIS ON THE OBJECTIVE COEFFICIENT OF VARIABLE A
                             OBJECTIVE      NEW VALUE
    ENTERING     DEPARTING    COEFFICIENT      OF        OBJECTIVE
    VARIABLE     VARIABLE       VALUE       VARIABLE       VALUE
       —            —            20            60           2100
    Slack(2)     Slack(5)       15            40           1800
    Slack(4)     Slack(3)       12            15           1680
    Slack(5)     Slack(6)        0            10           1500
    Slack(3)        A          -30             0           1200
```

18.4 Graphical Derivation of Parametric Profit Curve (Objective Coefficient)

Figure 18.4 shows the constraint set for our example problem. The dotted line shows the slope of the objective function $20A + 30C$. The line as drawn passes through the optimal solution $A = 60$, $C = 30$. As the coefficient of A is decreased, the relative appeal of C increases and the dotted line rotates or rolls counterclockwise around the boundary of the feasible region. When the coefficient of A is 15, the dotted line is parallel to the constraint line $A + 2C \le 120$. In this case, the point $A = 40$, $C = 40$ with profit 1800 becomes an optimal solution. Note that the point $A = 60$, $C = 30$ is also optimum. Indeed, at every breakpoint there will be alternate optima when objective coefficient parameterizing is done. Compare this with right-hand-side parameterizing, in which there is degeneracy at each breakpoint. When the coefficient of A is decreased to 12, the dotted line is parallel to the middle slanted line corresponding to the constraint $2A + 5C \le 280$. In this case, the point $A = 15$, $C = 50$ with profit 1680 becomes an optimal solution.

When the profit contribution of A is reduced to zero, the dotted line becomes horizontal and the point $A = 10$, $C = 50$ with profit 1500 becomes optimal.

Finally, when the profit contribution of A is reduced to -30, the point $A = 0$, $C = 40$ with profit 1200 becomes optimal.

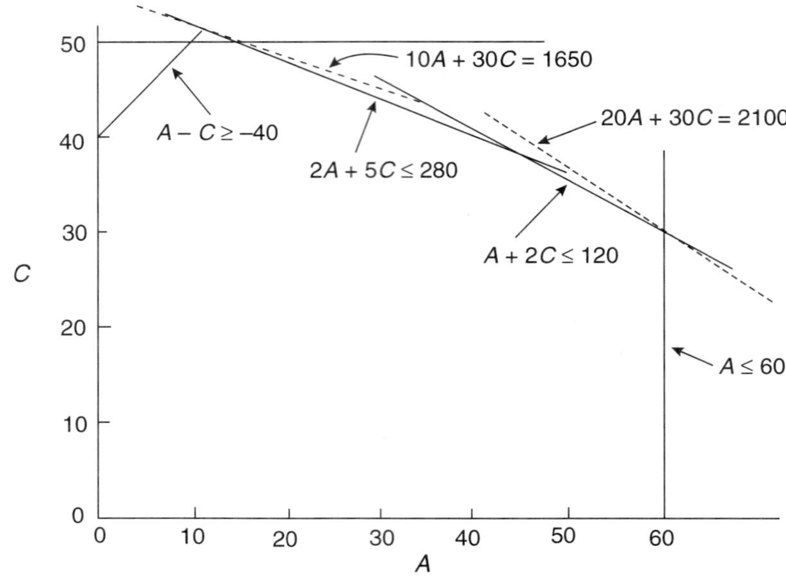

Figure 18.4
Parametric
Analysis of
Objective
Function
Coefficient

18.5 Changing Several Coefficients Simultaneously

Our discussion thus far has been in terms of changing only one coefficient at a time. One can additionally examine the effect of simultaneously varying several coefficients if the change in each parameter is linearly dependent upon a single parameter.

One application in which one might wish to consider changing several coefficients at once is in multiperiod planning. Each period might have a constraint defining plant capacity. Changing the plant capacity would entail changing the right-hand side of the plant capacity constraint in each of the periods in the model.

To illustrate simultaneous changes, suppose that in the Astro/Cosmo problem we want to examine the effect of simultaneously increasing the prices of both Astros and Cosmos. Specifically, for each dollar increase in Astro price we will increase the Cosmo price by three dollars. You can think of there being a second objective function that receives an adjustable weight f. The problem can be written

```
Max   20A + 30C + f(A + 3C)
s t
  A   <=   60
  C   <=   50
  A + 2C <= 120
```

When $f = 0$, the original problem is obtained. When $f = 1$, the profit contributions of A and C are 21 and 33, respectively. When $f = 2$, the profit contributions are 22 and 36, respectively, etc.

Some computer packages allow you to enter a second objective as above and then trace out the optimal solutions as f is varied. For this example, the row $A + 3C$ is known as a change row.

Alternatively, one can introduce a new variable, z, and the parametric problem can be written:

```
Max   20A + 30C + f z
s t
   A + 3C  - z =    0
   A    <=   60
   C    <=   50
   A + 2C   <= 120
```

This form is compatible with changing only one objective coefficient, f, at once. This illustrates the fact that the crucial feature for parametric analysis is the ability to vary a single coefficient. It is convenient, but not essential, to be able to specify a change row to be applied parametrically to the original objective.

A similar situation holds for simultaneously changing several right-hand-side coefficients. Suppose we want to examine the effect of decreasing capacities of both the Astro line capacity by two units and the Cosmo line by one unit.

We could write the problem as:

```
Max   20A + 30C
s t
   A    <=   60 - 2 f
   C    <=   50   - f
   A  + 2C   <=   120
```

Alternatively, one can introduce a new variable, Y, and the parametric problem can be written:

```
Max   20A + 30C
s t
   A   +   2Y   <=   60
   C   +   Y   <=   50
   A   +   2C   <= 120
   Y   =   f
```

where f is the parameter to be varied.

Again, the problem has been reduced to analyzing the effect of changing a single right-hand-side coefficient, f.

18.6 Supply and Demand Curves Derived via Parametric Analysis

Parametric analysis provides a way of approximating the supply and/or demand curve of a firm for a specific product. A demand (supply) curve specifies how much of a material a firm is willing to buy (sell) of the given material as a function of the material's price. A firm that is able to set the price of a product that it buys or sells will find it useful to know the supply or demand curve of its supplier or customer. Setting the price of a product it sells to the highest possible value will not necessarily maximize a firm's profit. The firm must know how much it can sell at a given price in order to maximize profits.

Suppose that firm X buys a specific product P from firm Y and that firm X uses an LP to make its allocation decisions. Firm Y can take this LP and if necessary add a constraint that puts an upper limit on how much of product P can be bought. If parametric analysis is performed on the right-hand side of this constraint, a curve such as in Figure 18.5 will be obtained. This curve is effectively firm X's demand curve for product P. There is some indication that petroleum companies have used this methodology occasionally to set the price of crude oil supplied to their refinery customers.

Similarly, if firm X sells a product S, a constraint could be added to its LP that places a lower limit on the amount produced of this product. Because this constraint is of $\geq$ type, it will have a nonpositive dual price. If parametric analysis is performed on the right-hand side of this constraint and the negative of the dual is plotted, a curve such as in Figure 18.6 is obtained. This curve is effectively firm X's supply curve for product S.

Economics texts usually draw supply and demand curves as smooth curves. This is for aesthetic and statistical reasons; e.g., conventional statistical regression produces smooth curves. The realities of technology suggest, however, that the curves have small steps as shown here. For example, there may be a threshold price for some product above which it is profitable to produce it by a different technology. Once this technology switch is made, a supplier may be willing to produce dramatically more of the product.

18.7 Parametric Programming and Tracing Out the Efficient Frontier in Multiobjective Problems

A cliché commonly heard in business decision making (and perhaps more in cocktail conversation) is, "What's the bottom line?" Implicit in this is that all considerations can be converted to a single unit of measure, dollars. The fact that this single measure of performance is frequently not an accurate measure of reality is borne out by the frequent repetition of another cliché: "You can't compare apples and oranges." In the latter case we say we have multiple criteria or multiple objectives.

Frequently, the multiple objectives are conflicting. Assembling an investment portfolio involves the conflicting objectives of minimizing risk and maximizing expected return. In a service organization, there are the conflicting objectives of minimizing costs and maximizing some measure of service. Planning in a typical firm involves the long-range objective of increasing market share, which conflicts with the short-range objective of maximizing profit. A key feature of the above examples is that the two objectives in each case were measured in different units, e.g., portfolio variance vs. dollars, dollars vs. service level, and percent share vs. dollars.

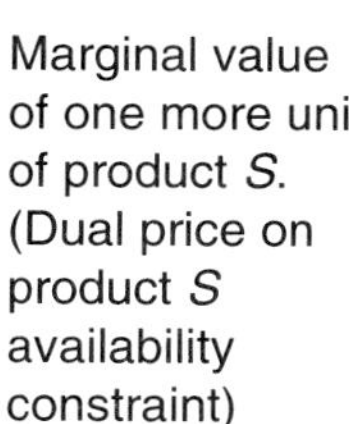

Figure 18.5
Stair-Step
Demand
Function

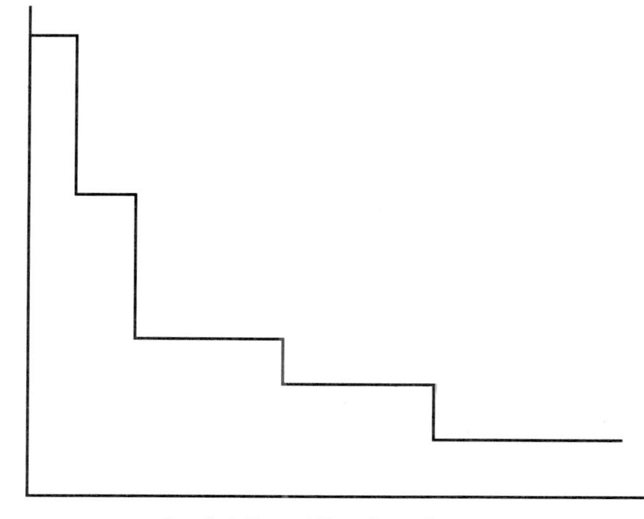

Figure 18.6
Stair-Step
Supply
Function

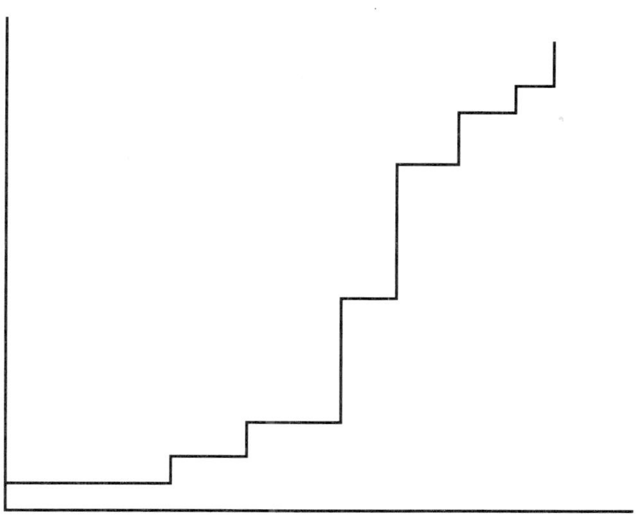

Parametric programming is frequently recommended in situations with two in-commensurate objectives. Loosely speaking, the objective is to:

Max (Objective 1) + $f \times$ (Objective 2).

Unfortunately, most people do not have an intuitive feel for an appropriate value for f. The parameter f is varied from 0 to infinity to produce a graph analogous to that in

Figure 18.7
Efficient
Frontier of
Two Objectives

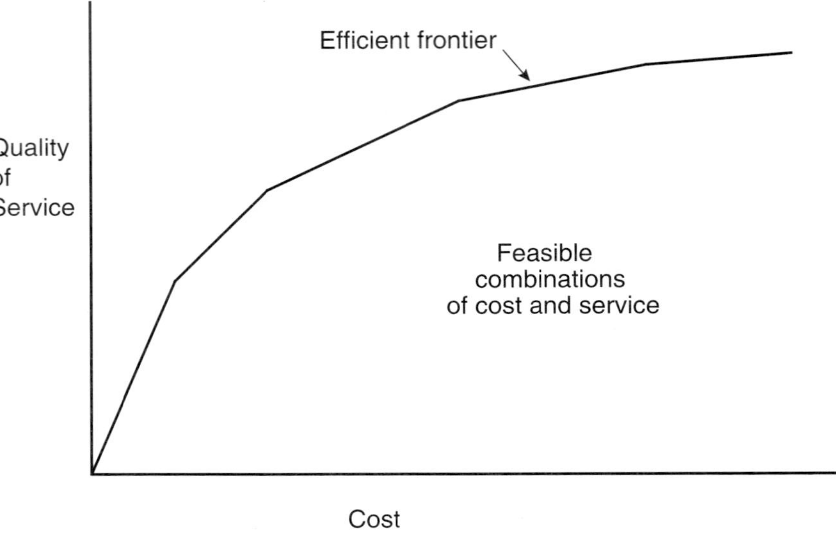

Figure 18.7. The one objective might be to minimize cost, whereas the other is to maximize the quality of service.

As the weight f applied to the service quality objective (e.g., measured as number of clients whose complaints were settled with no delay) is increased from zero to infinity, the piecewise linear curve is traced out from the origin.

Parametric programming has little to say about the exact compromise struck between service and cost, i.e., the best value of f. We can argue, however, that whatever compromise is struck, it should lie somewhere on the curve dubbed the "efficient frontier." This curve has the feature that for a given cost the curve specifies the highest achievable service level. Similarly, for a given service level, the curve gives the lowest cost that can achieve this service.

18.7.1 Parametric Analysis of Integer Programs

It is significantly more difficult to do parametric analysis of integer programs than of linear programs. Nevertheless, there are some useful things that can be said. For example, it is easier to do parametric analysis of the objective function of an IP than of the right-hand side of an IP. With regard to the former, Jenkins (1982) points out that for an IP with a maximize objective:

1. The optimal value is a convex piecewise linear function of the objective coefficient being altered.
2. One can completely determine the shape of this function by solving approximately k integer programs, where k is the number of breakpoints in the function. One need not know k beforehand.

To illustrate parametric objective analysis for an IP, consider the following IP.

```
Z(w)  = Max   (1 - w)  *  G0 + w * G1
s.t.
G0  =  21X1 + 22X2 + 16X3 + 31X4 + 15X5 + 12X6
G1  =  19X1 + 29X2 + 15X3 + 30X4 + 17X5 + 16X6
4X1 + 7X2 + 4X3 + 8X4 + 4X5 + 2X6 < 16

Xj = 0   or 1   for   j = 1, 2, 3, 4, 5, 6.
```

We want to compute $Z(w)$ as w varies from 0 to 1. When we solve this problem with $w = 0$, we get the solution: $Z(0) = 68$; $X1 = X3 = X4 = 1$ and the other Xs $= 0$. When we solve the problem with $w = 1$, we get the solution:

$Z(1) = 67$; $X1 = X3 = X5 = X6 = 1$ and the other Xs $= 0$.

If we fix the Xs in the $Z(0)$ solution, our objective value is a function of w according to the formula:

$Z = (1 - w)68 + w64$

Likewise, if we fix the Xs in the $Z(1)$ solution, our objective value is a function of w according to the formula:

$Z = (1 - w) 64 + w67.$

We can describe the current state of affairs with Figure 18.8.

The two curves intersect at the point $w = 4/7$; $Z = 65.71$. If the objective function value when $w = 4/7$ is in fact 65.71, we would be done and the maximum of just these two curves would define $Z(w)$.

To check, we solve the IP with $w = 4/7$. For efficiency, we could put in a bound on Z of 65.7 before solving. See the `BIP` command in LINDO for one way of doing this. Unfortunately, the solution has $Z = 66.4286$, corresponding to $X1 = X4 = X5 = 1$.

Figure 18.8
Parametric
Analysis of an IP
(Initial)

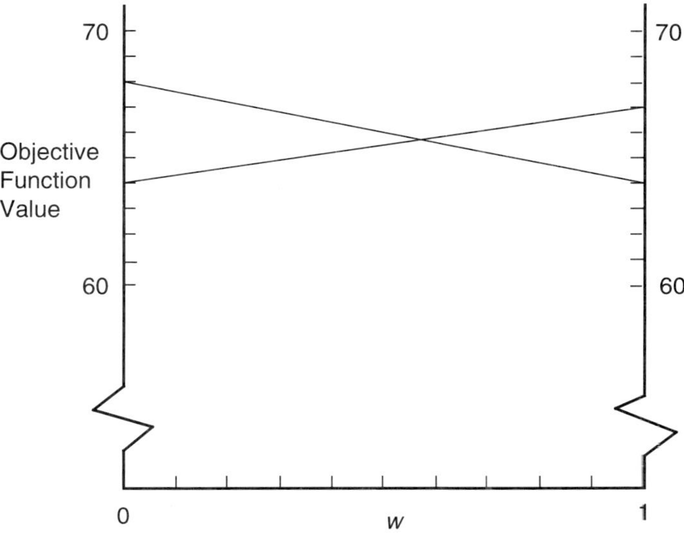

Figure 18.9
Parametric
Analysis of an IP
(Final)

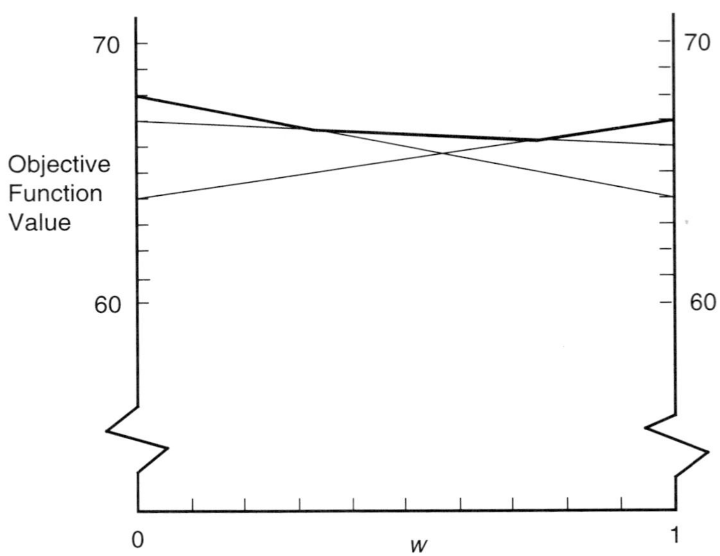

If we fix the Xs in the $w = (4/7)$ solution, our objective value is a function of w according to the formula:

$$Z = (1 - w)67 + w\,66.$$

Graphically, things now appear as in Figure 18.9. The third curve intersects with the two original curves at the points $w = 0.3333$ and $w = 0.75$. Solving the IP with $w = 0.3333$ gives the solution $Z(0.3333) = 66.67$; $X1 = X4 = X5 = 1$. Solving the IP with $w = 0.75$ gives the solution $Z(0.75) = 66.25$, $X1 = X3 = X5 = X6 = 1$ and the other $Xs = 0$. These two values match the values from the previous two curves, so we are done.

The results can be summarized as follows:

Range of w	Optimal Solution is
[0, 0.3333]	$X1 = X3 = X4 = 1$
[0.3333, 0.75]	$X1 = X4 = X5 = 1$
[0.75, 1]	$X1 = X3 = X5 = X6 = 1.$

18.8 PROBLEMS

Problem 1

For the example problem introduced at the beginning of this chapter, draw the graphs of total profit and the value of variable C as the profit contribution of C varies from 0 to 100, while the profit contribution of A remains at 20.

Problem 2

Add the constraint $C \geq b$ to the example problem introduced at the beginning of this chapter and draw the graph of total profit and the dual price of the constraint $C \geq b$ as b is increased from 0 to 50.

Problem 3

In a parametric LP analysis, it is possible for the optimal objective value to first increase and then decrease.

(a) Is this possible with a right-hand-side analysis? If yes, give an example.
(b) Is this possible with a parametric objective coefficient analysis? If yes, give an example.

Problem 4

Suppose that you have an LP procedure that can do parametrics on an arbitrary constraint coefficient but not on the right-hand-side or objective function row. Show by appending appropriate constraints or variables that this capability nevertheless allows one to indirectly do parametric analysis on either the right-hand side or the objective.

Problem 5

Suppose that variable y is zero in the optimal solution to a certain LP and has a reduced cost of 5. Now modify this LP by appending the constraint $y = 6$. What can you say about the dual price of this constraint in the optimal solution to the modified LP?

Problem 6

Consider the following variation on the Enginola Problem of chapter 1.

```
    MAX       20 A + 30 C + 47 V
    SUBJECT TO
       2)      A +            V <=   60
       3)            C              <=   50
       4)      A + 2 C + 3 V <=  119
    END
    GIN 3
```

Notice that all variables are required to be integer and the labor capacity is an odd number. We are not sure that the appropriate profit contribution for C is 30. Using the method described in this chapter, plot the optimal total profit as the profit contribution of C is varied from 0 to 50. How many integer programs did you have to solve to get the complete curve? How does the curve differ from that you would obtain if the integrality requirement were removed?

Methods for Solving Linear Programs

19.1 Introduction

The graphical method of solution outlined in Chapter 1 is an acceptable means of solution if there are only two decision variables. Its use in higher dimensions (more decision variables), however, must await further technologic advances in holography or other technology that will allow us to have three-dimensional or higher graphical systems.

The ideas of the graphical method have algebraic equivalents, however, that do in fact extend to an arbitrary number of variables. The algebraic method that has proven to be very successful is the Simplex method. It was developed by George Dantzig in approximately 1947 while he was working on Project Scoop for the Air Force. It is a tribute to the elegance and efficiency of the method that the essential steps of the Simplex as originally described by Dantzig are still incorporated in almost every LP solution procedure used today.

Recently, Khachian (1979) and Karmarkar (1985) proposed radically different algorithms for solving linear programs. The most notable feature of both algorithms is that their worst-case performance is considerably better than that of the Simplex method; that is, in contrast to the Simplex method, there are no problems that require an extremely long time to solve with new algorithms. Unfortunately, with Khachian's algorithm, it seems that essentially all problems require a long time to solve. It appears that Karmarkar's algorithm may be competitive with the Simplex method on certain very large problems with very few nonzero coefficients.

19.2 The Simplex Method

Most users of LP today get along quite nicely without knowing the steps of the Simplex method. Thus, the presentation here is mainly for the mathematically curious. You will discover, however, that the method is not difficult to comprehend. Further, understanding the Simplex method will help develop the skill of making correct formulations.

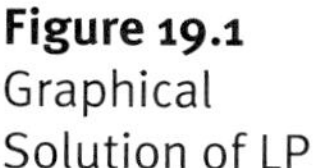

Figure 19.1
Graphical
Solution of LP

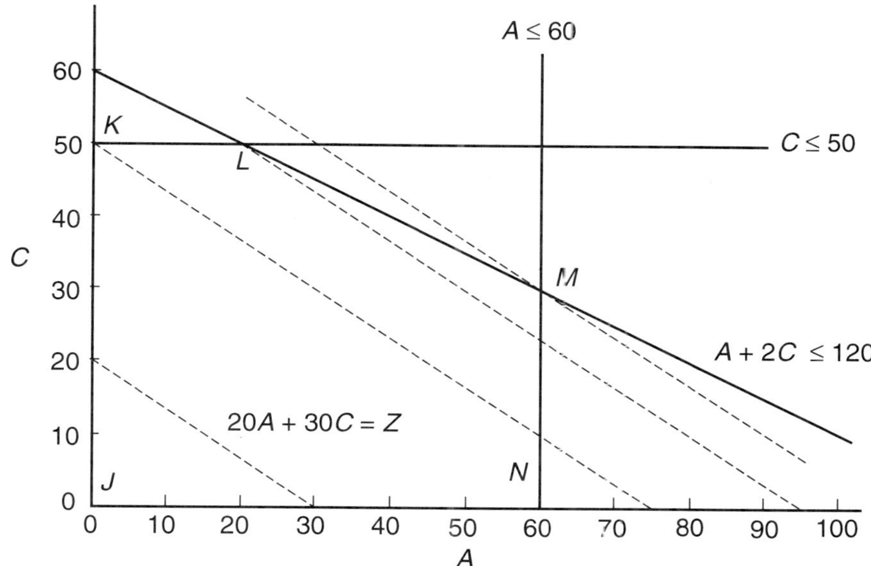

First, let us review how we would solve the Astro/Cosmo problem graphically. Recall that the problem is:

$$\text{Max:} \quad 20A + 30C$$

$$\text{Subject to:} \quad A \leq 60$$
$$C \leq 50 \qquad A \geq 0$$
$$A + 2C \leq 120 \qquad C \geq 0.$$

The problem can be described graphically as in Figure 19.1. The feasible region consists of those combinations of values for Astro production (A) and Cosmo production (C) that are in the area bounded by the lines JK, KL, LM, MN, and NJ. All points on a particular dotted line $20A + 30C = Z$ generate the same profit, Z. We want to shift the dotted line upward and to the right as much as possible. From the graph, it is obvious that the maximum shift occurs when the dotted line passes through the point M. Therefore, the point M, that corresponds to $A = 60$, $C = 30$, is the optimum.

It is apparent from the graph that you need only consider corner points as candidates for the optimum. A possible solution procedure is to enumerate every corner point, evaluate the profit at each, and select the best. This is not a good method if there are many corner points, and there will be many if there are lots of constraints and/or variables.

A myopic approach may do better. Suppose we start at the point J with $A = C = 0$, and consider the two possible paths along the feasible boundary for moving away from J. By increasing C, we move up toward point K. By increasing A, we move horizontally toward point N. If we are myopic, we note that we make \$30/unit increase in C versus only \$20/unit increase in A. We might use this as justification for moving to point K, which corresponds to $C = 50$, $A = 0$.

Once at K, the dotted line can be shifted further to the right if we move to the point L. Once at L, it is again obvious that profit can be improved by moving to M. Once at M, neither of the two paths out of M leads to an improvement and we stop.

The point N was not examined, so this method is more efficient than complete enumeration of all corner points. In retrospect, it would have been wiser at the outset to move to point N rather than K from point J. The next step would have been to point M, and the optimum would have been reached in only 2 instead of 3 steps. From the computer solution of this problem, you can take solace in the fact that the computer also took the longer, 3-step path.

The Simplex method proceeds from an initial feasible solution that need not be optimal, through a sequence of better and better feasible solutions, until finally the optimum solution is encountered. This is exactly what the graphical method does. Similarly, the Simplex method looks only at "corner point" solutions; further, it will generally consider only a very small fraction of all the corner points.

19.2.1 Equality Form, Slack, and Surplus Variables

For internal computations, the computer will convert every LP into one in which the objective is to maximize, and all constraints other than the nonnegativity constraints are equalities. This conversion is very easily executed by the following steps where necessary:

1. A "Minimize" objective is converted to a "Maximize" objective by multiplying the objective by -1. E.g.,

   Minimize $2x_1 - 2x_2$

   is equivalent to

   Maximize $-2x_1 + 2x_2$.

2. A "less than or equal to" constraint is converted to an equality constraint by adding a "slack" variable to the left-hand side. E.g., if row i is

   $$4x_1 + 5x_2 \leq 12,$$

   then it is equivalent to

   $$4x_1 + 5x_2 + s_i = 12$$
   $$s_i \geq 0.$$

   The nonnegativity constraint on the slack variable s_i prevents $4x_1 + 5x_2$ from exceeding 12.

3. A "greater than or equal to" constraint is converted to an equality constraint by subtracting a "surplus" variable from the left-hand side. E.g., if row k is

   $$6x_1 - 3x_2 \geq 9$$

   then it is equivalent to

   $$6x_1 - 3x_2 - s_k = 9$$
   $$s_k \geq 0.$$

When the Astro/Cosmo problem is converted to equality form we obtain:

$$\text{Max} \quad 20A + 30C$$

$$
\begin{aligned}
\text{subject to} \quad A \qquad\qquad + s_2 &= 60 \\
C \qquad + s_3 &= 50 \\
A + 2C \qquad + s_4 &= 120 \\
A &\geq 0 \\
C &\geq 0 \\
s_2,\, s_3,\, s_4 &\geq 0.
\end{aligned}
$$

19.2.2 Corner Points, Basic Solutions, and Number of Nonzero Variables

For a formulation in equality form, it is always true that in a corner point solution the number of nonzero variables will at most equal the number of constraints. Generally it will exactly equal the number of constraints. If it is less than the number of constraints, the solution is referred to as degenerate. For the time being, we will disregard the possibility of degenerate solutions.

An alternate and more frequently used term for a corner point solution is basic solution. Some standard terminology typically used is:

1. *Technological constraints:* constraints of the LP other than the nonnegativity constraints.
2. *Basic solution:* a solution that satisfies the technological constraints but not necessarily the nonnegativity constraints and has the number of nonzero variables less than or equal to the number of technological constraints.
3. *Degenerate solution:* a feasible solution in which the number of nonzero variables is strictly less than the number of technological constraints.
4. *Basic variable:* a variable that, in a nondegenerate basic solution, is nonzero.
5. *Basis:* the set of basic variables.
6. *Basic feasible solution:* a basic solution that also satisfies the nonnegativity constraints.

The validity of the Simplex method is based upon the following two facts, stated without proof:

1. If there is an optimal solution, there is a basic feasible optimal solution. E.g., if there are 12 technological constraints and you have an optimal solution with 14 variables nonzero, you can find another optimal solution with at most 12 variables nonzero.
2. For any nondegenerate basic feasible solution that is not optimum, there is an "adjacent" basic feasible solution (i.e., an adjacent corner point) that is strictly better.

Assuming that degeneracy does not rear its ugly head, facts (1) and (2) suggest the following procedure for finding the LP optimum:

1. Find an initial basic feasible solution.
2. Try to a find a better adjacent basic feasible solution. If none, go to (5).
3. Move to the new basic feasible solution.

4. Go to (2).
5. We have found an optimal solution because any basic feasible solution that is not optimal must have a better solution that is adjacent to it.

Now we can specify the steps of the Simplex method in slightly more detail:

1. Find an initial basic feasible solution.
2. Find a variable, call it j, which is zero in the current solution, that can be profitably increased. If none, go to (5).
3. Increase variable j while adjusting the values of the nonzero variables so as to maintain feasibility. The solution will temporarily be nonbasic, because there will be one too many nonzero variables. However, as variable j is increased, one of the nonzero variables will be driven to zero (if there is a finite optimum). At this point, we will have a new basic feasible solution.
4. Go to (2).
5. Stop. We have found an optimum solution.

19.2.3 Tableau Representation of the Equations

It is convenient to make one additional rearrangement before introducing the Simplex method. If we denote the profit by Z, we can write:

$$Z = 20A + 30C$$

Bringing all the variables to the left-hand side, the objective function appears just like any other constraint and the Astro/Cosmo problem appears as:

$$\begin{aligned} Z - 20A - 30C &= 0 \\ A \qquad\quad + s_2 &= 60 \\ C + s_3 &= 50 \\ A + 2C + s_4 &= 120 \end{aligned}$$

It is implicit that we wish to Maximize Z and keep A, C, s_2, s_3, and s_4 nonnegative.

For display purposes, these equations can be equally well described by the following tableau:

Z	A	C	s_2	s_3	s_4	RHS
1	−20	−30				
	1		1			60
		1		1		50
	1	2			1	120

That is, only the coefficients of the equations need be stored if we keep track of which row and which variable is associated with the coefficient. For computational purposes, the above format or tableau will be used.

19.2.4 Basic Variables

Because the number of basic variables will, barring degeneracy, be equal to the number of constraints, it is not surprising that each basic variable in a particular basic solution can be associated with exactly one constraint or equivalently one row of the tableau. The variable is said to be basic in that row. Intuitively, that row or constraint is used to solve for or compute the value of the variable basic in the row. To show this correspondence between basic variables and rows, we will augment the tableau with a column called "Basis"; e.g., for our example, the initial tableau with basis is:

Basis	Z	A	C	s_2	s_3	s_4	RHS
Z	1	-20	-30				
s_2		1		1			60
s_3			1		1		50
s_4		1	2			1	120

The value appearing under the "RHS" heading in a particular row will always be the value of the variable appearing under the "Basis" heading in that row. The initial basic feasible solution has $A = C = 0$, so $Z = 0$, $s_2 = 60$, $s_3 = 50$, and $s_4 = 120$. Thus, s_2, s_3, and s_4 constitute the basis.

19.2.5 Interpretation of Coefficients in the Tableau

The numbers in the columns of the tableau have the following interpretation:

(a) If the column is "RHS," the number in a specific row of the column is the value of the variable that is basic in that row.

(b) If the column corresponds to a nonbasic variable (say, j), the number in a specific row (say, row i), is the rate at which the variable that is basic in row i will decrease as variable j is increased. For our example problem at the initial solution, increasing C by 1 unit means that Z will decrease by -30 units; i.e., it will increase by 30 dollars. Similarly, the slack in the labor supply, s_4, will decrease by 2 hours if C is increased by 1 unit.

(c) If the column corresponds to a basic variable, the column will be all zero except for a 1 in the row in which the variable is basic.

At each step, the Simplex method will adjust the tableau so that the above three features are maintained.

We can now see how step (2) of the Simplex method is performed. Variable Z will always be basic in the first row. Thus, any variable that can be profitably increased will have a negative coefficient in the first row of the tableau. The tableau corresponds to an optimal solution if all the coefficients in the first row are nonnegative. If there are negative coefficients in the first row, the variable associated with the most negative is usually chosen to enter the basis.

Suppose we decide to increase C in our example. How much can we increase C before a basic variable is driven to 0? Considering column C of the initial tableau, we see that as C is increased:

s_2 remains at 60,
s_3 decreases 1 unit per unit increase of C,
s_4 decreases 2 units per unit increase of C.

Thus, $s_3 = 0$ when $s_3 = 50 - C = 0$ or when $C = 50$, and $s_4 = 0$ when $s_4 = 120 - 2C = 0$ or when $C = 120/2 = 60$. Therefore, s_3 reaches 0 first as C is increased.

At the new basic feasible solution, we will have $C = 50$, s_3 forced to 0, Z increased from 0 to $30 \times 50 = 1,500$, and s_4 decreased from 120 to $120 - 2 \times 50 = 20$.

19.2.6 Updating the Tableau/Pivoting

We have seen essentially half of the Simplex method by way of example. It remains to be demonstrated how the tableau is updated. This can be done if we recall that the tableau is simply a shorthand way of representing a set of equations. Further, when we say that variable x_j is basic in row i, it will mean that:

(a) equation i has been used to solve for x_j, and
(b) x_j has been substituted out of the other equations.

Updating the tableau corresponds to performing operations (a) and (b) for the entering variable. The row or equation that is used is the one in which the variable departing the basis has been basic. In the terminology of linear algebra or simultaneous linear equations, this operation is called pivoting.

In the first iteration, for example, variable C enters and the variable s_3 departs the basis. Substep (a) is easy to perform. The relevant row in equation form is:

$$C + s_3 = 50.$$

It is obvious that if $s_3 = 0$, $C = 50$. Step (b) requires us to use this equation to eliminate C from all the other equations (rows). The objective function row is:

$$Z - 20A - 30C = 0.$$

Multiplying the previous row by 30 and adding it to this row gives the new objective function row:

$$
\begin{aligned}
Z - 20 - 30C \quad &= \quad 0 \\
30C + 30s_3 &= 1,500 \\
\hline
Z - 20 \qquad + 30s_3 &= 1,500
\end{aligned}
$$

This makes sense; i.e., $C = 50$, $A = 0$ implies $Z = 30 \times 50 = 1,500$. The only other row containing C is the last row:

$$A + 2C + s_4 = 120.$$

The appropriate multiple in this case is -2, giving:

$$\begin{array}{rrrrr} A & +\,2C & & +\,s_4 & = & 120 \\ & -\,2C & -\,2s_3 & & = & -100 \\ \hline A & & -\,2s_3 & +\,s_4 & = & 20 \end{array}$$

The basic variable for this row is s_4, and it makes sense that the slack in the labor capacity is 20 if $C = 50$ and $A = 0$.

The entire tableau corresponding to this new basic feasible solution is:

Basis	Z	A	C	s_2	s_3	s_4	RHS
Z	1	−20			30		1500
s_2		1		1			60
C			1		1		50
s_4		1			−2	1	20

The TABLEAU and PIVOT commands of LINDO can be used alternately to show the successive steps and tableaux leading to the optimum.

From the second tableau, it is obvious that A should enter the solution. As A increases, Z will increase by \$20/unit, whereas both s_2 and s_4 will decrease at the same rate as A increases. Variable s_4 will decrease to 0 after A has increased by 20 units. Therefore, s_4 is the departing variable. The new tableau is:

Basis	Z	A	C	s_2	s_3	s_4	RHS
Z					−10	20	1900
s_2				1	2	−1	40
C			1		1		50
A		1			−2	1	20

In the third tableau, variable s_3 should enter; i.e., one should allow slack in the constraint $C \leq 70$. Each unit of increase in s_3 will increase profits by \$10. The tableau contains sufficient information to explain why this happens. A 1-unit increase causes C to decrease by 1 unit. This costs us \$30. However, A increases by 2 units, making us $2 \times \$20 = \$40$ for a net of \$10. Now we must determine which of s_2 or C reaches 0 first as s_3 increases. If s_2 is forced to zero, this corresponds to $2s_3 = 50$ or $s_3 = 50/2 = 25$. If C is forced to zero, this corresponds to $s_3 = 50$. Therefore, s_2 reaches 0 first as s_3 increases, so s_2 is the departing variable. The new tableau is:

Basis	Z	A	C	s_2	s_3	s_4	RHS
Z				5		15	2100
s_3				5	1	−5	20
C			1	−5		5	30
A		1		1			60

There are no variables with negative coefficients in the objective function row, so there is no variable that can be profitably entered, so this must be an optimal solution.

19.2.7 Other Difficulties

There are several minor difficulties with the Simplex method that our judiciously chosen example did not illustrate. A well-written LP code will handle these difficulties in matter-of-fact fashion. These difficulties are:

1. *An initial, basic feasible solution need not be obvious.* Thus, we must provide some way of getting a basic feasible solution if, in fact, one exists.
2. *Unboundedness.* The problem below has an unbounded solution:

   Max $3x$
   subject to
   $$4x \geq 12$$

   There is nothing to prevent us from making x arbitrarily large and making an infinite profit. An LP code should clearly identify such desirable but unrealistic situations.
3. *Degeneracy.* If the number of nonzero variables in a basic feasible solution is less than the number of constraints, the solution is said to be degenerate. In such a situation, the Simplex method need not find a strictly better solution at the next iteration. In fact, degeneracy is the major problem in solving large LPs. The Simplex method may iterate merrily away without improving the objective function value.

19.3 The Revised Simplex Method and Coefficient Sparsity

An LP with 2000 rows and 5000 columns can be represented by a matrix with 2000 $\times$ 5000 = 10,000,000 coefficients. This is a lot of storage space. In a typical real LP, less than 2% of these coefficients will be nonzero. There is, therefore, a temptation to exploit this coefficient sparsity. Ideally, you would like to get by with storing only 0.02 $\times$ 10,000,000 = 200,000 coefficients, rather than 10,000,000. This exploitation can be very valuable in large problems where the coefficient density is less than 1%.

The revised simplex method has been developed to exploit this sparsity. It follows the same path to the optimum; however, it stores the results of the computations in a way that exploits this sparsity. All commercial LP codes use the revised simplex method. Consider an LP with 500 rows and 1000 columns. The standard simplex method would require a matrix with 500 $\times$ 1000 = 500,000 elements to do the computations. On a typical computer, this would require at least 2,000,000 bytes of storage. This much storage may be expensive. Further, updating 500,000 elements at each pivot may be time consuming.

Fortunately, the real world is easier than the simple theory of the standard simplex method suggests. A typical real world LP has about four nonzero elements per column. Thus, a 500 $\times$ 1000 problem might have only 5000 nonzero elements out of the 500,000 possible. The revised simplex method with product form inverse exploits this sparsity so that the number of storage elements required is approximately twice the number of nonzeroes. The factor of 2 arises because we must store not only the nonzeroes but also the index of the row in which each occurs.

All commercial LP packages use the revised simplex method with product form inverse. Some of these packages use a variation of the product form inverse, which is called the elimination form of inverse. The essential idea is still the same.

We will first summarize the features of the revised simplex method with explicit inverse. The explicit inverse is conceptually simpler than the product form, but it does not exploit sparsity nearly as well as the product form.

Let E be the matrix or updated tableau as it would appear under the standard simplex method at any given iteration. The key observation that makes the revised simplex method attractive is that only a small fraction of the elements of E are needed to select the pivot at each iteration. Specifically:

(a) We need the first or objective function row of E in order to choose the entering variable.

(b) We need the column of E corresponding to the entering variable so we can choose the pivot row. Similarly, we need the updated right-hand side.

Thus, to choose the pivot element at an iteration we need examine at most 1000 + 500 = 1500 elements out of the 500,000 elements in E. This is an attractive reduction. The question of how to represent the effect of each pivot so that we need calculate only 1500 rather than 500,000 numbers at each pivot remains to be answered.

In general, suppose an LP has m rows and n columns. The revised simplex method with explicit inverse stores the original m by n LP matrix in sparse form and does not modify it from one pivot to the next. Rather, a smaller m by m matrix called B^{-1} is adjusted at each pivot.

If the original m by n LP matrix is denoted by T, the updated matrix or tableau can be obtained by doing a matrix multiply of B^{-1} and T, i.e., $E = B^{-1}T$. In particular, if we want the first row of E, we multiply the first row of B^{-1} times T. Because T is stored in sparse form and each column contains about four nonzeroes, the total of multiplications is about $4 \times n$, or 4000 for our 500×1000 example. Further, we do not have to "price out" every one of the 1000 columns at each iteration. In fact, it may be sufficient to examine just 200, say, in order to find a column with an attractive reduced cost in the first row. Thus, the work might involve some 800 multiplications to find the entering variable in our 500×1000 example.

Once the entering variable has been selected, the updated column in E corresponding to this variable can be generated by premultiplying the corresponding column in T by B^{-1}. The number of multiplications involved is approximately $4 \times m$ or 2000 for our example.

How is B^{-1} stored and how is it updated at each pivot? Here is where the explicit form inverse and product form differ. The explicit form simply stores a full m by m matrix. Updating at each iteration is simple. Pivots are done exactly as in the standard simplex method, except that the pivot operations are done on B^{-1} rather than on E. That is, the pivot row in B^{-1} is divided by the pivot element. Appropriate multiples of the pivot row are subtracted from the other rows in B^{-1}. Thus updating B^{-1} at a pivot requires about $m \times m$ multiplications and divisions. Mathematically, B^{-1} is the inverse of the matrix of (possibly permuted) columns of T corresponding to the basic variables.

Now let us compare the work required by the revised simplex method with explicit inverse and the standard simplex method for our example problem.

Operation	Standard	Revised with Explicit B^{-1}
(1) Select entering column	0 multiplications	800 multiplications
(2) Select pivot row	0 multiplications	2,000 multiplications
(3) Pivot	500,000 multiplications	250,000 multiplications
Total, One Iteration	500,000 multiplications	252,800 multiplications

We have reduced the work by about one-half, but it is still a lot of work, and the reduction is much less impressive if the number of columns approximately equals the number of rows.

19.3.1 Example of Revised Simplex Method with Explicit Inverse

We will illustrate the calculations under the revised simplex method with explicit inverse using the example that was used to illustrate the standard simplex method. The original tableau, T, is:

Row	Basis	Z	A	C	S_2	S_3	S_4	RHS
1	Z	1	−20	−30				
2	S_2		1		1			60
3	S_3			1		1		50
4	S_4		1	2			1	120

The initial B^{-1} is the identity matrix:

$$
\begin{matrix}
1 & 0 & 0 & 0 \\
0 & 1 & 0 & 0 \\
0 & 0 & 1 & 0 \\
0 & 0 & 0 & 1
\end{matrix}
$$

Multiplying the first row of B^{-1} times T gives the original objective function row:

A	C	S_2	S_3	S_4
−20	−30	0	0	0

We select C to enter. Multiplying C's column and the original RHS by B^{-1} gives the relevant part of E:

Row	Basis	C	RHS
(1)	Z	−30	0
(2)	S_2	0	60
(3)	S_3	1	50
(4)	S_4	2	120

The minimum ratio of 50/1 and 120/2 is 50, so the pivot row is (3). Adding 30 times row (3) to row (1) and subtracting 2 times row (3) from row (4) gives the new B^{-1}:

1	0	30	0
0	1	0	0
0	0	1	0
0	0	−2	1

Multiplying the first row of B^{-1} times T gives the updated objective function row:

A	C	S_2	S_3	S_4
−20	0	0	300	0

So A should enter. Multiplying A's original column and the original RHS by B^{-1} gives the relevant part of E:

Row	Basis	C	RHS
(1)	Z	−20	1500
(2)	S_2	1	60
(3)	S_3	0	50
(4)	S_4	1	20

The minimum of 60/1 and 20/1 is 20, so the pivot row should be (4). Adding 20 times row (4) to row (1) and subtracting row (4) from row (2) gives the new B^{-1}:

1	0	−10	20
0	1	2	−1
0	0	1	0
0	0	−2	1

Multiplying the first row of B^{-1} times T gives the updated objective function row of E:

A	C	S_2	S_3	S_4
0	0	0	−10	20

So S_3 should enter. Multiplying S_3's original column and the original RHS by B^{-1} gives:

Row	Basis	C	RHS
(1)	Z	−10	1900
(2)	S_2	2	40
(3)	C	0	50
(4)	A	−2	20

The minimum ratio of 40/2 and 50/1 is 20, so the pivot row is (2). Adding 5 times row (2) to row (1), subtracting 1/2 times row (2) from row (3), adding row (2) to row (4), and finally dividing row (2) by 2 gives the new B^{-1}:

$$
\begin{array}{cccc}
1 & 5 & 0 & 15 \\
0 & 1/2 & 1 & -1/2 \\
0 & -1/2 & 0 & 1/2 \\
0 & 1 & 0 & 0
\end{array}
$$

Multiplying the first row of B^{-1} gives the updated objective row of E:

A	C	S_2	S_3	S_4
0	0	5	0	15

All variables price out positive so we have an optimal solution. Multiplying B^{-1} times the original RHS gives:

Row	Basis	RHS
(1)	Z	2100
(2)	S_3	20
(3)	C	30
(4)	A	60

Thus, the optimal solution has $z = 2100$, $s_3 = 20$, $C = 30$, and $A = 60$. The dual prices are found in the first row of B^{-1}. Specifically, the dual prices of rows (2), (3), and (4) are 5, 0, and 15, respectively.

19.4 Revised Simplex Method with Product Form of Inverse

The revised simplex method with product form inverse uses a substantially different method for storing and updating B^{-1}. For most practical LPs, the density of B^{-1} under the explicit inverse method is approximately 50%; that is, about half the elements of B^{-1} are nonzero. Thus, the sparsity of the original data does not carry over to the explicit inverse. The product form inverse is able to retain much of the sparsity of the original data. This is true in particular for transportation or network LP problems.

The basic idea of the product form inverse is very simple. Namely, instead of performing the pivot at each iteration, simply append the column that should have been pivoted to a list of the (updated) columns that should have been pivoted. This contains all the information about a sequence of pivots. One of these "should have been pivoted" columns is usually called an eta vector. The entire list of eta vectors is called the eta file. We must now show that this information can be stored compactly and that it can be efficiently exploited. We can efficiently generate a column from E by simply starting with the corresponding original column from T and then applying the list of "should have been pivoted" columns to it. Thus, we already see how to create efficiently the information needed to select the pivot row, given that we know which variable is to enter.

Now we must show how to generate the objective function row of E with the product form inverse representation. Here, we recall how it was done with the explicit inverse: we simply multiplied the first row of B^{-1} times the original LP matrix. We will show how to construct the first row of B^{-1} from the eta file. The first row of E can then be reconstructed just as with the explicit inverse method.

For mathematical purposes, it is convenient to think of each eta vector as being stored in the following fashion:

(a) Divide each element in the column, except the pivot element, by the negative of the pivot element,
(b) replace the pivot element by its reciprocal,
(c) if the pivot element is in row k, embed the column in the kth column position of an identity matrix.

For example, suppose that the column that should have been pivoted was

Row

(1)	−10
(2)	2
(3)	1
(4)	−2

and the pivot was to be in row 2. Think of this being stored in the eta file as the matrix:

1	10/2	0	0
0	1/2	0	0
0	−1/2	1	0
0	1	0	1

Call this an eta matrix.

The reason for thinking of it in this form is that a pivot in row 2 of the column corresponds to premultiplying by the above matrix. For example, observe that premultiplying by this matrix corresponds to:

(a) adding 5 times the pivot row to row (1), subtracting 1/2 of the pivot row from row (3), adding the pivot row to row (4), and
(b) dividing the pivot row by 2.

Call the eta matrix corresponding to the kth pivot, h_k. Recalling how B^{-1} was updated at each pivot under the explicit form, we can then write B^{-1} at pivot k as the matrix product:

$$B^{-1} = h_k \times h_{k-1} \times h_{k-2} \ldots \times h_1 \times I$$

where I is the identity matrix.

We can get the first row of B^{-1} by the following procedure. Take the first row of h_k and multiply it times h_{k-1}. This gives a row vector as a result. This is multiplied times h_{k-2} etc. This process for getting the first row of B^{-1} may sound complicated, but it requires only about 20 FORTRAN statements to describe.

19.4.1 Example of Revised Simplex Method with Product Form Inverse

We shall illustrate the method with the example used earlier.

The original LP matrix, T, is:

Row	Basis	Z	A	C	S_2	S_3	S_4	RHS
1	Z	1	−20	−30				
2	S_2		1		1			60
3	S_3			1		1		50
4	S_4		1	2			1	120

The eta file is empty, so the first row of B^{-1} or the pricing vector is (1 0 0 0). C prices out at −30, so it is chosen to enter. Because the eta file is empty, the entering column and RHS of E are the same as in T, thus

Row	Basis	C	RHS
(1)	Z	−30	0
(2)	S_2	0	60
(3)	S_3	1	50
(4)	S_4	−2	120

The minimum ratio appears in row (3), so the pivot should be in row (3). Thus, we add the following eta vector to the eta file:

$$
\begin{array}{c}
h_1 \\
30 \\
0 \\
1 \\
\underline{-2} \\
\end{array}
$$

Pivot row   3

In practice, only the nonzeroes are stored.

At the start of the second iteration, we must find the first row of B^{-1}. This is simply the first row of the eta matrix corresponding to h_1, i.e.,

1   0   30   0

Multiplying this row vector times T gives the first row of E:

A	C	S_2	S_3	S_4
−20	0	0	30	40

Thus, variable A should enter.

The updated column of E corresponding to A is obtained by doing the matrix multiplication:

$$\begin{bmatrix} 1 & 0 & 30 & 0 \\ 0 & 1 & 0 & 0 \\ 0 & 0 & 1 & 0 \\ 0 & 0 & -2 & 1 \end{bmatrix} \times \begin{bmatrix} -20 \\ 1 \\ 0 \\ 1 \end{bmatrix} = \begin{bmatrix} -20 \\ 1 \\ 0 \\ 1 \end{bmatrix}$$

The relevant part of E is

Row	Basis	A	RHS
(1)	Z	−20	1500
(2)	S_2	1	60
(3)	C	0	50
(4)	S_4	1	20

The minimum ratio is in row (4), so the pivot is in row (4), and the new eta file is:

	h_2	h_1
	20	30
	−1	0
	0	1
	$\dfrac{1}{4}$	−2
Pivot row	4	3

The first row of B^{-1} is obtained by the matrix multiplication:

$$\begin{bmatrix} 1 & 0 & 0 & 20 \end{bmatrix} \times \begin{bmatrix} 1 & 0 & 30 & 0 \\ 0 & 1 & 0 & 0 \\ 0 & 0 & 1 & 0 \\ 0 & 0 & -2 & 1 \end{bmatrix} = \begin{bmatrix} 1 & 0 & -10 & 20 \end{bmatrix}$$

Multiplying this times T gives the first row of E:

A	C	S_2	S_3	S_4
0	0	0	−10	20

Thus, S_3 should enter. The updated column of E corresponding to S_3 is obtained by applying the eta file to S_3's column in T. The original column of S_3 was:

$$\begin{bmatrix} 0 \\ 0 \\ 1 \\ 0 \end{bmatrix}$$

Applying h_1 gives:

$$\begin{bmatrix} 30 \\ 0 \\ 1 \\ -2 \end{bmatrix}$$

Applying h_2 gives:

$$-10$$
$$2$$
$$1$$
$$-2$$

Thus, the relevant part of E is:

Row	Basis	A	RHS
(1)	Z	-10	1900
(2)	S_2	2	40
(3)	C	1	50
(4)	A	2	20

The minimum ratio occurs in row (2), so row (2) is the pivot row. The new eta file is:

	h_3	h_2	h_1
	5	20	30
	1/2	-1	0
	$-1/2$	0	1
	1	1	-2
Pivot row	2	4	3

The new first row of B^{-1} is constructed as follows: The first row of the h_3 matrix is:

$$1 \quad 5 \quad 0 \quad 0$$

Multiplying this times the h_2 matrix gives:

$$1 \quad 5 \quad 0 \quad 15$$

Multiplying this times the h_1 matrix gives:

$$1 \quad 5 \quad 0 \quad 15$$

Multiplying this times the T matrix gives the new first row of E:

A	C	S_2	S_3	S_4
0	0	5	0	15

There are no negative reduced costs, so this corresponds to the optimal solution:

Row	Basis	RHS
(1)	Z	2100
(2)	S_3	20
(3)	C	30
(4)	A	60

19.4.2 Revised Simplex Method: Summary of Computational Performance

We will now give a slightly optimistic estimate of the work per iteration using the revised simplex method with product form inverse. We will make the following slightly optimistic assumptions, which we will justify later.

(a) A problem with m rows has an eta file that contains m eta vectors on average.
(b) The density of nonzeroes in an eta vector is the same as the density of a column in the original LP matrix, e.g., four nonzeroes per column.

It is realistic to assume that only the nonzeroes in an eta vector are stored. In general, assume there are d nonzero elements per column in the original LP matrix. Now the steps in performing one iteration can be described as follows:

	Step	Number of Multiplications and Divisions
(i)	Get first row of B^{-1} (Get dual prices)	$d \times m$
(ii)	Get first row of E (Price out)	$d \times n$
		(less if not all columns are priced in each pass)
(iii)	Construct updated entering column	$d \times m$
(iv)	Select pivot row	m
(v)	Do the pivot and update RHS	m
	Total work per iteration	$2(1 + d)m + dn$

Compare this with approximately mn for the standard simplex method and m^2 for the revised simplex method with explicit inverse. For our example parameters with $m = 500$, $n = 1000$, and $d = 4$, the comparisons are approximately 9000 vs. 500,000 and 250,000.

Our analysis has been optimistic. Each iteration adds another eta vector. Thus, we might have more than m eta vectors in a problem requiring many iterations. We might realistically expect each eta vector added to be at least 50% dense. The key is that every few iterations (e.g., m) we may perform a process called reinversion. All the accumulated eta vectors are discarded. We then do at most m pivots to bring the current basis back into the solution. We can do these m pivots in any order. If the order is chosen wisely, for reasonable problems, the density of these at most m eta vectors will be about the same as for columns in the original LP matrix.

Let us illustrate reinversion for our example problem. The final basis consisted of the columns C, A, and s_3. The final eta file contained 10 nonzeroes. We discard this eta file and we decide to pivot A into row (2), C into row (4), and finally, s_3 into row (3). The corresponding eta file is:

	h_3	h_2	h_1
	0	−30	−20
	0	0	1
	1	1	0
	0	2	1
Pivot row	3	4	2

Note that h_3 corresponds to an identity matrix and thus has no effect. Therefore, it need not be stored. Thus, a judicious reinversion has reduced the eta file to two vectors from three and to six nonzeroes from ten, and regular inversion provides some justification for our earlier optimistic assumptions.

The motivation for the chosen order can perhaps be understood by considering the following permutation of the rows and columns in the basis.

Row	A	C	s_3
(2)	1		
(4)	1	2	
(3)	0	0	1
(1)	−20	−30	

The noticeable feature of this matrix is that it is lower triangular. Pivoting A into row (2) has no effect on columns C and s_3. Pivoting C into row (4) has no effect on column s_3. Thus, the density of each eta vector is exactly the same as the original column associated with that pivot.

The basic goal of a good reinversion routine is to find that triangular order if it exists. The revised simplex method with product form inverse tends to perform well on problems that have bases that can be permuted to this lower or almost lower triangular form. Basis matrices for network LPs can always be permuted to this lower triangular form.

You can observe the row and column permutation that LINDO uses to get an (almost) triangular basis configuration by executing the INVERT followed by BPIC commands. The latter command prints a basis picture that shows the locations of the nonzeroes in the permuted basis.

19.4.3 Getting an Initial Basic Feasible Solution

Our examples for illustrating the simplex method have had the property that the slack variables by themselves constituted a basic feasible solution. What do we do when this convenient property does not hold?

Consider the following problem:

$$
\begin{aligned}
\text{Max} \quad & 2X_1 + 7X_2 + 5X_3 \\
\text{s.t.} \quad & 2X_1 + X_2 + 4X_3 = 5 \\
& X_1 \qquad\quad - 2X_3 \geq 2
\end{aligned}
$$

There is no obvious initial basic feasible solution. A simple trick allows us still to use the simplex method. The trick consists of:

1. Add artificial variables as needed so that an initial basic feasible solution is obvious;
2. Give the artificial variables relatively unattractive coefficients in the objective function so that, if there is a solution with all the artificials zero, this solution will be found.

We will discuss three ways of doing part (2) of the trick:

(a) Big M method,
(b) Phase I/Phase II method,
(c) Little Epsilon method or composite method.

The Big M method is easiest to explain, so we will illustrate it first. Let M denote an arbitrarily large positive number. Our example with surplus and artificial variables added is:

$$
\begin{aligned}
\text{Max} \quad & 2X_1 + 7X_2 + 5X_3 - MA_2 - MA_3 \\
\text{s.t.} \quad & 2X_1 + X_2 + 4X_3 \qquad\qquad + A_2 \qquad = 5 \\
& X_1 \qquad\quad - 2X_3 - S \qquad\qquad + A_3 = 2
\end{aligned}
$$

An obvious initial solution is $A_2 = 5$, $A_3 = 2$.

Putting it in tableau form and making variables A_1 and A_3 basic gives:

Row	Basis	X_1	X_2	X_3	S	A_2	A_3	RHS
(1)	Z	$-2-3M$	$-7-M$	$-5-2M$	M			$-7M$
(2)	A_2	2	1	4		1		5
(3)	A_3	1		-2	-1		1	2

If a value is specified for M, the simplex method can be applied. There are two related difficulties, however, with the Big M method insofar as computer implementation is concerned:

(a) How do we know that we have chosen M sufficiently large? I.e., if termination occurs with some of the artificial variables still greater than zero, is it because there is no feasible solution or is it because we chose M too small?
(b) If we choose M too large, the true objective coefficients may be swamped or lost in the finite precision of computer arithmetic. The resulting "optimal" solution may be feasible but not optimal for the original objective, because of roundoff error.

The Phase I/Phase II methods allows us to effectively use an $M = \infty$ without incurring any of the roundoff difficulties of (b). This is achieved by separating the optimization into two phases:

(I) Minimize the sum of the infeasibilities and, thereby, either obtain a truly feasible initial basic solution or demonstrate unambiguously that there is no feasible solution,
(II) Optimize the true objective function, starting with the basic feasible solution supplied by Phase I.

It is convenient to think of appending an additional Phase I objective row to the tableau as shown below:

Row	Basis	X_1	X_2	X_3	S	A_2	A_3	RHS
(1)	Z_{II}	−2	−7	−5				
(2)	A_2	2	1	4		1		5
(3)	A_3	1		−2	−1		1	2
(4)	Z_I	−3	−1	−2	1			−7

The bottom row corresponds to the Phase I objective: Minimize $A_1 + A_2$. The bottom row of the tableau was obtained by pivoting A_2 in (2) and A_3 in (3), i.e., eliminating A_2 and A_3 from row (4). Thus, the Phase I objective would select X_1 as the first variable to enter, just as the Big M method would if M were ∞. As soon as all the artificial variables are driven to zero, we switch to the Phase II objective.

A misgiving that you might have about the Phase I/Phase II method is that it pays no attention to the true objective during Phase I. Thus, the first feasible solution may be far from optimal.

The Little Epsilon or Composite method combines the desirable features of both the Big M and the Phase I/Phase II methods. It uses a Phase I and a Phase II, but during Phase I it uses a composite or weighted combination of the Phase I and Phase II objectives, specifically, (Phase I objective) $+ \varepsilon \times$ (Phase II objective) where ε is a suitably small number. The Big M and Little Epsilon methods produce the same sequence of pivots if $M = 1/\varepsilon$.

A typical starting value for ε is 1. The value of ε is decreased towards 0 as needed until Phase I is complete. The hope is that when Phase I is complete, the solution will also be close to optimal for the Phase II objective.

Let us illustrate the Little Epsilon method with the previous tableau. Starting with $\varepsilon = 1$, variable X_2 prices out to −8 and it is chosen to enter. The departing variable is A_2 and the new tableau is:

Row	Basis	X_1	X_2	X_3	S	A_2	A_3	RHS
(1)	Z_{II}	12		23		7		35
(2)	X_2	2	1	4		1		5
(3)	A_3	1		−2	−1		1	2
(4)	Z_I	−1		2	1	1		−2

With $\varepsilon = 1$ no variable is attractive to enter, thus, ε must be decreased if it is not yet zero. We arbitrarily reduce ε to 0.01 and now X_1 prices out to $−1 + 0.12 = −0.88$, so it enters. The departing variable is A_3 and the new tableau is:

Row	Basis	X_1	X_2	X_3	S	A_2	A_3	RHS
(1)	Z_{II}			47	12	7	−12	11
(2)	X_2		1	8	2	1	−2	1
(3)	X_3	1		−2	−1		1	2
(4)	Z_I					1	1	

All artificial variables are at zero, so Phase I is finished. All nonartificial variables price out as unattractive in the Phase II objective so we are done. If the solution had not been optimal, we would have reset ε to 1 as Phase II began.

A number of other features of the Phase I/Phase II and Little Epsilon methods are important with regard to implementation. First, notice that the coefficient of a nonbasic variable in the Phase I objective is always the sum of its coefficients in rows in which an artificial variable is basic. Thus, the Phase I objective need never be stored. Portions of it can be easily constructed as needed. This construction is particularly easy with the revised simplex method. The essential modification is that an additional pricing vector corresponding to the Phase I objective is constructed. This "construct-as-needed" feature is also very compatible with partial pricing strategies, i.e., strategies that at each iteration consider but a small subset of the set of all columns as possible entering variables. Also notice that because an artificial variable will never be considered as an entering variable, these columns need never be stored. In our example, columns A_2 and A_3 never played a role once the initial tableau was constructed; thus, they could have been deleted. The net effect of all this is that the revised simplex method needs almost no modification to find an initial feasible solution. No columns or rows need be added to the problem. The only modifications are:

(a) Initially, rows that would otherwise be infeasible are marked as having an artificial variable basic in them,
(b) During Phase I the construction of the pricing vector is modified so that the price vector is a weighted sum of the first row and the infeasible rows of B^{-1}.

19.5 Barrier or Interior Path Methods for Solving LPs

Many people, after looking at a geometric view of how the simplex method follows a path around the exterior of the feasible region, have proposed an interior path method. Figure 19.2 illustrates this intuition.

Some people, after having proposed the use of a path through the interior, have realized that this approach is more easily proposed than implemented. The difficulty is that, unless chosen carefully, a path all the way through the interior will, as in the example in Figure 19.2, soon strike the exterior. Once on the exterior, the path very quickly follows a simplex-like path. Thus, we want to prevent the path from returning to the exterior until it reaches an optimum point. We will consider a problem of the following form:

$$\text{Min} \quad \sum_{j=1}^{n} c_j x_j$$

$$\text{subject to} \quad \sum_{j=1}^{n} a_{ij} x_j = b_i \quad \text{for } i = 1, 2, \ldots, m$$

$$x_j \geq 0 \quad \text{for } j = 1, 2, \ldots, n$$

We would like to encourage paths that stay away from the boundary. The device we will use is to replace the inequality constraints $x \geq 0$ by a "barrier" function that "repels" x if it gets close to 0.

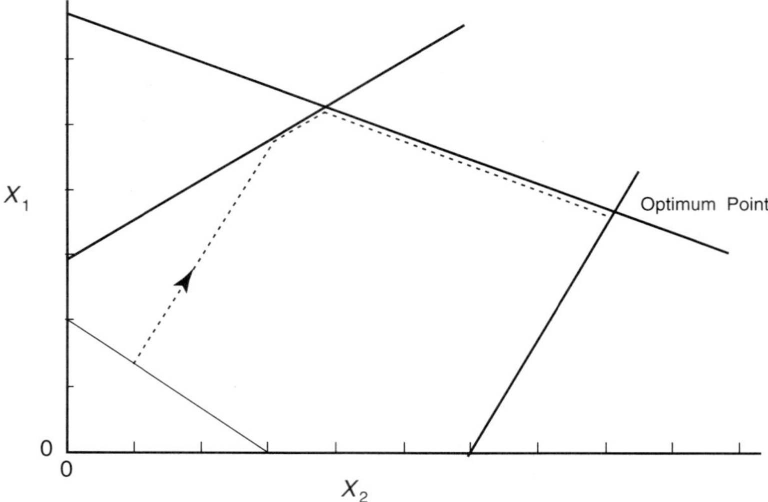

Figure 19.2
Path of Naive
Interior Path
Method

The "barrier" function we will use is the log barrier: $\ln(x)$. This function is illustrated in Figure 19.3. The key feature of the barrier function is that its cost approaches infinity as its argument approaches zero.

With the barrier function the problem becomes:

$$\text{Min} \quad u_1 \sum_{j=1}^{n} c_j x_j - u_2 \sum_{j=1}^{n} \ln\left(x_j\right)$$

$$\text{subject to} \quad \sum_{j=1}^{n} a_{ij} x_j = b_i \quad \text{for } i = 1, m$$

The parameters u_1 and u_2 allow us to express how strongly we wish to minimize the objective and how strongly we would like to stay away from the boundary. For u_2 large and positive, the barrier function will keep all x's > 0.

We can now describe in spirit how an interior path method works. If we hold u_1 fixed at some positive value and let u_2 approach zero, the solution to the above problem will approach the boundary of the feasible region at a point at which:

$$\sum_{j=1}^{n} c_j x_j \quad \text{is minimized.}$$

19.5.1 Example

The Astro-Cosmo problem when written in equality form is:

$$
\begin{array}{llll}
\text{Max} & 20A + 30C & & \\
\text{s.t.} & A & + s_2 & = 60 \\
& C & + s_3 & = 50 \\
& A + 2C & + s_4 & = 120 \\
& A, \quad C, \quad s_2, \quad s_3, \quad s_4 \geq 0
\end{array}
$$

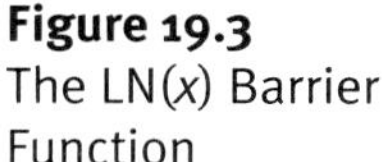

Figure 19.3
The LN(x) Barrier
Function

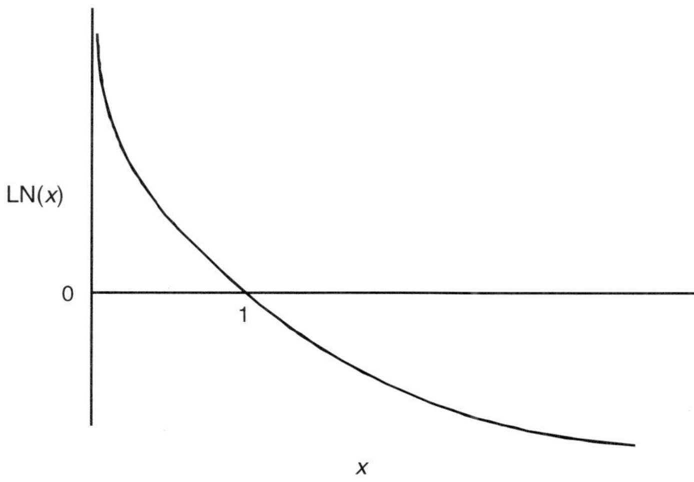

In barrier function form, the objective becomes:

$$\text{Max } u_1(20A + 30C) + u_2[\ln(A) + \ln(C) + \ln(s_2) + \ln(s_3) + \ln(s_4)]$$

This is a nonlinear program. We can solve it with a program such as LINGO.

If we let $u_1 = 0$, we get the point that in a sense is the center of the feasible region:

$$A = 23.3; \; C = 16.4; \; s_2 = 36.7; \; s_3 = 33.6; \; s_4 = 63.9.$$

If we let u_1 be some positive value and let u_2 approach zero, the solution will approach:

$$A = 60; \; C = 30; \; s_2 = 0; \; s_3 = 20; \; s_4 = 0.$$

The complete path that is traced out as u_1 is increased and u_2 is decreased is shown in Figure 19.4.

19.5.2 Eliminating the Nonlinear Feature

As stated, for a given value of u_2, we must solve a nonlinear problem. Further, it appears that we must solve infinitely many of these nonlinear problems as we let u_2 decrease to zero.

We will eliminate the nonlinear feature by using linear approximations. If we introduce Lagrange multiplier variables y_i for $i = 1, \ldots, m$, the Lagrange multiplier problem is:

$$\text{Min } \sum_{j=1}^{m} c_j x_j - u_2 \sum_{j=1}^{n} \ln\left(x_j\right) + \sum_{i=1}^{m} y_i \left(\sum_{j=1}^{n} a_{ij} x_j - b_i \right)$$

Figure 19.4
Continuous Path
Version of
Interior Path
Method

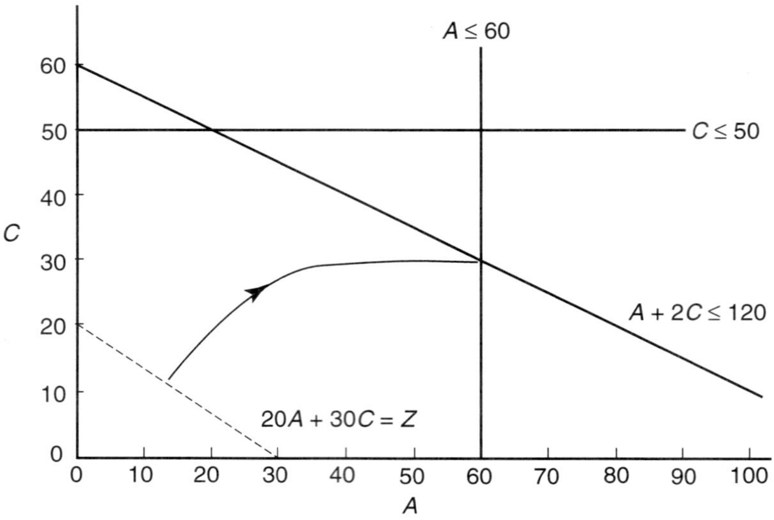

The first-order conditions are obtained by differentiating with respect to x_j and y_i to obtain:

for x_j :

$$c_j - u_2 / x_j + \sum_{i=1}^{m} y_i a_{ij} = 0 \tag{19.1}$$

for y_i :

$$\sum_{j=1}^{n} a_{ij} x_j = b_i \tag{19.2}$$

Suppose that we have a solution, $\{x_j\}$, that is feasible subject to the constraints (19.2). We want to find a new point $\{x_j\}$ that is better.

Define the differences:

$$d_j = x_j - \overline{x}_j$$

Dealing with the nonlinear terms u_2/x_j in 19.1 is a problem. A linear approximation based on a Taylor series first-order approximation to $1/x_j$ at $\overline{x}_j$ is $1/\overline{x}_j - d_j/\overline{x}_j^2$. Thus, a linear approximation to the first-order conditions is:

$$c_j - u_2 / \overline{x}_j + u_2 d_j / \overline{x}_j^2 + \sum_{i=1}^{m} y_i a_{ij} = 0$$

and

$$\sum_j a_{ij} x_j = b_i$$

or equivalently :

$$\sum_j a_{ij} d_j = 0$$

So for $\bar{x}_j$ given we want to solve for the d_js and y_js in the system of equations:
For $j = 1, \ldots, n$

$$u_2 d_j / \bar{x}_j^2 + \sum_{i=1}^{m} a_{ij} y_i = u_2 / \bar{x}_j - c_j \qquad (19.3)$$

and for $i = 1, m$

$$\sum_{j=1}^{n} d_j a_{ij} = 0 \qquad (19.4)$$

The general outline of the steps of an interior path method is then:

1. Obtain an initial solution that satisfies (19.1).
2. Based on the current point, solve the linearized first-order conditions system (19.3) and (19.4).
3. Using the d_j's obtained in step (2) as a direction, choose a step size to move to a new better solution if possible.
4. If a stopping criterion is satisfied, stop; else go to (2).

19.5.3 The Astro/Cosmo Problem Continued

Figure 19.5 shows the path followed by a "linearized and discretized" version of the interior path algorithm. For this particular version, we held $u_1 = u_2 = 1$ for each iteration. The values of the variables at each iteration were:

Iteration	A	C	s_2	s_3	s_4	Objective
0	1	1	59	49	117	50
1	21.96	31.94	38.04	18.06	34.16	1397.4
2	34.16	41.15	25.84	8.85	3.54	1917.7
3	49.33	35.19	10.67	14.81	0.28	2042.4
4	59.91	30.01	0.09	19.99	0.06	2098.6

At iteration 4, it is apparent that s_2 and s_4 are going to zero, and thus the solution should be $A = 60$, $C = 30$. At iteration 4, the three y variables, corresponding to the three dual prices, had values: 5.003, 0.006, and 14.998. Thus, they are close to the optimal dual prices of 5, 0, and 15.

19.5.4 Other Versions of Interior Path Algorithms

The interior path method we described is known as the primal affine method. The interior path method first popularized by Karmarkar (1985) required that the variables be scaled so that the constraint $\sum_{j=1}^{n} x_j = 1$ was satisfied. That approach has come to be known as the projective scaling approach.

One could also consider the dual of a problem and apply an interior path method to it. This has been the approach used by Marsten et al. (1989) in their successful implementation of an interior path algorithm.

The first suggestion of interior path methods of the kind described here is attributed to Dikin (1967).

Figure 19.5
Path of Piecewise
Linear Interior
Path Algorithm

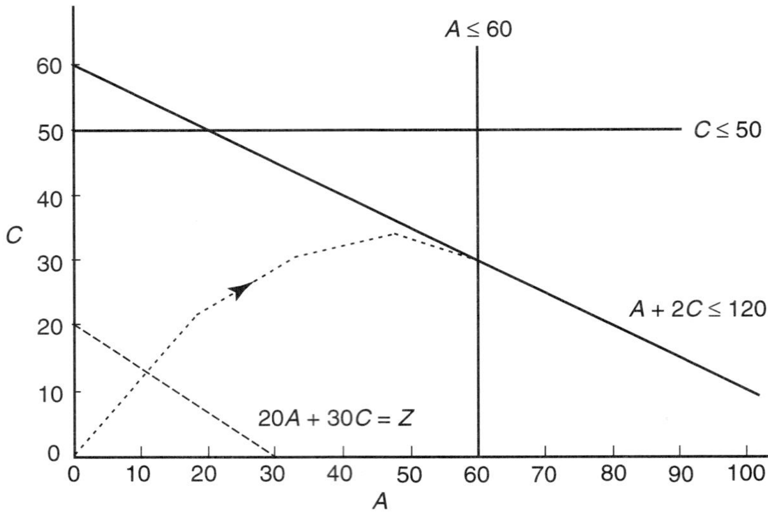

19.6 PROBLEMS

Problem 1

The following tableau arose during the application of the standard simplex method.

	x_1	x_2	x_3	x_4	x_5	x_6	RHS
Objective:	12	0	−15	0	5	0	1400
	4	0	2	1	1	0	12
	−2	1	−2	0	0	0	18
	5	0	3	0	−1	1	15

(a) Which variable should enter?
(b) In which row should the pivot occur?
(c) Which variables are basic in the above tableau and what are their values?
(d) Which variable goes to zero (departs) if the pivot mentioned in step (b) above is performed?
(e) Perform the pivot mentioned in step (b).
(f) Is the resulting solution optimal?

Problem 2

Consider the following problem:

$$\text{Max} \quad 4x_1 + 3x_2 - 9999a_1 - 9999a_2$$
s.t.
$$2x_1 + 4x_2 + a_1 \qquad = 6$$
$$6x_1 + x_2 \qquad + a_2 = 7$$

(a) Can you identify an initial feasible solution without doing any arithmetic? What variables are nonzero at which values?

(b) Temporarily disregard the simplex method rule for selecting entering variables and perform the two iterations necessary to bring these two variables into the solution.

(c) Now perform the regular simplex method to find the optimal solution.

Problem 3

Apply the simplex method to the following problem. In words, what can you say about the optimal solution?

$$\text{Max} \quad 5x + 4y + 3z$$

s.t.

$$
\begin{aligned}
x - 2y \quad &\le 5 \\
3x + y - z &\le 3 \\
+ 7y + z &\le 8
\end{aligned}
$$

Problem 4

Even though LINDO will not cycle on the following model:

```
MIN - 2 X1 - 3 X2 + X3 + 12 X4
  SUBJECT TO
     2)         - 2 X1 - 9 X2                  + X3   + 9 X4 <=   0
     3)   0.33333 X1   + X2 - 0.33333   X3   - 2 X4 <=   0
     4)           2 X1 + 3 X2                  - X3 - 12 X4 <=   2
  END
```

Show that if the straightforward simplex method is applied, in which the variable to enter at each pivot is chosen to be the one with the most negative reduced cost, cycling will occur.

References

Adams, J. L. (1986). *Conceptual Blockbusting.* Reading, MA: Addison-Wesley.

Ahuja, R. K., T. L. Magnanti, and J. B. Orlin. (1993). *Network Flows, Theory, Algorithms, and Applications.* Englewood Cliffs, NJ: Prentice Hall.

Arnold, L., and D. Botkin. (1978). "Portfolios to Satisfy Damage Judgement: A Linear Programming Approach." *Interfaces,* vol. 8, no. 2 (Feb.).

Aykin, T. (1996). "Optimal Shift Scheduling with Multiple Break Windows." *Management Science,* vol. 42, no. 4 (April), pp. 591–602.

Baker, E. K., and M. L. Fisher. (1981). "Computational Results for Very Large Air Crew Scheduling Problems." *Omega,* vol. 9, pp. 613–618.

Balas, E. (1979). "Disjunctive Programming." *Annals of Discrete Mathematics,* vol. 5, pp. 3–51.

Barnett, A. (1994). "How Numbers Can Trick You." *Technology Review,* vol. 97, no. 7 (October), pp. 38–45.

Bessent, A., W. Bessent, J. Kennington, and B. Reagan. (1982). "An Application of Mathematical Programming to Assess Productivity in the Houston Independent School District." *Management Science,* vol. 28, no. 12 (December), pp. 1355–1367.

Black, F. (1989). "How We Came Up with the Option Formula." *The Journal of Portfolio Management,* (winter), pp. 4–8.

Bland, R. G., and D. F. Shallcross. (1989). "Large Traveling Salesman Problems Arising in X-ray Crystallography: A Preliminary Report on Computation." *O.R. Letters,* vol. 8, no. 3, pp. 125–128.

Bradley, G. H., G. G. Brown, and G. W. Graves. (1977). "Design and Implementation of Large Scale Primal Transshipment Algorithms." *Management Science,* vol. 24, pp. 1–34.

Bradley, S. P., A. C. Hax, and T. L. Magnanti. (1977). *Applied Mathematical Programming.* Reading, MA: Addison-Wesley.

Braess, D. (1968). "Uber ein Paradoxon aus der Verkehrplanung." *Unternehmensforschung,* vol. 12, pp. 258–268.

Brearley, A. L., G. Mitra, and H. P. Williams. (1975). "An Analysis of Mathematical Programming Problems Prior to Applying the Simplex Algorithm." *Mathematical Programming,* vol. 8, pp. 54–83.

Brown, G. G., and D. S. Thomen. (1980). "Automatic Identification of Generalized Upper Bounds in Large-Scale Optimization Models." *Management Science,* vol. 26, no. 11, pp. 1166–1184.

Carino, D. R., T. Kent, D. H. Myers, C. Stacy, M. Sylvanus, A. L. Turner, K. Watanabe, and W. T. Ziemba. (1994). "The Russell-Yasuda Kasai Model: An Asset/Liability Model for a Japanese Insurance Company Using Multistage Stochastic Programming." *Interfaces,* vol. 24, no. 1, pp. 29–49.

Charnes, A., W. W. Cooper, and E. Rhodes. (1978). "Measuring the Efficiency of Decision Making Units." *European Journal of Operational Research,* vol. 2, pp. 429–444.

Ciriani, T. A., and R. C. Leachman. (1993). *Optimization in Industry.* New York: John Wiley & Sons.

Clarke, G., and J. W. Wright. (1964). "Scheduling of Vehicles from a Central Depot to a Number of Delivery Points." *Operations Research,* vol. 12, no. 4 (July–Aug.), pp. 568–581.

Clyman, D. R. (1995). "Unreasonable Rationality?" *Management Science,* vol. 41, no. 9 (Sept.), pp. 1538–1548.

Cunningham, K., and L. Schrage. (1991). *LINGO Optimization Modeling Language.* Chicago: LINDO Systems.

Dantzig, G. (1963). *Linear Programming and Extensions.* Princeton: Princeton University Press.

Dantzig, G., and B. Wolfe. (1960). "Decomposition Principle for Linear Programs." *Operations Research,* vol. 8, pp. 101–111.

Davis, L. S., and K. N. Johnson. (1987). *Forest Management.* 3rd ed. New York: McGraw-Hill.

Dembo, R. S., A. Chiarri, J. G. Martin, and L. Paradinas. (1990). "Managing Hidroeléctrica Española's Hydroelectric Power System." *Interfaces,* vol. 20, no. 1 (Jan.–Feb.), pp. 115–135.

d'Epenoux, F. (1963). "A Probabilistic Production and Inventory Problem." *Management Science,* vol. 10, no. 1 (Oct.), pp. 98–108.

DeWitt, C. W., L. Lasdon, A. Waren, D. Brenner, and S. Melhem. (1989). "OMEGA: An Improved Gasoline Blending System for Texaco." *Interfaces,* vol. 19, no. 1 (Jan.–Feb.), pp. 85–101.

Dikin, I. I. (1967). "Iterative Solution of Problems of Linear and Quadratic Programming." *Soviet Mathematics Doklady*, vol. 8, pp. 674–675.

Dutton, R., G. Hinman, and C. B. Millham. (1974). "The Optimal Location of Nuclear-Power Facilities in the Pacific Northwest." *Operations Research*, vol. 22, no. 3 (May–June), pp. 478–487.

Dyckhoff, H. (1981). "A New Linear Programming Approach to the Cutting Stock Problem." *Operations Research*, vol. 29, no. 6 (Nov.–Dec.), pp. 1092–1104.

Edie, L. C. (1954). "Traffic Delays at Toll Booths." *Operations Research*, vol. 2, no. 2 (May), pp. 107–138.

Eppen, G., K. Martin, and L. Schrage. (1988). "A Scenario Approach to Capacity Planning." *Operations Research*, vol. 37, no. 4 (July–August), pp. 517–530.

Eppen, G. D., and R. K. Martin. (1987). "Solving Multi-Item Capacitated Lot-Sizing Problems Using Variable Redefinition." *Operations Research,* vol. 35, no. 6 (Nov.–Dec.), pp. 832–848.

Fields, C., J. F. Hourican, and E. A. McGee. (1978). "Developing a Minimum Cost Feed Blending System for Intensive Use." Joint National TIMS/ORSA Meeting, New York.

Fillon, M. (1996). "Taming the Yangtze." *Popular Mechanics*, vol. 173, no. 7 (July), pp. 52–56.

Florian, M. (1977). "An Improved Linear Approximation Algorithm for the Network Equilibrium (Packet Switching) Problem." *Proceedings 1977 IEEE Conference Decision and Control.*

Geoffrion, A. M. (1976). "The Purpose of Mathematical Programming is Insight, Not Numbers." *Interfaces 7,* no. 1 (November), pp. 81–92.

Geoffrion, A. M., and G. W. Graves. (1974). "Multicommodity Distribution System Design by Benders Decomposition." *Management Science*, vol. 20, no. 5 (January), pp. 822–844.

Gomory, R. E. (1958). "Outline of an Algorithm for Integer Solutions to Linear Programs." *Bulletin of the American Mathematical Society*, vol. 64, pp. 275–278.

Grinold, R. C. (1983). "Model Building Techniques for the Correction of End Effects in Multistage Convex Programs." *Operations Research*, vol. 31, no. 3, pp. 407–431.

Grötschel, M., M. Jünger, and G. Reinelt. (1985). "Facets of the Linear Ordering Polytope." *Mathematical Programming*, vol. 33, pp. 43–60.

Gunawardane, G., S. Hoff, and L. Schrage. (1981)."Identification of Special Structure Constraints in Linear Programs." *Mathematical Programming*, vol. 21, pp. 90–97.

Hadley, G. (1962). *Linear Programming.* Reading, MA: Addison-Wesley.

Hane, C. A., C. Barnhart, E. L. Johnson, R. E. Marsten, G. L. Nemhauser, and G. Sigismondi. (1995). "The Fleet Assignment Problem: Solving a Large Scale Integer Program." *Mathematical Programming*, vol. 70, pp. 211–232.

Hansen, C. T., K. Madsen, and H. B. Nielsen. (1991). "Optimization of Pipe Networks." *Mathematical Programming,* vol. 52, pp. 45–58.

Hanson, W., and R. K. Martin. (1990). "Optimal Bundle Pricing." *Management Science,* vol. 36, no. 2 (February), pp. 155–174.

Infanger, G. (1994). *Planning Under Uncertainty: Solving Large-Scale Stochastic Linear Programs.* Danvers, MA: Boyd & Fraser.

Jenkins, L. (1982). "Parametric Mixed Integer Programming: An Application to Solid Waste Management." *Management Science,* vol 28, no. 11 (Nov.), pp. 1270–1284.

Jeroslow, R. G., K. Martin, R. L. Rardin, J. Wang. (1992). "Gainfree Leontief Substitution Flow Problems." *Mathematical Programming*, vol. 57, pp. 375–414.

Kall, P., and S. W. Wallace. (1994). *Stochastic Programming.* New York: John Wiley & Sons.

Karmarkar, N. K. (1985). "A New Polynomial Time Algorithm for Linear Programming." *Combinatorica,* vol. 4, pp. 373–395.

Khachian, L. G. (1979). "A Polynomial Algorithm in Linear Programming." *Soviet Mathematics Doklady,* vol. 20, no. 1, pp. 191–194.

King, R. H., and R. R. Love. (1980). "Coordinating Decisions for Increased Profits." *Interfaces*, vol. 10, no. 6 (December), pp. 4–19.

Konno, H., and H. Yamazaki. (1991). "Mean-Absolute Deviation Portfolio Optimization Model and Its Applications to Tokyo Stock Market." *Management Science*, vol. 37, no. 5 (May), pp. 519–531.

Kruskal, Jr., J. B. (1956). "On the Shortest Spanning Subtree of a Graph and the Traveling Salesman Problem." *Proc. Amer. Math. Soc.,* vol. 7, pp. 48–50.

Lasdon, L. S., and Terjung, R. C. (1971). "An Efficient Algorithm for Multi-Item Scheduling." *Operations Research,* vol. 19, no. 4, pp. 946–969.

Lawler, E. L. (1963). "The Quadratic Assignment Problem." *Management Science*, vol. 19, pp. 586–599.

Lawler, E. L., J. K. Lenstra, A. H. G. Rinnooy Kan, and D. B. Shmoys. (1985). *The Traveling Salesman Problem: A Guided Tour of Combinatorial Optimization.* New York: John Wiley & Sons.

Leontief, W. (1951). *The Structure of American Economy, 1919–1931.* New York: Oxford University Press.

Levy, F. K. (1978). "Portfolios to Satisfy Damage Judgements: A Simple Approach." *Interfaces,* vol. 9, no. 1 (Nov.), pp. 106–107.

Lin, S., and B. Kernighan. (1973). "An Effective Heuristic Algorithm for the Traveling Salesman Problem." *Operations Research,* vol. 21, pp. 498–516.

Madansky, A. (1962). "Methods of Solution of Linear Programs Under Uncertainty." *Operations Research,* vol. 10, pp. 463–471.

Manne, A. (1960). "Linear Programming and Sequential Decisions." *Management Science,* vol. 6, no. 3 (April), pp. 259–267.

Markowitz, H. M. (1959). *Portfolio Selection, Efficient Diversification of Investments.* New York: John Wiley & Sons.

Markowitz, H., and A. Perold. (1981). "Portfolio Analysis with Scenarios and Factors." *Journal of Finance,* vol. 36, pp. 871–877.

Marsten, R. E., M. P. Muller, and C. L. Killion. (1979). "Crew Planning at Flying Tiger: A Successful Application of Integer Programming." *Management Science,* vol. 25, no. 12 (Dec.), pp. 1175–1183.

Marsten, R. E., M. J. Saltzman, D. F. Shanno, G. S. Pierce, and J. F. Ballintijn. (1989). "Implementation of a Dual Affine Interior Point Algorithm for Linear Programming." *ORSA J. on Computing,* vol. 1, no. 4, pp. 287–297.

Maschler, M., B. Peleg, and L. S. Shapley. (1979). "Geometric Properties of the Kernel, Nucleolus, and Related Solution Concepts." *Mathematics of Operations Research,* vol. 4, no. 4 (Nov.), pp. 303–338.

Miller, H. E., W. P. Pierskalla, and G. J. Rath. (1976). "Nurse Scheduling Using Mathematical Programming." *Operations Research,* vol. 24, pp. 857–870.

Murchland, J. D. (1970). "Braess's Paradox of Traffic Flow." *Transportation Research,* vol. 4, pp. 391–394.

Nauss, R. M. (1986). "True Interest Cost in Municipal Bond Bidding: An Integer Programming Approach." *Management Science,* vol. 32, no. 7, pp. 870–877.

Nauss, R. M., and B. R. Keeler. (1981). "Minimizing Net Interest Cost in Municipal Bond Bidding." *Management Science,* vol. 27, no. 4 (April), pp. 365–376.

Nauss, R. M., and R. Markland. (1981). "Theory and Application of an Optimization Procedure for Lock Box Location Analysis." *Management Science,* vol. 27, no. 8 (August), pp. 855–865.

Neebe, A. W. (1987). "An Improved, Multiplier Adjustment Procedure for the Segregated Storage Problem." *Journal of the Operational Research Society,* vol. 38, no. 9, pp. 1–11.

Nemhauser, G. L., and L. A. Wolsey. (1988). *Integer and Combinatorial Optimization.* New York: John Wiley & Sons.

Orlin, J. B. (1982). "Minimizing the Number of Vehicles to Meet a Fixed Periodic Schedule: An Application of Periodic Posets." *Operations Research,* vol. 30, no. 4, pp. 760–776.

Padberg, M., and G. Rinaldi. (1987). "Optimization of a 532-City Symmetric Traveling Salesman Problem by Branch and Cut." *Operations Research Letters,* vol. 6, no. 1.

Perold, A. F. (1984). "Large Scale Portfolio Optimization." *Management Science,* vol. 30, pp. 1143–1160.

Plane, D. R., and T. E. Hendrick. (1977). "Mathematical Programming and the Location of Fire Companies for the Denver Fire Department." *Operations Research,* vol. 25, no. 4 (July–August), pp. 563–578.

Rigby, B., L. Lasdon, and A. Waren. (1995). "The Evolution of Texaco's Blending Systems: From Omega to StarBlend." *Interfaces,* vol. 25, no. 5, pp. 64–83.

Rogers, D. F., R. D. Plante, R. T. Wong, and J. R. Evans. (1991). "Aggregation and Disaggregation Techniques and Methodology in Optimization." *Operations Research,* vol. 39, no. 4 (July–August), pp. 553–582.

Ross, G. T., and R. M. Soland. (1975). "Modeling Facility Location Problems as Generalized Assignment Problems." *Management Science,* vol. 24, pp. 345–357.

Rothstein, M. (1985). "OR and the Airline Overbooking Problem." *Operations Research,* vol. 33, no. 2 (March–April), pp. 237–248.

Sankaran, J. (1989). Bidding Systems for Certain Nonmarket Allocations of Indivisible Items. Ph.D. dissertation, University of Chicago.

Schrage, L. (1975). "Implicit Representation of Variable Upper Bounds in Linear Programming." *Mathematical Programming.* Study 4, pp. 118–132.

Schrage, L. (1978). "Implicit Representation of Generalized Variable Upper Bounds in Linear Programming." *Mathematical Programming,* vol. 14, no. 1, pp. 11–20.

Schrage, L., and L. Wolsey. (1985). "Sensitivity Analysis for Branch and Bound Integer Programming." *Operations Research,* vol. 33, no. 5 (Sept.–Oct.), pp. 1008–1023.

Schrijver, A. (1986). *Theory of Linear and Integer Programming.* New York: John Wiley & Sons.

Sharpe, W. F. (1963). "A Simplified Model for Portfolio Analysis." *Management Science,* vol. 9 (Jan.), pp. 277–293.

Srinivasan, V. (1976). "Linear Programming Computational Procedures for Ordinal Regression." *Journal of ACM,* vol. 23, no. 3 (July), pp. 475–487.

Stigler, G. (1963). "United States vs. Loew's, Inc: A Note on Block Booking." *Supreme Court Review,* p. 152.

Stigler, G. J. (1945). "The Cost of Subsistence." *Journal of Farm Economics,* vol. 27, no. 2 (May), pp. 303–314.

Strevell, Michael, and Philip Chong. (1985). "Gambling on Vacation." *Interfaces,* vol. 15, no. 2 (March–April), pp. 63–67.

Subramanian, R. A., R. P. Scheff, J. D. Quillinan, D. S. Wiper, and R. E. Marsten. (1994). "Coldstart: Fleet Assignment at Delta Air Lines." *Interfaces,* vol. 24, no. 1 (Jan.-Feb.), pp. 104–120.

Tomlin, J., and J. S. Welch. (1985). "Integration of a Primal Simplex Algorithm with Large Scale Mathematical Programming System." *ACM Trans. Math. Software,* vol. 11, pp. 1–11.

Vickrey, William. (1961). "Counterspeculation, Auctions, and Competitive Sealed Tenders." *Journal of Finance* (March), vol. 16, no. 1, pp. 8–37.

Wall Street Journal. "UAL's United Alters Schedule, Cuts Costs, Boosts Flights in Face of Discount Fares." (19 June 1978), p. 8.

Wang, K. C. P., and J. P. Zaniewski. (1996). "20/30 Hindsight: The New Pavement Optimization in the Arizona State Highway Network." *Interfaces,* vol. 26, no. 3 (May–June), pp. 77–89.

Warner, D. M. (1976). "Scheduling Nursing Personnel According to Nursing Preference: A Mathematical Programming Approach." *Operations Research,* vol. 24, no. 5 (September–October), pp. 842–856.

Weingartner, H. M. (1972). "Municipal Bond Coupon Schedules with Limitations on the Number of Coupons." *Management Science,* vol. 19, no. 4 (Dec.), pp. 369–378.

What's Best User Manual. (1991). Chicago: LINDO Systems.

Index